Elisabeth PISAR

Medical Radiology

Diagnostic Imaging

Series editors

Maximilian F. Reiser
Hans-Ulrich Kauczor
Hedvig Hricak
Michael Knauth

Editorial Board

Andy Adam, London
Fred Avni, Brussels
Richard L. Baron, Chicago
Carlo Bartolozzi, Pisa
George S. Bisset, Durham
A. Mark Davies, Birmingham
William P. Dillon, San Francisco
D. David Dershaw, New York
Sam Sanjiv Gambhir, Stanford
Nicolas Grenier, Bordeaux
Gertraud Heinz-Peer, Vienna
Robert Hermans, Leuven
Hans-Ulrich Kauczor, Heidelberg
Theresa McLoud, Boston
Konstantin Nikolaou, Munich
Caroline Reinhold, Montreal
Donald Resnick, San Diego
Rüdiger Schulz-Wendtland, Erlangen
Stephen Solomon, New York
Richard D. White, Columbus

For further volumes:
http://www.springer.com/series/4354

Marc Lemmerling · Bert De Foer
Editors

Temporal Bone Imaging

Springer

Editors
Marc Lemmerling
Department of Radiology
Algemeen Ziekenhuis Sint-Lucas
Gent
Belgium

Bert De Foer
Department of Radiology
Sint-Agustinus Ziekenhuis
Wilrijk
Belgium

ISSN 0942-5373   ISSN 2197-4187   (electronic)
ISBN 978-3-642-17895-5   ISBN 978-3-642-17896-2   (eBook)
DOI 10.1007/978-3-642-17896-2
Springer Heidelberg New York Dordrecht London

Library of Congress Control Number: 2014952191

© Springer-Verlag Berlin Heidelberg 2015
This work is subject to copyright. All rights are reserved by the Publisher, whether the whole or part of the material is concerned, specifically the rights of translation, reprinting, reuse of illustrations, recitation, broadcasting, reproduction on microfilms or in any other physical way, and transmission or information storage and retrieval, electronic adaptation, computer software, or by similar or dissimilar methodology now known or hereafter developed. Exempted from this legal reservation are brief excerpts in connection with reviews or scholarly analysis or material supplied specifically for the purpose of being entered and executed on a computer system, for exclusive use by the purchaser of the work. Duplication of this publication or parts thereof is permitted only under the provisions of the Copyright Law of the Publisher's location, in its current version, and permission for use must always be obtained from Springer. Permissions for use may be obtained through RightsLink at the Copyright Clearance Center. Violations are liable to prosecution under the respective Copyright Law.
The use of general descriptive names, registered names, trademarks, service marks, etc. in this publication does not imply, even in the absence of a specific statement, that such names are exempt from the relevant protective laws and regulations and therefore free for general use.
While the advice and information in this book are believed to be true and accurate at the date of publication, neither the authors nor the editors nor the publisher can accept any legal responsibility for any errors or omissions that may be made. The publisher makes no warranty, express or implied, with respect to the material contained herein.

Printed on acid-free paper

Springer is part of Springer Science+Business Media (www.springer.com)

Preface

Over the past decades immense changes have occurred in medicine in general, and in the field of radiology more specifically. In radiology departments, some became more specialised in head and neck imaging in order to give better answers to referring ENT specialists. This collaboration between the referring physician and the radiologist created an even more focused interest on the temporal bone. In the 1980s, the fundamentals of temporal bone CT were established, and in the 1990s a comparable evolution was noted in the field of temporal bone MRI. Untill today, both imaging techniques have continuously evolved in the creation of temporal bone images. In the last years cone-beam CT has been added to the CT instrumentarium, and a growing importance was seen in the use of MRI in patients with cholesteatoma, by the application of non-EPI diffusion-weighted images. Both topics get an important place in this book. The purpose of the book is to provide a diverse view on temporal bone imaging issues, and is built around chapters focusing on a topographical basis on one hand, and on a pathological basis on the other hand. It was conceived that way to make the book easy to read and use. Without pretending to be complete it covers the broad spectrum of temporal bone imaging questions that the radiologist should be able to answer. Also some more exotic pathologies are illustrated, but this book does not have the ambition to bring a huge collection of castuistic examples.

Many authors coming from all over the world have collaborated on the book. We would like to thank them all for their enthusiasm for and contribution to this project despite their busy agendas. We are especially surprised by the excellent quality of the images that are presented throughout the different chapters. Radiological images are for the radiologist what paintings are for the painter. We hope that this book will be a museum worth repetitive visits. Last but not least, we like to acknowledge Nancy Verpoort who did a tremendous job in correcting illustrations and texts.

Marc Lemmerling
Bert De Foer

Contents

Indications for Temporal Bone Imaging: The Clinician's Approach 1
F. E. Offeciers

Temporal Bone Imaging Techniques 7
Marc Lemmerling, Bert De Foer, and Barbara Smet

Cross-Sectional Imaging Anatomy of the Temporal Bone 11
Marc Lemmerling, Barbara Smet, and Bert De Foer

External Ear Imaging 35
Robert Hermans

Acute Otomastoiditis and its Complications 53
Marc Lemmerling

Chronic Otomastoiditis without Cholesteatoma 61
A. Trojanowska and P. Trojanowski

Imaging of Cholesteatoma 69
Bert De Foer, Simon Nicolay, Jean-Philippe Vercruysse, Erwin Offeciers,
Jan W. Casselman, and Marc Pouillon

Otosclerosis 89
Marc Lemmerling

Temporal Bone Trauma 97
Sabrina Kösling and A. Noll

Temporal Bone Tumours 107
Cheng K. Ong, Eric Ting, and Vincent F. H. Chong

Congenital Malformations of the Temporal Bone 119
J. W. Casselman, J. Delanote, R. Kuhweide, J. van Dinther,
B. De Foer, and E. F. Offeciers

Imaging of Cerebellopontine Angle and Internal Auditory Canal Lesions 155
Bert de Foer, Ken Carpentier, Anja Bernaerts, Christoph Kenis,
Jan W. Casselman, and Erwin Offeciers

Inner Ear Pathology 219
Christoph Kenis, Bert De Foer, and Jan Walther Casselman

Imaging of Cochlear Implants 237
B. M. Verbist and J. H. M. Frijns

Petrous Apex Lesions. 249
Marc Lemmerling

Pathology of the Facial Nerve 257
Alexandra Borges

Imaging of the Jugular Foramen 307
Hervé Tanghe

Vascular Temporal Bone Lesions 329
Hervé Tanghe

Post-operative Temporal Bone Imaging 343
Luc van den Hauwe, Christoph Kenis, Bert De Foer, and Jan Walther Casselman

MultiPlanar Reformation in CT of the Temporal Bone 367
John I. Lane

Contributors

Anja Bernaerts Department of Radiology, GZA Hospitals Sint-Augustinus, Wilrijk, Belgium

Alexandra Borges Department of Radiology, Instituto Português de Oncologia Francisco Gentil- Centro de Lisboa, Lisbon, Portugal

Ken Carpentier Department of Radiology, GZA Hospitals Sint-Augustinus, Wilrijk, Belgium

Jan Walther Casselman Department of Radiology, AZ Sint Jan Hospital, Brugge, Belgium; Department of Radiology, GZA Sint Augustinus Hospital, Wilrijk, Belgium; Department of Radiology and Medical Imaging, AZ Sint-Jan Brugge-Oostende, Bruges, Belgium; Ghent University, Ghent, Belgium

Vincent F. H. Chong Department of Diagnostic Radiology, National University Hospital, Singapore, Singapore; Yong Loo Lin School of Medicine, National University of Singapore, Singapore, Singapore

Bert De Foer Department of Radiology, AZ Sint-Augustinus, Antwerp, Belgium; Department of Radiology, GZA Hospitals Sint-Augustinus, Wilrijk, Belgium

J. Delanote Department of Radiology and Medical Imaging, AZ Sint-Jan Brugge-Oostende, Bruges, Belgium

J. H. M. Frijns Department of Otolaryngology, Leiden University Medical Center, Leiden, The Netherlands

Robert Hermans Department of Radiology, University Hospitals Leuven, Leuven, Belgium

Christoph Kenis Department of Radiology, Sint-Franciskus Hospital, Heusden-Zolder, Belgium; Department of Radiology, AZ Sint Jan Hospital, Brugge, Belgium

Sabrina Kösling Martin Luther Universität Halle-Wittenberg, Universitätsklinik für Diagnostische Radiologie, Halle, Germany

R. Kuhweide Department of ENT, AZ Sint-Jan Brugge-Oostende, Bruges, Belgium

John I. Lane Division of Neuroradiology, Department of Radiology, Mayo Clinic College of Medicine, Rochester, MN, USA

Marc Lemmerling Department of Radiology, AZ Sint-Lucas Hospital, Gent, Belgium; Department of Radiology, Ghent University Hospital, Gent, Belgium

Simon Nicolay Department of Radiology, GZA Hospitals Sint-Augustinus, Wilrijk, Belgium

A. Noll Martin Luther Universität Halle-Wittenberg, Universitätsklinik für Diagnostische Radiologie, Halle, Germany

E. F. Offeciers Department of ENT, AZ Sint-Augustinus, Antwerp, Belgium; European Institute for ENT-Head and Neck Surgery, AZ Sint-Augustinus, Antwerp, Belgium

Cheng K. Ong Department of Diagnostic Radiology, National University Hospital, Singapore, Singapore; Yong Loo Lin School of Medicine, National University of Singapore, Singapore, Singapore

Marc Pouillon Department of Radiology, GZA Hospitals Sint-Augustinus, Wilrijk, Belgium

Barbara Smet Department of Radiology, AZ Sint-Lucas Hospital, Gent, Belgium

Hervé Tanghe Department of Radiology, Section of Neuroradiology and ENT Radiology, Erasmus Medical Centre, Erasmus University Rotterdam, CE, Rotterdam, The Netherlands

Eric Ting Department of Diagnostic Radiology, National University Hospital, Singapore, Singapore; Yong Loo Lin School of Medicine, National University of Singapore, Singapore, Singapore

A. Trojanowska Department of Radiology and Nuclear Medicine, University Medical School, Lublin, Poland

P. Trojanowski Chair and Department of Otolaryngology Head and Neck Surgery, University Medical School, Lublin, Poland

Luc van den Hauwe Department of Radiology, AZ Klina, Brasschaat, Belgium; Department of Radiology, Antwerp University Hospital, Edegem, Belgium

J. van Dinther Department of ENT, AZ Sint-Augustinus, Antwerp, Belgium; European Institute for ENT- Head and Neck Surgery, AZ Sint-Augustinus, Antwerp, Belgium

B. M. Verbist Department of Radiology, Leiden University Medical Center, Leiden, The Netherlands; Department of Radiology, Radboud University Nijmegen Medical Center, Nijmegen, The Netherlands

Jean-Philippe Vercruysse Department of ENT, Heilig Hartziekenhuis, Mol, Belgium

Indications for Temporal Bone Imaging: The Clinician's Approach

1 Introduction 1
2 Which Information Does the Clinician Need from the Radiologist? 2
2.1 How Does the Clinician Decide Which Imaging to Ask for? 2
3 How the Clinician Should Approach the Indication for Imaging? 3
3.1 Let Us Now See Which Elements of the Diagnostic Work-up Should Urge the Clinician to Ask for Imaging 3
3.2 Family History for Hearing Loss and Ear Surgery 3
3.3 Personal History and Symptoms 3
3.4 Clinical Examination and Otoscopy 4
4 Conclusion 5

Abstract

Recent progress in imaging technology has greatly improved the diagnostic quality and the therapeutic safety in the field of otology and neurotology. This makes imaging one of the cornerstones in the diagnostic work-up and follow-up of temporal bone pathology. By confirming the clinically and audiometrically suspected diagnosis, imaging helps to select the best and safest diagnostic option. It allows the ear surgeon to prepare for surgery in the most efficient way, it identifies contraindications and concomitant ear pathology and warns against potential surgical complications. This allows the clinician to counsel the patient in an honest and a realistic way. The chapter describes how the clinician can decide which imaging sequences to ask for, taking as a starting point the conventional diagnostic aids such as personal and family medical history, symptoms and clinical signs, micro-otoscopy, and audiological work-up. Two pathological situations are described in detail as examples: (1) the patient with conductive or mixed hearing loss with an intact tympanic membrane; (2) the pre-operative work-up and post-operative follow-up of the cholesteatoma patient. A close collaboration between clinician and radiologist is crucial to ensure a correct understanding of the indications for imaging by the clinician, and the selection and application of the correct sequences by the radiologist.

1 Introduction

While imaging since its early days has been an important diagnostic tool in the diagnosis of temporal bone disease, due to the hidden nature and limited accessibility of its structures to the clinician's unaided or even microscope-aided eye, recent progress in imaging technology has greatly improved the diagnostic quality and the therapeutic safety in the field of otology and neurotology.

F. E. Offeciers (✉)
European Institute for ORL, Sint-Augustinus Hospital, Wilrijk, Belgium
e-mail: erwin.offeciers@GZA.be

The advent of new therapeutic possibilities necessitated improved image resolution and a better discrimination of structures and tissues within the temporal bone.

As a consequence, recent MRI sequences open the door to the routine application of imaging in the diagnostic work-up and post-operative follow-up of cholesteatoma, in the latter case even replacing routine exploratory second stage surgery for residual disease. Because of its enhanced resolution and lower radiation dose, Cone beam CT (CBCT) is finding its place in the pre-operative work-up of conductive and mixed hearing loss (HL), facilitating patient counseling and preventing erroneous indications for surgery as well as helping to avoid per-operative complications. The overall effect is a more focussed, safer, more successful and cost-effective intervention.

Within the context of the very variable regional socio-economic conditions throughout the world, otologists and neurotologists need to adapt to these new possibilities, broadening their indications for imaging for the pre-operative work-up and post-operative follow-up. The close collaboration between clinician and otoneuroradiologist is the cornerstone for success, necessitating frequent contacts and discussion of the cases: a real on-going clinico-radiological conversation. The clinician should provide follow-up feedback to his radiologist in order to corroborate or invalidate radiological protocols, thus offering to the radiologist the opportunity of fine-tuning his technique and skills. The radiologist must keep the clinician informed on the development of new imaging sequences and techniques, thus allowing the clinician to identify new clinical applications.

The importance of an intense collaboration between clinician and radiologist cannot be sufficiently emphasised. It is part of a culture of interaction and cross-fertilisation between different specialties.

Therefore, I urge my ENT trainees to take their questions about imaging to their colleagues in the imaging department. Vice versa, young radiologists should ask the clinicians for regular feedback on their imaging protocols and take every opportunity to attend a number of surgical interventions connected to the cases they imaged, in order to familiarise themselves with the work and language of their clinical colleagues.

A common complaint by radiologists is the often very limited clinical information they receive from the clinician. A closer collaboration automatically resolves this important communication flaw, which often leads to either incomplete or superfluous examinations. It is the clinician's task to amend this.

The various chapters in this book will provide details related to specific pathological entities. This introductory chapter aims to inform the reader on the questions the clinician puts to his radiologist, or in other words, on the kind of information the clinician will expect from his radiological colleagues. As cases in point, two clinical situations will be discussed in some detail: (1) the diagnostic challenge of a conductive or mixed HL with an intact tympanic membrane (TM); (2) the important role of imaging in the pre-operative work-up and post-operative follow up of cholesteatoma cases.

2 Which Information Does the Clinician Need from the Radiologist?

Imaging confirms or contradicts a diagnosis suspected on the basis of the information acquired from: (1) the personal and family history; (2) the clinical examination (otoscopy, vestibular tests); (3) the audiometry and vestibular test battery.

It helps to select the best and safest therapeutic option. If this means surgery, it helps to prepare the operation in the most efficient way: define the urgency of the intervention (e.g., the timing of cholesteatoma surgery in a school attending child); select the best surgical approach; prepare the necessary instruments and surgical aids (e.g., LASER, micro-drill, biological glue, facial nerve monitor, etc.); identify some potential contraindications (e.g., cochleo-vestibular anomalies in stapedotomy for otosclerosis); identify concomitant pathology of the temporal bone (e.g. vestibular schwannoma in mixed HL); warn the surgeon about potential anatomical risk factors which could lead to per- or post-operative complications (e.g., a dehiscent facial canal with herniation of the facial nerve impacting on the stapes in functional middle ear surgery). This information will allow the surgeon to counsel the patient in an honest and realistic way. As such, pre-operative imaging (or the absence of it) has important medicolegal implications.

2.1 How Does the Clinician Decide Which Imaging to Ask for?

A new case starts with the patient's personal and family history.

We listen to the complaints and symptoms: HL (time of onset: congenital, early childhood, abrupt, progressive, posttraumatic or iatrogenic, linked to inflammation/infection), tinnitus (occupational or leisure noise exposure, pulsating, objective versus subjective, etc.), balance problems (time line), ear discharge, otalgia, facial paresis or palsy (spontaneous, posttraumatic, recurrent).

This often already focuses the attention in a specific diagnostic direction.

We then examine the patient: otoscopy (status and structure of the external ear, external meatus and ear canal—dysplasia, skin lesions, bone lesions, fracture lines; status of the TM—normal, retracted, tympanosclerosis, colour change or pulsation—vascular lesions, bulging, blunting or lateralisation, perforation, cholesteatoma, suspect lesion—tumour, malignant external otitis, aeration of the middle ear).

Key information is also provided by the audiometry—conductive HL, mixed HL or sensorineural HL—unilateral or bilateral, symmetric or asymmetric loss (caveat cerebellopontine angle lesions in asymmetric bone conduction levels)—and by the vestibular test battery.

The above information usually suffices to decide which kind of imaging information we will need, in order to confirm or contradict the suspected diagnosis.

CT is still the method of excellence to visualise bony lesions and air—bone and soft tissue—bone contrast. Today, CBCT is preferred to multi-detector CT because of its lower radiation dose and better resolution. Thus, in most cases concerning functional middle ear surgery (conductive HL), CT will suffice. However, in case of asymmetric bone conduction thresholds, MRI will be needed to exclude, e.g., a vestibular schwannoma in the internal acoustic meatus, the cerebellopontine angle (CPA) or the cochleovestibular labyrinth. In case of a history of congenital sensorineural HL, MRI is the best tool for evaluation.

For the work-up of cochlear implant candidates, MRI is the main tool to determine the accessibility and implantibility of the cochlea, the presence of a normally sized cochlear nerve branch, the absence of lesions at the level the auditory pathways or the auditory cortex and the absence of unexpected concomitant pathology which could eventually jeopardize the long-term safety or function of the cochlear implant. However, CT remains important to provide the surgeon with a reliable roadmap to execute the surgery.

So in many pathological entities of the temporal bone, both MRI and CT have their specific roles.

It is clearly the clinician's responsibility to instruct the radiologist which imaging examination is needed, to indicate for what purpose and to define what he wants to see. This will direct the radiologist in selecting the correct imaging sequences.

The various chapters in this book will elaborate in detail how best to visualise the various temporal bone pathologies, thus instructing the clinicians which examinations to ask for.

3 How the Clinician Should Approach the Indication for Imaging?

The following is an illustration of how the clinician should think about the help he can get from imaging to make the right decisions.

Example 1: The patient with conductive or mixed HL with an intact tympanic membrane Patients suffering from conductive or mixed HL usually seek better hearing, preferably by surgery instead of having to use a hearing aid.

The main questions for the clinician thus are: (1) Can surgery improve the hearing? (2) Can the operation be performed in a safe way?

Until quite recently most such cases would not be sent for pre-operative imaging. However, the recent improvement in resolution and the lower radiation dose offered by CBCT is rapidly changing this attitude. The pre-operative imaging work-up is indeed a key factor in providing an answer to these questions.

3.1 Let Us Now See Which Elements of the Diagnostic Work-up Should Urge the Clinician to Ask for Imaging

The diagnostic methods available in patients with conductive HL with an intact TM are: personal and family history, otoscopy, audiology, imaging and surgical inspection. However, surgical inspection is only performed as a last resort, when all diagnostic efforts have failed to yield a plausible pre-operative diagnosis. Today this should be rather the exception.

3.2 Family History for Hearing Loss and Ear Surgery

The usual suspect is otosclerosis. CBCT can confirm the diagnosis in over 90 % of the cases. However, osteogenesis imperfecta can present with similar symptoms and audiograms. Imaging is needed to evaluate the operability of these cases, because they can be difficult and sometimes impossible to improve (e.g., in case of round window obliteration). Also, Enlarged Vestibular aqueduct (EVA) can present with a seemingly mixed HL. These cases warrant MRI for their diagnosis, and present a definite contraindication to functional stapes surgery.

3.3 Personal History and Symptoms

The *time of onset of the hearing loss* is a crucial diagnostic element. If it is congenital or has an early childhood onset, it necessitates MRI to exclude EVA or congenital cochlear dysplasia, which are both contraindications to stapes surgery.

A *history of head trauma* warrants CBCT to exclude or identify traumatic ossicular luxation or subluxation.

A fluctuating pattern of HL contradicts the nature of an ossicular fixation. It necessitates repeated audiometry for confirmation. Repeated otoscopy and tympanometry should rule out otitis media with effusion. If connected with an early onset, MRI should be asked for to rule out EVA.

Autophony coupled with vestibular symptoms warrants CBCT to rule out superior semicircular canal dehiscence (SSCD).

Recurrent dizziness coupled with a history of head trauma or barotrauma can point to a labyrinthine fistula.

A *history of recurrent inflammatory middle ear disease* can suggest incus lysis or tympanosclerotic fixation of the ossicles. CBCT can provide the diagnosis.

A *history of previous middle ear surgery* warrants CBCT to evaluate the condition of the ossicles (integrity, presence of ossicular prosthesis) and the middle ear (aeration, scar tissue formation).

3.4 Clinical Examination and Otoscopy

Congenital facial abnormalities coupled with congenital conductive HL can be associated with minor middle ear dysplasia. It needs CBCT work-up.

Otoscopic signs of TM or middle ear disease necessitate pre-operative CT imaging (incus lysis, tympanosclerotic fixation of the ossicles, aeration of the middle ear?). *Bulging and whitish discolouration* of an intact TM, or deep retraction of the pars flaccida can suggest congenital or respectively acquired cholesteatoma. Non-EPI DW MRI can confirm the diagnosis. A pulsating TM suggests a vascular abnormality. A colour change in a bulging part of the TM can suggest a tympanic glomus tumour. Full imaging work-up is needed.

The most *important audiological findings* that predict trouble and thus necessitate pre-operative imaging are: fluctuating thresholds (EVA), unusual form of the audiogram (malleus fixation, LVA, SCCD) and stapedial reflex presence (posttraumatic ossicular luxation). In case of asymmetric bone conduction thresholds MRI is mandatory to exclude a concomitant CPA or intralabyrinthine lesion (e.g. schwannoma).

CT can be used to detect causes like otosclerosis, tympanosclerosis, posttraumatic ossicular lesions, incus lysis, minor ear dysplasias and SCCD. MRI must be used to exclude a vestibular or intralabyrinthine schwannoma, to detect labyrinth dysplasia, and is used when there is a suspicion of cholesteatoma. Hence, imaging must be performed whenever something is 'out of tune'. The most important reasons to ask for diagnostic imaging are: atypical history, cases suspect for congenital HL, suspect otoscopic image, asymmetric BC thresholds and surgical revision cases. However, given the amount of valuable pre-operative information provided, which allows for efficient planning and comprehensive patient counseling, a thorough pre-operative imaging work-up is advocated.

Example 2: The pre-operative work-up and post-operative follow-up of cholesteatoma cases The diagnosis of a middle ear cholesteatoma is usually based on the otoscopic evaluation of the patient. For the pre-operative work-up of a middle ear cholesteatoma, prior to first stage surgery, CT scan is still the imaging evaluation tool of choice. It can nicely demonstrate the erosion of the ossicles and the bony spur of the epitympanic space. It delineates the bony tegmen and the capsula otica (e.g. to exclude intracranial involvement or a fistula of the lateral semicircular canal). However, in some cases adding MR sequences is indicated. When there is doubt concerning the diagnosis or concerning the extent of the cholesteatoma (e.g. intracranially when the tegmen is absent on CT scan), the non-EPDW sequence provides the diagnosis. In case of a labyrinthine fistula, adding T2-weighted MR sequences to the CT scan can inform the surgeon on the presence or absence of scar tissue in the intralabyrinthine space. This knowledge helps to counsel the patient on the degree of risk for sensory HL as a consequence of the surgical dissection of the pathology (the presence of scar tissue between the cholesteatoma matrix and the membraneous labyrinth makes the dissection less dangerous and thus protects function).

The radiologist should have a basic understanding of the various types of *surgical techniques* that are used in chronic ear disease. There are two main classes of techniques. In the canal wall down (*CWD*) tympanoplasty, the middle ear cavities are cleared of pathology by taking down the superior and posterior bony wall of the external auditory canal, thus creating a large resection cavity as an end result. The mastoid and attic space are thus left open, in continuity with the external auditory canal, while a small middle ear is created by restoring the TM on a more medial level. (The CWD techniques are also called 'open techniques'.) The main advantage of CWD is that the cavity can be monitored for residual disease by otoscopy, thus obviating routine exploratory second stage surgery. The main disadvantages of the CWD technique are the usually worse results on the functional and hygienic level (non-self cleaning nor waterresistant ear) and a higher comorbidity (regular cleaning needed, and recurrent inflammation due to a lack of self cleaning capacity of keratine).

In the canal wall up (*CWU*) tympanoplasty (also called 'closed techniques'), the external auditory canal is kept intact or is surgically restored. This increases the risk for residual cholesteatoma which cannot be seen by otoscopy and until recently (before the advent of the non-EPDW MR sequence) necessitated routine surgical staging in many cases.

However, in recent years the bony obliteration tympanoplasty (*BOT*) technique is quickly gaining ground, because it combines the advantages of CWD and CWU tympanoplasty without their respective disadvantages. In the BOT the mastoid, antrum and attic (the so-called paratympanic space) are cleared of disease and soft tissue, keeping the bony canal wall intact. Then the tympano-attical barrier and posterior tympanotomy are blocked by sculpted cortical bone, thus effectively separating the middle ear space from the paratympanic space. Subsequently, the paratympanic space is completely filled with bone pâté up to the cortical level. Finally the TM and ossicular chain are reconstructed. The major advantage of the BOT is the low rate of residual and very low rate of recurrent disease. This technique obviates the need for routine exploratory second stage surgery, on condition that imaging can reliably diagnose residual disease in a non-invasive way. The non-EPDW MR sequence provides an excellent tool to rule out or confirm residual cholesteatoma.

Over the past few years *MR imaging* has gained an increasing importance for the pre-operative diagnosis and post-operative follow-up of middle ear cholesteatoma.

Whereas CT is regarded as the primary imaging tool in the clinically clear-cut middle ear cholesteatoma to evaluate the extension of the cholesteatoma, MRI found its place in the diagnostic work-up of the clinically doubtful cholesteatoma and as a non-invasive screening tool for residual disease in the follow-up after primary surgery.

Mainly two types of MR imaging techniques have been used: the delayed gadolinium-enhanced T1-weighted sequences (*DgeT1*) and the non-echo-planar diffusion-weighted MR sequences (*non-EPDW*).

The rationale of the DgeT1 is based on the fact that scar tissue and inflammation require time to enhance and that early scanning might result in false-positive results. The echo-planar diffusion-weighted MR sequences (*EPDW*) have been abandoned in favour of the non-EPDW thanks to a higher resolution, the thinner slice thickness and the complete lack of susceptibility artefacts of the latter sequences. On diffusion-weighted sequences, cholesteatoma lights up as a hyperintense lesion on b-1,000 images. It has been proven that the combination of DgeT1 and non-EPDW yields no higher sensitivity, specificity, negative and positive predictive value than the non-EPDW alone. Imaging of middle ear cholesteatoma can hence be performed using non-echo-planar diffusion-weighted sequences alone. The association to T2-weighted sequences will allow the surgeon to locate a hyperintensity seen on diffusion-weighted sequences more exactly with respect to the anatomical landmarks of the temporal bone.

Exception should be made in case of an infected cholesteatoma and in case of suspicion of associated complications. In those cases, the combined protocol including DgeT1 and non-EPDW should be used.

Screening for residual cholesteatoma by imaging should be performed by MRI using solely non-EPDW. This prevents unwarranted routine exploratory second stage surgery as well as irradiation from repeated CT scans. The MR controls are usually scheduled at 1 and 5 years post-operatively.

4 Conclusion

Imaging is one of the cornerstones in the diagnostic work-up and follow-up of temporal bone pathology.

A close collaboration between clinician and radiologist is crucial to ensure a correct understanding of the indications for imaging by the clinician, and the selection and application of the correct sequences by the radiologist.

Temporal Bone Imaging Techniques

Marc Lemmerling, Bert De Foer, and Barbara Smet

Contents

1 CT Techniques for Temporal Bone Imaging 7
1.1 CBCT of the Temporal Bone 7
1.2 MSCT of the Temporal Bone 8
2 MR Techniques for Temporal Bone Imaging 8
2.1 Imaging of the Cerebellopontine Angle and Inner Ear 8
2.2 Cholesteatoma Imaging 8

Abstract

Multi-slice CT and Cone Beam CT are actually both used to image the temporal bone. Two completely different MR protocols are used to respectively image the inner ear and middle ear.

1 CT Techniques for Temporal Bone Imaging

Multi-slice CT (MSCT) has been used for many years to image the temporal bone. However, the last couple of years Cone Beam CT (CBCT) is taking over that role.

1.1 CBCT of the Temporal Bone

CBCT uses a rotating gantry on which an X-ray tube and detector is attached. A cone-shaped X-ray beam is directed through the middle of the temporal bone onto a two-dimensional X-ray detector. Because CBCT uses the entire FOV of the two-dimensional X-ray detector, only a single 360° gantry rotation is necessary to acquire a 3D-volumetric data set. Of this data reconstructions can be made in any desired plane.

The advantages of CBCT over MSCT are the shorter examination time, high spatial resolution, and low radiation dose. It is also less sensitive for metallic and beam hardening artifacts because image acquisition is based on conventional radiographic images. The most important disadvantage of CBCT is its high sensitivity for motion artifacts because the patient has to hold the head perfectly still during the acquisition time of approximately 40 s.

Many manufacturers construct cone beam scanners, and their parameters will differ. In some scanners the patients are in a sitting position. We chose a scanner with supine patient position. Fixation of the patient's head is done to

M. Lemmerling (✉) · B. Smet
Department of Radiology, AZ St-Lucas Hospital,
Groenebriel 1, 9000 Gent, Belgium
e-mail: marc.lemmerling@azstlucas.be

B. De Foer
Department of Radiology, GZA Hospitals Sint-Augustinus,
Oosterveldlaan 24, 2610 Wilrijk, Belgium

prevent motion artifacts. We use the following parameters (only suggestive because scanner specific):
- 110 kV
- ±140 mAs
- Field of view 15 × 5 cm High Resolution
- Slice thickness 0.15 mm
- Scan time 40 s

Reconstructions in the axial and coronal planes are made of the axial raw data images with a slice thickness of respectively 0.3 and 1 mm using special software.

The technicians are instructed to make this reconstruction in a plane parallel to the lateral semicircular canal. This is the axial imaging set. The coronal imaging set is reconstructed exactly perpendicular to this axial set of images. On the most cranial axial image the superior semicircular canal is shown. The most anterior coronal image is made just anterior to the geniculate ganglion of the facial nerve. This procedure is repeated for both the right and left temporal bones separately, and images are viewed using a window width of 3050 HU and a window level of 525 HU. These parameters for windowing only have an indicative value, as each radiologist has to make his/her own choice. Systematic visualization of both stapes crura and of the suspensory ligaments in the middle ear cavity can be a helpful indicator when choosing the windowing parameters.

1.2 MSCT of the Temporal Bone

The images are acquired in a single imaging plane using a multi-slice detector scanner. The patient is lying on his/her back and the gantry of the scanner is not tilted. We use the following imaging parameters (only indicative because scanner and user-specific):
- 120 kV
- 250 mAs
- Collimation 0.5 mm or 0.625 mm
- Scan time 1.0 s

Postprocessing is done in a similar way as data acquired with CBCT. After acquiring the raw dataset images are reconstructed with a slice thickness of 1 mm and by using an ultra high resolution reconstruction mode. The technicians are instructed to make this reconstruction in a plane parallel to the lateral semicircular canal. This is the axial imaging set. The coronal imaging set is reconstructed exactly perpendicular to this axial set of images. On the most cranial axial image the superior semicircular canal is shown. The most anterior coronal image is made just anterior to the geniculate ganglion of the facial nerve. This procedure is repeated for both the right and left temporal bones separately, and the images are viewed using a window width of 4000 HU and a window level of 200 HU.

These parameters for windowing only have an indicative value, as each radiologist has to make his/her own choice. Systematic visualization of both stapes crura and of the suspensory ligaments in the middle ear cavity can be a helpful indicator when choosing the windowing parameters.

2 MR Techniques for Temporal Bone Imaging

Since many years MR is used for inner ear imaging. During the last years, an increasing role is reserved for MR in the detection of cholesteatoma.

2.1 Imaging of the Cerebellopontine Angle and Inner Ear

A lot of discussion exists on which MR imaging protocol should be used for the temporal bone. Controversy exists on which sequences should be used, what the exact slice thickness of the images should be and even the eventual use of contrast agents. The following imaging protocol can be considered as an example of how a good protocol can look like, but each radiologist can tailor them according to personal experiences or according to different indications. The following sequences are standard in our department:

1. 5 mm thick axial TSE T2-weighted images of the brain, brain stem, and posterior fossa, performed to study the brain for cerebral anomalies causing hearing loss, tinnitus, vertigo, … (e.g., cerebral arteriovenous malformations, brain stem ischemia, …)
2. 1–3 mm thick axial SE T1-weighted images of the temporal bone
3. 0.4–0.7 mm thick axial high resolution T2-weighted images of the inner ear structures
4. 1–3 mm thick axial SE T1-weighted images of the temporal bone after intravenous injection of gadolinium
5. 1–3 mm thick coronal SE T1-weighted images of the temporal bone after intravenous injection of gadolinium

The following changes are currently made:
- Performing T1-weighted images in 3D technique with the use of thin slices (e.g., 1 mm). This is especially interesting to study the relationship between small tumors and the cranial nerves in the internal auditory meatus
- Performing reconstructions of the 3D TSE T2-weighted sequence in other planes than the axial one. This is most often done to study the relationship between different small structures in the cerebellopontine angel and internal auditory meatus, such as cranial nerves, vessels, and small tumors
- Performing additional MR angiographic sequences, especially interesting if vascular lesions are detected

- Performing specific sequences for detection of endolymphatic hydrops (see chapter on inner ear pathology)

2.2 Cholesteatoma Imaging

Since the introduction of MR for cholesteatoma imaging, two completely different techniques have been introduced, the one basically using diffusion-weighted images (DW), the other performing T1-weighted images before and after intravenous injection of gadolinium. Non-echoplanar (non-EP) DW proved to be better than echoplanar DW images.

Following scan protocol can be used for cholesteatoma imaging:

1. 2 mm thick coronal b0 and b800 or b1000 non-EP DW images with ADC map
2. 2 mm thick axial TSE T2-weighted images
3. 2 mm thick coronal T2-weighted images

If complications (such as middle cranial fossa invasion, facial nerve paralysis, or membranous labyrinth invasion) are suspected, following protocol is performed 45 min after intravenous injection of gadolinium:

1. 2 mm thick coronal b0 and b800 or b1000 non-EP DW images with ADC map
2. 0.4–0.7 mm thick axial high resolution T2-weighted images
3. 2 mm thick coronal TSE T2-weighted images
4. 2 mm thick coronal SE T1-weighted images
5. 2 mm thick axial SE T1-weighted images

Cross-Sectional Imaging Anatomy of the Temporal Bone

Marc Lemmerling, Barbara Smet, and Bert De Foer

Contents

1 Anatomy 11
1.1 External Ear 11
1.2 Middle Ear 11
1.3 Inner Ear 15
2 Cross Sectional Imaging Anatomy 17
2.1 Axial CT Images 17
2.2 Coronal CT Images 17
2.3 Axial T2-weighted MR Images 26
2.4 Axial T1-weighted MR Images 18
References 23

Abstract

The temporal bone contains the external, middle and inner ear. In the middle ear the ossicles and a suspensory apparatus transfer the acoustic energy. In the inner ear the membranous labyrinth is embedded in the osseous labyrinth. The inner ear is responsible for hearing and balance. In this chapter we focus on the anatomy and radiologic anatomy of the temporal bone.

1 Anatomy

1.1 External Ear

The external ear consists of an ovoid auricula or pinna and an oval, cylindrical meatus acusticus externus, or external auditory canal. Its function is to collect and amplify air vibration by the auricula and conduct them through the external auditory canal to the tympanic cavity or middle ear.

The auricula is the appendage that projects from the lateral surface of the head and is composed of fibrocartilage, covered with thin skin continuous with the lining of the external auditory canal. The auricula is attached to the skull by muscles and ligaments, and to the external auditory canal by fibrous tissue. The auricula has a complex shape that causes delays in the path of sound and helps in sound localization.

The external auditory canal measures approximately 4 cm in length and is curved in an S-shape. It consists of fibrocartilage laterally and of bone medially, and is also lined with thin skin. The medial border of the external auditory canal is closed by the tympanic membrane that attaches superiorly to the scutum and inferiorly to the tympanic annulus. The mandibular condyle and the mastoid cells and respectively located anterior and posterior to the osseous portion of the external auditory canal.

M. Lemmerling (✉) · B. Smet
Department of Radiology, AZ St-Lucas Hospital, Groenebriel 1, 9000 Gent, Belgium
e-mail: marc.lemmerling@azstlucas.be

B. De Foer
Department of Radiology, GZA Hospitals Sint-Augustinus, Oosterveldlaan 24, 2610 Wilrijk, Belgium

1.2 Middle Ear

The middle ear or tympanic cavity is an air-filled space located in the temporal bone between the air-filled external ear and the fluid-filled inner ear. The middle ear contains a chain of three movable auditory ossicles, the malleus, incus, and stapes. They are supported by the tympanic membrane, the anterior, superior and lateral malleal ligaments, the posterior incudal ligament, the tendons of the tensor tympani and stapedius muscles, and the annular ligament.

The primary function of the middle ear is to act as an impedance element between the air-filled external ear and the fluid-filled inner ear. When sound waves hit the tympanic membrane, their energy is converted into mechanical vibrations that sets the ossicular chain in motion, transducing kinetic energy to the stapedial footplate, thus generating a wave in the cochlea. The frequency of this wave determines which hair cells are stimulated, which in turn emit a neural signal to the brain, resulting in hearing perception.

1.2.1 Tympanic Cavity

The middle ear is a six-sided cavity containing the three auditory ossicles supported by the tympanic membrane, the auditory ligaments, the tendons of the tensor tympani and stapedius muscles, and the annular ligament (Fig. 1). The roof of the tympanic cavity is formed by a thin bony plate, the tegmen tympani. The floor is also formed by a thin plate of bone, the fundus tympani, that separates the tympanic cavity from the jugular fossa. The lateral wall is mainly formed by the tympanic membrane and partly by a ring of bone on which the membrane inserts. The ring is incomplete at its upper portion, forming the notch of Rivinus. The medial wall is formed by the lateral wall of the inner ear. The posterior boundaries are defined by the mastoid and the anterior boundaries by the carotid canal.

The tympanic cavity can be divided into three subdivisions in the coronal plane: the epi-, meso-, and hypotympanum. The epitympanum is the attic, formed by an imaginary line drawn between scutum and tympanic segment of the facial nerve. The mesotympanum is the middle part delineated by the line between scutum and tympanic segment of the facial nerve on one hand, and a line connecting the tympanic annulus and the base of the cochlear promontoryon the other hand. The hypotympanum is the lowest part of the tympanic cavity and lies below the line between tympanic annulus and the base of the cochlear promontory.

1.2.2 Auditory Ossicles

The tympanic cavity contains three auditory ossicles: the malleus, the incus, and the stapes (Fig. 2). The ossicles act as a lever transforming the large and weak motion of the tympanic membrane into a small and forceful movement of

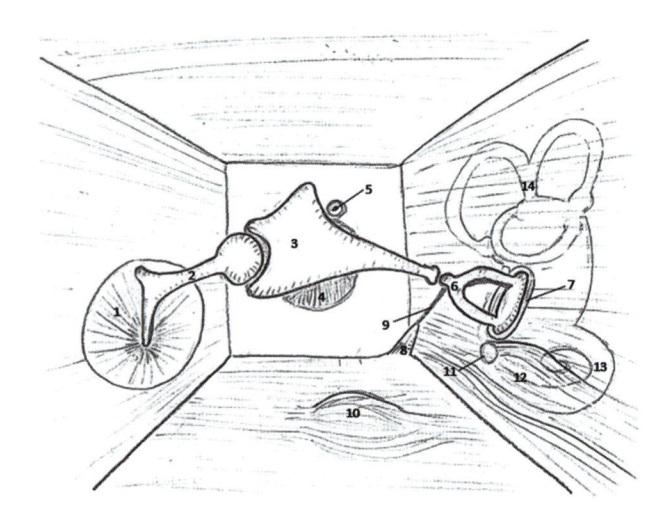

Fig. 1 A schematic visualization of the tympanic cavity as a box after removal of the posterior wall with tympanic membrane (*1*) and malleus (*2*) on the lateral wall, incus (*3*), Eustachian tube (*4*) and tensor tympani tendon (*5*) at the level of the cochleariform process on the anterior wall, stapes (*6*) at the oval window (*7*) on the medial wall, pyramidal eminence (*8*) with stapedius tendon (*9*) attached to the neck of the stapes, jugular bulb (*10*), round window (*11*), cochlear promontory (*12*) with cochlea (*13*) and semicircular canals (*14*) shining trough the medial wall of the tympanic cavity

the stapes. The malleus is attached to the tympanic membrane and the stapes is connected to the fenestra vestibuli, traditionally referred to as the oval window. In between the incus is suspended by delicate articulations, the incudomalleal and incudostapedial joints.

The malleus, named after the resemblance to a hammer, consists of a head, neck, and three processes:, the manubrium, the anterior and lateral processes.

The incus resembling an anvil consists of a corpus and 2 crura (processes). The anterior part of the corpus articulates with the head of the malleus in a saddle-shaped diarthrosis. The two processes are positioned perpendicular to each other with the short process running almost horizontally backward and the long process descending nearly vertically and bending medially, ending in a little notch covered by cartilage, the lenticular process, articulating with the head of the stapes.

The stapes similar to a stirrup, consists of a head, neck, 2 crura and a base. In between the 2 crura lies the foramen obturatorium. The 2 crura diverge from the neck and are at their end connected to an oval plate that is fixed to the fenestra vestibuli by a ring of ligamentous fibers, the annular ligament.

1.2.3 Suspensory Apparatus

The malleus, incus, and stapes are situated between the tympanic membrane and oval window, and are supported by the tympanic membrane, the anterior, superior, and lateral malleal ligaments, the posterior incudal ligament, the tendons of the tensor tympani and stapedius muscles, and the annular ligament (Fig. 3).

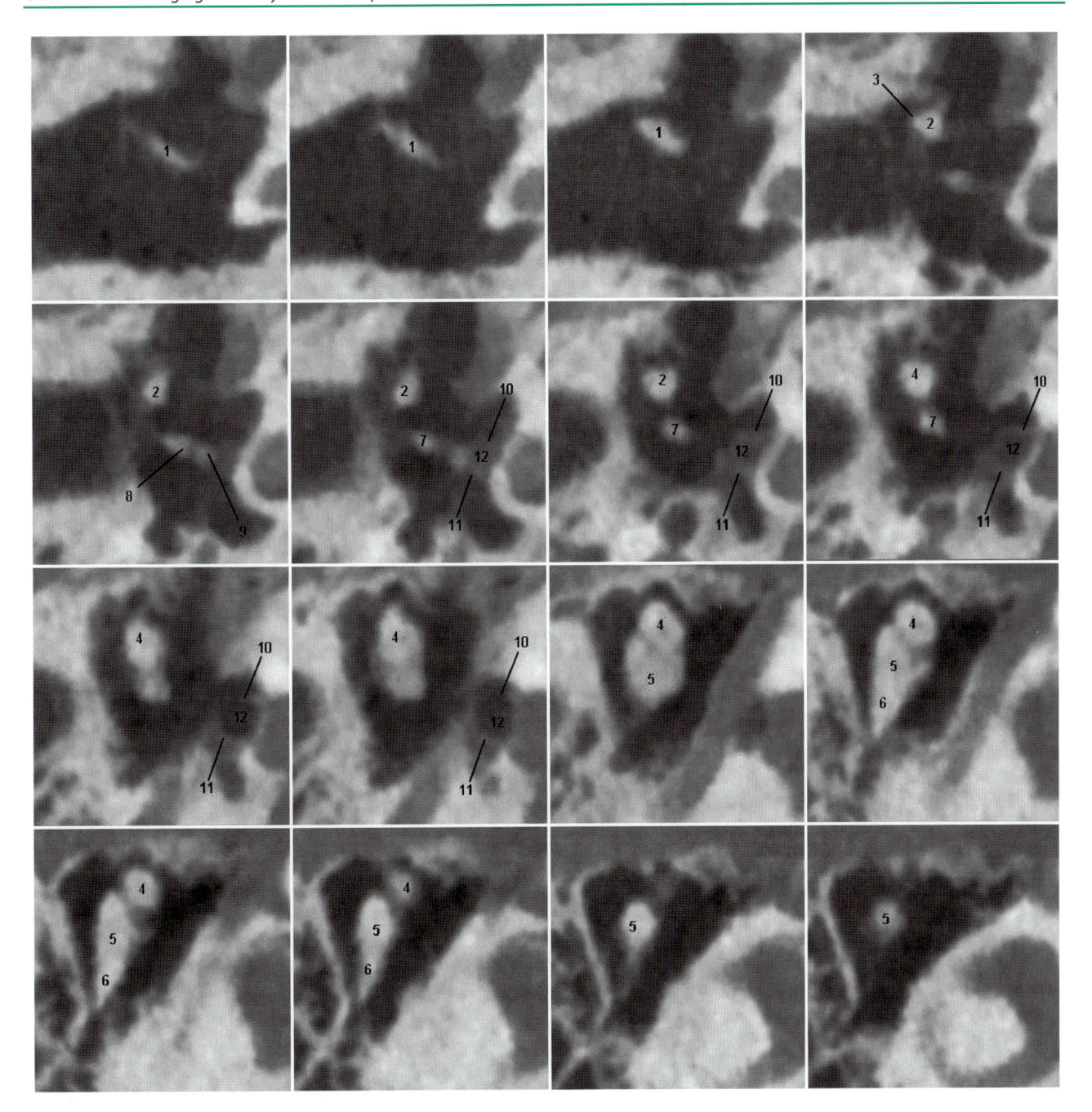

Fig. 2 Consecutive axial 0.3 mm thick CBCT images through a normal middle ear showing the ossicular chain with malleus manubrium (*1*), neck (*2*), lateral process (*3*) and head (*4*); incus body (*5*) with short (*6*) and long process (*7*) and its lenticular process (*8*) articulating with the head of the stapes (*9*); anterior (*10*) and posterior crus (*11*) of the stapes and the foramen obturatorium (*12*)

The malleus is supported by the superior, anterior, and lateral malleal ligaments, the tensor tympani muscle tendon, the tympanic membrane, and the incudomalleal joint. The incus is supported by the posterior incudal ligament and two joints, the incudomalleal and incudostapedial joints. The stapes is supported by the stapedius muscle tendon and the incudostapedial joint.

Axial CBCT images are excellent to see the anterior malleal ligament (AML), posterior incudal ligament (PIL), and the stapedius muscle tendon. Coronal images are excellent to see the superior malleal ligament (SML) and the lateral malleal ligament (LML). The tensor tympani muscle tendon can be appreciated on both axial and coronal images (Table 1).

The AML is attached at one end to the malleal neck, just above the anterior process, and to the anterior tympanic wall by the other end. The PIL connects the incus short process to the incudal fossa (Fig. 4). The SML runs from the roof of the epitympanic recess to the malleus head

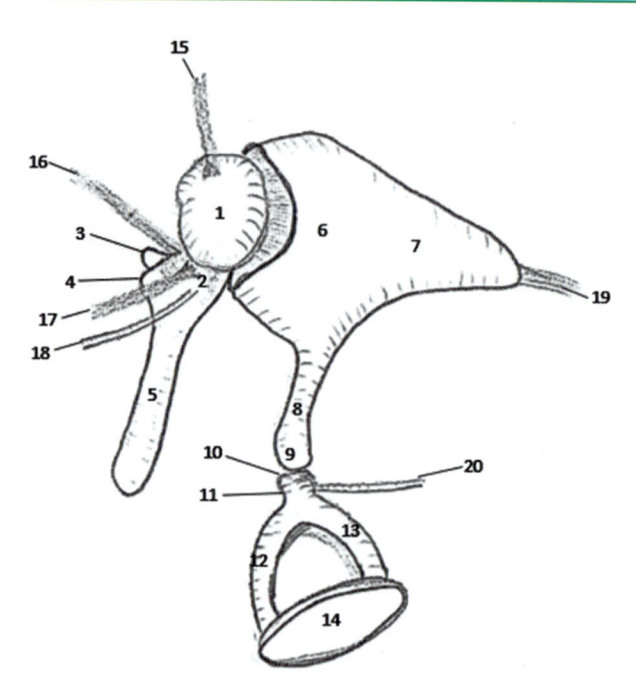

Fig. 3 A schematic visualization of the ossicular chain and its suspensory apparatus with malleus and its head (*1*), neck (*2*), lateral (*3*) and anterior process (*4*) and manubrium (*5*); incus with body (*6*), short (*7*) and long process (*8*) ending in the lenticular process (*9*); stapes with head (*10*), neck (*11*), anterior (*12*) and posterior crus (*13*), and footplate (*14*). The superior malleal ligament (*15*) inserts on the malleal head (*1*); the lateral malleal ligament (*16*), anterior malleal ligament (*17*), and tensor tympani tendon (*18*) insert on the malleal neck (*2*); the posterior incudal ligament (*19*) inserts on the incus short process (*7*); and the stapedius muscle tendon (*19*) mostly inserts on the stapes neck (*11*)

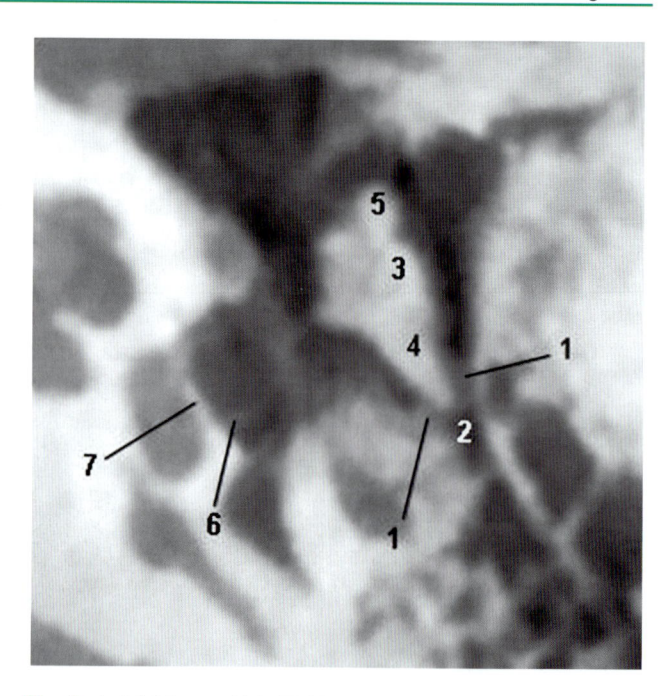

Fig. 4 Axial 0.3 mm thick CBCT image through a normal middle ear showing the posterior incudal ligament (*1*), fossa incudis (*2*), incus body (*3*) and its short process (*4*), malleus head (*5*), crus posterior of the stapes (*6*), and foramen ovale (*7*)

Table 1 Origin and insertion of suspensory middle ear ligaments and tendons

	ORIGIN → INSERTION
Axial	
AML	Anterior epitympanic wall → malleus neck
PIL	Incudal fossa → incus short process
Stapedius tendon	Pyramidal eminence → stapes neck
Tensor tympani tendon	Cochleariform process → malleus neck
Coronal	
SML	Epitympanic roof → malleus head
LML	Notch of rivinus → malleus neck
Tensor tympani Tendon	Cochleariform process → malleus neck

AML anterior malleal ligament; *PIL* posterior incudal ligament; *SML* superior malleal ligament; *LML* lateral malleal ligament

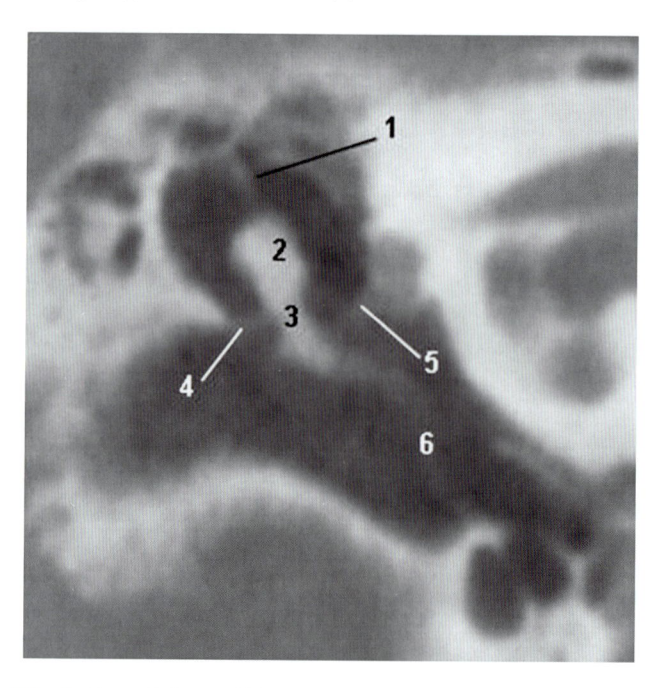

Fig. 5 Coronal 1 mm thick CBCT image through a normal middle ear showing the superior malleal ligament (*1*), malleus head (*2*), malleus neck (*3*), lateral malleal ligament (*4*), tensor tympani tendon (*5*), and tympanic membrane (*6*)

(Fig. 5). The LML extends from the posterior part of the notch of Rivinus to the malleus neck (Fig. 6).

The tensor tympani muscle arises from the cartilaginous (upper) portion of the auditory tube in which it is contained, then swerves around the cochleariform process resulting in a tendon that attaches to the neck of the malleus (Fig. 7).

The muscle belly of the tensor tympani muscle is located antero-inferior to the tympanic segment of the facial nerve.

The smallest muscle in the human body is the stapedius muscle, arising from the apex of the pyramidal eminence immediately behind the oval window, runs forward and

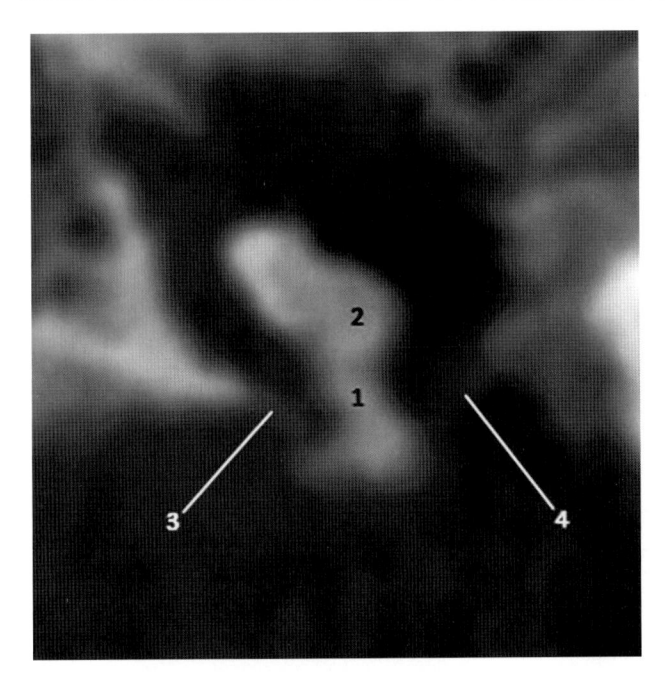

Fig. 6 Coronal 1 mm thick CBCT image through a normal middle ear showing the malleus neck (*1*), malleus head (*2*), lateral malleal ligament (*3*), and tensor tympani tendon (*4*)

inserts onto the posterior surface of the neck of the stapes in the majority of patients (Fig. 8). Occasionally, it inserts on the head or on the posterior crus of the stapes due to the persistence of a greater or lesser degree of angulation between the tendon and the belly of the stapedius muscle during embryological development.

The ligaments of the middle ear solely act as a suspensory apparatus, whereas the muscles of the middle ear also exert a protective function. Contraction of the tensor tympani muscle pulls the malleus anteromedially, while contraction of the stapedius muscle pulls the stapes posteriorly. Both muscles pull in more or less opposite directions, applying forces perpendicular to the motion of the ossicular chain. Their contraction, stimulated by the acoustic reflex, is a protective mechanism that stiffens the ossicular chain, thereby protecting the inner ear of being overwhelmed by exuberant sound wave vibrations. This mechanism is also responsible for the improvement of signal-to-noise ratio.

1.3 Inner Ear

The inner ear is a fluid-filled labyrinthine space in the temporal bone called the labyrinth, named after its complexity in shape. It consists of two parts, the bony osseous labyrinth and the membranous labyrinth. The osseous labyrinth consists of five structures: cochlea, vestibule, three semicircular canals, and the cochlear and vestibular aqueduct. The osseous labyrinth contains perilymph in which the membranous labyrinth is bathing. The membranous labyrinth is a collection of interconnecting sacs and ducts that follow the form of the osseous labyrinth and contain fluid called endolymph.

The inner ear is responsible for hearing and balance. The cochlea contains distal fibers of the cochlear nerve that alter mechanical vibrations into nerve signals that are sent to the brain, resulting in hearing. The vestibule and semicircular canals are responsible for balance. The utricle and saccule, both parts of the vestibule, determine the orientation relative to gravity by detecting linear accelerations. The semicircular canals deliver information about turning by detecting rotational movements.

1.3.1 The Osseous Labyrinth

The osseous labyrinth consists of three parts: cochlea, vestibule, and three semicircular canals. It is lined by a thin fibro-serous membrane covered with a layer of epithelium that secretes perilymph.

The cochlea resembles a snail-shell and forms the anterior part of the inner ear. The base of the cochlea connects with the internal auditory canal by numerous perforations through which the cochlear division of the acoustic nerve passes. The cochlea measures about 5 mm in axial length and makes approximately two and a half turns around a central axis named the modiolus. The osseous lamina spiralis subdivides the spiral canal into the scala vestibuli and scala tympani, which meet each other at the apex of the modiolus in the helicotrema. From the free border of the osseous lamina spiralis, the basilar membrane stretches to the outer wall of the bony cochlea. The basilar membrane contains hair cells that are essential for hearing.

The basal first turn of the cochlea opens in the tympanic cavity in the round window and is closed by a secondary tympanic membrane or round window membrane. When sound waves reach the stapes, an inward movement of the stapes in the oval window causes an outward bulging of the round window membrane in the round window, allowing free movement of inner ear fluids. This sets in motion a wave form that stimulates the hair cells on the basilar membrane, exciting the sensory mechanism, which results in a flow of nerve impulses to the higher centers, resulting in hearing.

The cochlear aqueduct also extends from the basal turn of the cochlea—more specific from the scala tympani—and runs parallel and posteriorly to the internal auditory canal. It opens in the inferior surface of the petrous part of the temporal bone near the jugular fossa, lateral of the jugular foramen. It forms a communication between the subarachnoid cavity and the labyrinth and is a possible entryway for micro-organisms, although in human the lumen is small and often not patent. Its function is not clear but some authors believe that a stapes footplate gusher, leakage of perilymph through an opening in the stapes footplate, may result when the cochlear aqueduct is abnormally patent.

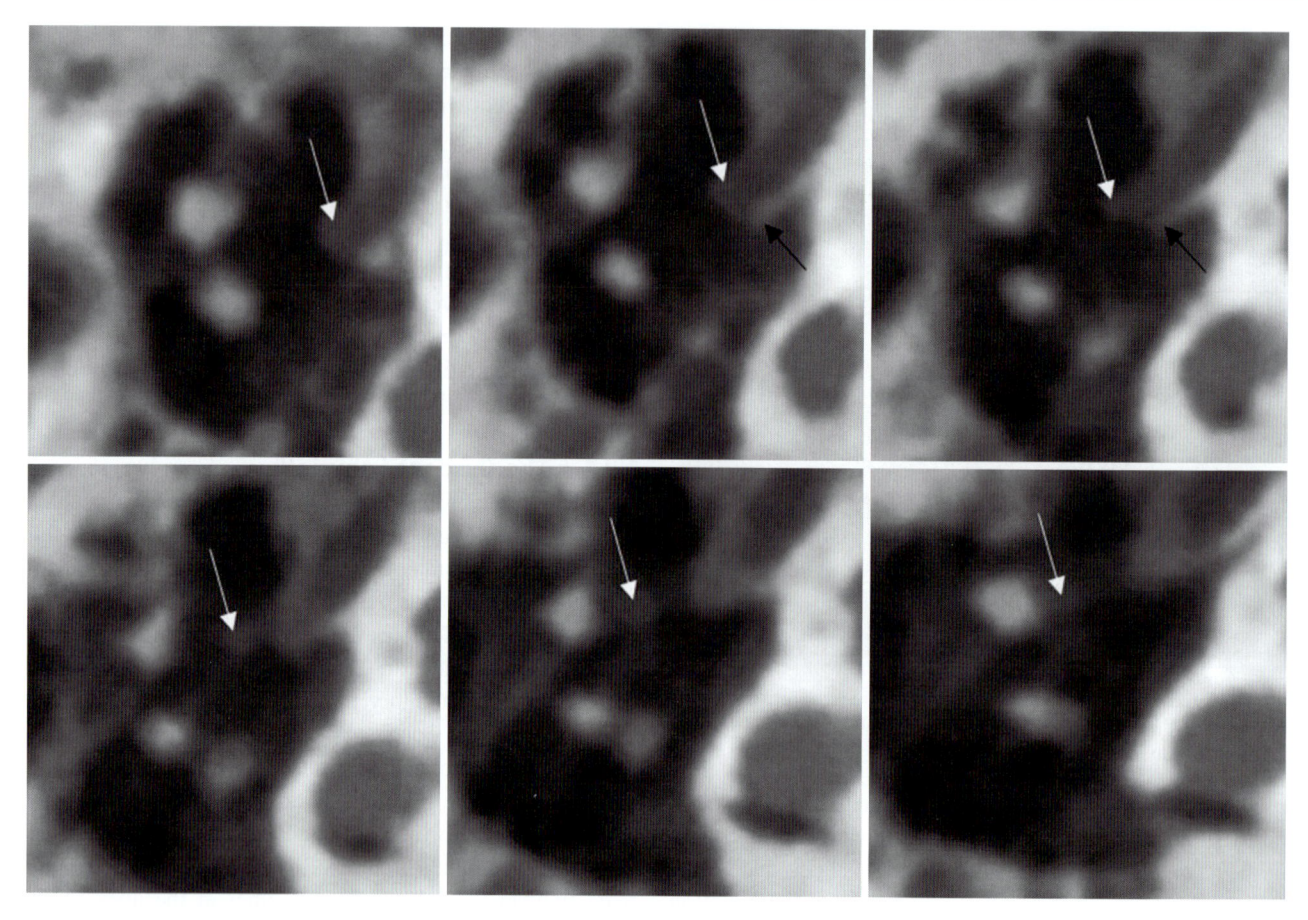

Fig. 7 Consecutive axial 0.3 mm thick CBCT images through a normal middle ear showing the tensor tympani muscle tendon (*white arrow*) passing around the cochleariform process (*black arrow*) and inserting on the malleal neck

The vestibule forms the central part of the osseous labyrinth and is somewhat oval in shape and measures approximately 4–5 mm. It is situated medial to the tympanic cavity and leads anteriorly to the cochlea and posteriorly to the semicircular canals. In its lateral wall, the oval window is closed by the footplate of the stapes. There are two depressions in its medial wall, the inferiorly spherical recess and the superiorly elliptical recess. They correspond with the saccule and utricule, both parts of the membranous vestibule. The recesses are perforated by several small holes forming the lamina cribrosa, which separates the vestibule from the fundus of the internal auditory canal and contains filaments of the acoustic nerve. Other openings in the vestibule are the five orifices of the semicircular canals and the vestibular aqueduct. The latter is a bony canal between the vestibule and the posterior surface of the petrous bone and contains the endolymphatic duct, which ends posteriorly in a blind pouch between the layers of the dura mater within the cranial cavity, the endolymphatic sac. The endolymphatic duct and sac play an important role in the normal metabolic activity of the inner ear. A loss of function results in a progressive increase in volume and biochemical degradation of endolymph. The vestibular aqueduct is enlarged when it measures more than 1.5 mm in diameter halfway between the vestibule on one hand and the posterior temporal bone surface on the other hand. An enlarged vestibular aqueduct is one of the most common inner ear deformities that results in hearing loss during childhood, and its presence should always warrant a search for cochlear deficiency.

There are three bony semicircular canals, the vertical and opposite to each other placed superior and posterior semicircular canal and the horizontal placed lateral semicircular canal. They measure about 1 mm in diameter and each stands at right angles to the other two. The upper bony margin of the superior semicircular canal forms a convexity in the petrous roof, the arcuate eminence. The lateral semicircular canal slightly protrudes into the epitympanum where it is vulnerable for fistulizing epitympanic cholesteatomas. It is in close contact with the midtympanic portion of the facial nerve, which passes along the undersurface of the lateral semicircular canal. Each semicircular canal has an enlargement at one end, forming a bony ampulla that contains the cristae with the vestibular sensory epithelium and that opens in the vestibule. The other nonampullary sides also open in the vestibule but the superior and posterior semicircular canals join to form a common crus, thus resulting in five orifices in the vestibule (Fig. 9).

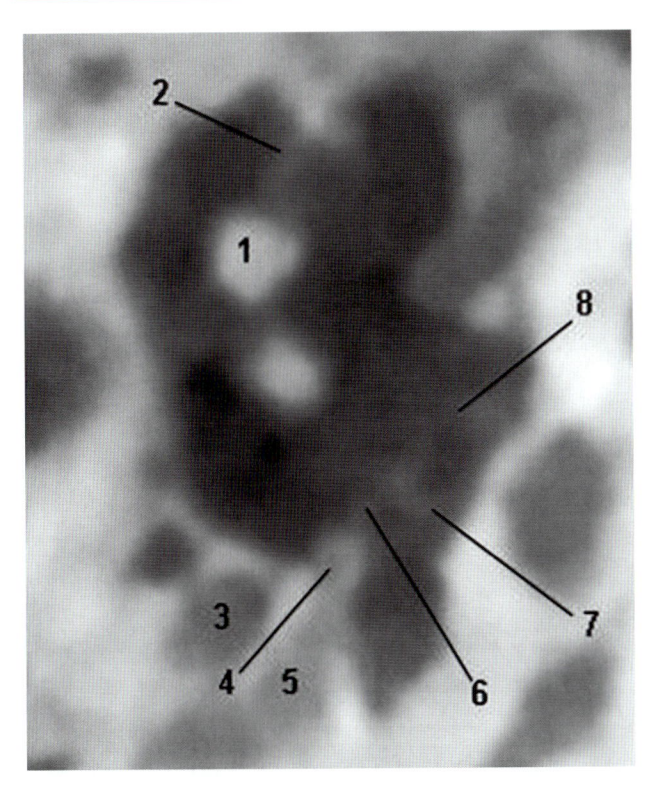

Fig. 8 Axial 0,3 mm thick CBCT image through a normal middle ear showing the malleus head (*1*), anterior malleal ligament (*2*), posterior genu of the facial nerve (*3*), pyramidal eminence (*4*), stapedius muscle (*5*), stapedius muscle tendon (*6*), and the stapes with its posterior (*7*) and anterior crus (*8*)

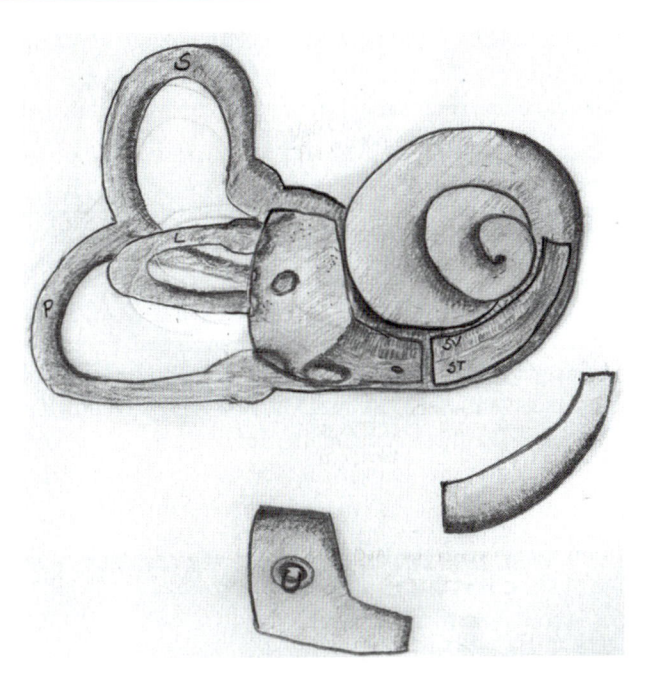

Fig. 9 The bony osseous labyrinth consisting of the snail-shell shaped cochlea, the central vestibule and the three semicircular canals (superior (*S*), posterior (*P*) and lateral (*L*) canal). The lateral wall of the vestibule and the anterior wall of the basal turn of the cochlea are taken out showing the opening of the basal turn of the cochlea in the round window, the cochlear aqueduct that extends from the scala tympani (*ST*), the scala vestibuli (*SV*) and the vestibular aqueduct in the posterior wall of the vestibule. The lateral wall of the vestibule shows the oval window closed by the stapes

1.3.2 The Membranous Labyrinth

The membranous labyrinth is suspended in the osseous labyrinth, and is separated from its bony walls by perilymph except for some places where it is fixed to the walls of the cavity by fibrous bands. The membranous labyrinth also contains fluid, endolymph.

The membranous labyrinth more or less follows the form of the osseous labyrinth except for the vestibule that consists of two membranous sacs, the utricle and saccule. The utricle lies in contact with the bony elliptical recess and communicates with the semicircular ducts by five orifices. From its anterior wall runs the utriculosaccular duct, which opens in the endolymphatic duct. The saccule is smaller and globular in shape and lies in contact with the spherical recess. From its posterior wall, the endolymphatic duct is given off, which joins the utriculosaccular duct and passes along the vestibular aqueduct to end in the endolymphatic sac. Both utricle and saccule show a thickening near the elliptical and spherical recess respectively forming the utricular and saccular macula which receive the utricular and saccular filaments of the acoustic nerve.

The semicircular ducts are about one-fourth of the diameter of the osseous canals but are otherwise similar in number and shape. In the ampulla, the wall is thickened forming the transverse septum that also receives the filaments of the acoustic nerve.

Both vestibule and semicircular canals play an important role in the vestibular functions of the inner ear. In the maculae of the utricle and saccule and in the transverse septa of the ampullae of the semicircular ducts, we find hair cells connected to the filaments of the vestibular nerve, a division of the acoustic nerve. The utricle and saccule that are respectively more or less in the horizontal and parasagittal plane have—beside hair cells—also otoliths which allow linear acceleration detection respectively in the axial and coronal imaging planes and generate otolith-ocular reflexes and otolith-body or righting reflexes. The semicircular canals detect angular acceleration and exert direct control over the eyes to compensate for head movement by the vestibulo-ocular reflex.

The ductus cochlearis or scala media also follows the bony canal of the cochlea as a spirally arranged tube. It consists of the basilar membrane that extends from the osseous lamina spiralis and the more delicate vestibular membrane or Reissner's membrane, forming the floor and the roof of the duct, respectively. The scala media lies between the superiorly scala vestibuli and the inferiorly scala tympani and contains the spiral organ of Corti. This complex organ consists of thousands of auditory nerve receptors, each with their own hair cell which transforms mechanical pressure vibrations into action potentials leading to electrical signaling to the auditory cortex, resulting in hearing (Gray 1918; Harnsberger 1995; Lane 2006; Lemmerling 1997).

2 Cross Sectional Imaging Anatomy

2.1 Axial CT Images

The images are shown from a left temporal bone, from cranially to caudally. The last image is not a part of the previous series. The last image is an enlarged view at oval window level in another person, showing the anterior and posterior stapes crurae. All images have a 1 mm slice thickness.

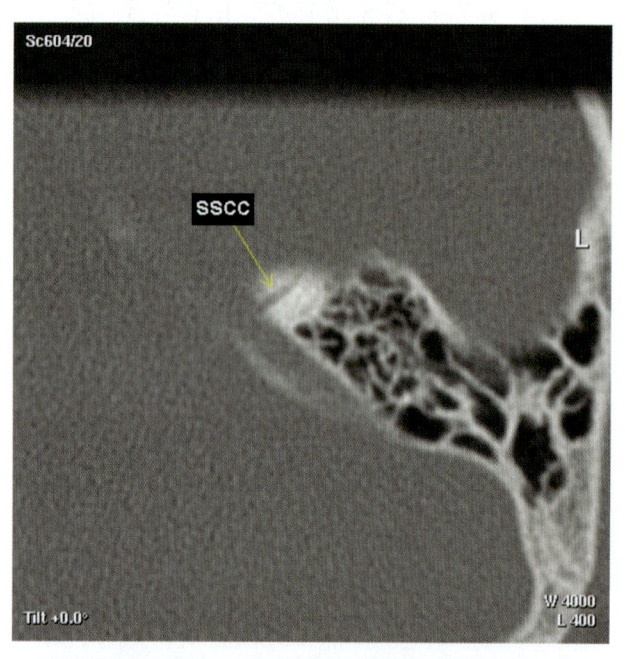

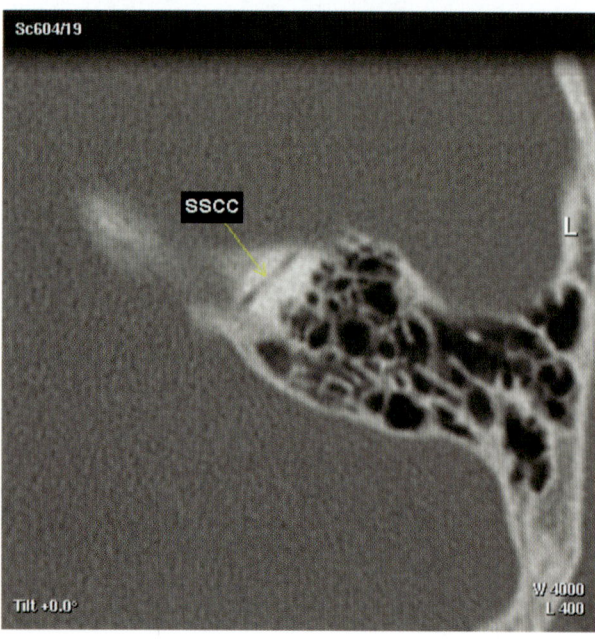

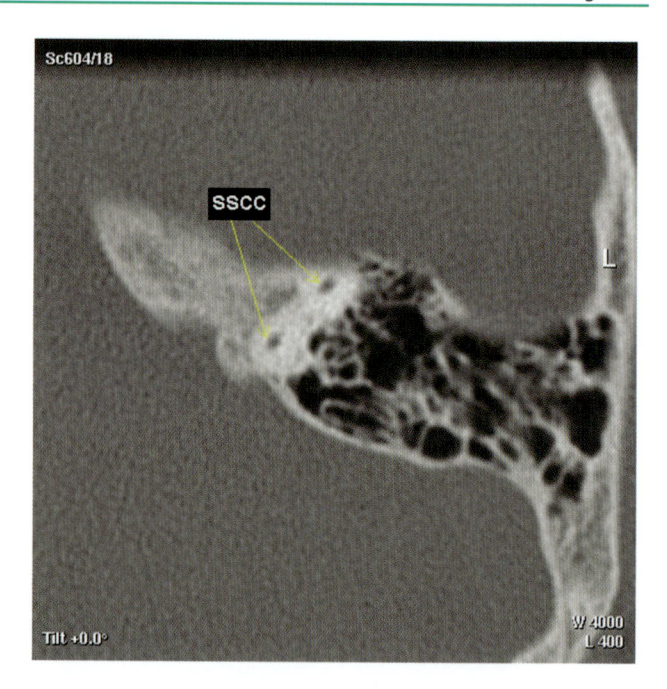

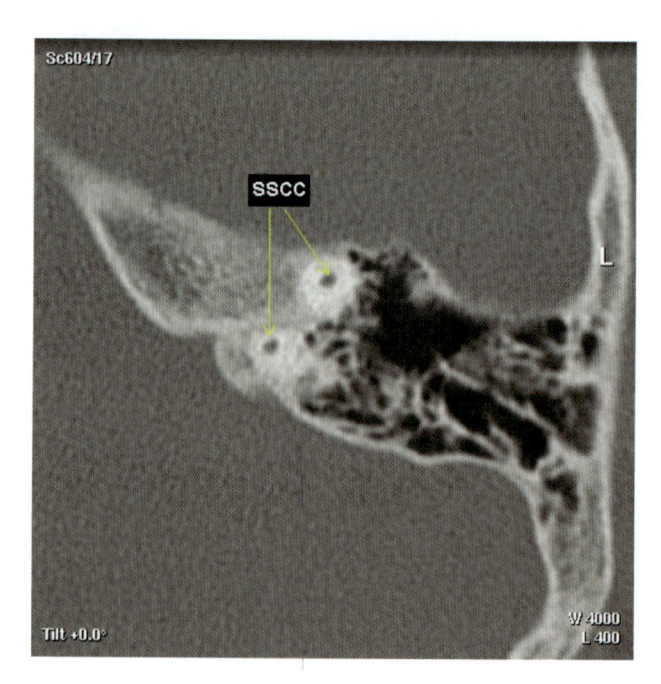

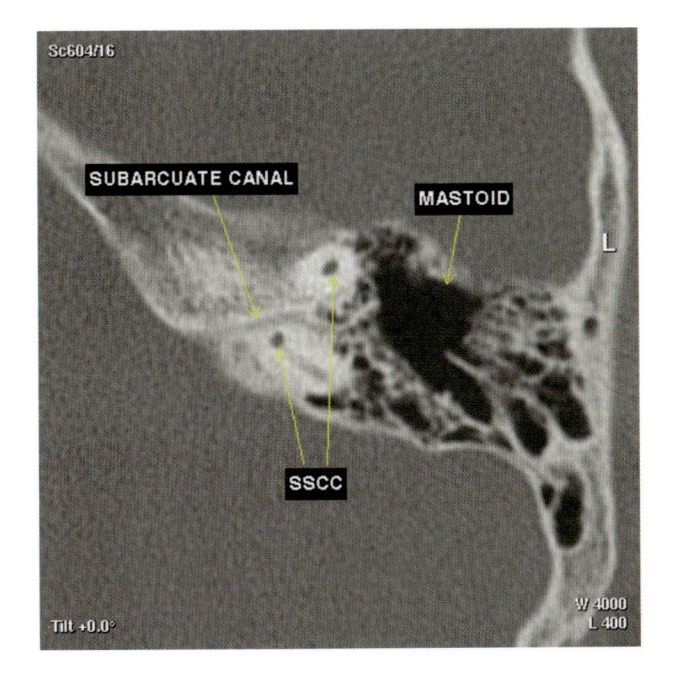

Cross-Sectional Imaging Anatomy of the Temporal Bone

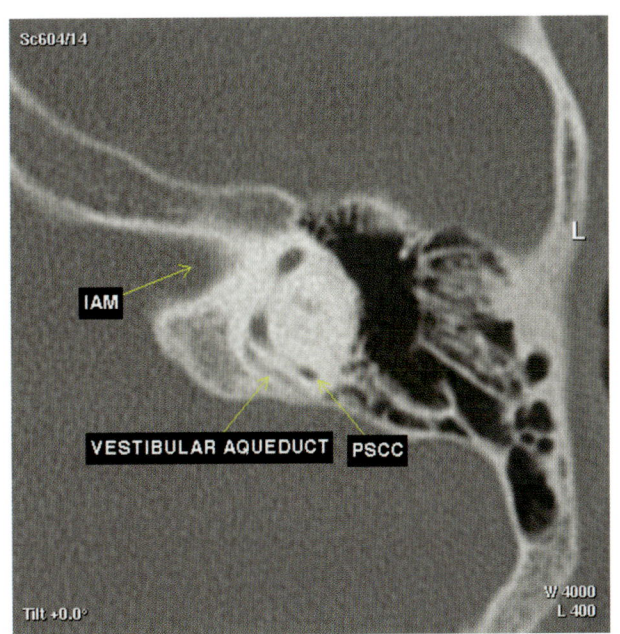

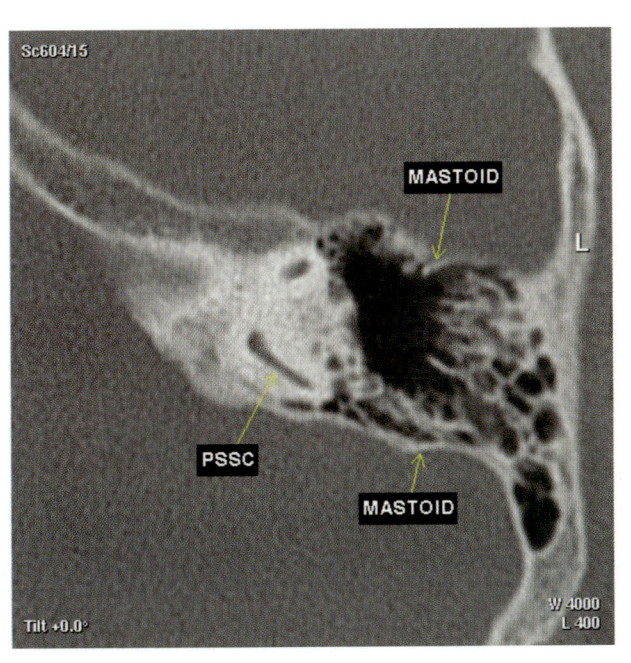

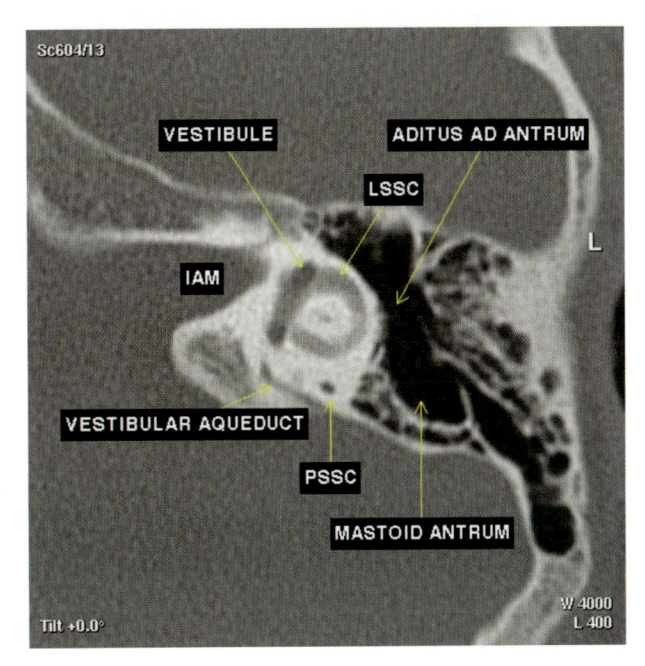

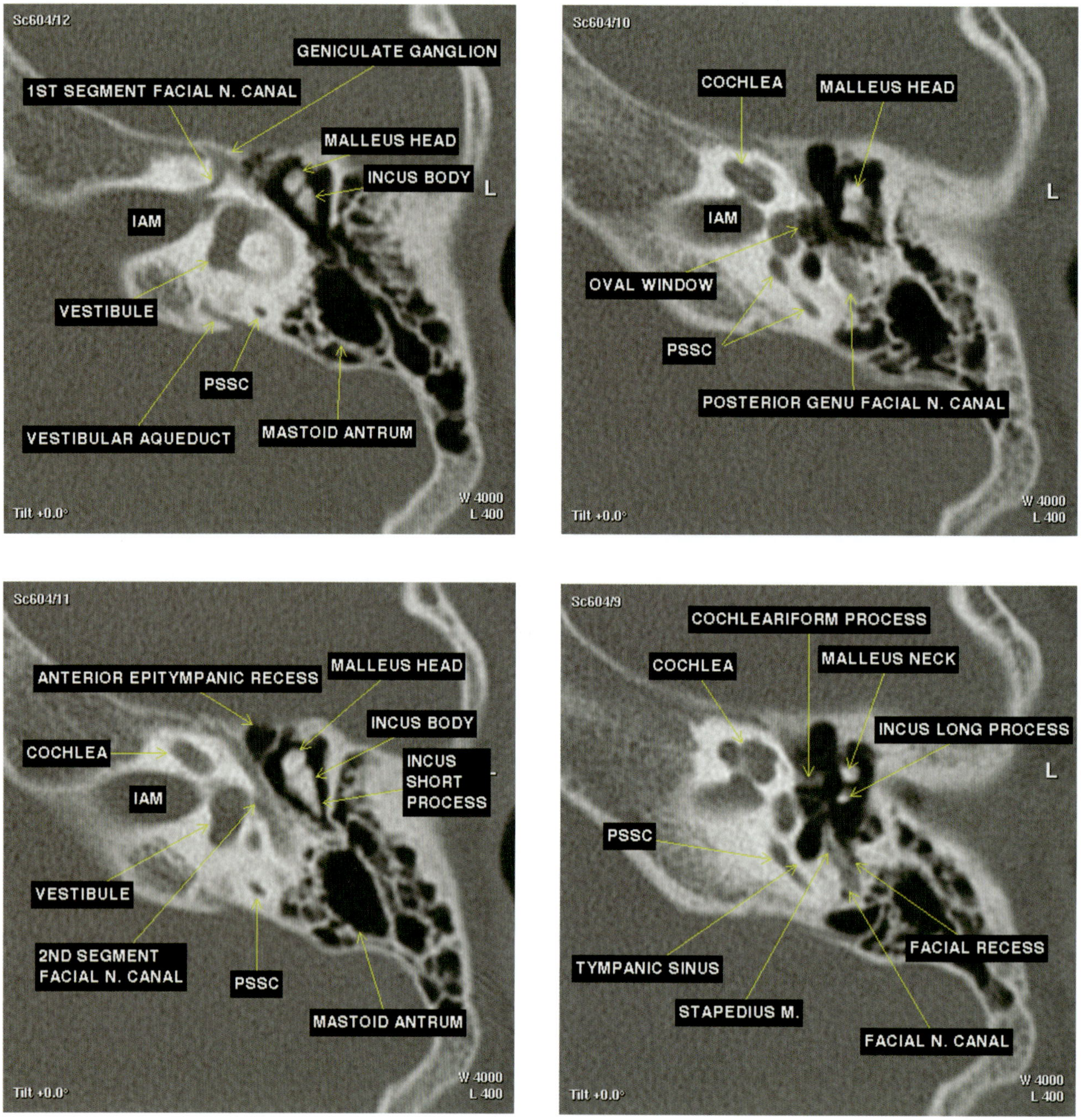
Sc604/12
GENICULATE GANGLION
1ST SEGMENT FACIAL N. CANAL
MALLEUS HEAD
INCUS BODY
L
IAM
VESTIBULE
PSSC
VESTIBULAR AQUEDUCT
MASTOID ANTRUM
W 4000
L 400
Tilt +0.0°
Sc604/10
COCHLEA
MALLEUS HEAD
L
IAM
OVAL WINDOW
PSSC
POSTERIOR GENU FACIAL N. CANAL
W 4000
L 400
Tilt +0.0°
Sc604/11
MALLEUS HEAD
ANTERIOR EPITYMPANIC RECESS
INCUS BODY
COCHLEA
INCUS SHORT PROCESS
IAM
VESTIBULE
2ND SEGMENT FACIAL N. CANAL
PSSC
MASTOID ANTRUM
W 4000
L 400
Tilt +0.0°
Sc604/9
COCHLEARIFORM PROCESS
COCHLEA
MALLEUS NECK
INCUS LONG PROCESS
L
PSSC
FACIAL RECESS
TYMPANIC SINUS
STAPEDIUS M.
FACIAL N. CANAL
W 4000
L 400
Tilt +0.0°

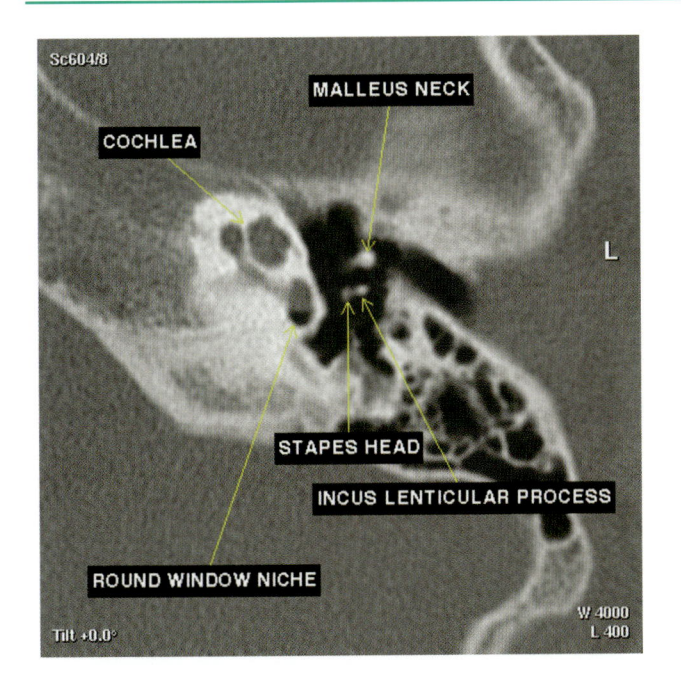

Cross-Sectional Imaging Anatomy of the Temporal Bone

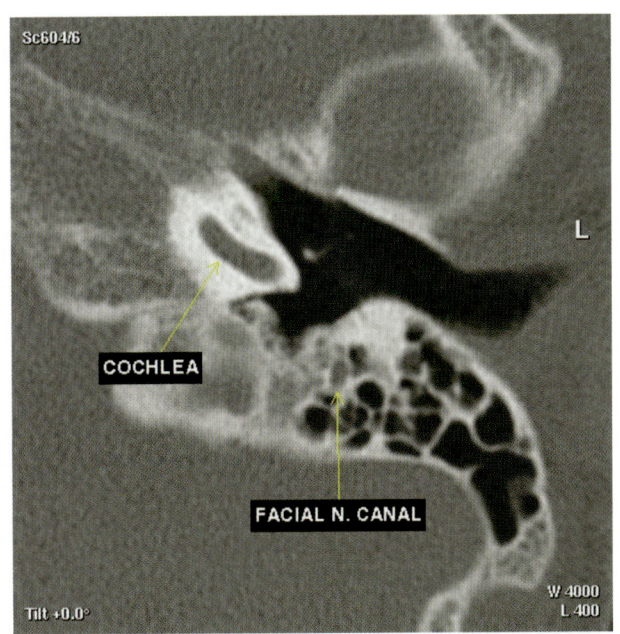

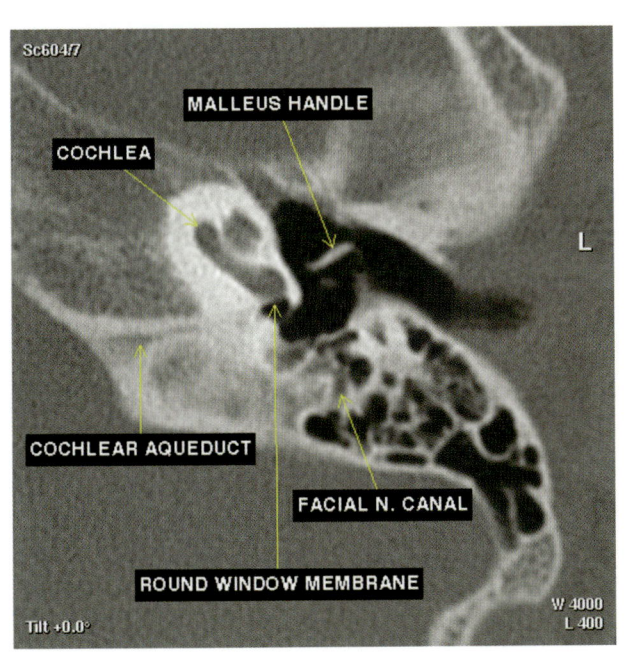

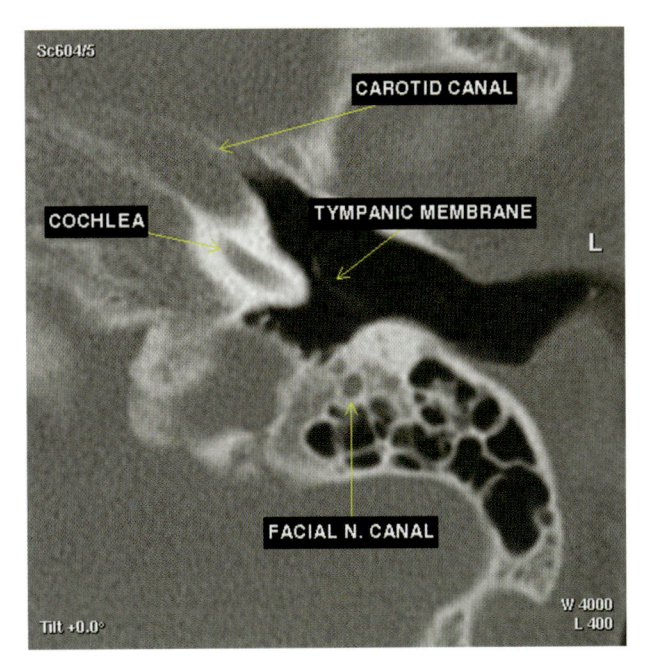

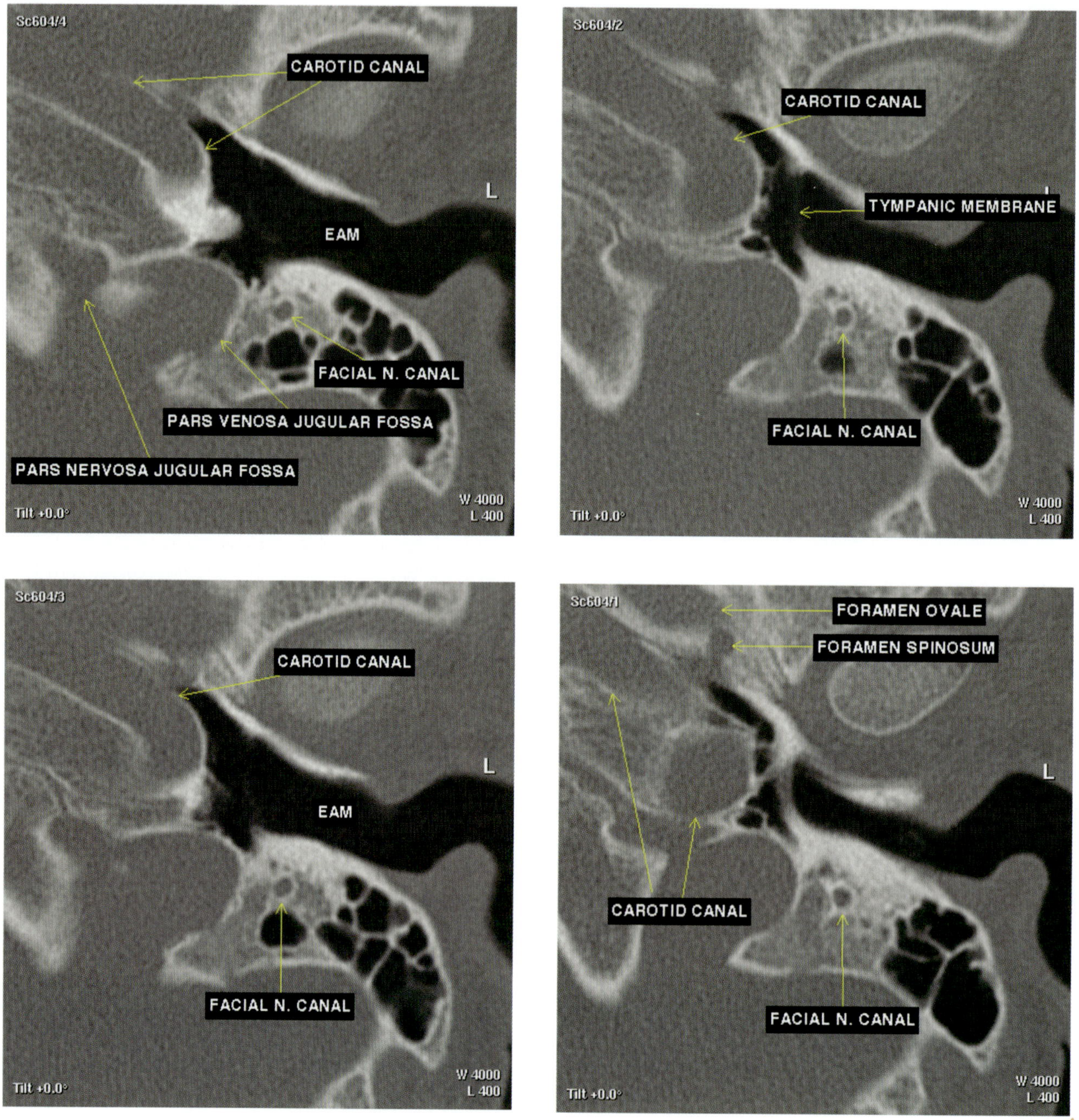
Sc604/4
CAROTID CANAL
L
EAM
FACIAL N. CANAL
PARS VENOSA JUGULAR FOSSA
PARS NERVOSA JUGULAR FOSSA
Tilt +0.0°
W 4000
L 400
Sc604/2
CAROTID CANAL
TYMPANIC MEMBRANE
FACIAL N. CANAL
Tilt +0.0°
W 4000
L 400
Sc604/3
CAROTID CANAL
L
EAM
FACIAL N. CANAL
Tilt +0.0°
W 4000
L 400
Sc604/1
FORAMEN OVALE
FORAMEN SPINOSUM
L
CAROTID CANAL
FACIAL N. CANAL
Tilt +0.0°
W 4000
L 400

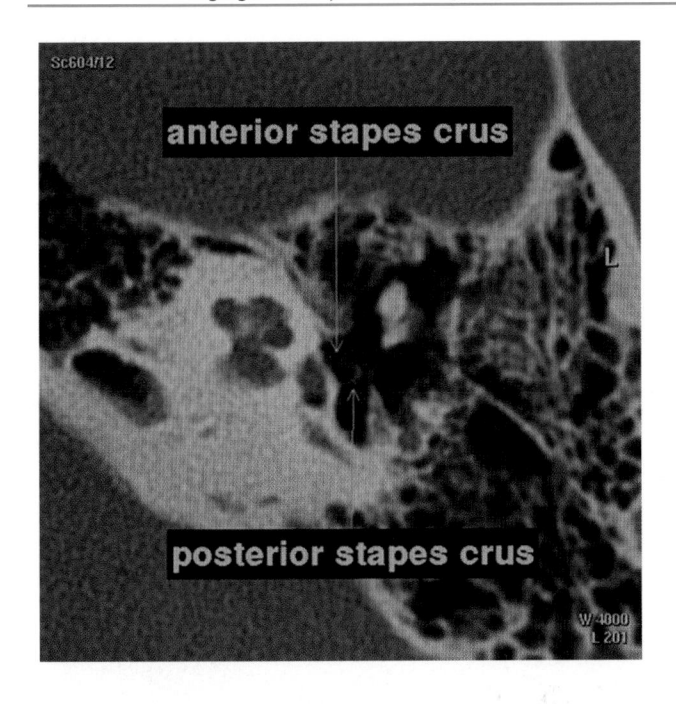

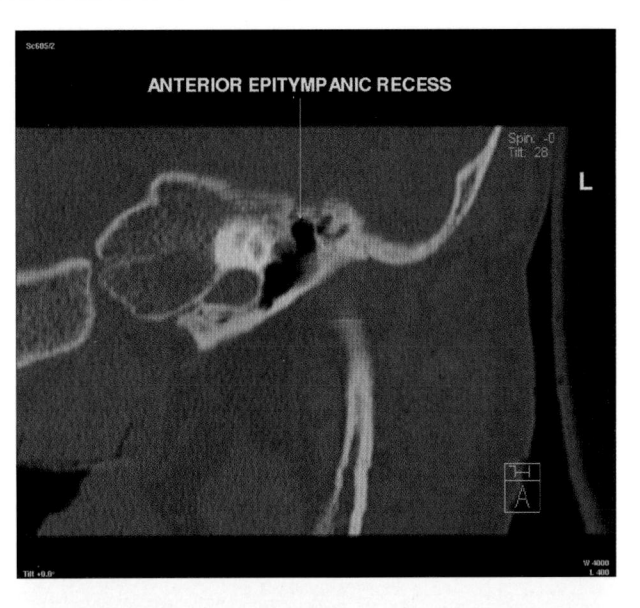

2.2 Coronal CT Images

The images are shown from a left temporal bone, from anteriorly to posteriorly. All images have a 1 mm slice thickness.

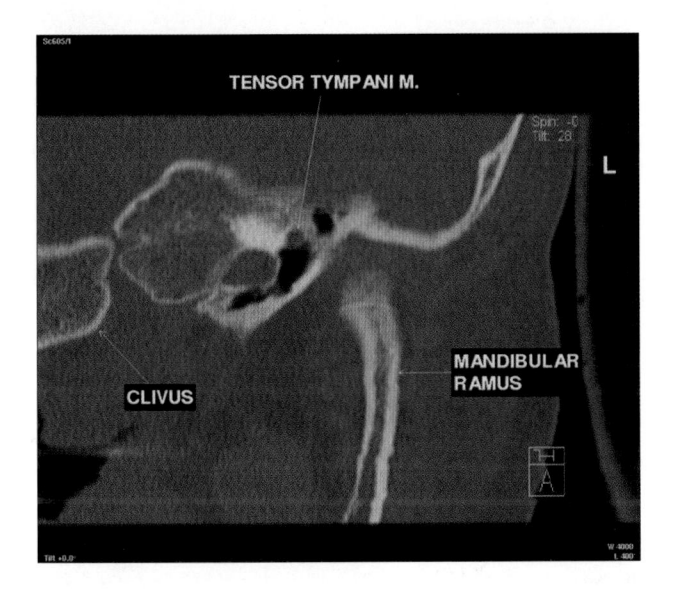

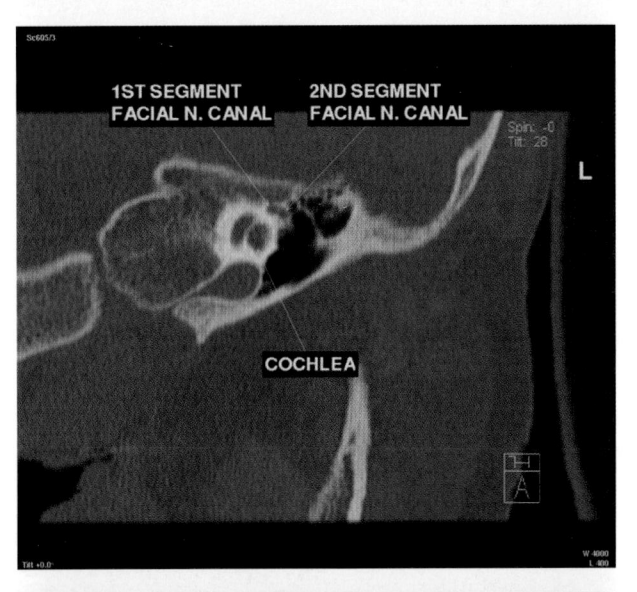

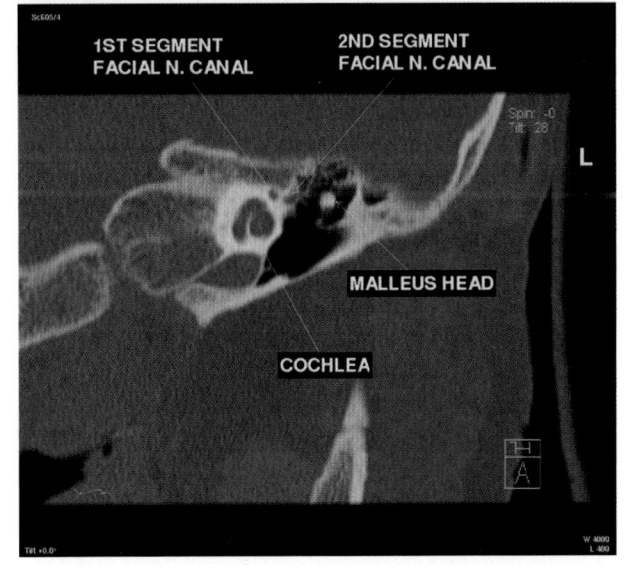

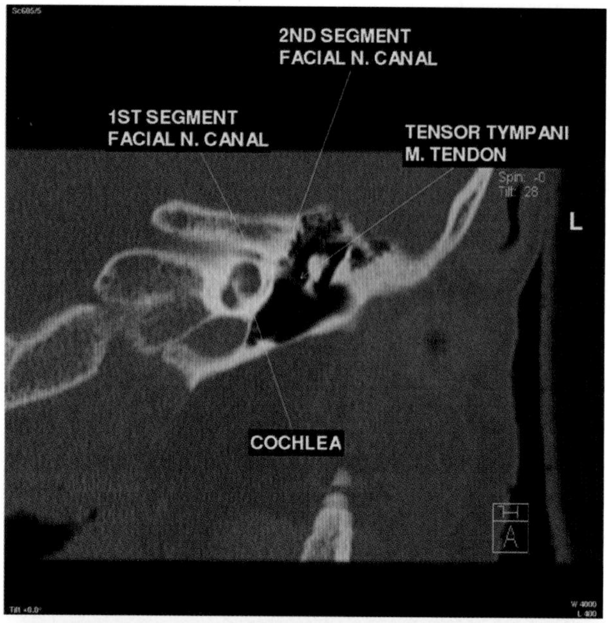
2ND SEGMENT
FACIAL N. CANAL
1ST SEGMENT
FACIAL N. CANAL
TENSOR TYMPANI
M. TENDON
L
COCHLEA

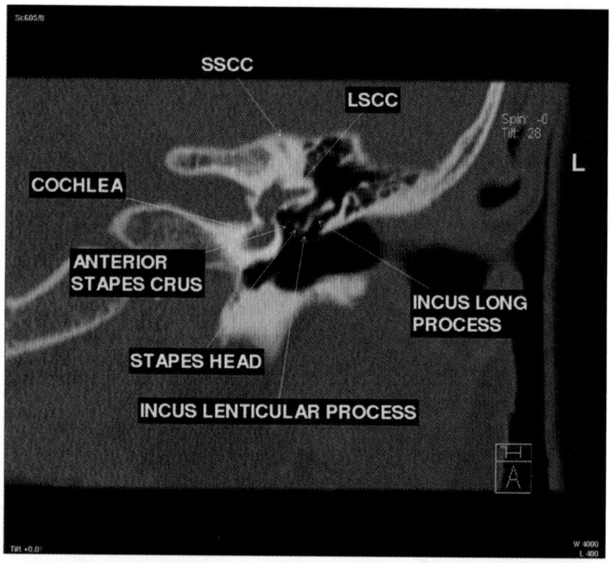
SSCC
LSCC
L
COCHLEA
ANTERIOR
STAPES CRUS
INCUS LONG
PROCESS
STAPES HEAD
INCUS LENTICULAR PROCESS

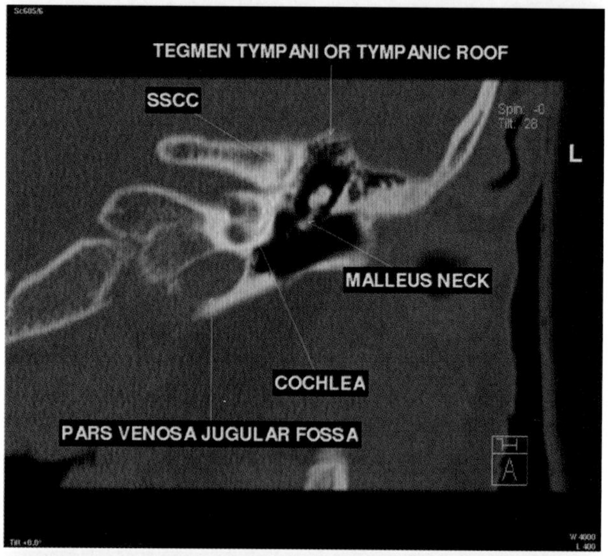
TEGMEN TYMPANI OR TYMPANIC ROOF
SSCC
L
MALLEUS NECK
COCHLEA
PARS VENOSA JUGULAR FOSSA

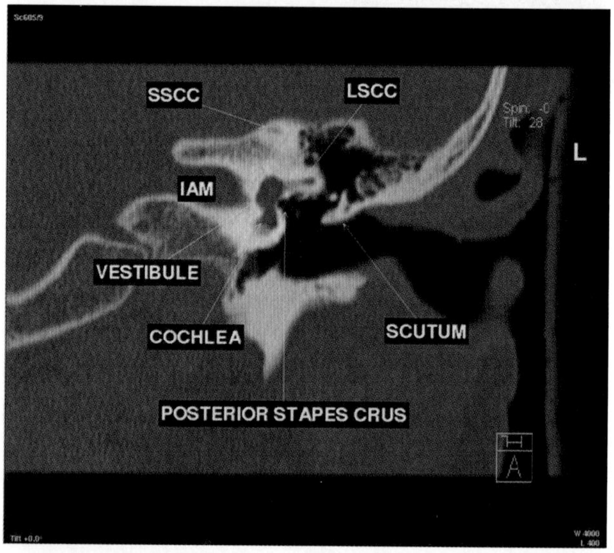
SSCC
LSCC
L
IAM
VESTIBULE
COCHLEA
SCUTUM
POSTERIOR STAPES CRUS

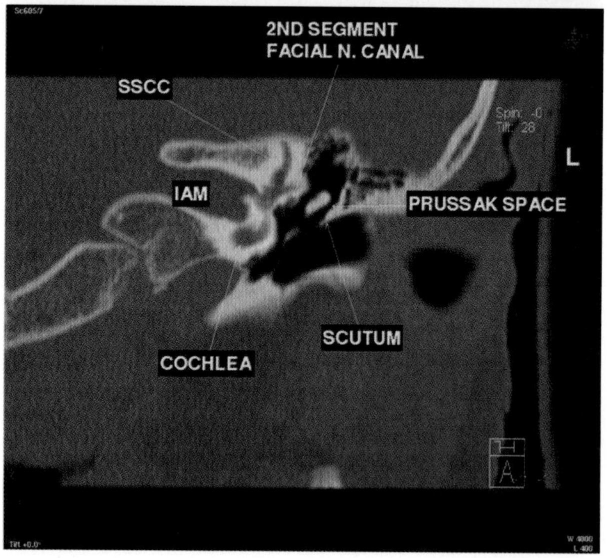
2ND SEGMENT
FACIAL N. CANAL
SSCC
L
IAM
PRUSSAK SPACE
SCUTUM
COCHLEA

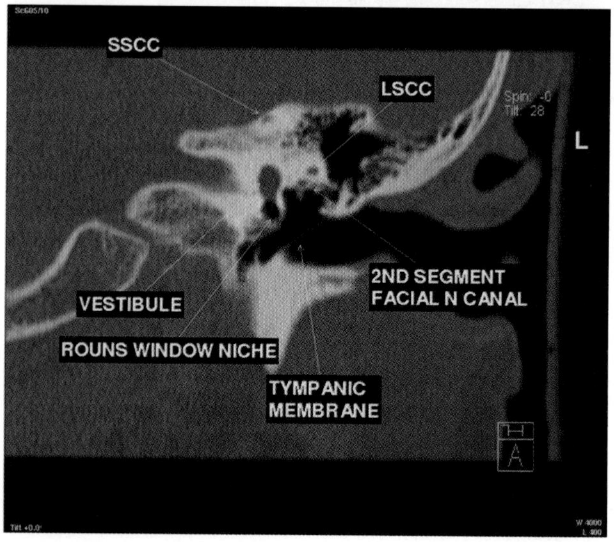
SSCC
LSCC
L
2ND SEGMENT
FACIAL N CANAL
VESTIBULE
ROUNS WINDOW NICHE
TYMPANIC
MEMBRANE

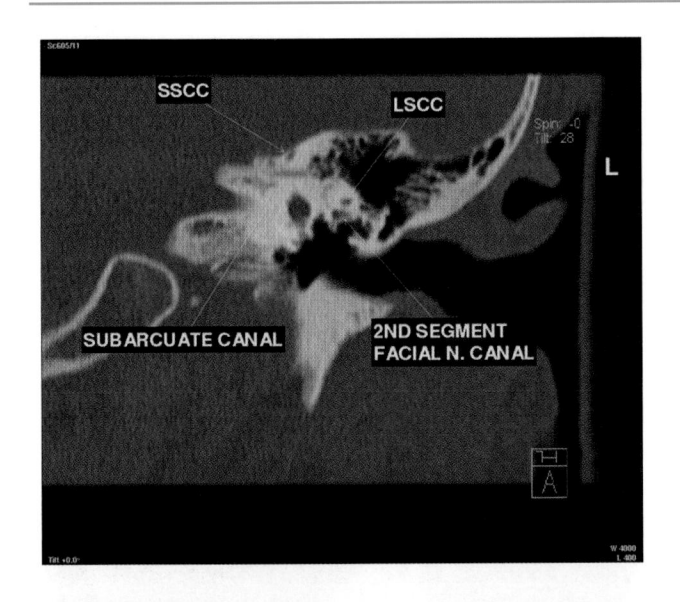

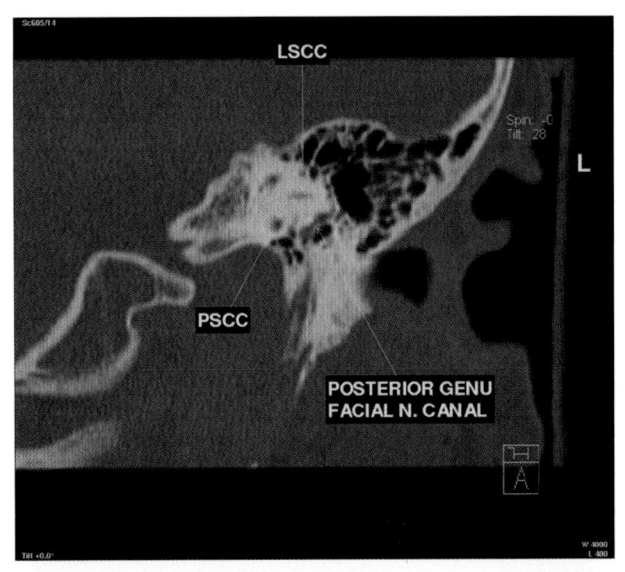

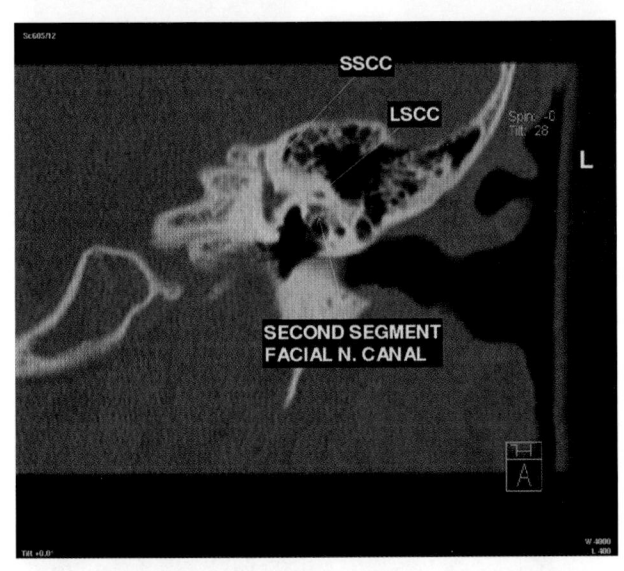

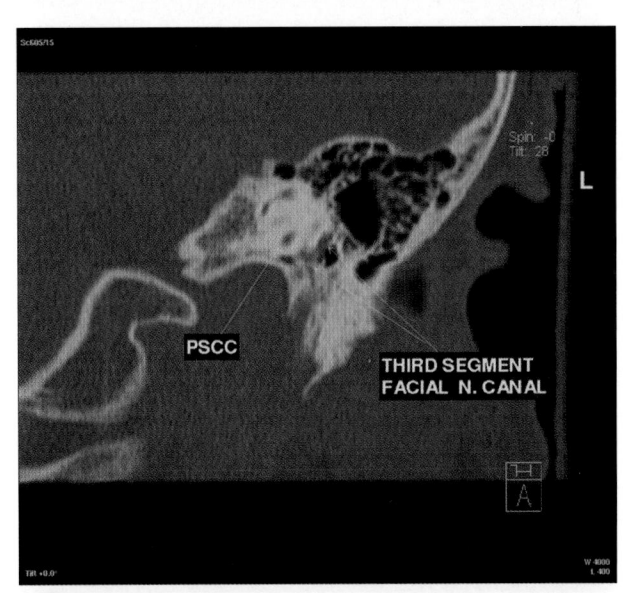

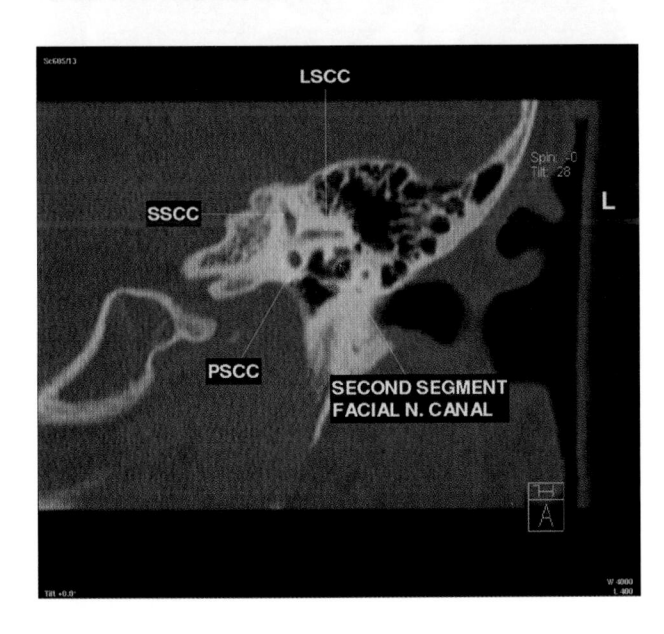

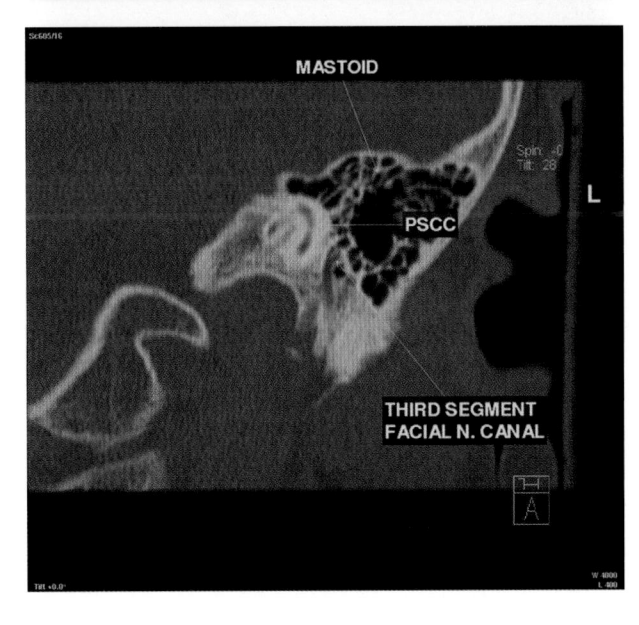

Cross-Sectional Imaging Anatomy of the Temporal Bone

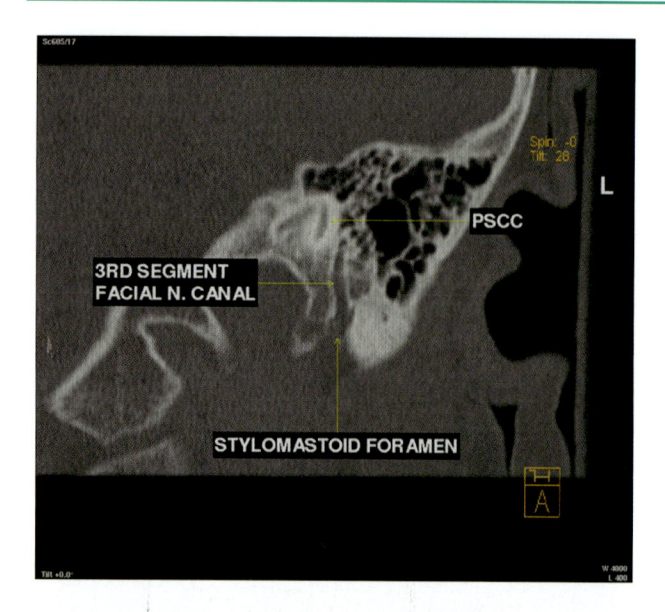

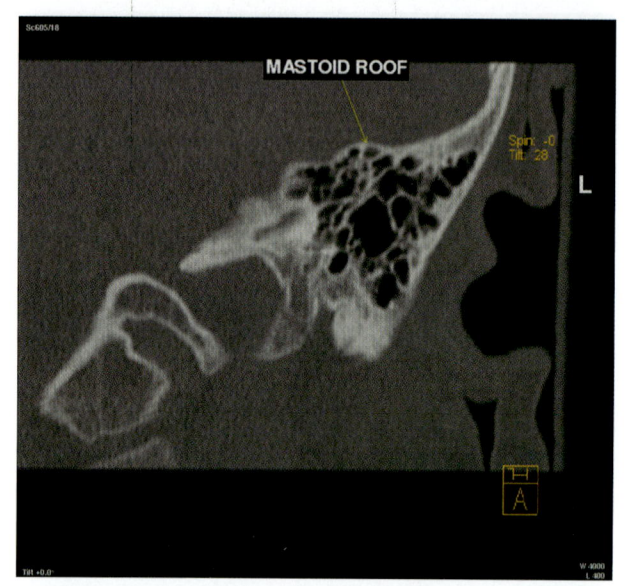

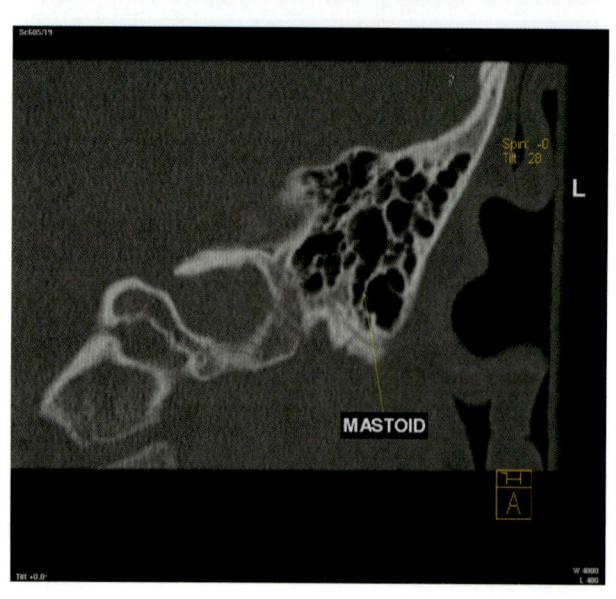

2.3 Axial T2-weighted MR Images

The images are shown from a left temporal bone, from cranially to caudally. All images have a 0.7 mm slice thickness.

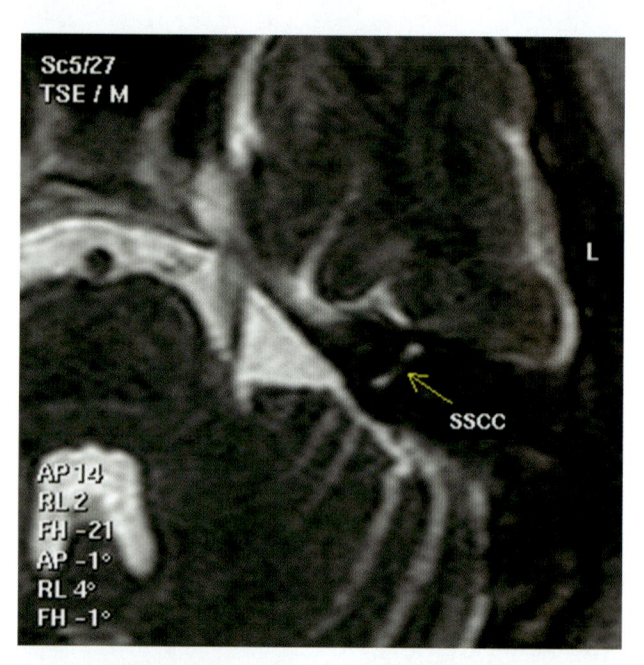

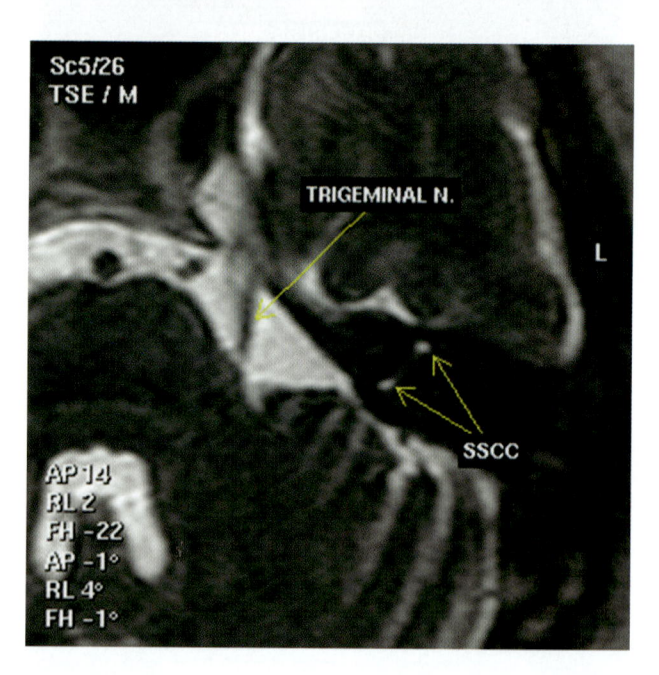

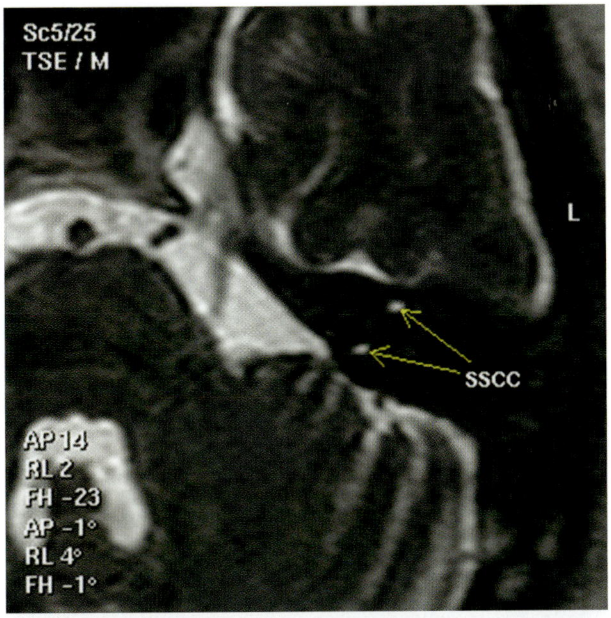
Sc5/25
TSE / M
L
SSCC
AP 14
RL 2
FH -23
AP -1°
RL 4°
FH -1°

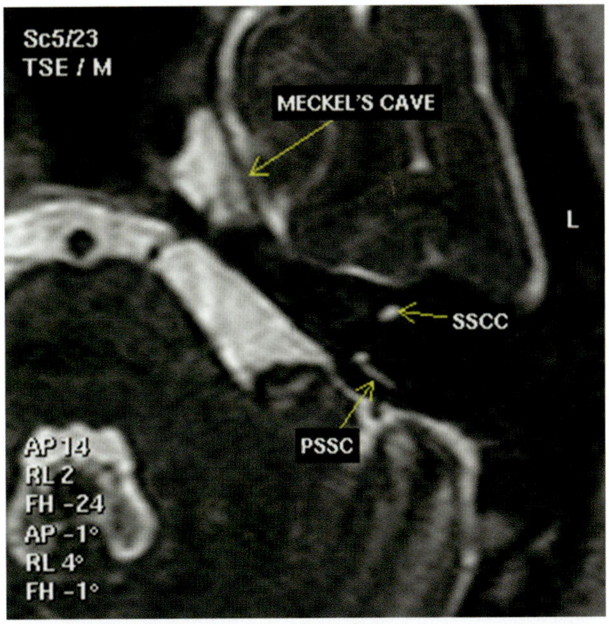
Sc5/23
TSE / M
MECKEL'S CAVE
L
SSCC
PSSC
AP 14
RL 2
FH -24
AP -1°
RL 4°
FH -1°

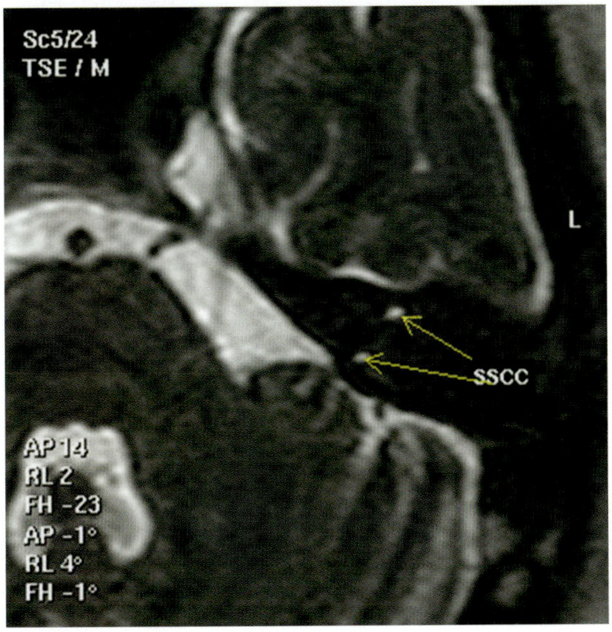
Sc5/24
TSE / M
L
SSCC
AP 14
RL 2
FH -23
AP -1°
RL 4°
FH -1°

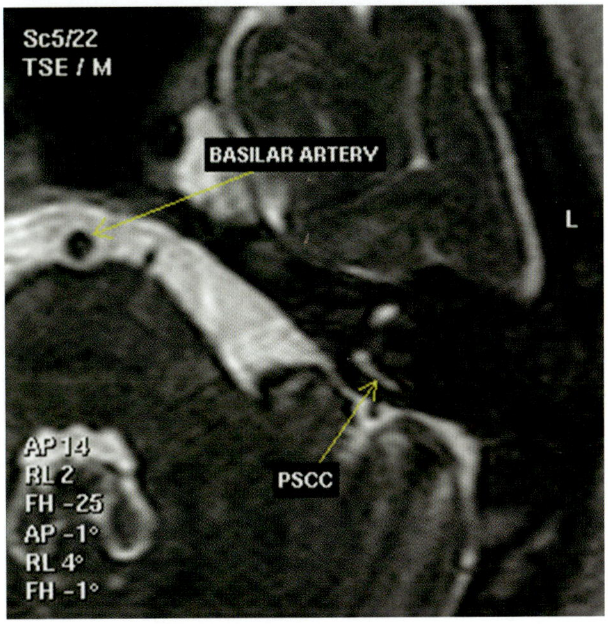
Sc5/22
TSE / M
BASILAR ARTERY
L
PSCC
AP 14
RL 2
FH -25
AP -1°
RL 4°
FH -1°

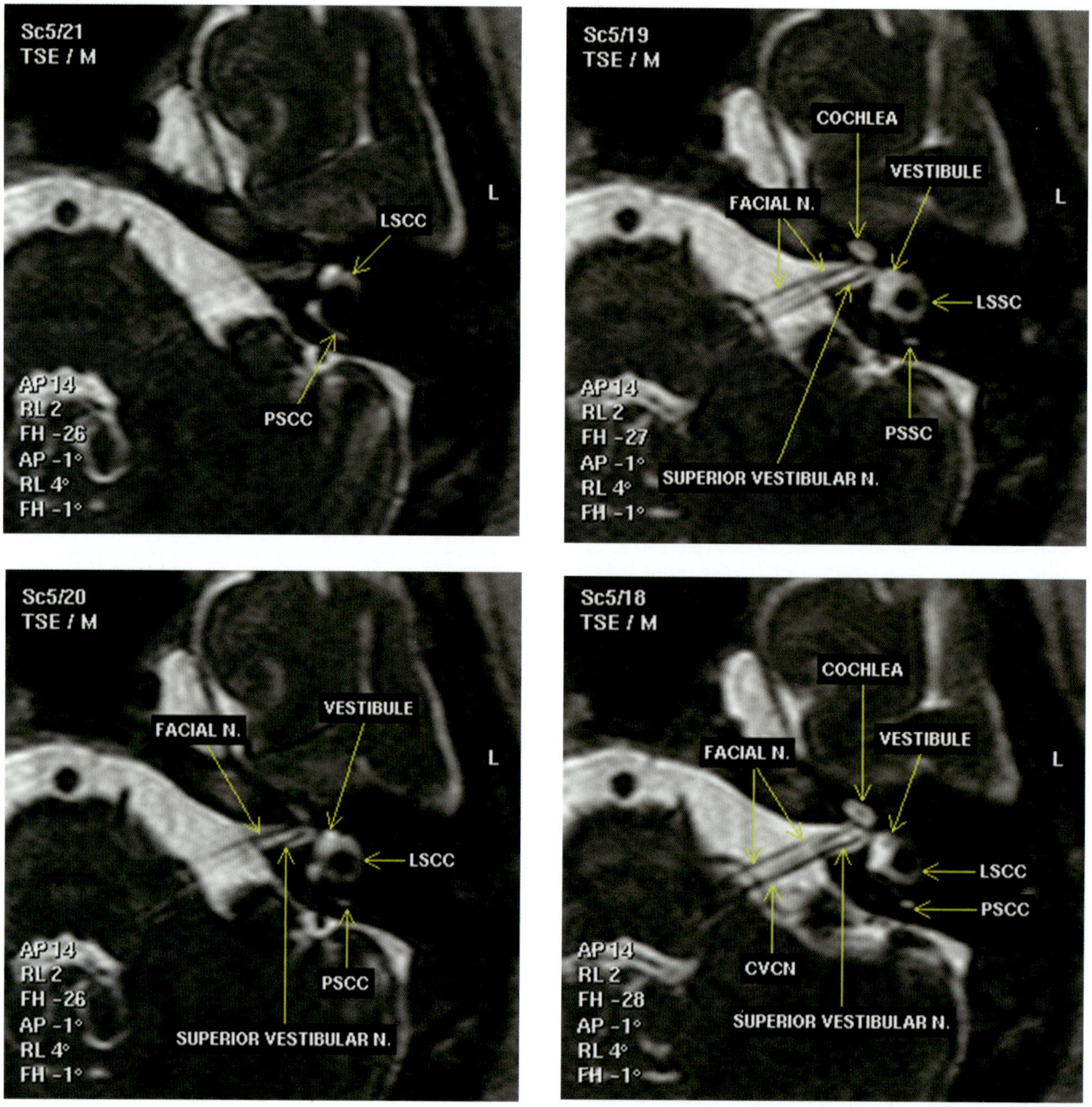
Sc5/21
TSE / M
L
LSCC
PSCC
AP 14
RL 2
FH -26
AP -1°
RL 4°
FH -1°
Sc5/19
TSE / M
COCHLEA
VESTIBULE
FACIAL N.
L
LSSC
PSSC
SUPERIOR VESTIBULAR N.
AP 14
RL 2
FH -27
AP -1°
RL 4°
FH -1°
Sc5/20
TSE / M
VESTIBULE
FACIAL N.
L
LSCC
PSCC
SUPERIOR VESTIBULAR N.
AP 14
RL 2
FH -26
AP -1°
RL 4°
FH -1°
Sc5/18
TSE / M
COCHLEA
VESTIBULE
FACIAL N.
L
LSCC
PSCC
CVCN
SUPERIOR VESTIBULAR N.
AP 14
RL 2
FH -28
AP -1°
RL 4°
FH -1°

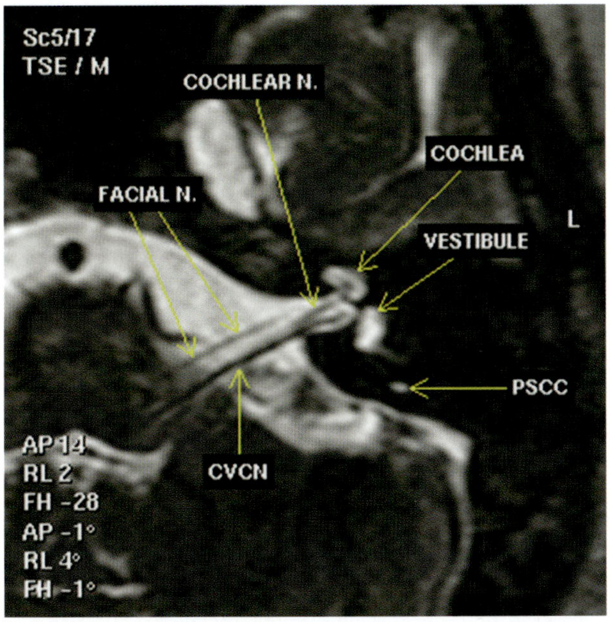
Sc5/17
TSE / M
COCHLEAR N.
COCHLEA
FACIAL N.
VESTIBULE
L
PSCC
CVCN
AP 14
RL 2
FH -28
AP -1°
RL 4°
FH -1°

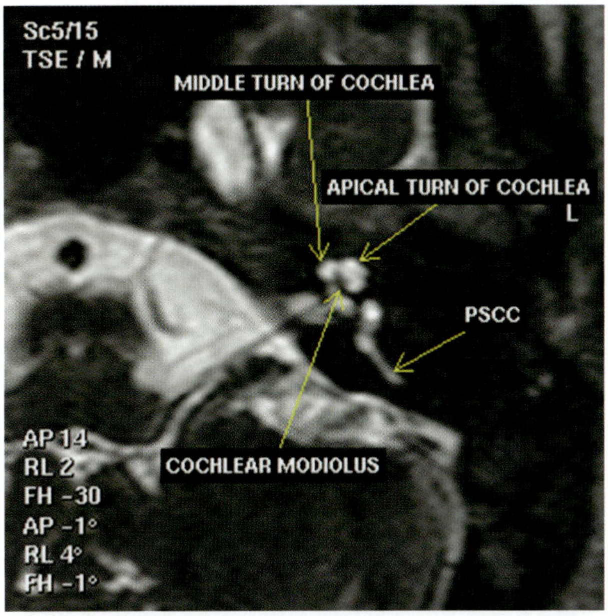
Sc5/15
TSE / M
MIDDLE TURN OF COCHLEA
APICAL TURN OF COCHLEA
L
PSCC
COCHLEAR MODIOLUS
AP 14
RL 2
FH -30
AP -1°
RL 4°
FH -1°

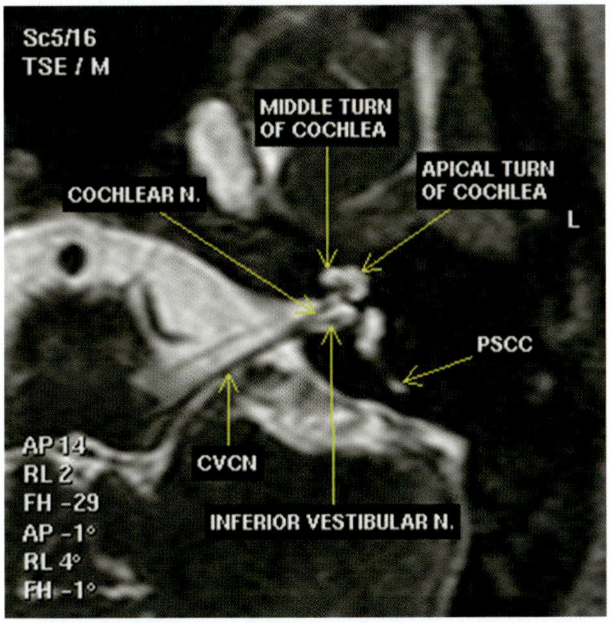
Sc5/16
TSE / M
MIDDLE TURN
OF COCHLEA
APICAL TURN
OF COCHLEA
COCHLEAR N.
L
PSCC
CVCN
INFERIOR VESTIBULAR N.
AP 14
RL 2
FH -29
AP -1°
RL 4°
FH -1°

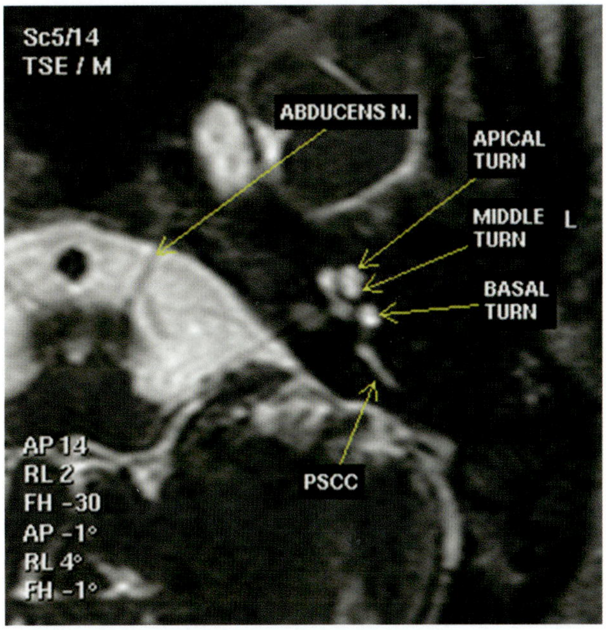
Sc5/14
TSE / M
ABDUCENS N.
APICAL
TURN
MIDDLE
TURN
L
BASAL
TURN
PSCC
AP 14
RL 2
FH -30
AP -1°
RL 4°
FH -1°

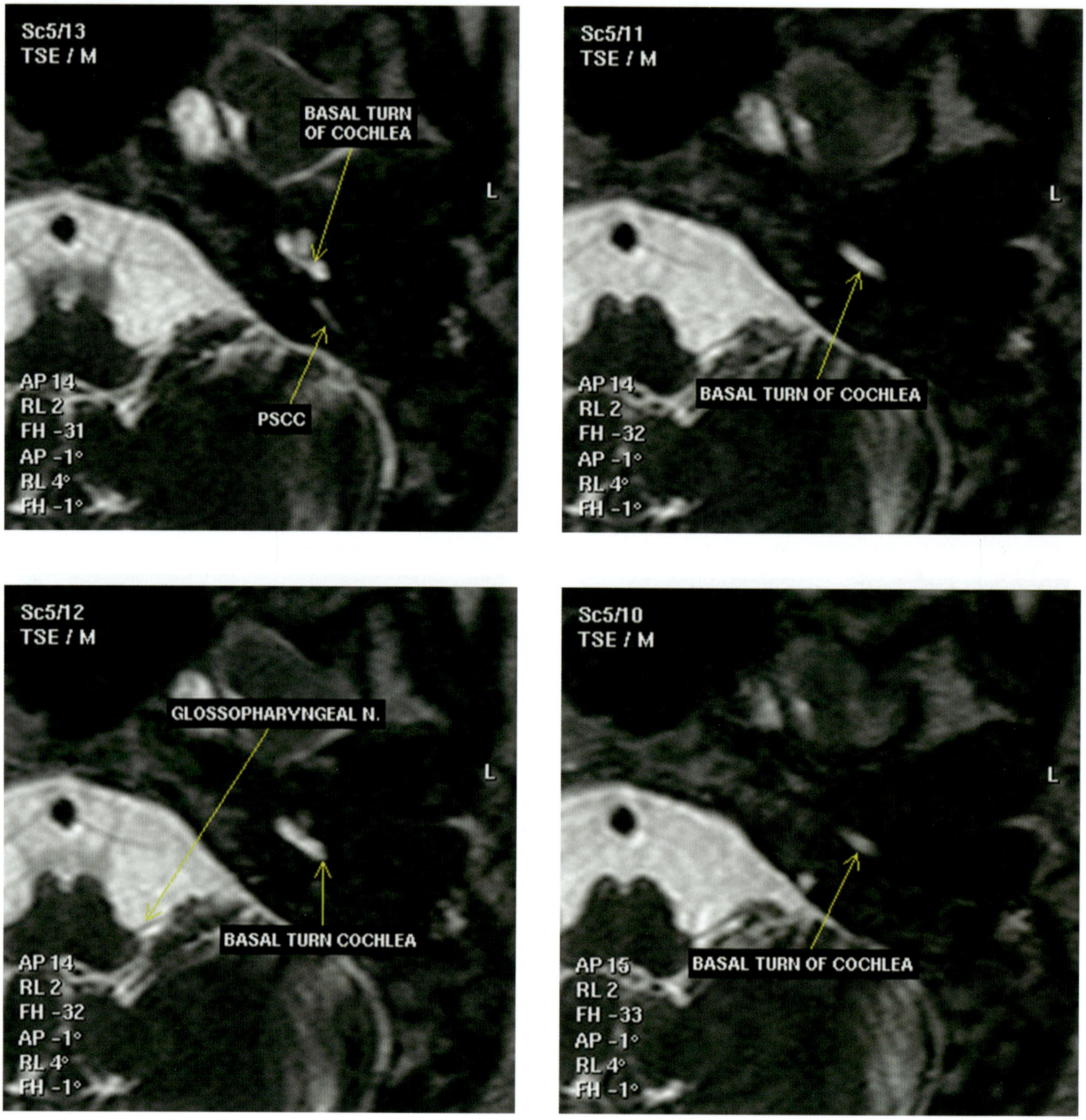
Sc5/13
TSE / M
BASAL TURN OF COCHLEA
L
PSCC
AP 14
RL 2
FH -31
AP -1°
RL 4°
FH -1°
Sc5/11
TSE / M
L
BASAL TURN OF COCHLEA
AP 14
RL 2
FH -32
AP -1°
RL 4°
FH -1°
Sc5/12
TSE / M
GLOSSOPHARYNGEAL N.
L
BASAL TURN COCHLEA
AP 14
RL 2
FH -32
AP -1°
RL 4°
FH -1°
Sc5/10
TSE / M
L
BASAL TURN OF COCHLEA
AP 15
RL 2
FH -33
AP -1°
RL 4°
FH -1°

Cross-Sectional Imaging Anatomy of the Temporal Bone

2.4 Axial T1-weighted MR Images

The images are shown from a right temporal bone, from cranially to caudally. All images have a 3.0 mm slice thickness.

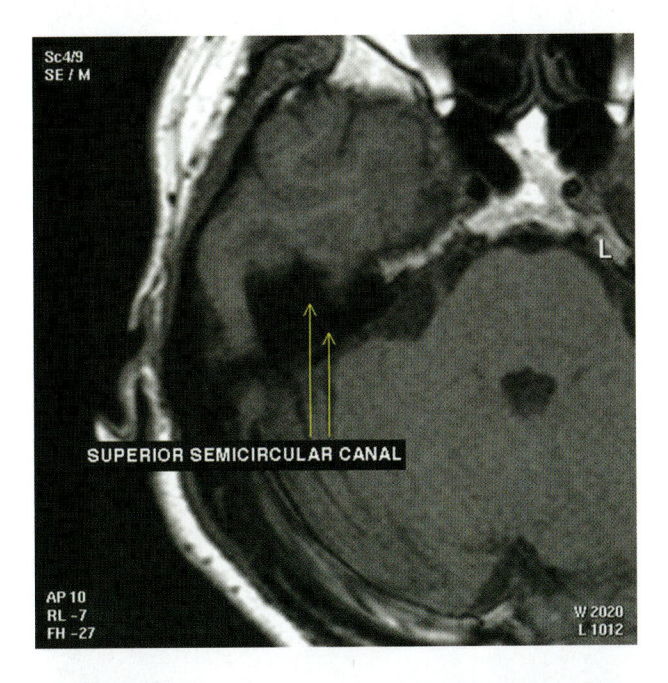

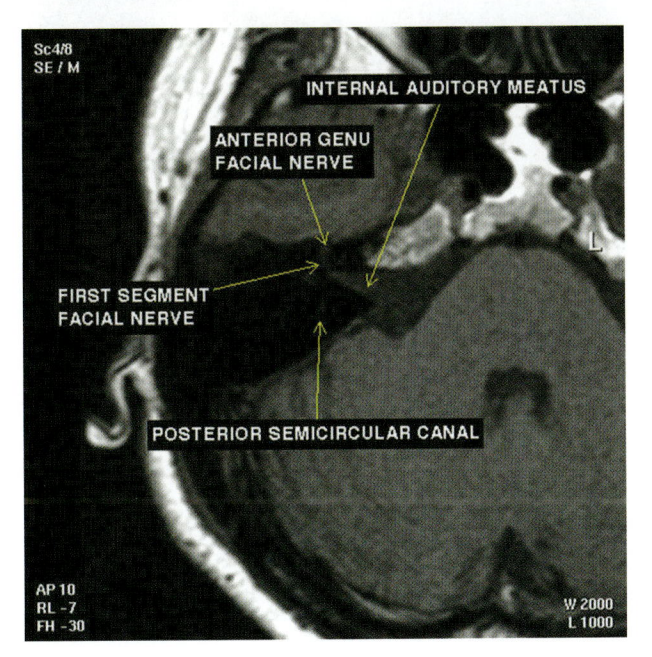

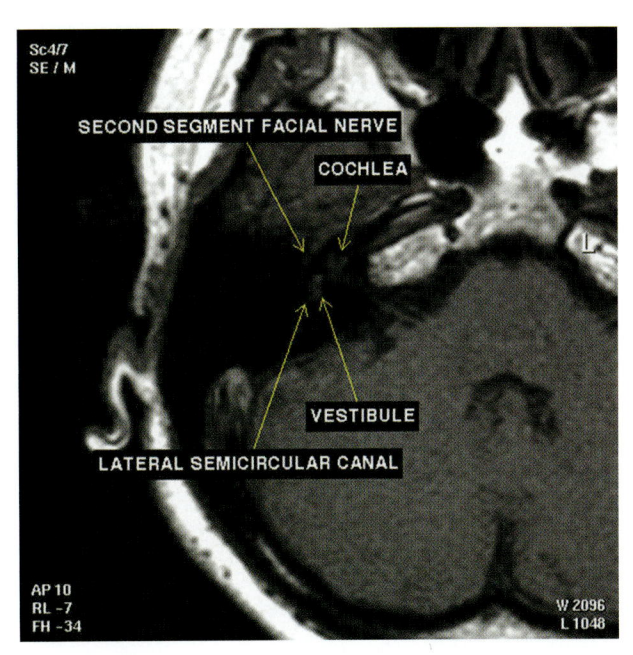

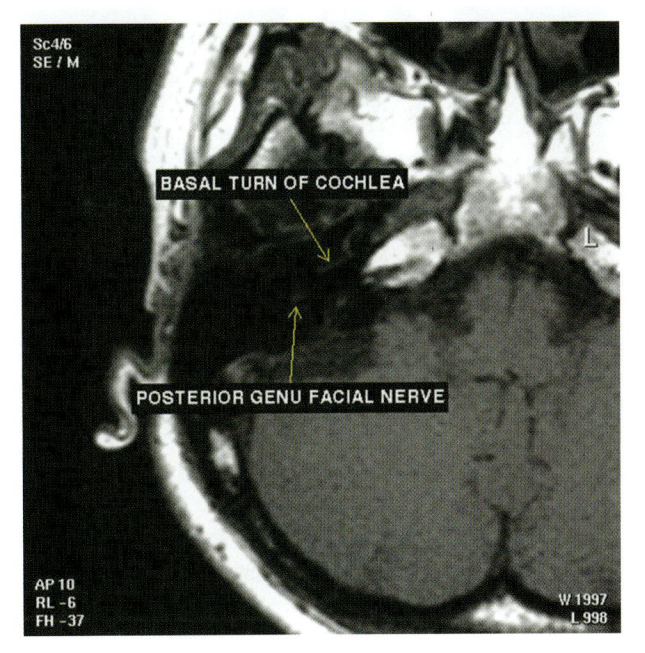

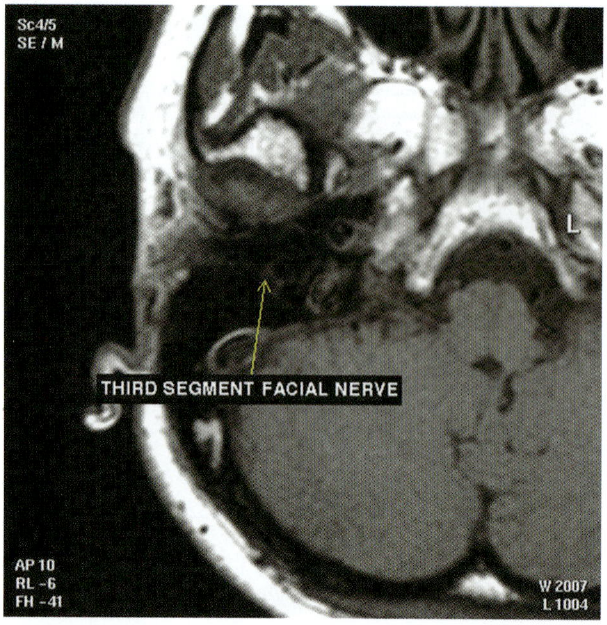
Sc4/5
SE / M
L
THIRD SEGMENT FACIAL NERVE
AP 10
RL -6
FH -41
W 2007
L 1004

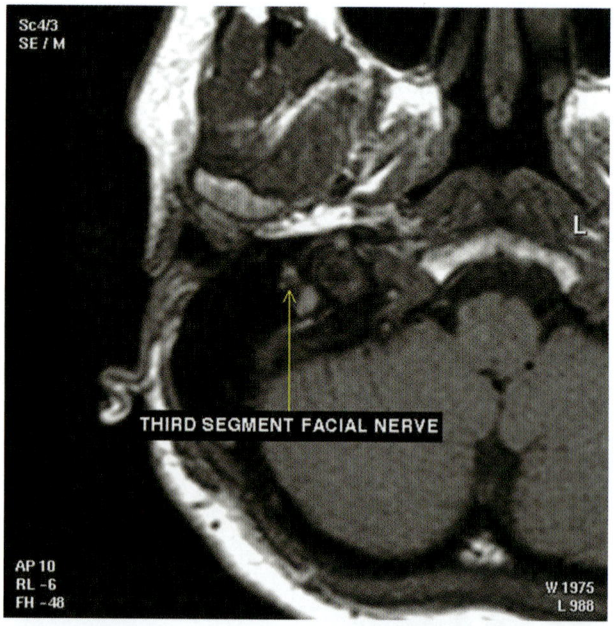
Sc4/3
SE / M
L
THIRD SEGMENT FACIAL NERVE
AP 10
RL -6
FH -48
W 1975
L 988

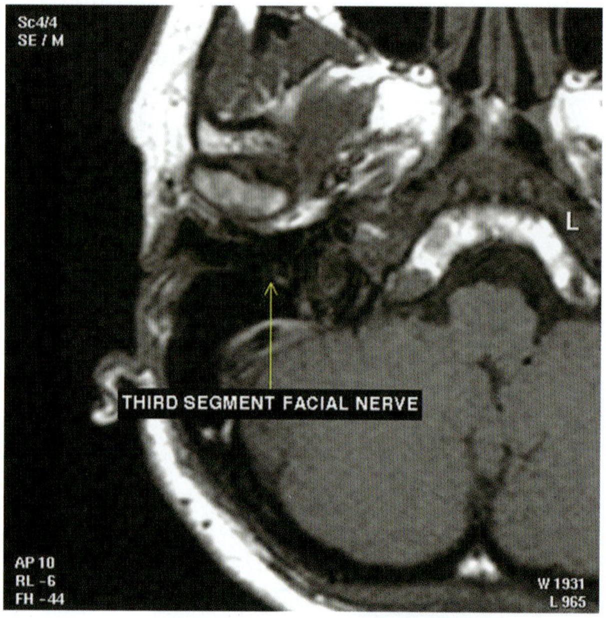
Sc4/4
SE / M
L
THIRD SEGMENT FACIAL NERVE
AP 10
RL -6
FH -44
W 1931
L 965

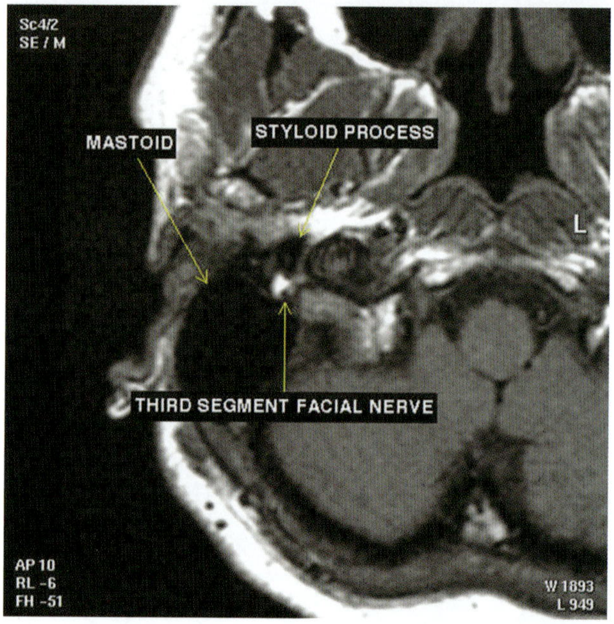
Sc4/2
SE / M
MASTOID
STYLOID PROCESS
L
THIRD SEGMENT FACIAL NERVE
AP 10
RL -6
FH -51
W 1893
L 949

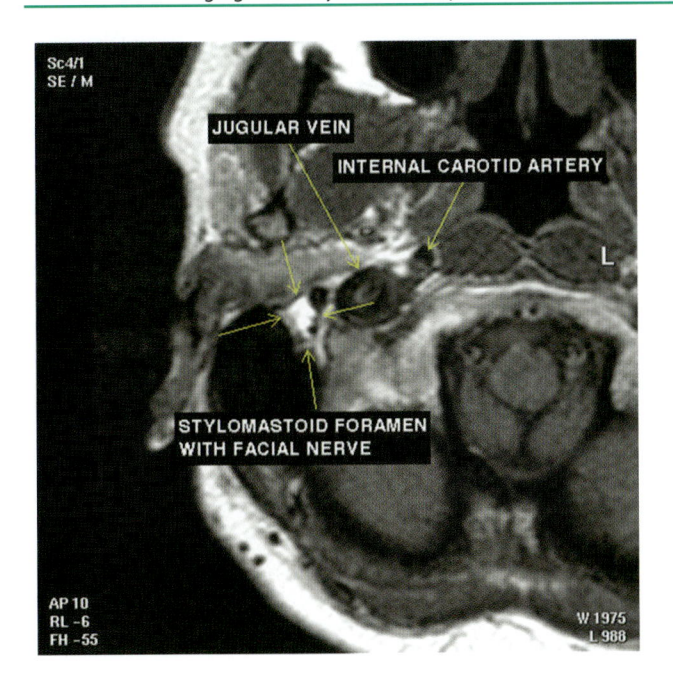

References

Gray H (1918) Anatomy of the Human Body. Philadelphia: Lea & Febiger (2000) Bartleby.com, www.bartleby.com/107/

Harnsberger HR (1995) Handbook of Head and Neck Imaging, 2nd edn. p 426–458

Lane JI(2006). Middle and Inner Ear: Improved Depiction with Multiplanar Reconstruction of Volumetric CT Data. Radiographics Jan-Feb (1)26: 115–124

Lemmerling M (1997) CT of the Normal Suspensory Ligaments of the Ossicles in the Middle Ear. AJNR 18(3):471–477

External Ear Imaging

Robert Hermans

Contents

1	Introduction	35
2	Congenital Malformations	35
2.1	Aural Dysplasia	35
2.2	Branchiogenic Anomalies	37
2.3	Preaurical Sinus	37
3	Inflammatory Conditions	38
3.1	External Otitis	38
3.2	Necrotizing External Otitis	39
4	Trauma	43
5	Fibrous Dysplasia	44
6	Benign Neoplasms	45
6.1	Cholesteatoma	45
6.2	Keratosis Obturans	47
6.3	Exostoses and Osteoma	48
6.4	Other Tumours	48
7	Malignant Neoplasms	50
	References	50

Abstract

The external ear can be affected by various congenital, inflammatory, traumatic, or tumoral conditions. CT and MRI can be of complementary value to the clinical examination. This chapter reviews the CT and MRI features of different external ear abnormalities.

1 Introduction

The external ear is easy to examine clinically; therefore, in most cases, imaging has no or only a minor role to play. However, if the external auditory canal is severely deformed or obstructed, clinical inspection is more difficult, making the role of imaging studies more important in patient management.

2 Congenital Malformations

2.1 Aural Dysplasia

The incidence of aural dysplasia is between 1/3300 and 1/10000 births. Failure of the first branchial cleft to canalise will cause stenosis or absence (atresia) of the external auditory canal. Very often, these patients have a small, abnormally shaped auricle; this is called microtia. The degree of microtia is associated to the severity of the external canal deformation; in cases of minor microtia, stenosis of the external auditory canal is most common, while in patients with major microtia, atresia is predominant (Mayer et al. 1998).

Aural dysplasia is usually unilateral and not associated with other deformities; however, it may be associated with a number of syndromes, such as hemifacial microsomia. Commonly, congenital anomalies of the external and middle ear are associated, as these structures have a common embryological origin, namely the first branchial apparatus.

R. Hermans (✉)
Department of Radiology, University Hospitals Leuven,
Herestraat 49, B-3000 Leuven, Belgium
e-mail: robert.hermans@uzleuven.be

Fig. 1 9-year-old child showing microtia on *left* side. **a, b** *Coronal* CT-images. The *right* external auditory canal appears normal, while on the *left* side it is narrowed and has a steeper slope (*asterisks*). **c, d** *Axial images*. Normally developed middle ear cavity on *right* side. On the *left* side, the epitympanon is very small, only containing the head of the malleus (*arrow*). The incus and stapedial superstructure are absent on the *left* side, while the *left* footplate (*arrowhead*) is well developed, although somewhat turned towards the coronal plane compared to the *right* side. The *left* mastoid is not pneumatized. The inner ear structures appeared normal on both sides

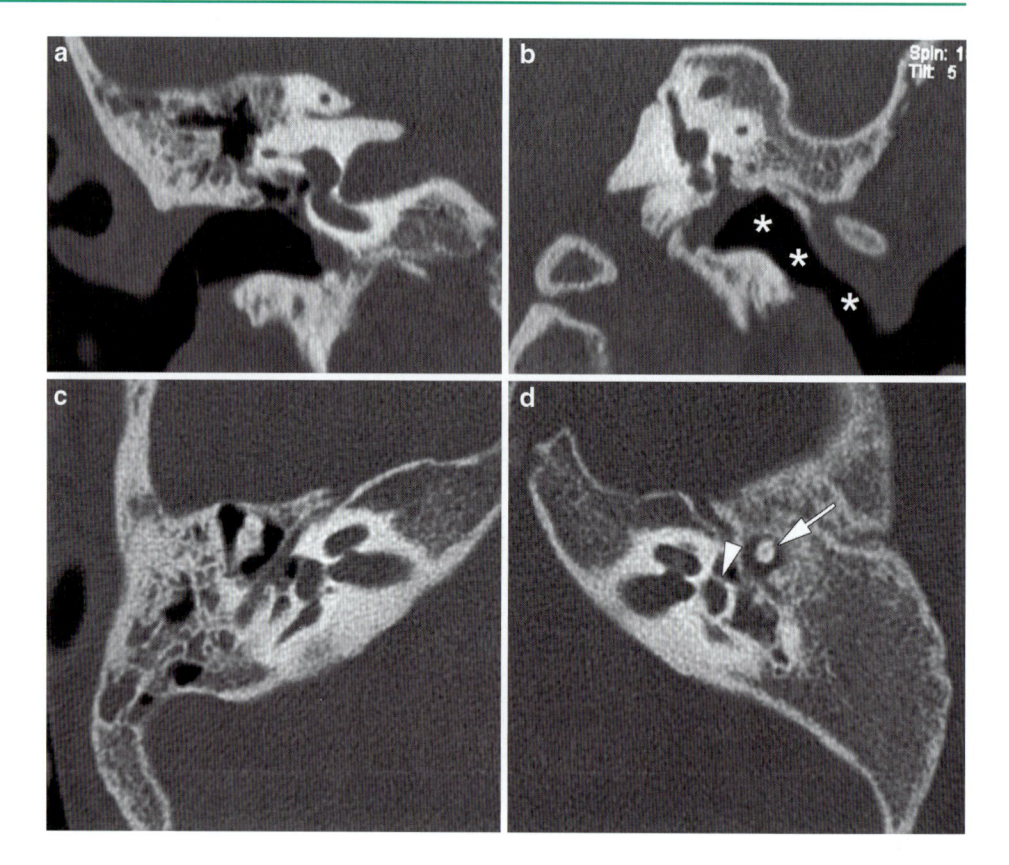

The inner ear has a different origin, and therefore it is usually normal in these patients.

A congenitally narrowed external auditory meatus is associated with dysplasia of the tympanic bone. Such a canal often runs in an abnormal direction, sloping more upwards than usual (Fig. 1). Apart from narrowing of the bony portion of the external canal, associated fibrosis may further narrow or completely obstruct the external ear canal. The tympanic membrane may be present or absent.

When no external auditory canal is formed, the tympanic bone is aplastic. The lateral wall of the middle ear consists of soft tissue (Fig. 2), or a bony plate which is situated at the expected level of the tympanic membrane (Fig. 3). Such a bony plate is called an atresia plate, and this may correspond to a 'frust' tympanic bone or to downward extension of the squamous part of the temporal bone, meeting the floor of the middle ear.

The size of the tympanic cavity is often diminished, making surgery more difficult. The tegmen may have a low position, which may also complicate the surgical approach. The air content of the mastoid is often reduced, correlating with the degree of abnormality of the external ear.

The size of the bony Eustachian tube may be reduced, but sometimes this structure appears enlarged (Mayer et al. 1998).

Ossicular chain abnormalities are very frequently associated with aural dysplasia. Aplasia of the tympanic bone is associated with fusion of the neck of the malleus to the lateral epitympanic wall or atresia plate (Figs. 2 and 3). In addition, other ossicular anomalies may be present: fusion of the malleus and incus, with absence of the normal malleoincudal joint, is common, and the long process of the incus may have an abnormal orientation or be hypoplastic or absent. The most important ossicular structure to look for on CT is the stapes; absence of the stapes makes surgical reconstruction more complex. Furthermore, the presence and width of the oval window should be checked; on coronal images, it should have a diameter of about 2 mm (Yeakley and Jahrsdoerfer 1996).

The tympanic segment of the facial nerve canal is often displaced caudally, sometimes reaching as low as the round window (Mayer et al. 1998). The second genu and mastoid portion of the facial nerve typically are more anteriorly positioned than normal, which is important for the surgeon to know, as this may severely hinder surgical reconstruction. The mastoid portion of the facial nerve may curve anteriorly toward the area of the temporomandibular joint, or leave the temporal bone in a more lateral direction. Determining the exact course of the facial nerve is of utmost importance to avoid postoperative facial paralysis (Fig. 4).

When the tympanic bone is aplastic, the position of the temporomandibular joint is frequently more posterior than normal, because of lack of a posterior bony support. Confluence of the temporomandibular joint soft tissue with the middle ear is regarded unfavourable for surgery, as

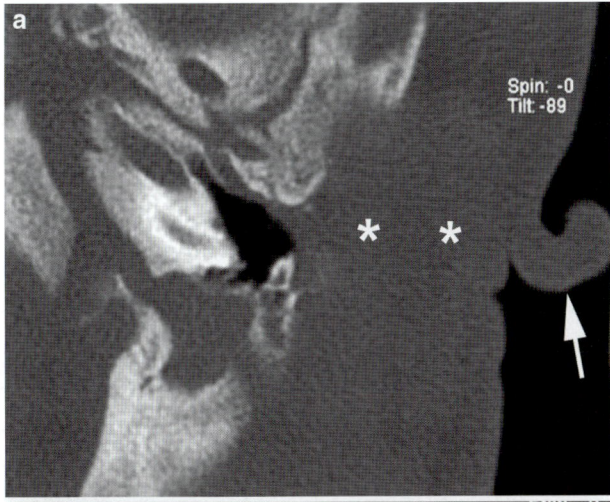

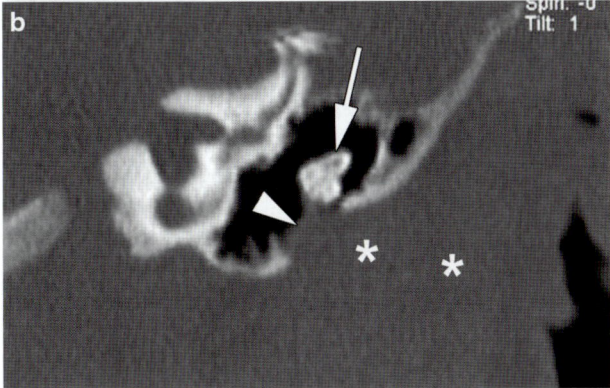

Fig. 2 *Axial* and *coronal* CT-image of *left* temporal bone in a neonatus. Abnormal auricle (*arrow*, **a**) The external ear canal is absent: only soft tissue is seen (*asterisks*). The lateral wall of the middle ear consists of soft tissue (*arrowhead*, **b**) no tympanic membrane is identified. The malleus and incus appear deformed and fused (*arrow*, **b**)

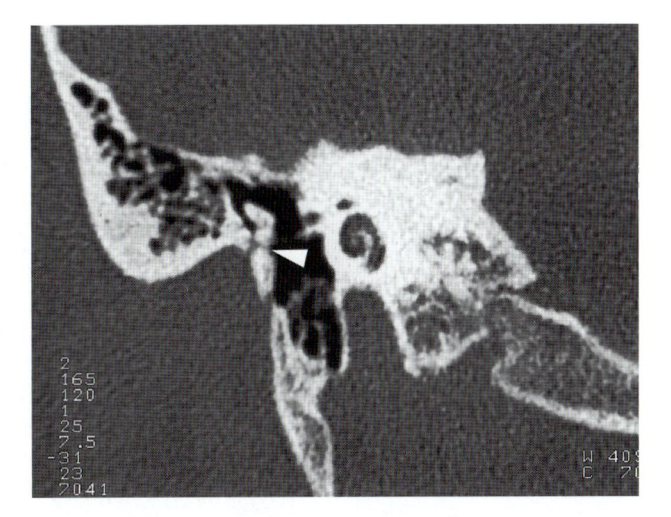

Fig. 3 *Coronal* CT image through *right* temporal bone in an adult patient. Atresia of the external auditory canal. The neck of the malleus is fused with the atresia plate (*arrowhead*)

maintaining support for the surgically created hearing apparatus is more difficult (Yeakley and Jahrsdoerfer 1996).

A 10-point scale has been devised based on the CT-findings, predicting the risk of complications and postoperative hearing results (Yeakley and Jahrsdoerfer 1996).

The CT study should also exclude the presence of a congenital or acquired cholesteatoma: atresia or stenosis of the external ear canal may hinder the normal migration of epithelium, leading to the accumulation of keratinized debris and hence formation of a cholesteatoma.

Although rare, abnormalities of the inner ear should be looked for. Usually, when associated with aural dysplasia, these inner ear malformations are minor; the labyrinthine function is not necessarily abnormal. The internal auditory canal may appear widened and more angled than normal.

2.2 Branchiogenic Anomalies

Although aural dysplasia can be regarded as a branchiogenic anomaly (see above), other anomalies arising from the branchiogenic apparatus may occur around the external ear.

Defects of the branchial apparatus manifest as a cyst, a sinus, or a fistula. Anomalies of the branchial complex are vestigial remnants, resulting from incomplete obliteration of the branchial apparatus or buried epithelial cell rests.

As indicated above, the first branchial apparatus is involved in the development of the external and middle ear, but also the Eustachian tube, maxilla, and mandible.

First branchial cleft anomalies lie close to, or have a connection with the external ear canal. Various classifications have been proposed, such as that described by Work (Work 1972). A Work type I anomaly corresponds to a lesion in the preauricular region, running more or less parallel to the external ear canal, embedded within the parotid gland, and lateral to the facial nerve (Fig. 5).

A Work type II anomaly extends downward to the angle of the mandible; it may be lying medial or lateral to the facial nerve branches, or between these nerve branches (Fig. 6). At the level of the mandibular angle an inflammatory mass lesion may be produced (Fig. 7). Demonstration of a connection to the external ear canal, typically at the junction of the cartilaginous and bony part, allows confirming the diagnosis.

2.3 Preaurical Sinus

The auricle develops from six mesenchymal proliferations surrounding the first pharyngeal cleft. These swellings fuse

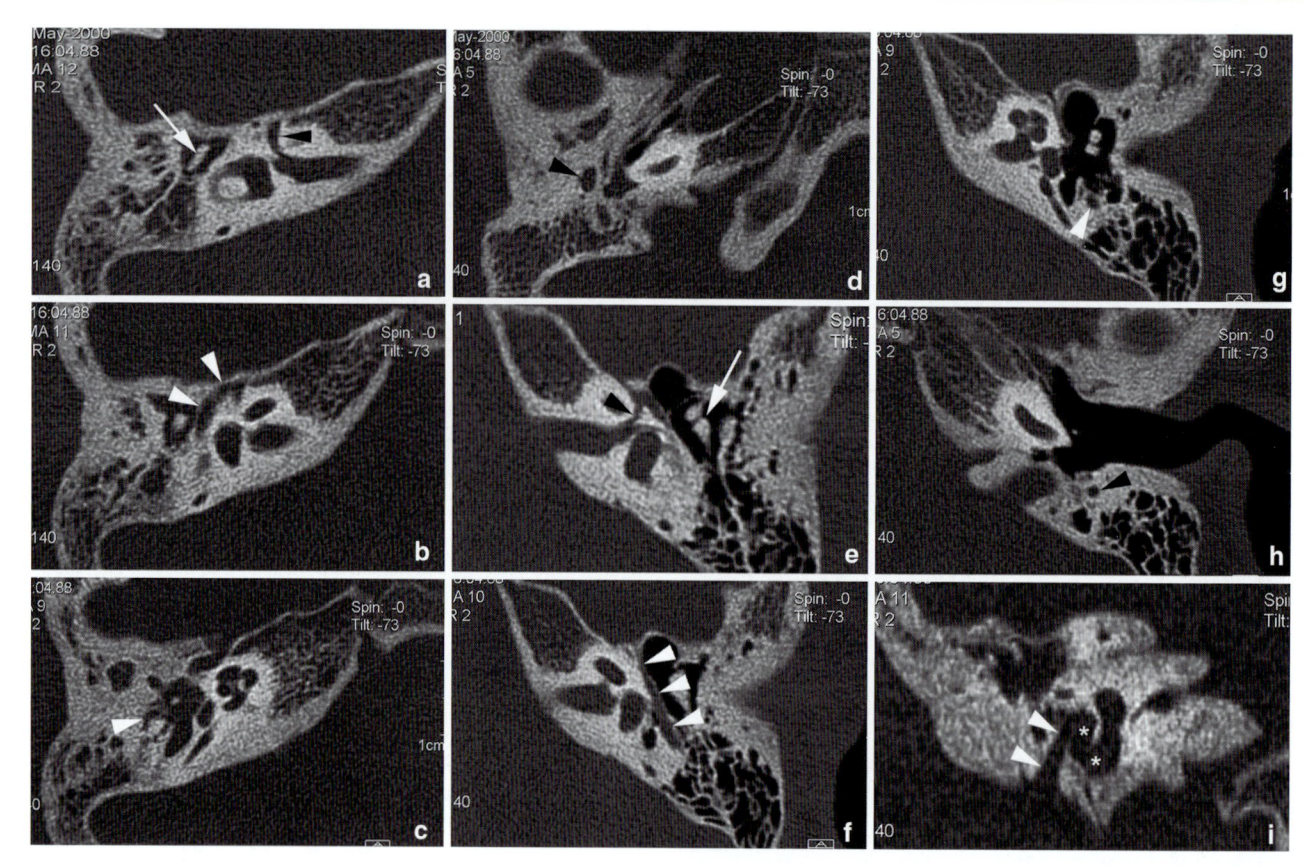

Fig. 4 *Right*-sided Goldenhar syndrome in a 12-year-old patient. **a–d** *Axial* CT images through *right* temporal bone. The facial nerve canal shows a relatively long labyrinthine segment (**a**, *arrowhead*); note the associated hypoplastic appearance of the ossicular chain (**a**, *arrow*). Short tympanic segment of facial nerve (**b**, *arrowheads*); a second genu cannot be clearly identified, but the mastoid segment of the facial canal is running posterolaterally to the tympanic cavity (**c**, *arrowhead*). At a lower level, the mastoid segment of the facial nerve can be seen to run lateral to the middle ear cavity (**d**, *arrowhead*). **e–h** For comparison, the corresponding heterolateral structures are labelled on *axial* CT images of the normal *left* temporal bone at similar levels. **i** Coronal CT image through *right* temporal bone. The short mastoid segment of the facial nerve canal (*arrowheads*) can be seen to run inferolaterally, just lateral from the middle ear cavity (*asterisks*) (the opacification of the *right* middle ear cavity is presumably caused by chronic dysfunction of the Eustachian tube)

and gradually form the definitive auricle. As this fusion is a rather complicated process, developmental abnormalities may arise (Langman 1981). A sinus results when one of the sulci between the auricular hillocks incompletely disappears. Most authors believe that a preauricular sinus is not an anomaly of the first branchial apparatus.

A preauricular sinus is a relatively common congenital abnormality. It consists of a blind-ending opening in the external ear, often located at or near the anterior crus of the helix. The diagnosis is made clinically. Most of these sinuses remain asymptomatic, but repeat infection may cause chronic discharge, repeated abscess formation and scarring, making surgical excision of the sinus and its possible ramifications necessary. Recurrences may follow incomplete resection (Currie et al. 1996).

Preoperative visualisation of the extent of the lesion may be helpful to prevent incomplete resection. Usually, injection of the sinus tract with contrast medium is not successful, as the lumen is often blocked by epithelial debris (Lau 1983). Forced injection of methylene blue, followed by surgery a few days later has also been suggested. A noninvasive method is high-resolution ultrasound, allowing to visualise the sinus, its branches, and any associated cystic component in the subcutaneous tissues; also the relationship of the lesion to the auricular cartilage and parotid gland can be demonstrated (Ahuja et al. 2000).

3 Inflammatory Conditions

3.1 External Otitis

In most cases of external otitis, imaging studies are not required as the disease can be well inspected and followed up by clinical examination.

External otitis, also known as swimmer's ear, is a common condition; maceration by water or trauma is often the etiologic factors. Also dermatologic and endocrinologic

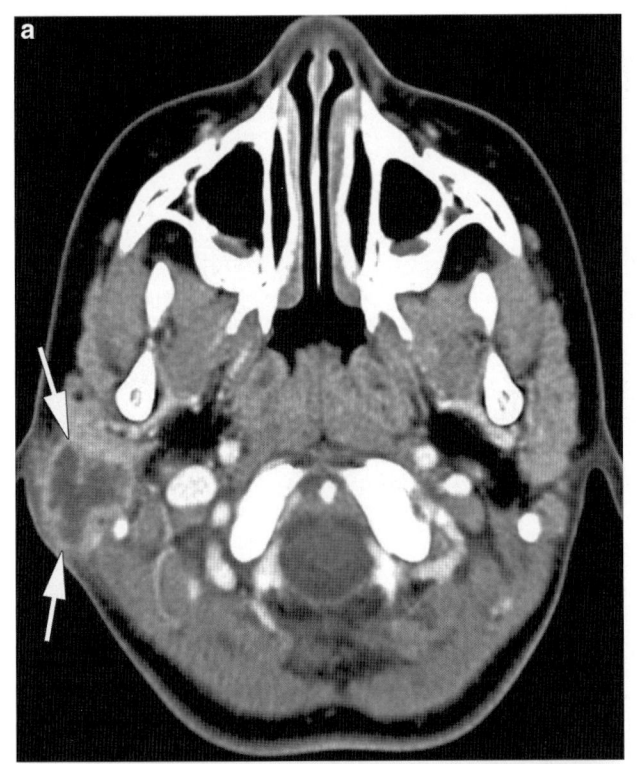

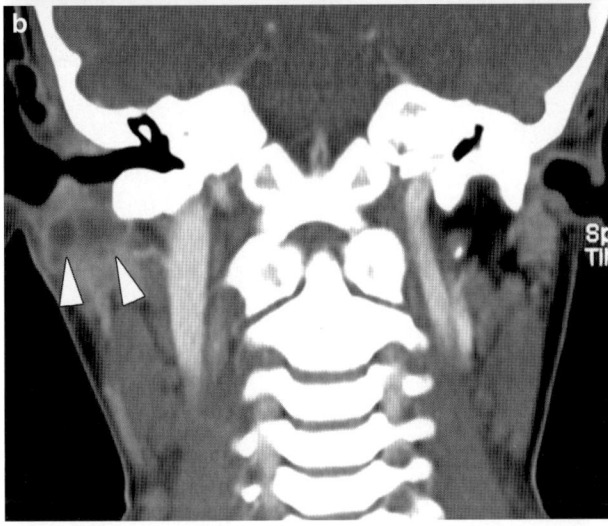

Fig. 5 7-year-old child presenting with a painful infra-auricular swelling. *Axial* (**a**) and *coronal* CT-image (**b**) show a cystic lesion with a thick enhancing wall, embedded in the parotid gland (**a**, *arrows*) and running parallel to the external ear canal (**b**, *arrowheads*). Infected first branchial cleft cyst (type I)

is by drainage of fluctuant areas and topical antibiotics; systemic antibiotics are needed when there is cellulitis or systemic symptoms.

Chronic external otitis may lead to acquired stenosis of the external auditory canal (Keohane et al. 1993), as recurrent inflammation with formation of granulation tissue may eventually lead to fibrosis and obliteration of the canal. Treatment is either by surgical correction or by a hearing aid.

Ramsay–Hunt syndrome (also known as herpes zoster oticus) corresponds to acute facial neuritis, causing facial paralysis, otalgia, and vesicles in the external ear. It is thought to be a cranial polyneuropathy caused by the herpes zoster virus (De and Pfleiderer 1999). Sometimes also hearing loss, tinnitus, or vertigo may be present. MRI shows enhancement of the facial nerve, similar as in Bell's palsy; enhancement of the intracanalicular portion of the vestibulocochlear nerve and the labyrinth may sometimes be seen.

Relapsing polychondritis is a rare inflammatory disease of cartilage of unknown origin, producing a bizarre form of arthritis. It may involve the cartilages of the ear, nose, and respiratory tract. Involvement of the auricle and cartilaginous portion of the external auditory canal is clinically apparent. Imaging is not required for evaluation of the external ear. Also the inner ear may be involved in this condition; enhancement of the labyrinthine structures on MRI has been reported (Vourtsi et al. 1998).

3.2 Necrotizing External Otitis

Necrotizing external otitis is a severe infection of the external ear, almost exclusively caused by *Pseudomonas aeruginosa*. Because of the aggressive clinical course, it has also been called 'malignant external otitis' (Chandler 1968). However, the disease is not neoplastic, and also does not remain limited to the external ear. Generally, 'necrotizing external otitis' is considered the most accurate descriptive name of this disease process.

Most patients are suffering from diabetes, or otherwise immunocompromised; the disease also occurs in elderly patients. It usually occurs unilateral, but bilateral cases have been described. Severe otalgia is the most common symptom; the patients may also suffer from purulent otorrhea. Clinical examination shows inflammatory changes and the presence of granulation tissue at the junction of the bony and cartilaginous part of the external auditory canal.

The exact pathogenesis is unknown. Pseudomonas is not a commensal of the external auditory canal, but may colonise this structure; colonisation may occur after non-discriminant use of broad spectrum antibiotics for ear infection or after irrigation of the ears with nonsterile tap water containing Pseudomonas (Rubin and Yu 1988).

conditions may give rise to external otitis. External otitis presents with itching, sometimes severe pain, and a cheesy discharge. The ear canal is diffusely swollen and tender. Most cases are controlled with topical treatment. In severe cases, cellulitis of the surrounding structures may be present, requiring systemic antibiotic treatment.

External ear furuncles are also common; they appear as localized, tender, and possibly fluctuant swellings. Treatment

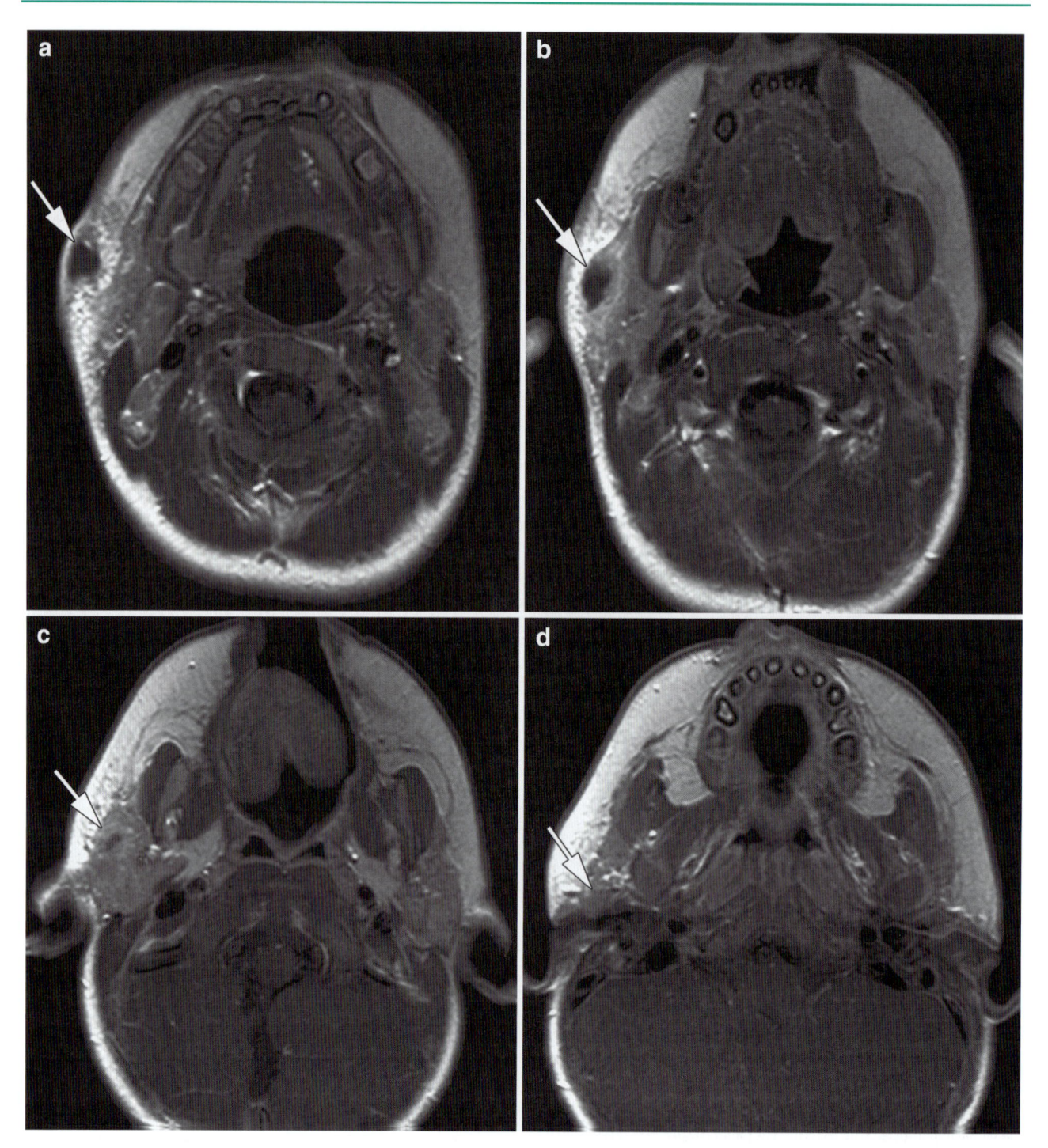

Fig. 6 18-month-old child initially presenting with a *right*-sided preauricular abscess and a sinus opening at the level of the right mandibular angle. This opening was present since birth. *Axial* contrast-enhanced T1-weighted spin echo images (**a–d**) show a tubular enhancing structure (*arrows*), partially fluid-filled, extending from the skin at the level of the mandibular angle (**a**), through the superficial lobe of the parotid gland (**b, c**), eventually reaching the external ear canal (**d**). This sinus was excised, including its connection with the external ear canal. First branchial cleft anomaly (type II)

Ischaemic conditions, related to diabetic microangiopathy or the effect of ageing, result in hypoperfusion and may increase susceptibility to infection. Also decreased activity of white blood cells may be a contributing factor.

The infection rapidly spreads to involve surrounding bone and soft tissues. The disease may erode into the bone of the mastoid. Anterior extension into the temporomandibular joint may occur, possibly causing destructive

External Ear Imaging

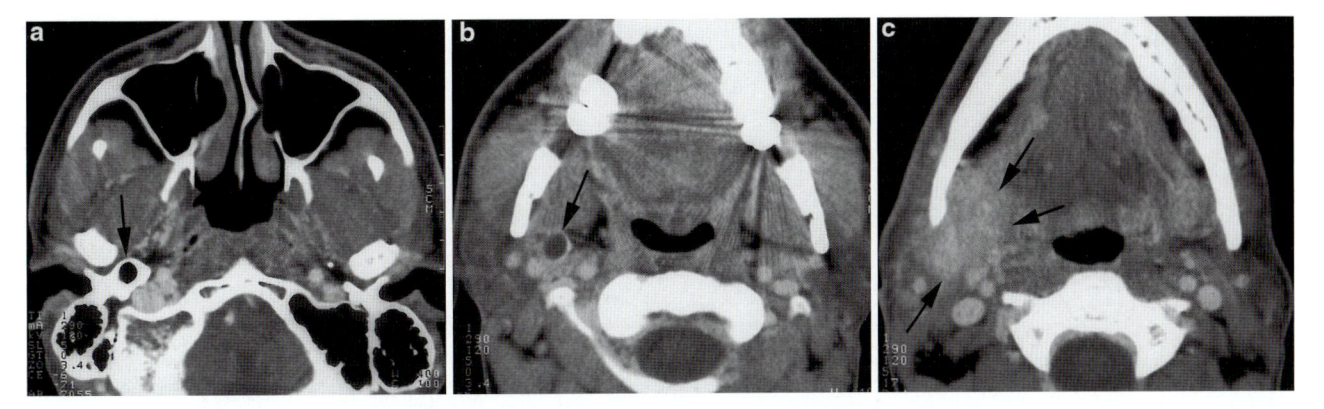

Fig. 7 *Axial* contrast-enhanced CT images. *Right* sided tubular anomaly communicating with the malformed tympanic bone (**a**, *arrow*), extending inferiorly just deep to the parotid gland (**b**, *arrow*), ending in an inflammatory mass in the submandibular space (**c**, *arrows*). First branchial cleft anomaly (type II)

Fig. 8 *Axial* CT-images through skull base show destruction of the bony external auditory canal, erosion of the mastoid bone and invasion of the temporomandibular joint (**a**). The contrast-enhanced image reveals extension of the infection into the soft tissues of the infratemporal fossa (**b**, *arrows*). Necrotising external otitis

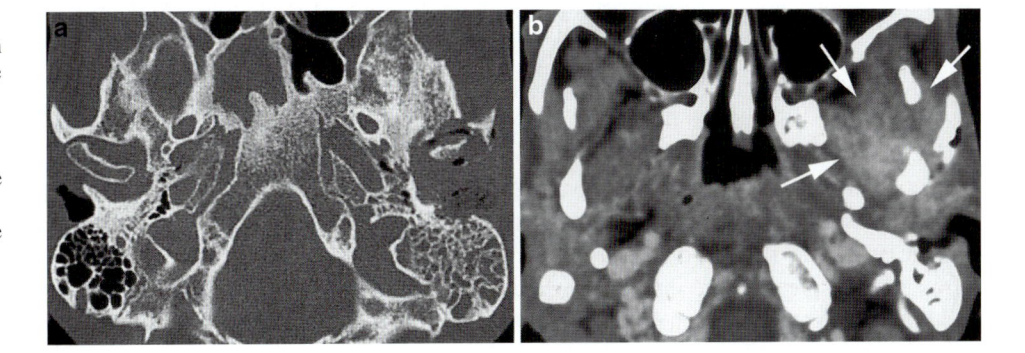

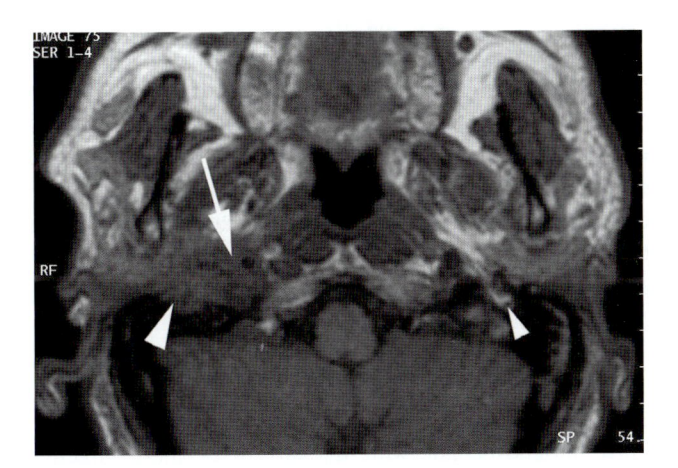

Fig. 9 *Axial* T1-weighted MR image. Diabetic patient suffering from *right* sided external otitis and facial palsy. In continuity with the external auditory canal, an infratemporal soft tissue infiltration is seen, extending in the fat pad below the stylomastoid foramen (large *arrowhead*), and into the carotid space (*arrow*). On the *left*, note normal facial nerve just below the stylomastoid foramen (small *arrowhead*). Necrotising external otitis

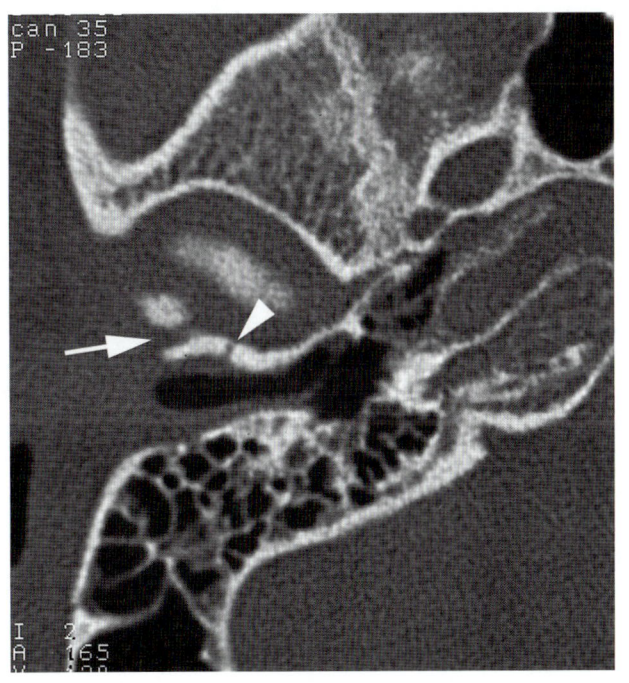

Fig. 10 *Axial* CT-image in a patient with post-traumatic ear bleeding. A nondisplaced fracture of the right tympanic bone is seen (*arrowhead*); no other temporal bone fractures were apparent. Normal squamotympanic suture (*arrow*)

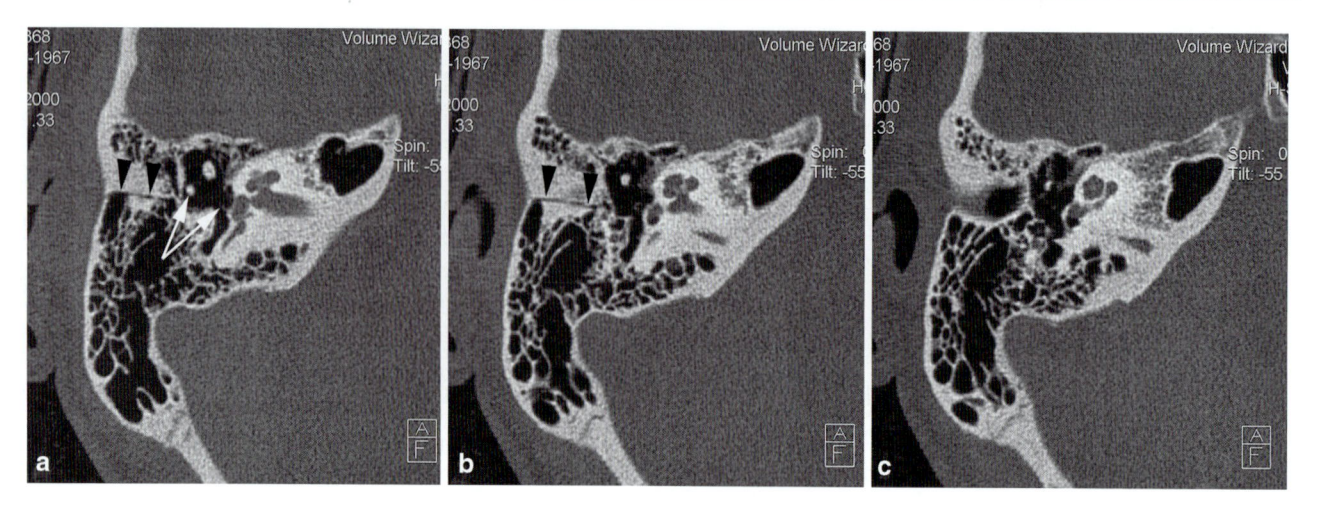

Fig. 11 *Axial* adjacent CT-images in a patient with post-traumatic conductive hearing loss. A longitudinal temporal bone fracture (*arrowheads*) is extending in the lateral wall of the middle ear (**a–c**), as well as in the superior wall of the external auditory canal. The incus is luxated; dissociation is seen between long process of incus and stapedial superstructure (**a**, *arrows*)

osteomyelitis (Midwinter et al. 1999); anterior spread may also involve the parotid gland.

Anteromedial extension into the infratemporal space may occur. Facial nerve palsy develops in 24–43 % of the cases, and is considered to be bad prognostic sign (Rubin and Yu 1988). The facial nerve usually becomes affected by infratemporal spread of the infection toward the stylomastoid foramen. As the infection spreads below the skull base, other cranial neuropathies can result. Intracranial extension may occur in advanced cases.

CT and MRI are excellent techniques to visualise the disease extent. MRI is the preferred modality if intracranial spread is suspected (Grandis et al. 1995).

CT shows thickening of the soft tissues in the external ear canal, possibly with erosion of the tympanic bone. Erosion and destruction of the temporomandibular joint may occur (Fig. 8). Typically, subtemporal extension begins at the junction of the osseous and cartilaginous part of the external auditory canal. Soft tissue infiltration and abnormal enhancement may be seen underneath the temporal bone, extending into the stylomastoid foramen; this infiltration may further progress into the parapharyngeal space (including the carotid space) and masticator space. Soft tissue infiltration and/or abnormal enhancement of the parotid gland may be observed. Hypodense regions with thick and/or irregular rim enhancement, corresponding to abcedation, may be present.

The disease may extend toward the clivus and apex of the petrous bone. A discontinuous pattern of bone destruction, with 'skip' areas, may be seen. In severe cases, not only cortical erosion, but also trabecular alterations in the medullary bone space may be observed; these medullary changes may appear osteosclerotic, osteolytic, or mixed.

The disease may extend posteriorly and erode into the mastoid, possibly causing destruction of the mastoid portion of the facial nerve canal.

The most common finding on MRI is infiltration of the fat behind the mandibular condyle (Kwon et al. 2006). Other common findings are parapharyngeal fat infiltration, skull base bone marrow infiltration, lateral nasopharyngeal wall thickening, and preclival soft tissue infiltration (Fig. 9).

An abnormal flow void in the internal carotid artery, which may be displaced, and intracranial dural enhancement (in the middle or posterior cranial fossa, in severe cases extending into the foramen magnum) may be present.

Necrotizing external otitis occasionally causes central skull base osteomyelitis. Atypical cases of central skull base osteomyelitis, arising from the sphenoid or occipital bone, without obvious external otitis, are much less frequently seen (Chang et al. 2003). Inadequately treated necrotizing external otitis may also give rise to contralateral skull base osteomyelitis (Singh et al. 2005).

The radiographic differentiation from true malignant neoplasia may be difficult; rarely both conditions are present at the same time (Rubin et al. 1990). In cancer, the bone involvement is expected to display a more contiguous pattern of destruction, while in necrotizing otitis media 'skip' areas may be present. The clinical picture in external ear cancer is different, without or with only minimal pain. However, cancer may rarely mimic necrotizing otitis media in its clinical appearance (Mattuci et al., 1986; Al-Shihabi 1992).

The treatment consists of surgical debridement of the external auditory canal, drainage of collections, and intravenous antibiotics. Malignant otitis externa used to have a grave prognosis, but with the advent of more effective antibiotics, the infection can be controlled in the majority of cases. Cranial nerve involvement is often quoted as a bad prognostic sign. It does reflect more extensive disease, and the mortality rate is higher in these patients. However, recovery of facial nerve function after successful treatment has been observed.

Fig. 12 *Left*-sided conductive hearing loss after soft tissue injury to external ear canal. Clinical examination shows complete soft tissue obliteration of the *right* external ear canal. *Axial* and *coronal* CT images (**a**, **b**) confirm soft tissue obliteration of this structure (*arrows*); normal aeration of the middle ear cavity. Posttraumatic fibrosis and stenosis

Fig. 13 **a**, **b** *Axial* CT-images through skull (magnified on *left* temporal bone) in a child involved in a traffic accident. A longitudinal temporal bone fracture (*arrows*), running through the external ear canal (*arrowheads*) is present. **c**, **d** The patient presents 6 years later with *left*-sided otorrhea. *Axial* (**c**) and *coronal* (**d**) CT-image show complete opacification of the external ear canal and middle ear cavity (*asterisks*). The external ear canal appears widened, with eroded margins (*arrowheads*). Taking into account the previous history, this appearance is very suggestive for a posttraumatic cholesteatoma. This was surgically confirmed

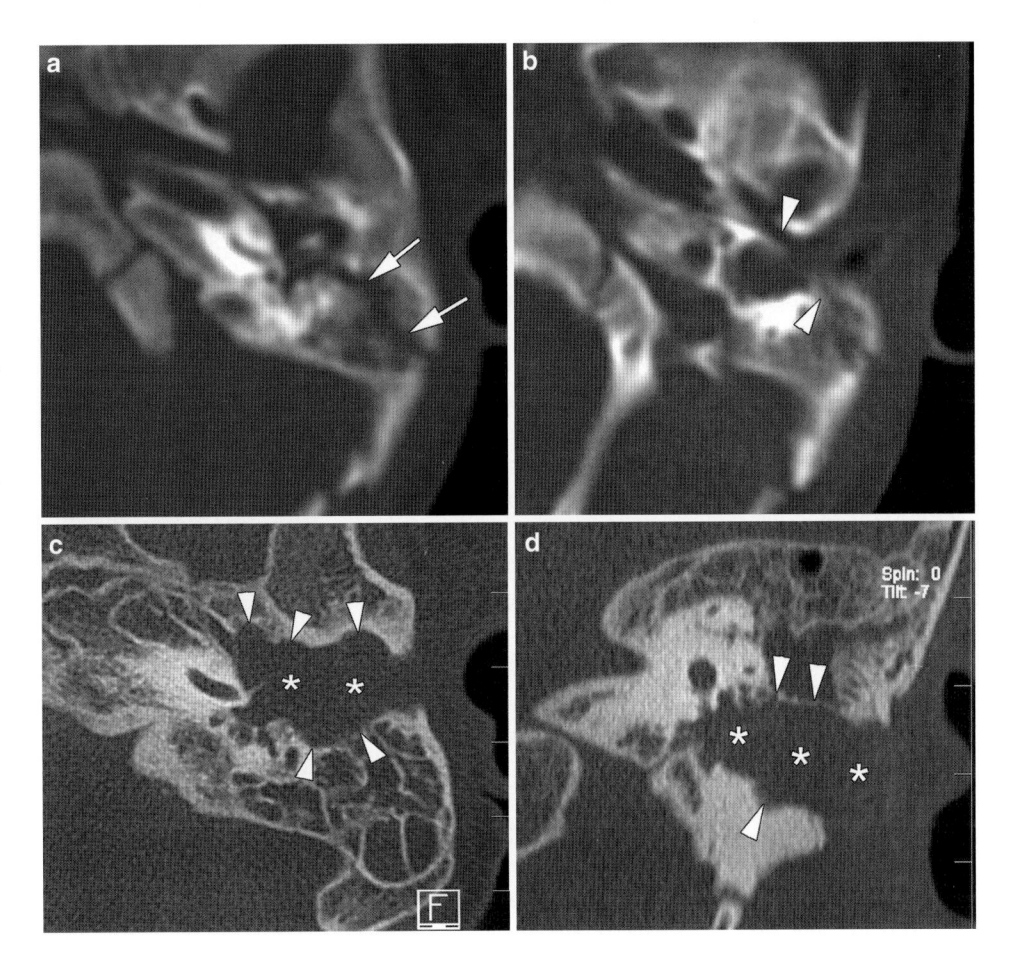

4 Trauma

Trauma to the external canal is most commonly caused by instrumentation, either by the patient itself, or by a physician. Most of these smaller lacerations or canal haematomas can be handled with antibiotic drops, but more complex lacerations need temporary packing of the ear canal, in order to avoid fibrotic stenosis.

Fractures of the tympanic bone are quite frequent; they are usually caused by the impact of a posteriorly displaced mandibular condyle, itself resulting from a blow to the chin region. Care should be taken not to misinterpret the normal squamotympanic suture as a fracture line (Fig. 10).

Longitudinal fractures of the temporal bone run more or less along the long axis of the temporal bone. Such a fracture typically originates from a blow to the temporoparietal portion of the skull, with inferior propagation of the

Fig. 14 Patient treated by irradiation for a *right*-sided lateral oropharyngeal squamous cell cancer, 6 years earlier. During the follow-up, the patient mentioned *right*-sided otalgia; clinical examination showed some debris in the external ear canal. *Axial* (**a**) and *sagittal* CT-image (**b**) through the *right* external ear show irregular osteolysis of the tympanic bone, with some small bone sequesters embedded in soft tissue swelling (*arrowheads*). Also some osteolysis is seen in the mandibular head. This was interpreted as osteoradionecrosis of the tympanic bone and mandibular head. Conservative treatment was initiated

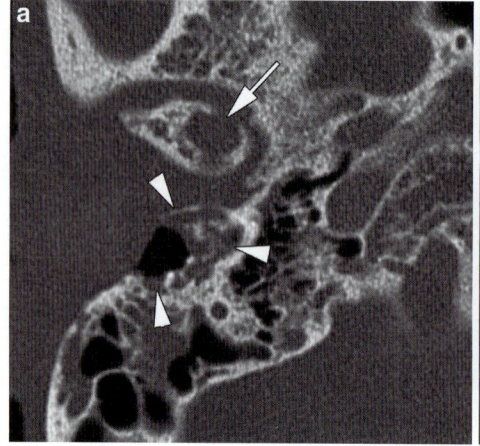

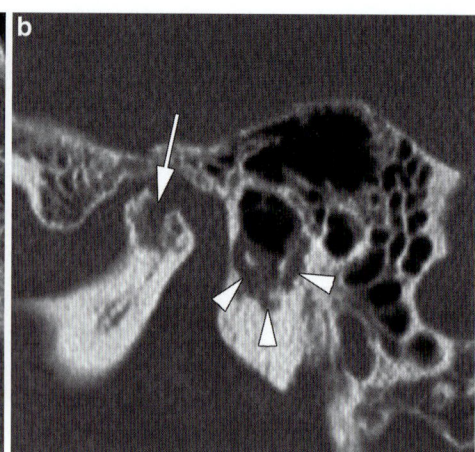

fracture line through the mastoid into the lateral wall of the middle ear, passing behind, through, or in front of the external auditory canal (Fig. 11).

Fractures through the external auditory canal are treated by temporary packing of the canal to prevent canal stenosis.

Soft tissue trauma to the external ear canal, without recognisable fracture, may lead to fibrosis and stenosis of the external auditory canal (Fig. 12).

Post-traumatic canal stenosis may lead to accumulation of debris deep to the stenosis, and formation of a cholesteatoma (McKennan and Chole 1992). A post-traumatic cholesteatoma may also develop as a result of implantation of ear canal squamous epithelium into the fracture line (McKennan and Chole 1989). Entrapment of epithelium may occur because of complex displacement of bony fragments or diastasis of suture lines. A tear of the tympanic membrane is also believed to be a possible origin for cholesteatoma formation (Freeman 1983). Post-traumatic cholesteatoma of the external ear may only become symptomatic after a delay of several years. Imaging shows the presence of a soft tissue mass, possibly associated with surrounding bone erosion. A close topographic relationship to a fracture line usually exists (Franssens et al. 1993) (Fig. 13). As these patients have no prior history of ear disease, a well-pneumatised mastoid air cell complex usually is present, allowing extensive growth of the lesion. Histologically, there is no difference with the nontraumatic type of cholesteatoma. Treatment consists in removal of the cholesteatoma and restoration of a wide patent ear canal (Freeman 1983).

Osteoradionecrosis of the external ear canal is a rare complication of radiotherapy of head and neck neoplasms. Often there is a delay of several years after the end of therapy before symptoms occur. Usually, the patient

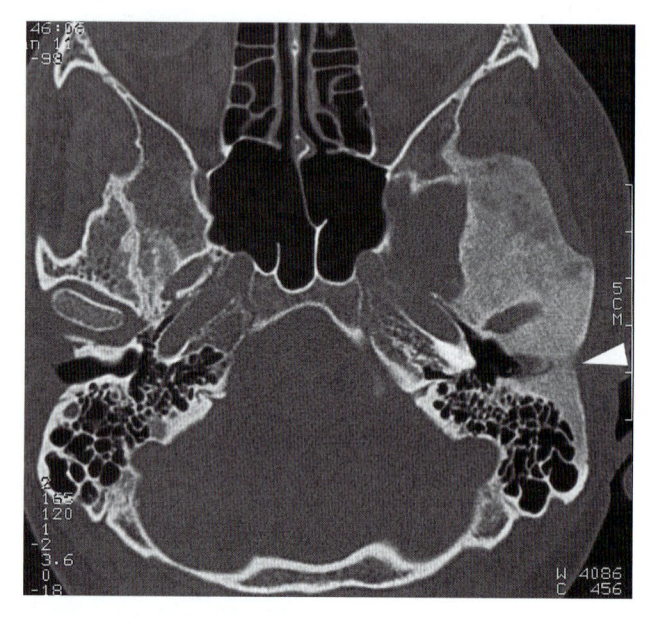

Fig. 15 *Axial* CT-image. Enlargement of the squamous part of the *left* temporal bone, showing the typical ground-glass appearance of fibrous dysplasia; the enlargement of the bone causes stenosis of the external ear canal (*arrowhead*) (courtesy by Bert De Foer, MD, Antwerp, Belgium)

complains of otalgia and/or otorrhea. Imaging shows variable amounts of bone fragmentation and soft tissue thickening (Fig. 14) (Guida et al. 1990).

5 Fibrous Dysplasia

Fibrous dysplasia is a condition in which normal medullary bone is replaced by an abnormal proliferation of fibrous tissue, resulting in asymmetric distortion and expansion of

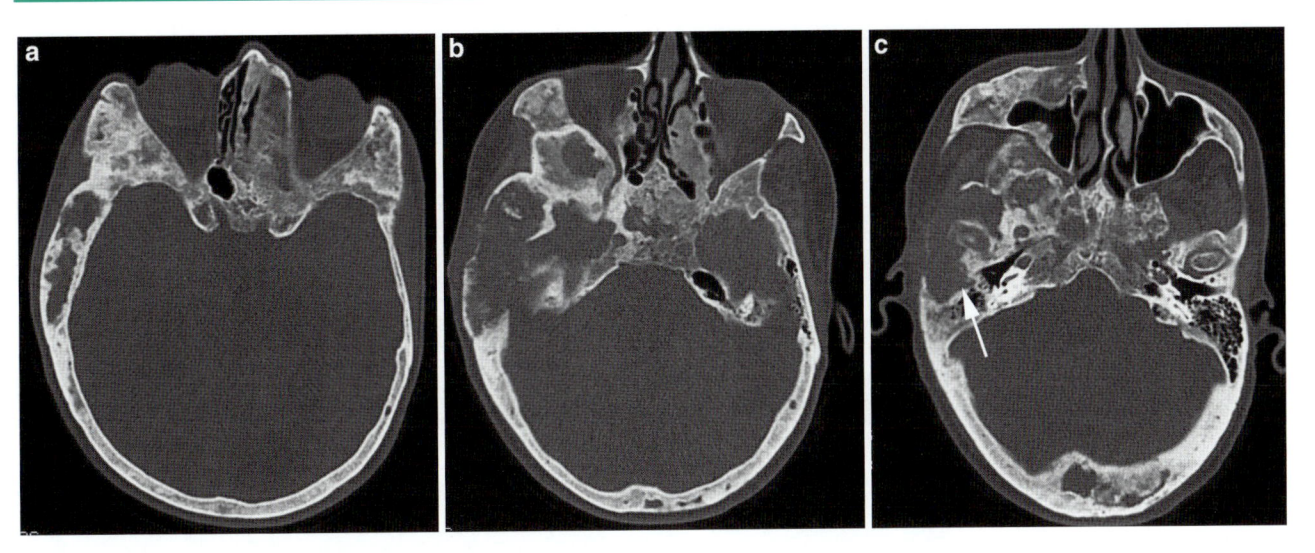

Fig. 16 McCune–Albright syndrome. Both sides of the sphenoid bone, *left* ethmoid bone, and squamous part of the *right* temporal bone show expansion of the bone, with a mixed osteolytic appearance, areas of dense calcifications and partly a ground-glass appearance (**a**, **b**). Stenosis of the *right* external ear canal by the bone expansion (**c**, *arrow*)

bone. It may be confined to a single bone (monostotic fibrous dysplasia) or involve multiple bones (polyostotic fibrous dysplasia). The monostotic form may involve any of the facial bones, but is most commonly seen in the maxilla. The association of the polyostotic form with sexual precocity and cutaneous pigmentation in a female patient is known as McCune–Albright syndrome.

Fibrous dysplasia is a disease of young patients. It may be an incidental finding. In the temporal bone, fibrous dysplasia most commonly involves the squamous portion. The most common symptom in temporal bone involvement is stenosis of the external auditory canal, resulting in conductive hearing loss. As in any stenosis of the external canal, a secondary cholesteatoma may develop deep to the stenosis (Vrabec and Chaljub 2000). Rarely, other parts of the temporal bone may be involved by fibrous dysplasia.

Usually, no new lesions appear after the cessation of skeletal growth. The lesions become more sclerotic with time but may continue to grow slowly into adulthood. Occasionally, reactivation of the lesions occurs during pregnancy. Secondary malignant degeneration into a sarcoma (about 0.5 % of cases) should be considered when stable or recurrent fibrous dysplasia produces pain or soft tissue extension (Schwartz and Alpert 1964).

Radiologically, fibrous dysplasia usually appears as enlarged bone with a dense 'ground-glass' aspect (Fig. 15); sometimes the lesions have a more osteolytic aspect with regions of dense calcification within them (Fig. 16) (Brown et al. 1995).

On CT, the bone remodelling associated with a middle fossa meningioma may roughly mimic fibrous dysplasia. However, in meningioma the thickened and sclerotic bone appears irregularly delineated; the bone delineation in fibrous dysplasia usually is sharply defined. In case of doubt, a complementary MRI study should be performed (see below).

On MRI, the lesions usually have a low signal intensity on T1-weighted images and either high or low signal intensity on T2-weighted images. The signal intensity on T1- and T2-weighted images and the degree of contrast enhancement on T1-weighted images depends on the amount of bony trabeculae, degree of cellularity and presence of cystic and haemorrhagic changes (Jee et al. 1996). Incidentally found fibrous dysplasia may be confused with a neoplastic lesion on an MR study.

The treatment of fibrous dysplasia affecting the external ear has traditionally been conservative, directed towards the management of the external canal stenosis (Megerian et al. 1995).

6 Benign Neoplasms

6.1 Cholesteatoma

Cholesteatoma is an expansive mass of exfoliated keratin within a sac of stratified squamous epithelium, most often occurring in the middle ear. Cholesteatoma is usually an acquired disease ('secondary cholesteatoma'), but may be congenital ('primary cholesteatoma'). Congenital cholesteatoma is an ectoblastic derived mass, originating from epithelial rests; as such lesions may be found everywhere in the temporal bone, they may also occur in the external auditory canal.

Cholesteatoma most commonly occurs within the middle ear. External auditory canal cholesteatoma is rare.

Fig. 17 *Coronal* (**a**) and *sagittal* (**b**) CT-images. Soft tissue thickening in the external ear canal (*arrowheads*), causing erosion of its inferior bony wall. A small calcification is present (*arrow*). External auditory canal cholesteatoma

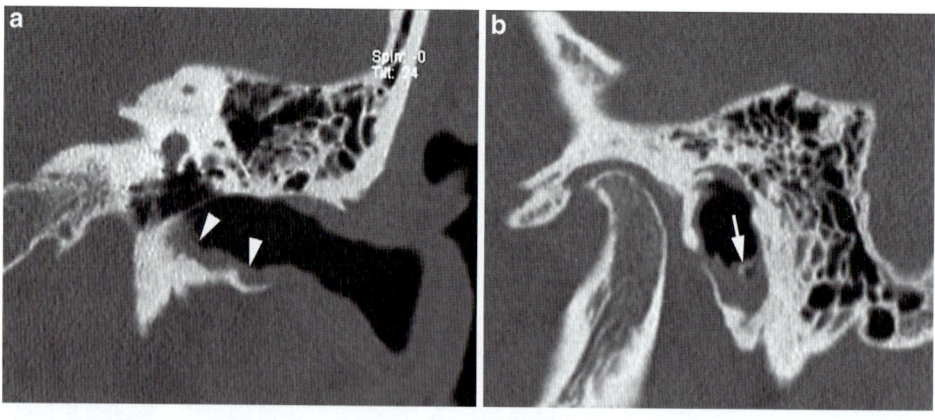

Fig. 18 *Axial* (**a**) and *coronal* (**b**) CT-images of *left* temporal bone. Soft tissue mass eroding through the posterocranial wall of the external auditory canal into the mastoid (*arrows*). External auditory canal cholesteatoma

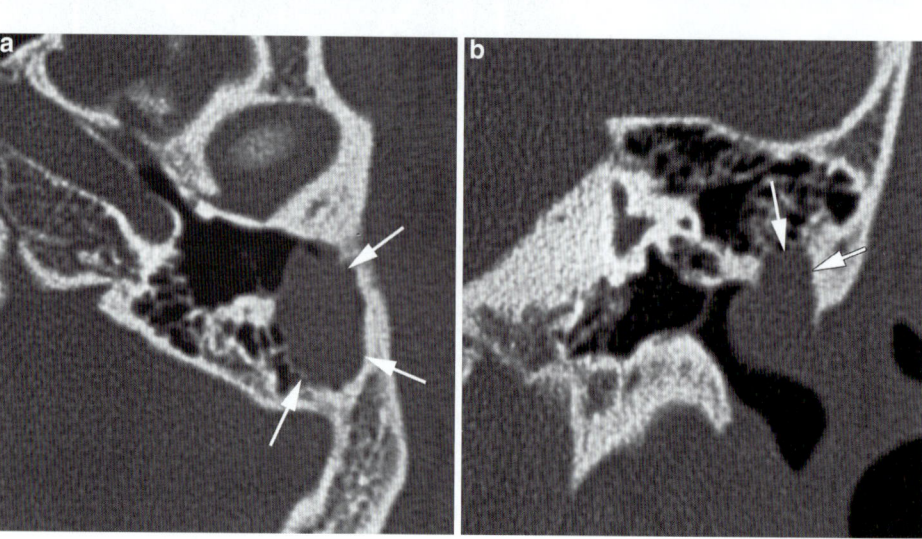

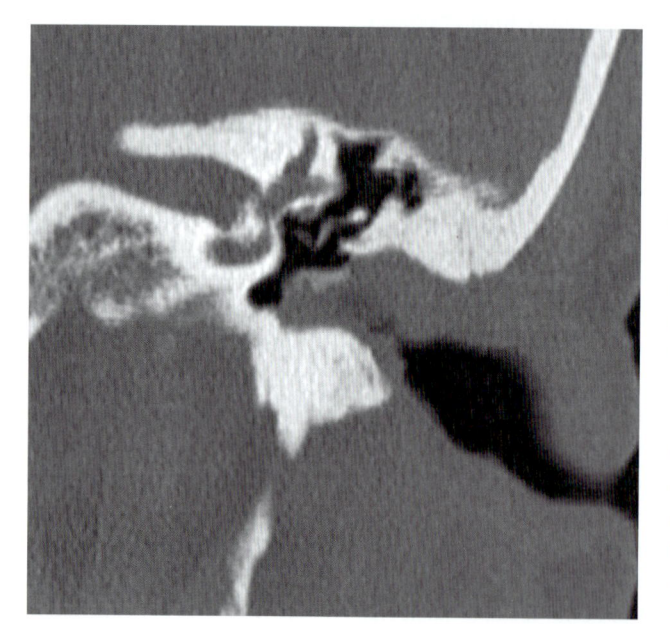

Fig. 19 *Coronal* CT-image shows obliteration of the external auditory canal by soft tissue. The walls of the canal appear intact. Keratosis obturans. The tympanic membrane contains calcifications, not being a typical finding in this condition (courtesy by Marc Lemmerling, MD, PhD, Gent, Belgium)

Patient with external canal cholesteatoma may present with itching, pain, and foul-smelling otorrhea (Heilbrun et al. 2003).

In a review of 39 external canal cholesteatomas, Vrabec and Chaljub (2000) identified several possible causes. In their practice, most cases were seen after tympanomastoid surgery, and therefore classified as 'iatrogenic'. These cases present as invagination of skin through a defect in the posterior canal wall or as a subepithelial mass lesion. Imaging revealed destruction of the canal wall lateral to the scutum. The second more common cause was described as 'spontaneous' external canal cholesteatomas, and believed to be related to focal osteitis, minor trauma to the external canal skin, or retention of hard cerumen. Presumably, they may also arise from ectopic epithelium. Trauma was believed to be the third most common cause; post-traumatic cholesteatoma is described more extensively above.

In some of the patients described by Vrabec and Chaljub (2000), stenosis of the external auditory canal caused cholesteatoma (two patients had congenital stenosis, the other patient suffered from acquired stenosis due to fibrous dysplasia). Any process causing occlusion or narrowing of

Fig. 20 *Sagittal* CT-images (**a**, **b**) through *right* and *left* external ear canal in same patient, showing multiple nodular bony structures (*arrowheads*) arising from the bony canal wall: exostoses

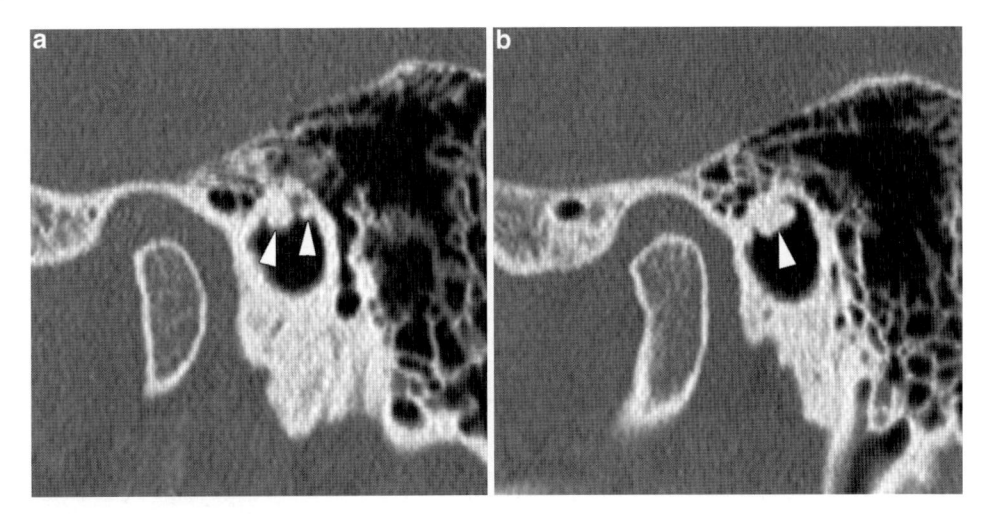

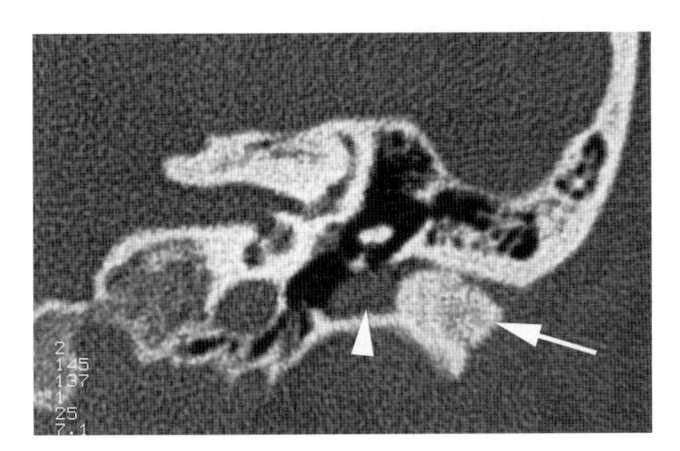

Fig. 21 *Coronal* CT-image through *left* temporal bone. Solitary bony outgrowth, attached to the tympanic bone, corresponding to an osteoma (*arrow*). Some retro-obstructive debris or inflammation is present between the osteoma and the tympanic membrane (*arrowhead*)

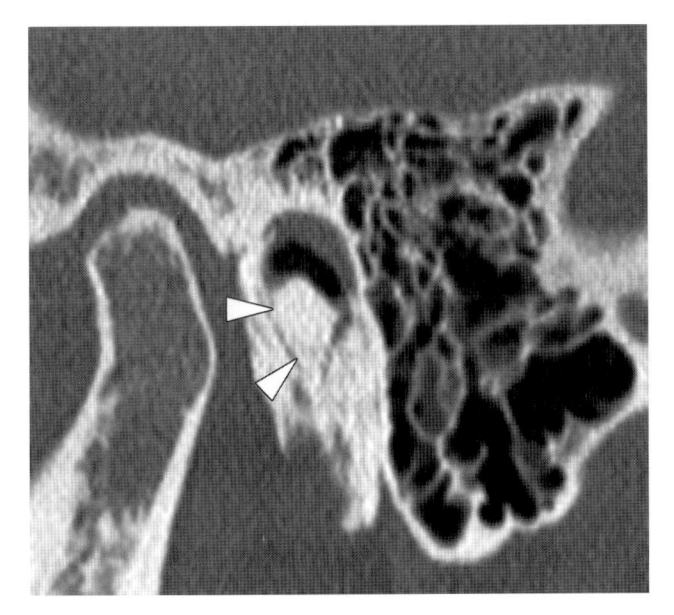

Fig. 22 *Sagittal* CT-image showing small osteoma (*arrowheads*) attached to anterior and inferior wall of bony external ear canal

the external canal may result in retention of squamous debris medial to the stenosis; this has also been described in Paget's disease and with external canal osteoma. It may also occur with acquired stenosis due to external otitis, if such stenosis is located rather laterally in the canal.

Imaging shows soft tissue thickening and erosion of the bony EAC wall; some calcifications may be seen within the soft tissue mass (Fig. 17). In patients with EAC cholesteatoma, the middle ear and mastoid may be extensively pneumatised; once such a cholesteatoma has gained access to these cavities, it may become quite large (Fig. 18). Reported complications include facial nerve paralysis, ossicular erosions and labyrinthine fistula (Brookes and Graham 1984; Vrabec and Chaljub 2000; Heilbrun et al. 2003).

6.2 Keratosis Obturans

Keratosis obturans is a condition in which an epidermal keratin plug is found in the external auditory canal, often bilateral. The presenting symptoms are pain and conductive hearing loss; these symptoms may be acute, caused by swelling of the plug when moistured (e.g. after swimming) (Persaud et al. 2004).

There is evidence that keratosis obturans is caused by abnormal epithelial migration across the tympanic membrane and out of the external ear canal (Corbridge et al. 1996).

The accumulation of large plugs of desquamated epithelium may lead to a greatly widened bony canal; however, the tympanic membrane is usually spared. In young patients, an association with sinusitis and/or bronchiectasis has been noted in up to 77 % of cases, but this concurrence is less often found in adult patients (about 20 %). Also, bilateral involvement is more frequently seen in juvenile cases than in adults.

On CT, soft tissue thickening is seen in the external auditory canal (Fig. 19), possibly with ballooning and erosion of its bony borders. Very rarely, keratosis obturans

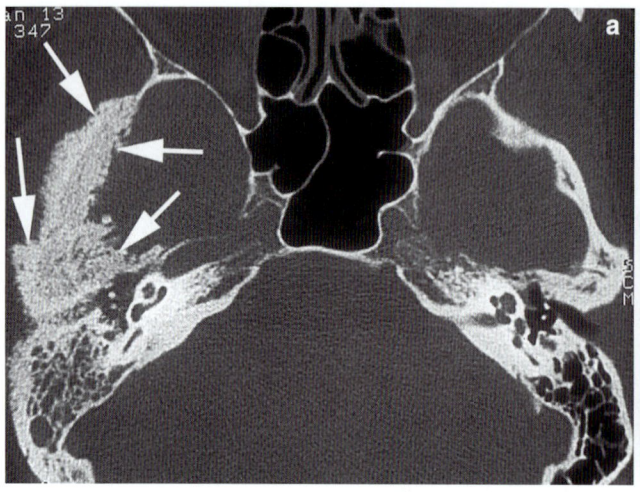

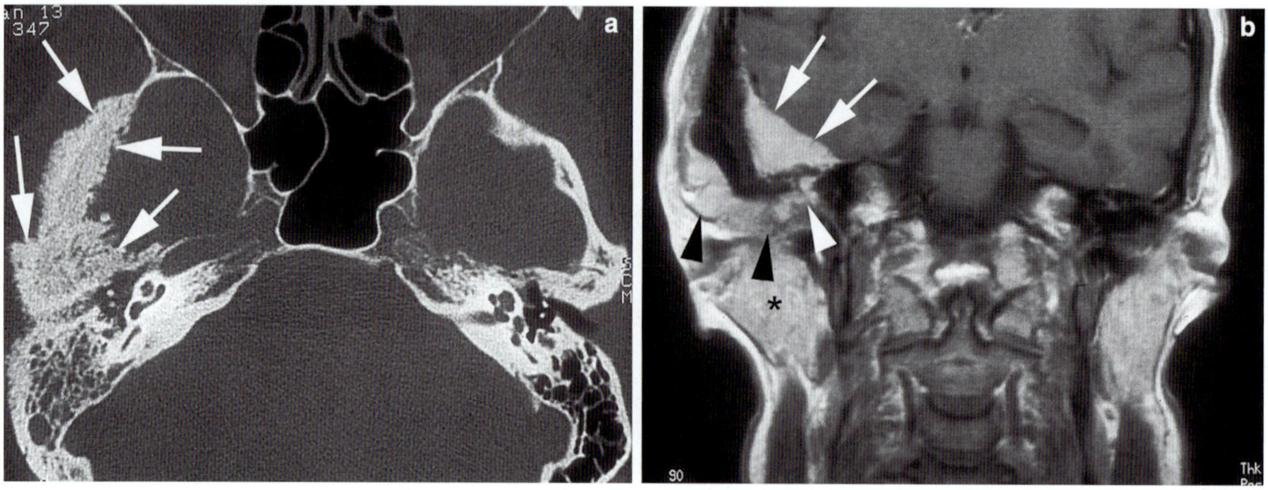

Fig. 23 Patient with acquired soft tissue stenosis of the *right* external ear canal. Axial CT-image (**a**) shows extensive sclerotic bone remodelling of the squamous part of the right temporal bone (*arrows*); although somewhat reminiscent of the ground-glass aspect seen in fibrous dysplasia (see Fig. 15), the irregular surface should rise the suspicion of hyperostosis induced by a meningioma. Opacification of the *right* middle ear cavity is seen. Coronal enhanced T1-weighted spin echo image (**b**). A strongly enhancing mass lesion is seen in the middle cranial fossa (arrows), with transosseous extension into the middle ear, external ear canal and along the outside of the squamous bone (*arrowheads*). Biopsy of the external ear mass revealed meningioma. Parotid gland (*asterisk*)

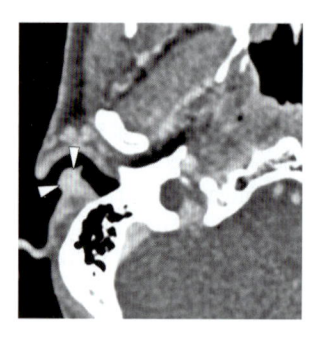

Fig. 24 *Axial* CT-images. A small, exophytic enhancing soft tissue mass is seen on the posterior wall of the right external ear canal (*arrowheads*). Small squamous cell carcinoma may be seen to extend into the middle ear cavity and facial nerve canal (Persaud et al. 2003; Glynn et al. 2006).

The differential diagnosis is external auditory canal cholesteatoma, which is usually a unilateral disease, presenting as otorrhea and a more chronic, dull pain (Piepergerdes et al. 1980).

6.3 Exostoses and Osteoma

Exostoses are multiple, usually bilateral, nodular elevations of bone involving the tympanic bone (Kemink and Graham 1982; Tran et al. 1996). They develop because of prolonged irritation of the EAC, most commonly secondary to excessive contact with cold sea water (surfer's ear). Patients may present with conductive hearing loss.

CT shows multiple, usually bilateral and more or less symmetrical, broad based nodular bony elevations in the EAC. The overlying soft tissues may appear normal, or thickened in case of associated external otitis (Fig. 20).

An osteoma is a solitary, unilateral and pedunculated bony growth in the outer half of the bony EAC. It is usually asymptomatic, but symptoms can arise if obstruction occurs (Kemink and Graham 1982; Tran et al. 1996). CT shows a solitary, unilateral and pedunculated bony growth of the bony external ear canal. The underlying bone appears normal, as well as the overlying soft tissues (Figs. 21 and 22). Medial to the stenosis, debris may accumulate; erosion of the surrounding bone at this level suggests a secondary cholesteatoma (Lee et al. 2005).

6.4 Other Tumours

Different other kinds of benign tumours may be encountered within the external auditory canal. All of these lesions are rare.

Chronic external otitis may be associated with the formation of a non-neoplastic aural polyp. Several types of tumours arising from the ceruminous glands may be seen. Vascular malformations, haemangiomas, smooth muscle tumours and tumours of neural origin have been described. Rarely, the external auditory canal may become invaded by a meningioma originating from the middle cranial fossa (Tsunoda and Fukaya 1997) (Fig. 23).

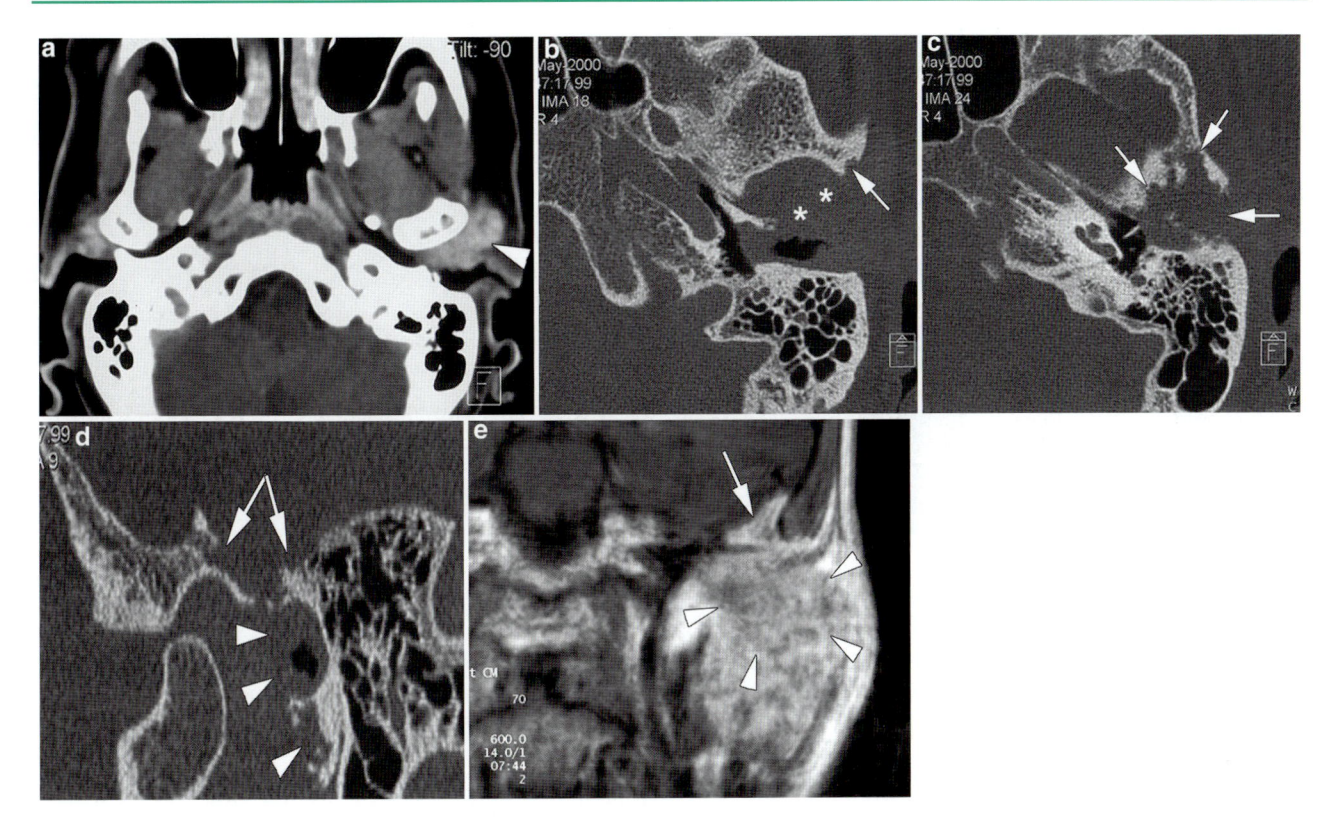

Fig. 25 Patient with squamous cell carcinoma of left external ear canal. **a** *Axial* CT-image (soft tissue window) shows enhancing mass lesion originating from the anterior wall of the canal (*arrow*), growing against the mandibular condyle. **b, c** *Axial* CT-images (bone window). Soft tissue thickening in the canal is seen, with lysis of the anterior wall of the tympanic bone (expected position is indicated by asterisks, **b**). Some osteolysis is seen at the origin of the zygomatic process (*arrow*, **b**). More superiorly, lysis of the roof of the external ear canal and adjacent part of the squamous portion (*arrowheads*, **c**). **d** *Sagittal* CT-image (bone window) confirms extensive osteolysis of the tympanic bone (*arrowheads*) and superior extension in the squamous portion of the temporal bone (*arrows*). **e** Coronal gadolinium-enhanced T1-weighted image shows extension into middle cranial fossa (*arrow*) and into parotid gland (*arrowheads*)

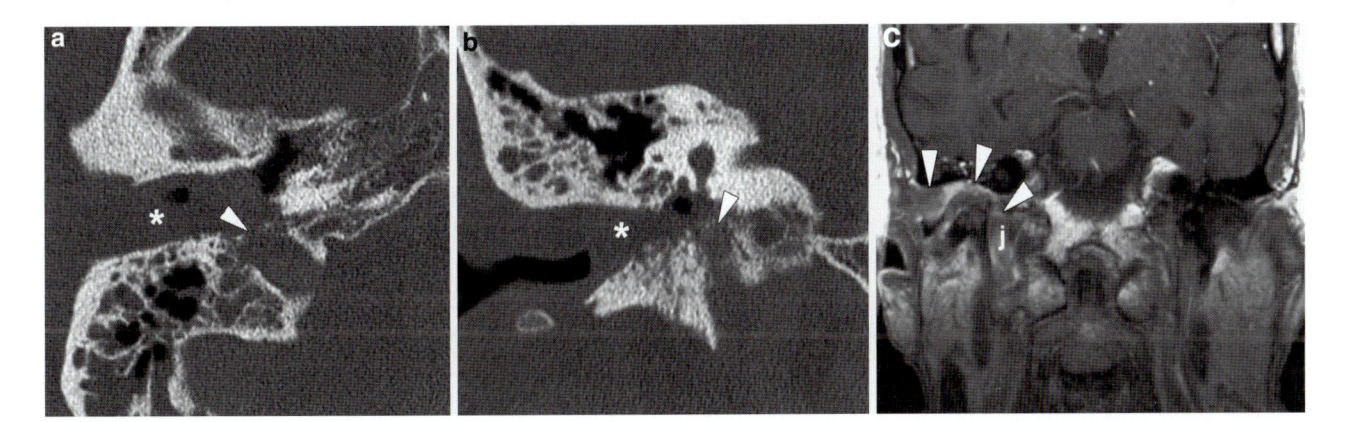

Fig. 26 Patient with squamous cell carcinoma of right external ear canal. **a, b** Axial and *coronal* CT-image. Soft tissue thickening in the external ear canal (*asterisk*), extending into the middle ear and eroding the jugular plate, covering the jugular fossa (*arrowhead*). **c** Coronal gadolinium-enhanced T1-weighted spin echo image. The tumour mass (*arrowheads*) grows from the external ear canal into the middle ear, and appears to extend above the jugular bulb (**j**). During surgery, the tumour was invading the wall of the jugular vein

Fig. 27 Patient suffering from squamous cell carcinoma of right external ear canal. **a** *Axial* T2-weighted spin echo image shows large, relatively hypointense mass, extending posteriorly into the mastoid cells (*arrow*). Anteriorly, the mass (*arrowhead*) cannot be separated from the superior pole of the parotid gland. **b** Coronal gadolinium-enhanced T1-weighted spin echo image. The tumour (*arrows*) grows deep into the external ear canal (*asterisk*), reaching the tympanic membrane. The ossicular chain is visible as it is surrounded by enhancing tissue (*arrowhead*); this corresponded histologically to granulation tissue

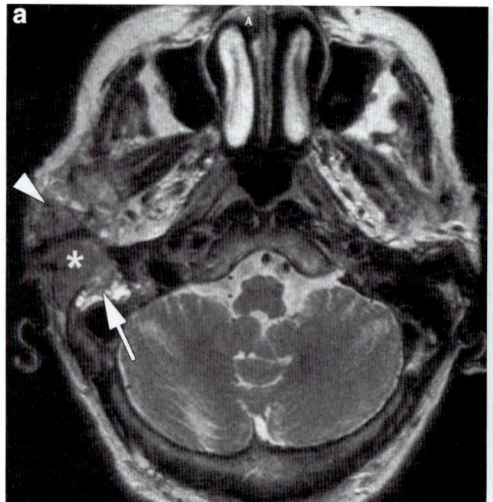

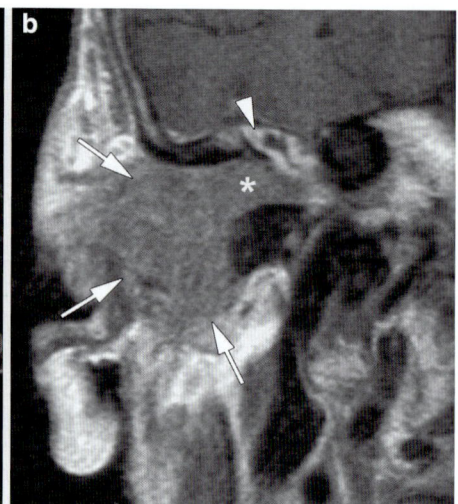

7 Malignant Neoplasms

Primary external ear malignant neoplasms are not common. External ear cancer initially appears as a painless lesion; enlarging lesions cause minor bleeding, itching, pain and intermittent drainage of serous fluid. Often, these symptoms are attributed to external otitis. Eventually, as the clinical situation progressively becomes worse, further exploration will reveal the true nature of the lesion. More advanced cancer may cause stenosis of the external auditory canal, trismus, conchal and preauricular swelling, and facial nerve palsy (Million et al. 1994). Spread towards the middle ear, and more rarely inner ear, may occur (Breau et al. 2002).

Histologically, external ear malignancies usually correspond to squamous cell carcinoma or basocellular carcinoma. On rare occasions, adenocarcinoma, developing from the ceruminous glands, lymphoma or malignant melanoma is encountered in the external canal.

As assessment of bone detail is critical to treatment planning, CT is the first study to perform (Gillespie et al. 2001).

The tumour appears as an enhancing soft tissue thickening or mass centred in the EAC (Fig. 24). Assessment of associated bone destruction is critical to treatment planning. The tympanic bone is usually the first bony structure to be invaded. With further tumour growth, surrounding structures, such as the parotid gland, temporomandibular joint and middle ear are likely to become involved. Also intracranial spread is possible (Figs. 25 and 26). Tumour spread to the neck lymph nodes may occur; the parotid and upper parajugular lymph nodes are at risk and an imaging study of the neck is therefore desirable.

MRI is frequently used as an adjunct to CT when intracranial, perineural and/or perivascular tumour spread is suspected (Fig. 25). The tumour appears as a soft tissue mass with variable intensities on T2-weighted and T1-weighted images, and shows homogeneous or heterogeneous enhancement (Figs. 26 and 27).

Treatment is by radiotherapy, surgery or a combination of both. After radical treatment of extensive neoplasms, it is useful to obtain a baseline imaging study (optimal timing probably about 4 months after completion of treatment), and to perform periodical follow-up imaging studies, in order to detect recurrent tumour at an as early as possible stage (Million et al. 1994).

Malignant neoplasms secondarily invading the external auditory canal may arise from neighbouring structures, such as the periauricular skin or parotid gland. Rarely, haematogenous spread to the external auditory canal from a distant site is encountered; it may be seen with breast cancer, but also metastatic lung cancer or urogenital cancer has been reported at this site.

References

Ahuja AT, Marshall JN, Roebuck DJ, King AD, Metreweli C (2000) Sonographic appearances of preauricular sinus. Clin Radiol 55:528–532

al-Shihabi BA (1992) Carcinoma of temporal bone presenting as malignant otitis externa. J Laryngol Otol 106:908–910

Breau RL, Gardner EK, Dornhoffer JL (2002) Cancer of the external auditory canal and temporal bone. Curr Oncol Rep 4:76–80

Brookes GB, Graham MD (1984) Post-traumatic cholesteatoma of the external auditory canal. Laryngoscope 94:667–670

Brown EW, Megerian CA, McKenna MJ, Weber A (1995) Fibrous dysplasia of the temporal bone: imaging findings. AJR Am J Roentgenol 164:679–682

Chandler JR (1968) Malignant external otitis. Laryngoscope 78:1257–1294

Chang PC, Fischbein NJ, Holliday RA (2003) Central skull base osteomyelitis in patients without otitis externa: imaging findings. AJNR Am J Neuroradiol 24:1310–1316

Corbridge RJ, Michaels L, Wright T (1996) Epithelial migration in keratosis obturans. Am J Otolaryngol 17:411–414

Currie AR, King WW, Vlantis AC, Li AK (1996) Pitfalls in the management of preaurciular sinuses. Br J Surg 83:1722–1724

De S, Pfleiderer AG (1999) An extreme and unusual variant of Ramsay Hunt syndrome. J Laryngol Otol 113:670–671

Franssens Y, Hermans R, Feenstra L, Baert AL (1993) Posttraumatic external auditory canal cholesteatoma. J Belge Radiol 76:320–321

Freeman J (1983) Temporal bone fractures and cholesteatoma. Ann Otol Rhinol Laryngol 92:558–560

Gillespie MB, Francis HW, Chee N, Eisele DW (2001) Squamous cell carcinoma of the temporal bone: a radiographic-pathologic correlation. Arch Otolaryngol Head Neck Surg 127:803–807

Glynn F, Keogh IJ, Burns H (2006) Neglected keratosis obturans causing facial nerve palsy. J Laryngol Otol 120:784–785

Grandis JR, Curtin HD, Yu VL (1995) Necrotizing (malignant) external otitis: prospective comparison of CT and MR imaging in diagnosis and follow-up. Radiology 196:499–504

Guida RA, Finn DG, Buchalter IH, Brookler DH, Kimmelman CP (1990) Radiation injury to the temporal bone. Am J Otol 11:6–11

Heilbrun ME, Salzman KL, Glastonbury CM, Harnsberger HR, Kennedy RJ, Shelton C (2003) External auditory canal cholesteatoma: clinical and imaging spectrum. AJNR Am J Neuroradiol 24:751–756

Jee WH, Choi KH, Choe BY, Park JM, Shinn KS (1996) Fibrous dysplasia: MR imaging characteristics with radiopathologic correlation. AJR Am J Roentgenol 167:1523–1527

Kemink JL, Graham MD (1982) Osteomas and exostoses of the external auditory canal—medical and surgical management. J Otolaryngol 11:101–106

Keohane JD, Ruby RR, Janzen VD, MacRae DL, Parnes LS (1993) Medial meatal fibrosis: the University of Western Ontario experience. Am J Otol 14:172–175

Kwon BJ, Han MH, Oh SH, Song JJ, Chang KH (2006) MRI findings and spreading patterns of necrotizing external otitis: is a poor outcome predictable? Clin Radiol 61:495–504

Langman J (1981) Ear. In: Medical embryology, 4th edn. Williams & Wilkins, Baltimore, pp 303–304

Lau JT (1983) Towards better delineation and complete excision of preauricular sinus. Aust N Z J Surg 53:267–269

Lee DH, Jun BC, Park CS, Cho KJ (2005) A case of osteoma with cholesteatoma in the external auditory canal. Auris Nasus Larynx 32:281–284

Mattuci KF, Setzen M, Galantich P (1986) Necrotizing otitis externa occurring concurrently with epidermoid carcinoma. Laryngoscope 96:264–266

Mayer TE, Brueckmann H, Siegert R et al (1998) High-resolution CT of the temporal bone in dysplasia of the auricle and external auditory canal. Am J Neuroradiol AJNR 18:53–65

McKennan KX, Chole RA (1989) Posttraumatic cholesteatoma. Laryngoscope 99:779–782

McKennan KX, Chole RA (1992) Traumatic external auditory canal atresia. Am J Otol 13:80–81

Megerian CA, Sofferman RA, McKenna MJ, Eavey RD, Nadol JB Jr (1995) Fibrous dysplasia of the temporal bone: ten new cases demonstrating the spectrum of otologic sequelae. Am J Otol 16:408–419

Midwinter KI, Gill KS, Spencer JA, Fraser ID (1999) Osteomyelitis of the temporomandibular joint in patients with malignant otitis externa. J Laryngol Otol 113:451–453

Million RR, Cassisi NJ, Mancuso AA, Stringer SP (1994) Temporal bone. In: Million RR, Cassisi NJ (eds) Management of head and neck cancer: a multidisciplinary approach, 2nd edn. J.B. Lippincott Company, Philadelphia, pp 751–764

Persaud R, Chatrath P, Cheesman A (2003) Atypical keratosis obturans. J Laryngol Otol 117:725–727

Persaud RA, Hajioff D, Thevasagayam MS, Wareing MJ, Wright A (2004) Keratosis obturans and external ear canal cholesteatoma: how and why we should distinguish between these conditions. Clin Otolaryngol Allied Sci 29:577–581

Piepergerdes JC, Kramer BM, Behnke EE (1980) Keratosis obturans and external auditory canal cholesteatoma. Laryngoscope 90:383–391

Rubin J, Yu VL (1988) Malignant external otitis: insights into pathogenesis, clinical manifestations, diagnosis and therapy. Am J Med 85:391–398

Rubin J, Curtin HD, Yu VL, Kamerer DB (1990) Malignant external otitis: utility of CT in diagnosis and follow-up. Radiology 174:391–394

Schwartz DT, Alpert M (1964) The malignant transformation of fibrous dysplasia. Am J Med Sci 247:35–54

Singh A, Al KM, Hyder MJ (2005) Skull base osteomyelitis: diagnostic and therapeutic challenges in atypical presentation. Otolaryngol Head Neck Surg 133:121–125

Tran LP, Grundfast KM, Selesnick SH (1996) Benign lesions of the external auditory canal. Otolaryngol Clin North Am 29:807–825

Tsunoda R, Fukaya T (1997) Extracranial meningioma presenting as a tumour of the external auditory meatus: a case report. J Laryngol Otol 111:148–151

Vourtsi A, Papadopoulos A, Golfinopoulos S et al (1998) Abnormal enhancement of the membranous labyrinth in a case of relapsing polychondritis. Ann Otol Rhinol Laryngol 107:81–82

Vrabec JT, Chaljub G (2000) External canal cholesteatoma. Am J Otol 21:608–614

Work WP (1972) Newer concepts of first branchial cleft defects. Laryngoscope 82:1581–1593

Yeakley JW, Jahrsdoerfer RA (1996) CT evaluation of congenital aural atresia: what the radiologist and surgeon need to know. J Comp Ass Tomogr 20:724–731

Acute Otomastoiditis and its Complications

Marc Lemmerling

Contents

1 Introduction 53
2 Coalescent Mastoiditis and Mastoid Subperiosteal Abscess 54
3 Complications 56
3.1 Otogenic Intracranial Abscess 56
3.2 Sinus Thrombosis 56
3.3 Labyrinthitis 58
3.4 Meningitis 59

References 59

Abstract

Acute otomastoid disease is most frequently seen in the pediatric population. An appropriate therapy traditionally leads to healing. Occasionally the disease can advance to a stage of coalescent mastoiditis that can cause a breakthrough of the mastoid wall with development of a mastoid subperiostal abscess. CT is an excellent technique to investigate this coalescence with subsequent abscess formation. Many other even rarer complications of acute otomastoid disease are better studied with MRI: formation of an otogenic intracranial abscess, sigmoid and transverse sinus thrombosis, labyrinthitis, and meningitis.

1 Introduction

The middle ear and mastoid constitute an extension of the upper respiratory tract. Via the aditus ad antrum, the mastoid antrum, which is the largest mastoid cell, communicates with the epitympanic portion of the middle ear cavity. The middle ear and adjacent pneumatized portions of the temporal bone are subject to bacterial invasion via the eustachian tube. When a mild infection occurs, pain will be present for a short period, the tympanic membrane will be hyperemic, and an appropriate therapy leads to healing without functional alterations. However, if an acute infection persists for more than a few days, resorption of the ossicles will occur as well as of the mastoid by a process of demineralization and osteoclastic activity. In case of more pronounced disease, the tympanic cavity wall and/or mastoid wall can be destructed and a subperiosteal abscess, Bezold's abscess (break through the mastoid tip), sigmoid sinus thrombosis, or otogenic brain abscess is formed. In rare cases, bacterial labyrinthitis can complicate acute infectious middle ear disease. Meningitis is another rare complication of acute infectious otomastoid disease and is most often hematogeneous in nature (Friedman et al. 1990).

M. Lemmerling (✉)
AZ St Lucas Hospital Gent, Groenebriel 1, 9000 Gent, Belgium
e-mail: marc.lemmerling@azstlucas.be

Fig. 1 CT in a patient with coalescent mastoiditis on the right side obviously shows coalescence of the mastoid cells and resorption of the lateral mastoid wall (*arrows*) (**a**, **c**). The contralateral normal ear is shown (**b**, **d**)

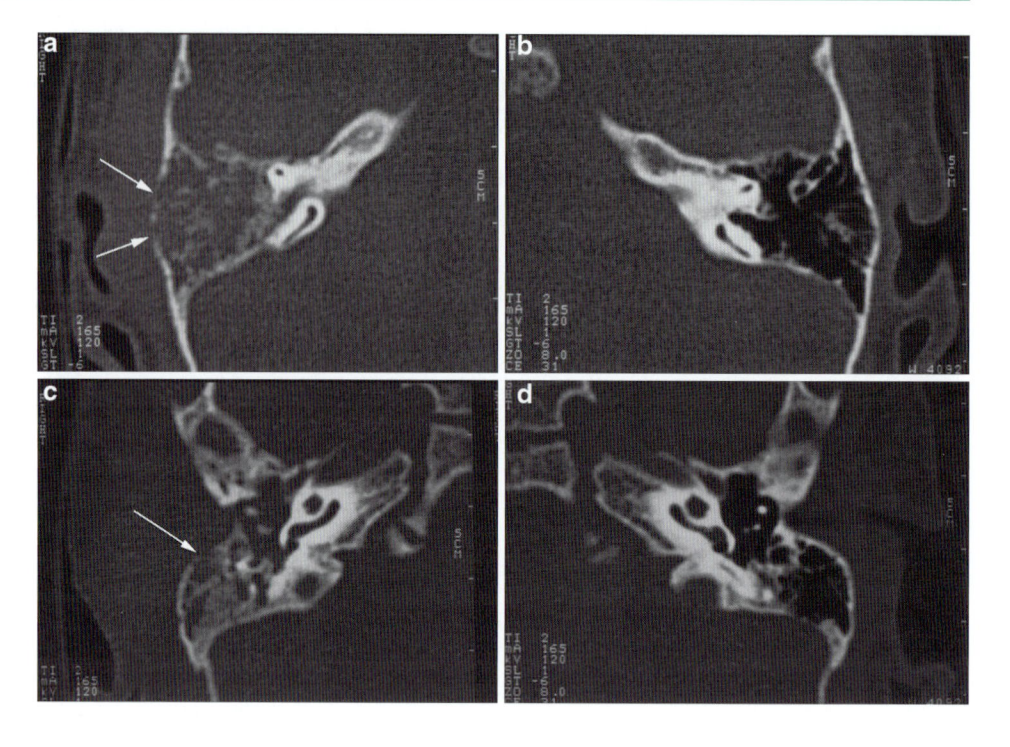

The clinical picture of mastoiditis has changed a lot with the advent of antibiotics. A delay is consequently noted in the recognition of the intracranial complications in children and in the institution of appropriate therapy (Kuczkowski and Mikaszewski 2001). Data suggest that the suppurative complications of acute otitis media are increasing due to an increasing incidence of resistant streptococcus pneumoniae (Bach et al. 1998; Zapalac et al. 2002). Despite the use of specialized imaging modalities, antibiotics, and microsurgical procedures, the resulting mortality of intracranial otogenic complications is still about 10 % (Kaftan and Draf 2000).

Streptococcus pneumoniae is the most common pathogen causing intracranial-complicating acute otitis media (meningitis, brain abscess, and subdural empyema) (Kaftan and Draf 2000). Streptococcus pyogenes is another important pathogen (Bahadori et al. 2000; Dobben et al. 2000). Fungal mastoiditis is almost exclusively seen in immunocompromised patients (Slack et al. 1999; Yates et al. 1997). Massive granulations and proliferation of fungi can create fistula to the inner ear, mimicking cholesteatoma on imaging studies (Chen et al. 1999; Ohki et al. 2001). Early surgical debridement followed by antimicrobial therapy may be life preserving in this patient population (Chen et al. 1999). Other unusual pathogens, such as Rhodococcus equi should be included in the differential diagnosis of the immunocompromised patient with aggressive otitis (Ibarra and Jinkins 1999). Otomastoiditis is a rare but important manifestation of tuberculosis and should be considered if a history of chronic otorrhea resistant to conventional therapy is found in a patient with widespread temporal bone destruction on CT examinations (Cavallin and Muren 2000). Nontuberculous mycobacterial mastoiditis presents in the same manner, but is often resistant to antituberculous agents, so the preferred treatment is mastoidectomy (Stewart et al. 1995).

2 Coalescent Mastoiditis and Mastoid Subperiosteal Abscess

The local clinical manifestations of advancing acute mastoiditis are pain and erythema in the mastoid region, tenderness, swelling in the postauricular region with protrusion of the auricle, and edema of the posterosuperior wall of the external auditory canal. All four signs are present in about 40 % of the cases (Cohen-Kerem et al. 1999). Postauricular erythema and protrusion of the auricle are the two most frequent clinical signs of acute mastoiditis for some authors (Cohen-Kerem et al. 1999; Bahadori et al. 2000), while other groups mention that these two specific signs were rather rare in their population (Dhooge et al. 1998). In 95 % of these patients, a concomitant ipsilateral, inflamed, bulging, and immobile eardrum is seen (Bahadori et al. 2000).

If an acute otomastoid infection persists for more than a few days, resorption of the ossicles and mastoid can occur by a process of demineralization and osteoclastic activity. In such circumstances, mastoid cells will coalesce and the term 'coalescent mastoiditis' is used (Fig. 1). Studies suggest that coalescent mastoiditis has a current incidence of 0.24 % patients with suppurative otitis media (Spiegel et al. 1998).

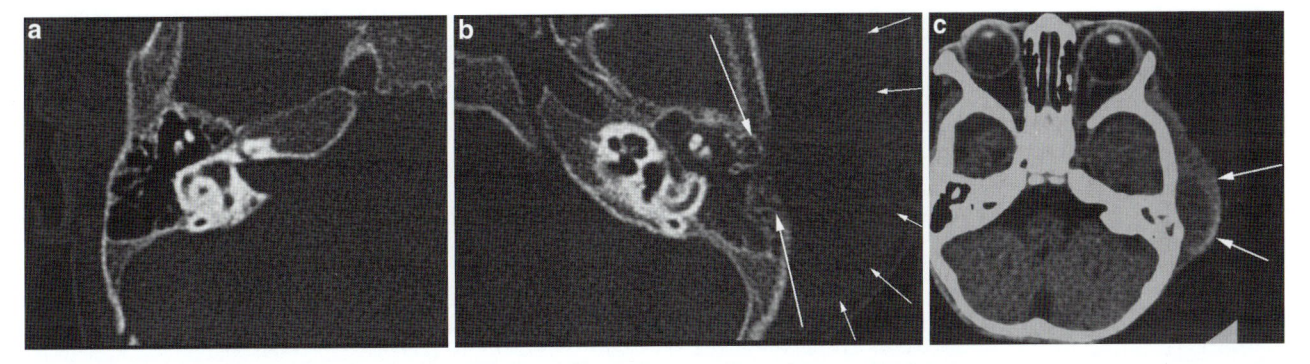

Fig. 2 CT of the normal right temporal bone shows a normal lateral otomastoid cortex (**a**), while on the contralateral side (**b**) the lateral cortex of the opacified otomastoid is fragmented (*large arrows*) and soft tissue swelling is seen (*small arrows*). This subperiosteal abscess (*arrows*) is best evaluated on images in soft tissue setting (**c**)

The sensitivity and accuracy of temporal bone CT findings was evaluated for the diagnosis of acute coalescent mastoiditis, by scoring for mastoid bone integrity on three points, the air cell septae, the sigmoid cortical plate, and the lateral cortical wall. CT turned out to be a valuable technique, and the erosion of the cortical plate that overlies the sigmoid sinus was the most sensitive and specific CT finding for distinguishing coalescent from noncoalescent mastoiditis (Antonelli et al. 1999).

Mastoid subperiosteal abscess develops when the process of coalescence of the mastoid cells leads to a breakthrough of the mastoid cortex and pus collection appears in the postauricular soft tissues. At this moment, clinical examinations and imaging studies, CT as well as MR, become very important, since the difference between the periostitis stage and the abscess stage cannot be deducted from the initial body temperature of the patient, the number of polymorphonuclears, or the CRP values (Francois et al. 2001). Subperiosteal abscess is seen in nearby 50 % of patients diagnosed with coalescent mastoiditis (Spiegel et al. 1998). The destructed lateral cortical otomastoid wall is easily visualized on CT examinations, and the images in soft tissue setting will show the present abscess (Figs. 2 and 3). MRI is able to show the same findings.

Occasionally, the infection can spread to the temporomandibular joint. When this spread pattern happens to be undertreated severe complications can occur, such as postarthritis ankylosis (Fig. 4).

In a retrospective study of 48 children with postauricular swelling and otoscopic signs of acute otitis media, the mastoid pus and the otorrhea were sterile whereas Streptococcus pneumoniae was the most frequent pathogen (Francois et al. 2001). While traditionally in children mastoid subperiosteal abscess required mastoidectomy, the improvement of antibiotic therapy has now changed this approach. It is accepted that uncomplicated acute mastoiditis is treated with myringotomy and intravenous antibiotics (Cohen-Kerem et al. 1999), and that in case of mastoid subperiosteal abscess formation treatment consists of tympanostomy tube insertion, intravenous antibiotics, and postauricular incision with abscess drainage. Such procedure avoids morbidity and complications of mastoid surgery in children (Bauer et al. 2002).

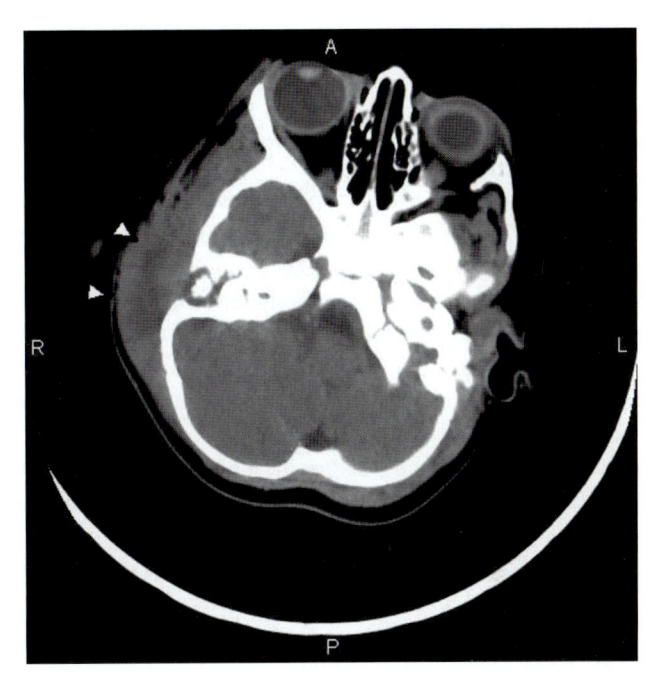

Fig. 3 In this child with severe fever, this axial CT image in soft tissue setting well-demonstrates the interruption in the lateral cortical wall of the mastoid with subsequent abscess formation

In rare cases, the pus escapades the mastoid near the incisura digastrica and tracks along the digastric and sternocleidomastoid muscles into the neck. Such abscesses are classically referred to as Bezold's abscess (Spiegel et al. 1998). Reports of Bezold's abscess in children are rare, since their mastoid pneumatization is not yet completed (Marioni et al. 2001). Most Bezold's abscesses are seen in adults and are associated with a history of cholesteatoma and mastoidectomy (Castillo et al. 1998).

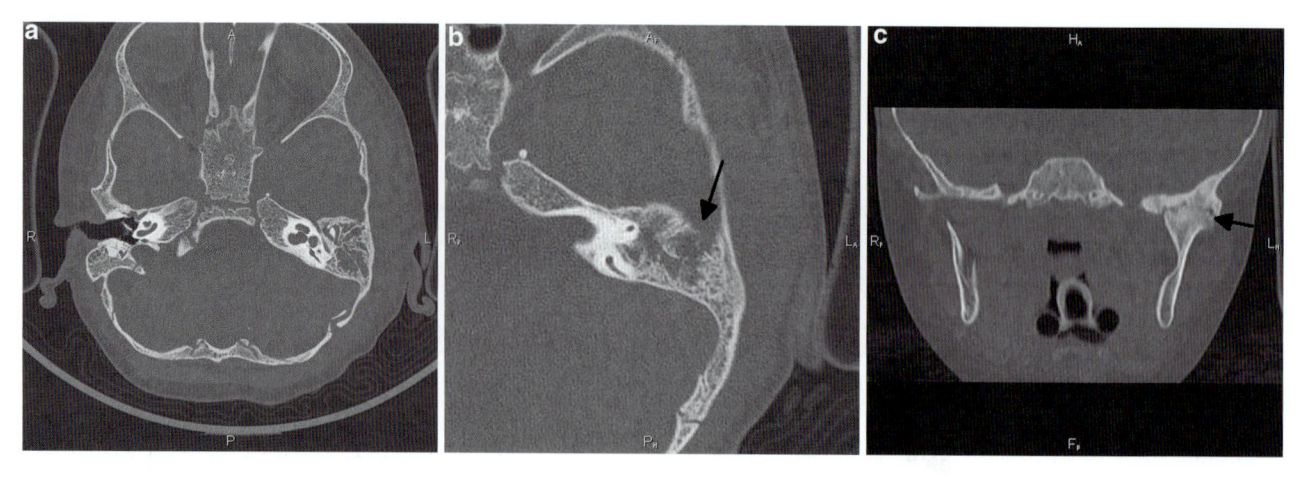

Fig. 4 In another child with left side soft tissue swelling and subperiosteal abscess formation (**a**) in combination with coalescent mastoiditis with erosion of the mastoid cortex (**b**) imaging of the left temporomandibular joint performed 6 months later shows ankylosis as a delayed complication of arthritis (**c**)

3 Complications

The clinical course of acute otitis media is often short and the process terminates because of the host's immune system, the infection-resistant properties of the mucosal linings, and the susceptibility of the major organisms to penicillin. About 1–5 % of untreated or inadequately treated patients may experience complications. Prior to these complications, warning symptoms or signs may be evident: severe earache and/or headache, vertigo, chills and fever, and meningeal symptoms or signs (Dobben et al. 2000).

If complications of inflammatory otomastoid disease are suspected, CT permits accurate diagnosis (Dobben et al. 2000), but MR is the imaging modality of choice (Dobben et al. 2000; Maroldi et al. 2001).

3.1 Otogenic Intracranial Abscess

Increasing temporoparietal headache, near the affected ear, is often the only indication of otogenic brain abscess formation (Dobben et al. 2000). Although rarely seen, among all intracranial complications of middle ear disease, epidural abscess formation is the commonest one (Bizakis et al. 1998). It is most frequently seen as a severe complication of the untreated cholesteatoma, but is also noted in patients suffering from acute mastoiditis. Its therapy depends on the importance of the abscess formation and ranges from high-dosed antibiotics to drainage (Kempf et al. 1998).

MR is the modality of choice to image these abscesses. In view of imaging characteristics, an otogenic intracranial abscess is not different from nonotogenic intracranial abscesses, but its location is typically in the temporal lobe or cerebellum, and the ipsilateral middle ear and mastoid are opacified. The mass generally has a mixed high signal on the T2-weighted images, a mixed low signal on the T1-weighted images and is surrounded by edema. After intravenous injection of gadolinium ring enhancement is seen. Hemorrhage may be present in some parts of the abscess (Fig. 5).

3.2 Sinus Thrombosis

Among all complications of mastoiditis, sigmoid and transverse sinus thrombosis are the least frequent ones (Rocha et al. 2000). It is described to be occasionally complicated by cerebellar venous infarction (Nayak et al. 1994; Ram et al. 2001). Sinus thrombosis is a difficult entity to diagnose. To my personal experience, the disease is easiest to recognize on T1-weighted images before intravenous injection of gadolinium, where the thrombus has an increased signal (Fig. 6). MR angiographic techniques with phase contrast are another valuable alternative.

The exact relationship between sinus thrombosis and mastoid disease remains a point of debate in the literature. In many of these thrombosis patients no signs of mastoid infection were present, because is it believed that the mastoid changes are likely due to venous congestion as a consequence of the sinus thrombosis and not of mastoiditis (Fink and McAuley 2002). In a study of 27 children (of which 61 % were neonates) with cerebral venous thrombosis, the most common risk factors were mastoiditis, persistent pulmonary hypertension, cardiac malformation, and dehydration. Many authors suggest to always test these children and young adults for protein C and antithrombin III deficiency, since these were the most common coagulopathies found in this population (Carvalho et al. 2001; Ram et al. 2001).

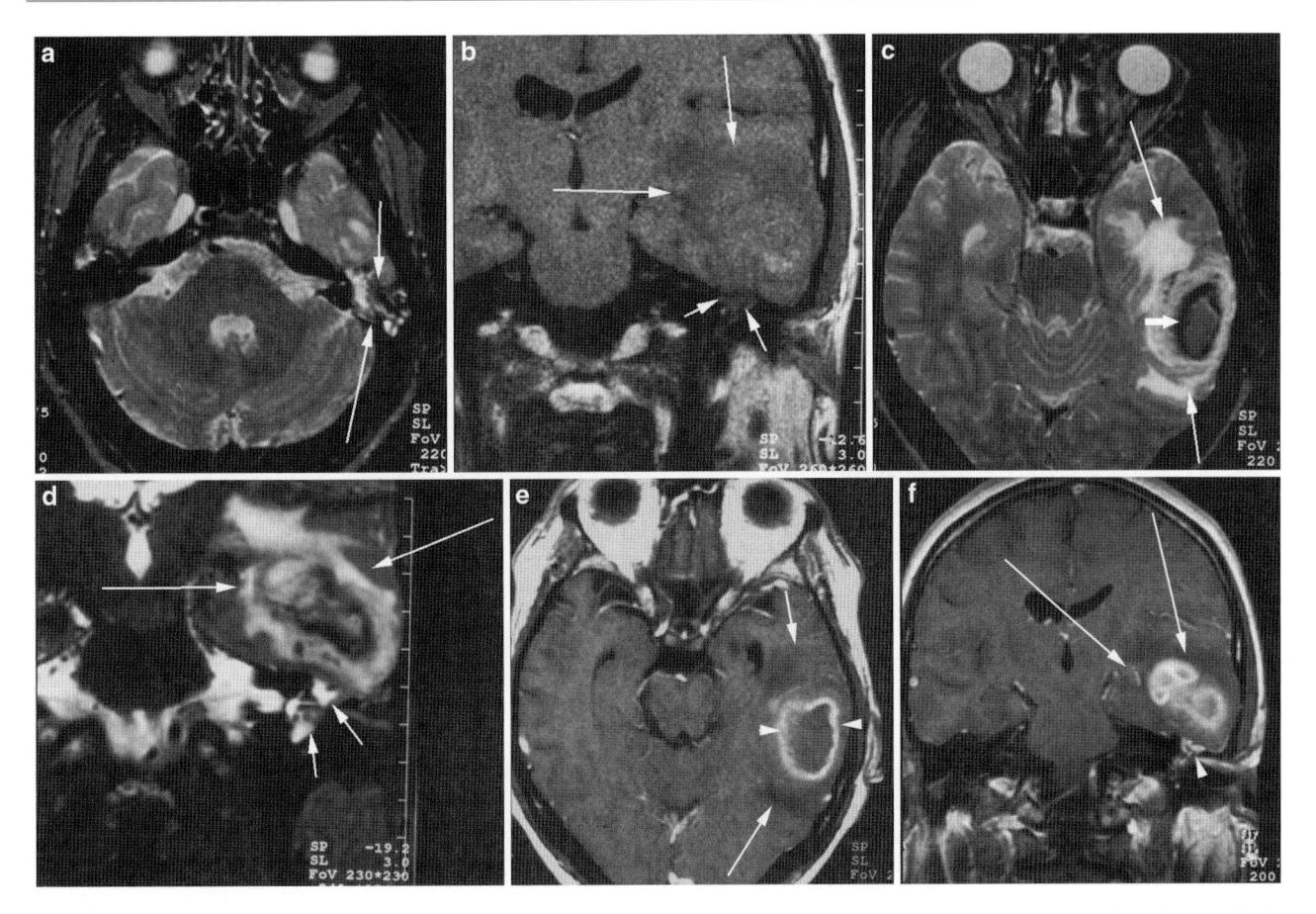

Fig. 5 In this patient with acute otomastoiditis on the left side, the axial T2-weighted image (**a**) at temporal bone level shows the opacified left otomastoid (*arrows*). The coronal T1-weighted image before injection of gadolinium (**b**) shows a large hypointense region (*large arrows*) in the temporal lobe of the brain, with some hyperintense (hemorrhagic) components, and the opacified otomastoid is also shown (*small arrows*). On the axial T2-weighted image at temporal lobe level (**c**) an abscess is visualized (*small arrow*), surrounded by vasogenic edema (*large arrows*). The coronal T2-weighted image (**d**) shows the continuity between the abscess and its surrounding edema on one hand (*large arrows*) and the inflammatory/infectious otomastoid disease (*small arrows*) on the other hand. The continuity is realized through an interrupted tegmen tympani. Ring enhancement (*small arrow*) is demonstrated on the T1-weighted image after intravenous injection of gadolinium (**e**). The perilesional edema is not enhancing (*large arrows*). The coronal T1-weighted image after gadolinium injection (**f**) confirms the findings noted on the coronal T2-weighted image, with the enhancing abscess and the nonenhancing edema (*large arrows*) in the temporal lobe region, and the enhancing otomastoid disease (*small arrows*). Note that no linear signal void is present between both enhancing regions, indicating that the normal tegmen tympani is absent

Fig. 6 On the T1-weighted image before gadolinium injection in a patient with right-sided otomastoid opacification (*small arrows*) a high signal is present in the sigmoid sinus (*large arrows*) (**a**) and is also seen in the transverse sinus (*arrows*) (**b**). Sigmoid and transverse sinus thrombosis

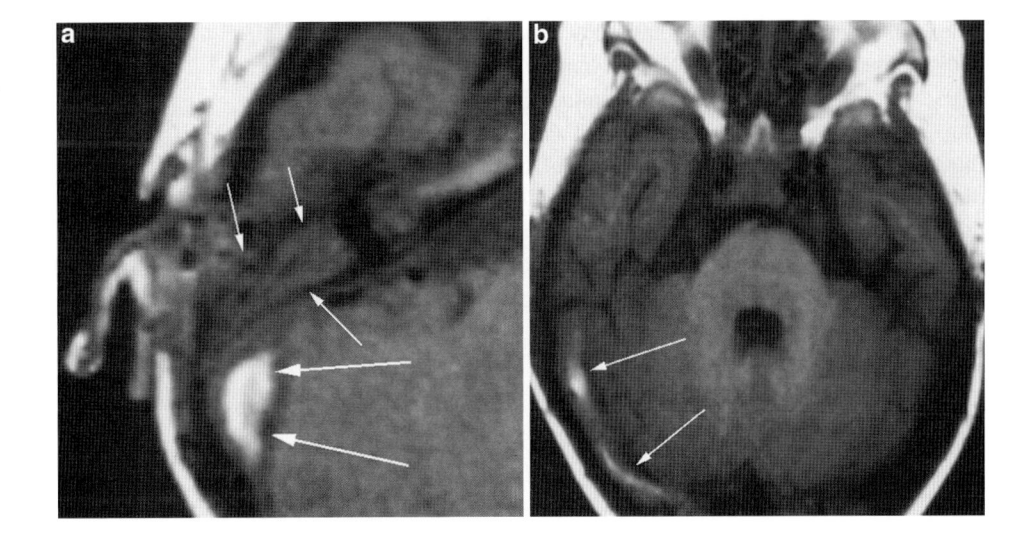

Fig. 7 The axial T2-weighted image in a patient with otomastoiditis shows hyperintense opacification (**a**). The 1 mm thick T2-weighted image through the inner ear (**b**) shows a normal hyperintense signal on the right side in the vestibule (*small arrow*), cochlea (*large arrow*), and lateral semicircular canal (*arrow head*), indicating the normal presence of endo- and perilymph. The corresponding contralateral signal intensity is decreased in all these inner ear components. The axial post-gadolinium T1-weighted image on the right side (**c**) shows a normal signal in the inner ear (*arrows*), whereas the left inner ear (**d**) enhances strongly (*large arrows*), as well as the opacified left otomastoid (*small arrows*)

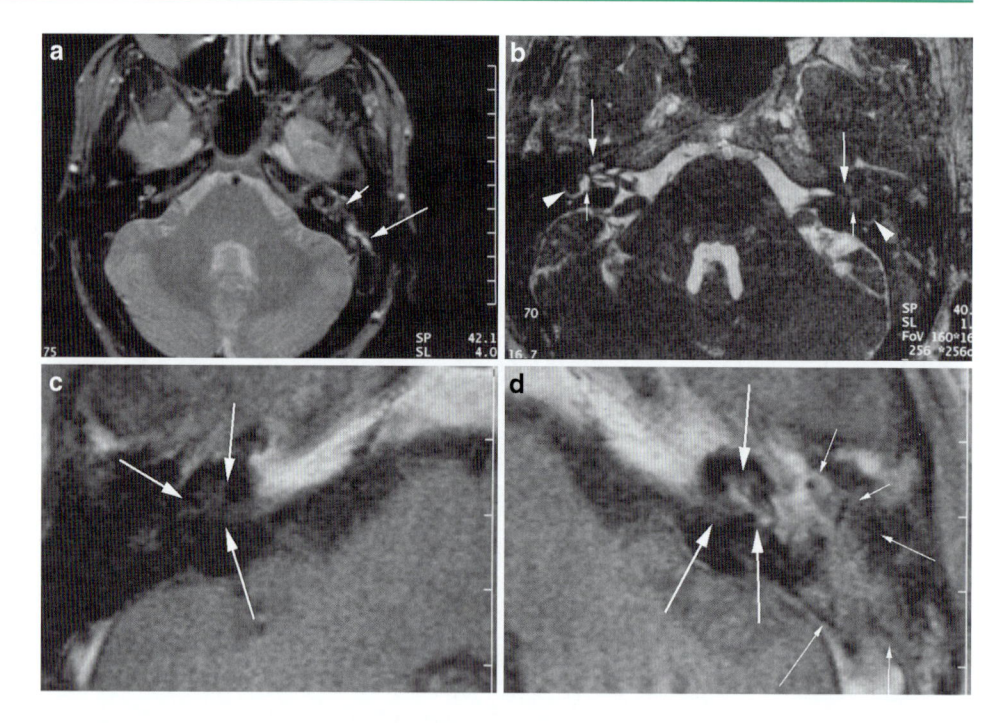

Fig. 8 In a patient with acute otomastoiditis, the coronal T1-weighted image after gadolinium injection shows the enhancing middle ear cavity and mastoid (**a**). The axial T1-weighted image after gadolinium injection in the same patient shows linear enhancement along the walls of the internal auditory meatus, indicating the presence of meningeal thickening and inflammation (**b**)

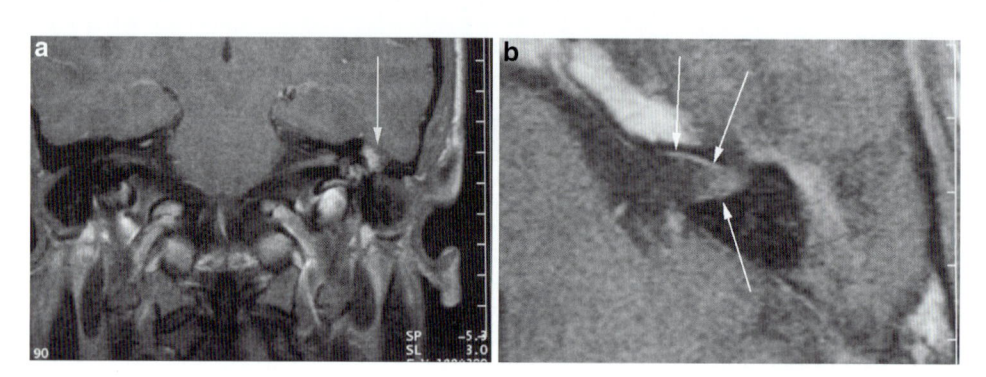

Sigmoid sinus thrombosis has become increasingly uncommon, while in the preantibiotic era the condition was mortal in over 90 % of the cases. Consequently, a high index of suspicion is actually required to make the diagnosis and choose for early surgical intervention (Keogh et al. 2001; Rocha et al. 2000). The presenting signs and symptoms are often subtle or nonspecific and not in proportion to the magnitude of the problem, leading to a common delay in diagnosis (Fritsch et al. 1990; Ram et al. 2001). It is suggested that imaging studies are performed in all mastoiditis patients with pain or vertigo that is not rapidly resolving after appropriate antibiotic treatment (Keogh et al. 2001). Patients may present with otorrhoea, otalgia, neck pain, fever, and chills (See et al. 2000). The therapeutic strategy is a point of debate, and ranges from internal jugular vein ligation, over anticoagulant therapy to the administration of less conventional antibiotic therapy (Dallari et al. 1997).

3.3 Labyrinthitis

Bacterial labyrinthitis that complicates otomastoid disease appears to happen via the round window. More often the involvement of the labyrinth is a reaction to bacterial exotoxins rather than bacterial invasion. This so-called tympanogenic labyrinthitis is unilateral in contrast with meningogenic labyrinthitis. MRI is the study of choice and shows that the endo- and perilymphatic spaces are filled with purulent material. The inner ear enhances on the T1-weighted images performed after gadolinium injection (Fig. 7).

3.4 Meningitis

Meningitis is another rare complication of acute infectious otomastoid disease and is most often hematogenous in nature (Friedman et al. 1990). The enhancing thickened meningeal structures are best visualized on T1-weighted images after intravenous injection of gadolinium (Fig. 8).

References

Antonelli PJ, Garside JA, Mancuso AA, Strickler ST, Kubilis PS (1999) Computed tomography and the diagnosis of coalescent mastoiditis. Otolaryngol Head Neck Surg 120(3):350–354

Bach KK, Malis DJ, Magit AE, Pransky SM, Kearns DB, Seid AB (1998) Acute coalescent mastoiditis in an infant: an emerging trend? Otolaryngol Head Neck Surg 119(5):523–525

Bahadori RS, Schwartz RH, Ziai M (2000) Acute Mastoiditis in children: an increase in frequency in Northern Virginia. Pediatr Infect Dis J 19(3):212–215

Bauer PW, Brown KR, Jones DT (2002) Mastoid subperiosteal abscess management in children. Int J Pediatr Otorhinolaryngol 63(3):185–188

Bizakis JG, Velegrakis GA, Papadakis CE, Karampekios SK, Helidonis ES (1998) The silent epidural abscess as a complication of acute otitis media in children. Int J Pediatr Otorhinolaryngol 45(2):163–166

Carvalho KS, Bodensteiner JB, Connolly PJ, Garg BP (2001) Cerebral venous thrombosis in children. J Child Neurol 16(8):574–580

Castillo M, Albernaz VS, Mukherji SK, Smith MM, Weissman JL (1998) Imaging of Bezold's abscess. Am J Roentgenol 171(6):1491–1495

Cavallin L, Muren C (2000) CT findings in tuberculous otomastoiditis. A case report. Acta Radiol 41(1):49–51

Chen D, Lalwani AK, House JW, Choo D (1999) Aspergillus mastoiditis in acquired immunodeficiency syndrome. Am J Otol 20(5):561–567

Cohen-Kerem R, Uri N, Rennert H, Peled N, Greenberg E, Efrat M (1999) Acute mastoiditis in children: is surgical treatment necessary? J Laryngol Otol 113(12):1081–1085

Dallari S, Zaccarelli SC, Sintini M, Gatti G, Balli R (1997) Acute mastoiditis with complications: a report of two cases. Acta Otorhinolaryngol Belg 51(2):113–118

Dhooge IJ, Vandenbussche T, Lemmerling M (1998) Value of computed tomography of the temporal bone in acute otomastoiditis. Rev Laryngol Otol Rhino (Bord) 119(2):91–94

Dobben GD, Raofi B, Mafee MF, Kamel A, Mercurio S (2000) Otogenic intracranial inflammations: role of magnetic resonance imaging. Top Magn Reson Imaging 11(2):76–86

Fink JN, Mcauley DL (2002) Mastoid air sinus abnormalities associated with lateral venous sinus thrombosis: cause or consequence? Stroke 33(1):290–292

Francois M, Van den Abbeele T, Viala P, Narcy P (2001) Acute external mastoiditis in children: report of a series of 48 cases. Arch Pediatr 8(10):1050–1054

Friedman EM, Mc Gill TJI, Healy GB (1990) Central nervous system complications associated with acute otitis media in children. Laryngoscope 100:149–151

Fritsch MH, Miyamoto RT, Wood TL (1990) Sigmoid sinus thrombosis diagnosis by contrasted MRI scanning. Otolaryngol Head Neck Surg 103(3):451–456

Ibarra R, Jinkins JR (1999) Severe otitis and mastoiditis due to Rhodococcus equi in a patient with AIDS. Case report. Neuroradiology 41(9):699–701

Kaftan H, Draf W (2000) Intracranial otogenic complications: inspite of therapeutic progress still a serious problem. Laryngorhinootologie 79(10):609–615

Kempf HG, Wiel J, Issing PR, Lenarz T (1998) Otogenic brain abscess. Laryngorhinootologie 77(8):462–466

Keogh IJ, Hone SW, Colreavy M, Gaffney R (2001) Sigmoid sinus thrombosis: an old foe revisited. Ir Med J 94(4):117–118

Kuczkowski J, Mikaszewski B (2001) Intracranial complications of acute and chronic mastoiditis: report of two cases in children. Int J Pediatr Otorhinolaryngol 60(3):227–237

Marioni G, de Filippis C, Tregnaghi A, Marchese-Ragona R, Staffieri A (2001) Bezold's abscess in children: case report and review of the literature. Int J Pediatr Otorhinolaryngol 61(2):173–177

Maroldi R, Farina D, Palvarini L, Marconi A, Gadola E, Menni K, Battaglia G (2001) Computed tomography and magnetic resonance imaging of pathologic conditions of the middle ear. Eur J Radiol 40(2):78–93

Nayak AK, Karnad D, Mahajan MV, Shah A, Meisheri YV (1994) Cerebellar venous infarction in chronic suppurative otitis media. A case report with review of four other cases. Stroke 25(5):1058–1060

Ohki M, Ito K, Ishimoto S (2001) Fungal mastoiditis in an immunocompetent adult. Eur Arch Otorhinolaryngol 258(3):106–108

Ram B, Meiklejohn DJ, Nunez DA, Murray A, Watson HG (2001) Combined risk factors contributing to cerebral venous thrombosis in a young woman. J Laryngol Otol 115(4):307–310

Rocha JL, Kondo W, Gracia CM, Baptista MI, Buchele G, da Cunha CA, Martins LT (2000) Central venous sinus thrombosis following mastoiditis: report of 4 cases and literature review. Braz J Infect Dis 4(6):307–312

See KC, Leong JL, Tan HK (2000) Otogenic lateral sinus thrombosis—a case report. Ann Acad Med Singap 29(6):753–756

Slack CL, Watson DW, Abzug MJ, Shaw C, Chan KH (1999) Fungal mastoiditis in immunocompromised children. Arch Otolaryngol Head Neck Surg 125(1):73–75

Spiegel JH, Lustig LR, Lee KC, Murr AH, Schindler RA (1998) Contemporary presentation and management of a spectrum of mastoid abscesses. Laryngoscope 108(6):822–828

Stewart MG, Troendle-Atkins J, Starke JR, Coker NJ (1995) Nontuberculous mycobacterial mastoiditis. Arch Otolaryngol Head Neck Surg 121(2):225–228

Yates PD, Upile T, Axon PR, de Carpentier J (1997) Aspergillus mastoiditis in a patient with acquired immunodeficiency syndrome. J Laryngol Otol 111(6):560–561

Zapalac JS, Billings KR, Schwade ND, Roland PS (2002) Suppurative complications of acute otitis media in the era of antibiotic resistance. Arch Otolaryngol Head Neck Surg 128(6):660–663

Chronic Otomastoiditis without Cholesteatoma

A. Trojanowska and P. Trojanowski

Contents

1 Introduction 61
2 Indications for imaging 62
3 Pathophysiology of Inflammatory Changes
   in the Middle Ear and Mastoid 62
4 CT Features in Chronic Otomastoiditis 62
4.1 Mastoid Process Changes 62
4.2 Tympanic Membrane Changes 62
4.3 Ossicular Chain Fixation 63
4.4 Ossicular Chain and Tympanic Cavity Erosion 65
5 COM management—what the surgeon
   needs to know 65

References 67

Abstract

Chronic otomastoiditis usually causes fixation or damage to the middle ear ossicles and tympanic membrane, resulting in conductive hearing loss. In such cases computed tomography is regarded to be the examination of choice, and imaging studies are performed to evaluate the reasons of conductive hearing loss—either ossicular chain fixation or erosion. Thin slice, high-resolution CT permits diagnosis of the various stages of chronic otomastoiditis and associated complications. However, this method is unable to differentiate between different types of effusions in tympanic cavity; also evaluation of cholesteatoma is challenging in many cases.

1 Introduction

Chronic otomastoiditis (COM) is a persistent or recurrent inflammation of the middle ear and mastoid, lasting usually for a minimum of 12 weeks, and resulting in permanent perforation of the tympanic membrane. Chronic otomastoiditis is marked by the presence of irreversible inflammatory changes within the middle ear and mastoid; it usually causes ongoing damage to the middle ear ossicles and tympanic membrane, resulting in conductive hearing loss (Chole 1986). Other symptoms include otorrhea, pain, vertigo.

The pathology itself is usually first estimated on otoscopic examination and diagnosis is made upon clinical findings, patient's history, and results of audiological tests, but further questions concerning the extent of the disease, its exact location, structures involved, and possible bone erosion will be addressed in detail only with imaging studies (Mafee et al. 1986).

Computed tomography is regarded to be the examination of choice in cases of chronic middle ear and mastoid inflammation, because of its superior bone detail and high resolution (Swartz et al. 1998).

A. Trojanowska (✉)
Department of Radiology and Nuclear Medicine,
University Medical School, Lublin, Poland
e-mail: agnieszka30@yahoo.com

P. Trojanowski
Chair and Department of Otolaryngology Head and Neck
Surgery, University Medical School, Lublin, Poland

Thin slice, high-resolution CT permits diagnosis of the various stages of chronic otomastoiditis and its associated complications. However, this method is unable to differentiate between different types of effusions in tympanic cavity; also evaluation of cholesteatoma may be challenging (Lemmerling et al. 2008, 2009).

2 Indications for imaging

Majority of patients with COM should undergo diagnostic imaging studies. Most important indications include (Maroldi et al. 2001):
- longstanding inflammation, unresponsive to medical treatment
- evaluation of possible causes of conductive hearing loss (ossicle erosion or fixation)
- clinical suspicion of cholesteatoma
- suspected temporal bone complications, such as petrositis, labyrinthitis, subperiosteal abscess, labyrinthine fistula
- suspected intracranial complications like brain abscess, meningitis.

From the clinical point of view, in cases of chronic inflammation, if there is no clinical suspicion of cholesteatoma, imaging studies are basically performed to evaluate the reasons for conductive hearing loss—either ossicular chain fixation or erosion (Bonafe 1999).

3 Pathophysiology of Inflammatory Changes in the Middle Ear and Mastoid

The most common finding in temporal bones with chronic otomastoiditis is osteitis. In a review of 123 temporal bones with chronic otomastoiditis, Meyerhoff et al. found osteitis in 90.2 %, mucoperiosteal fibrosis in 76.4 %, granulation tissue in 69.1 %, tympanosclerosis in 27.6 %, and cholesterol granuloma in 13 % (Meyerhoff 1978).

Aeration of the middle ear and mastoid depends on the free movement of air from the Eustachian tube into the mastoid air cells, via antrum. Since middle ear is separated from the antrum not only by the ossicles but also by mucosal folds, there are only two constant openings: between tensor tympani tendon and the stapes and another—between the short process of the incus and stapedial tendon. Oedema and inflammation, also the presence of granulation tissue may block these openings, preventing drainage of the antrum and mastoid. Prolonged obstruction of these openings may lead to characteristic changes in the mucosa and bone. Granulation tissue within the temporal bone may lead to bone erosion; osteoclastic bone resorption is frequent in chronic otitis media.

As a consequence of otitis media sequelae, in almost 40 % of patients subepithelial connective tissue of the middle ear and tympanic membrane becomes hyalinized or calcified; new bone formation also occurs. This process, leading to ossicular chain fixation concerns most frequently the head of the malleus and incus. Sometimes calcifications of the connective tissue occur within the tympanic membrane. Pathophysiology of these changes is still unclear to some extent. Most probably longstanding inflammation or infection causes degeneration of collagen and with this mechanism dystrophic calcifications occur (Chole 1986).

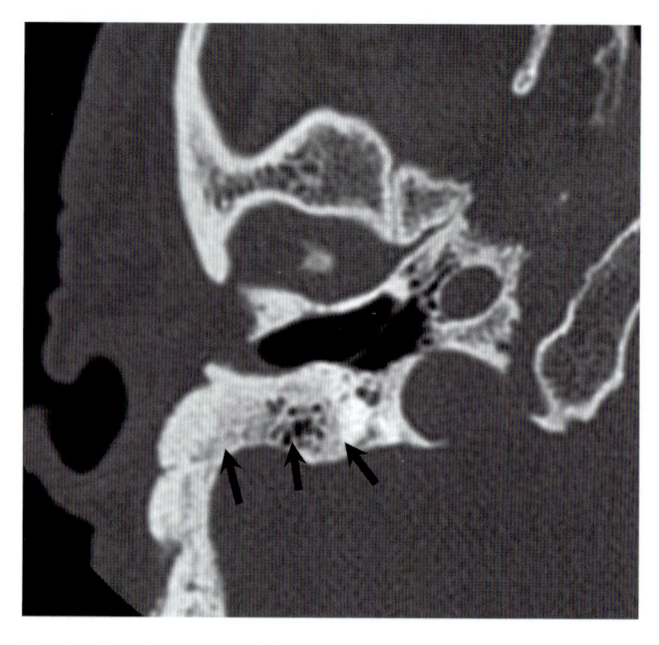

Fig. 1 Chronic otomastoiditis. On this axial CT scan a small, underdeveloped, poorly pneumatized mastoid is visible (*arrows*)

4 CT Features in Chronic Otomastoiditis

4.1 Mastoid Process Changes

Chronic otitis media is frequently accompanied by underdeveloped mastoid pneumatization (Fig. 1).

Opacification of mastoid air cells and sclerosis of mastoid are typical imaging findings (Fig. 2). Evidence of bone erosion (mastoid septae and rarely, cortex) is characteristic for chronic suppurative otitis media (Veillon 2000; Pandey et al. 2009).

4.2 Tympanic Membrane Changes

Visualization and evaluation of the tympanic membrane is best performed with otoscopy. However, some findings which are typical for chronic inflammation, are well visible with CT and they usually inform the radiologist of some more profound changes within the middle ear and mastoid.

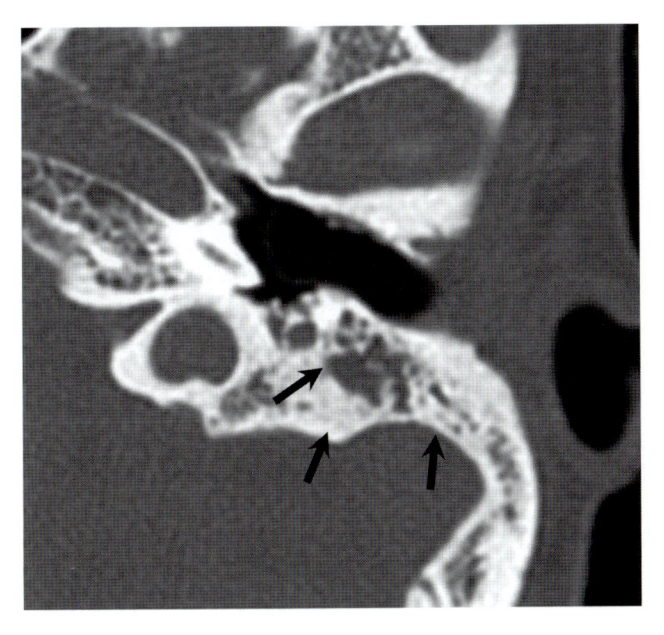

Fig. 2 This axial CT scan shows sclerotic mastoid process with opacified air cells (*arrows*)

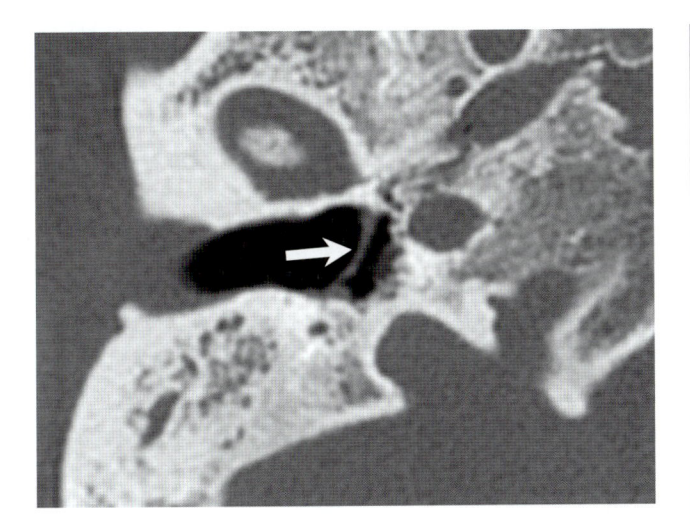

Fig. 3 Axial CT scan of the right middle ear. Thick tympanic membrane (*arrow*)

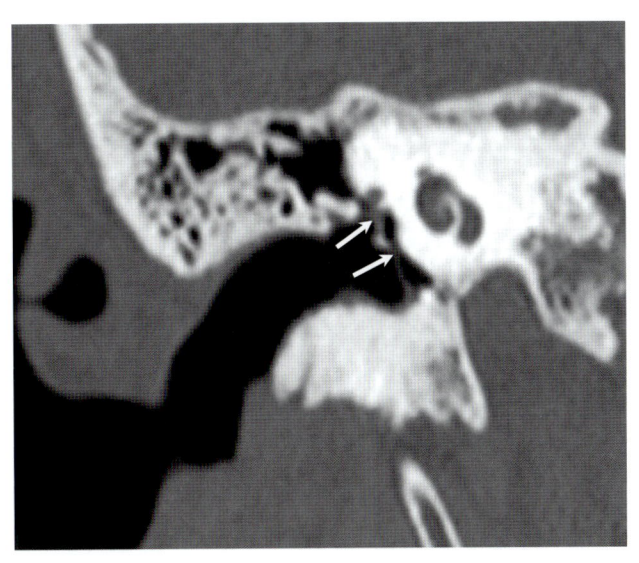

Fig. 4 In this patients axial CT scan of the right ear reveals deep retraction of the thickened and calcified tympanic membrane, which almost touches stapes head

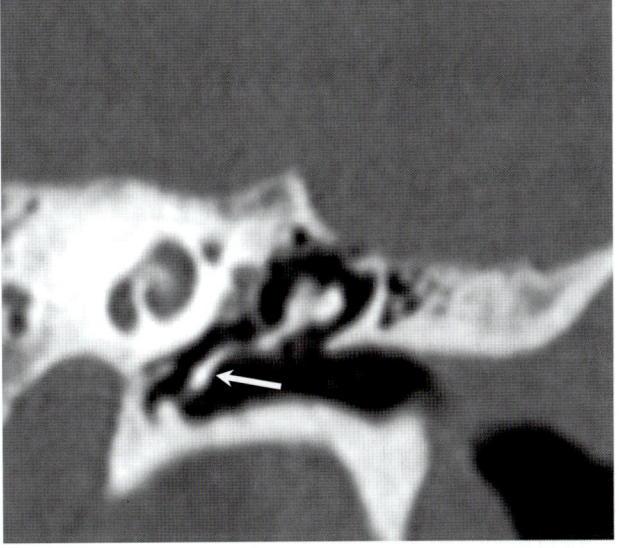

Fig. 5 In this patient a thick calcified plaque is visible in the tympanic membrane (*arrow*). This finding is typical for myringosclerosis

Tympanic membrane thickening and/or perforation is pathognomonic for chronic inflammation. It is evaluated with otoscopic imaging; on CT thickened membrane is visible as grey line of soft tissue density (Fig. 3).

Tympanic membrane retraction is the condition, when a part of the tympanic membrane is pulled inwards within the middle ear, usually due to negative pressure in the middle ear. It is also best evaluated with otoscopy. If the retraction is profound, it may become adherent to the stapes head (Fig. 4) (Mafee et al. 1986).

The term *Myringosclerosis* stands for the formation of the hyalinized collagen in the tympanic membrane. In most cases changes are clinically significant and cause little or no hearing loss. On CT myringosclerosis is visible as thickened and calcified (Fig. 5) tympanic membrane (Lemmerling et al. 2009).

4.3 Ossicular Chain Fixation

Post-inflammatory ossicular chain fixation (PIOF) is a common problem in patients with COM and in many cases it results with conductive hearing loss. It usually takes three

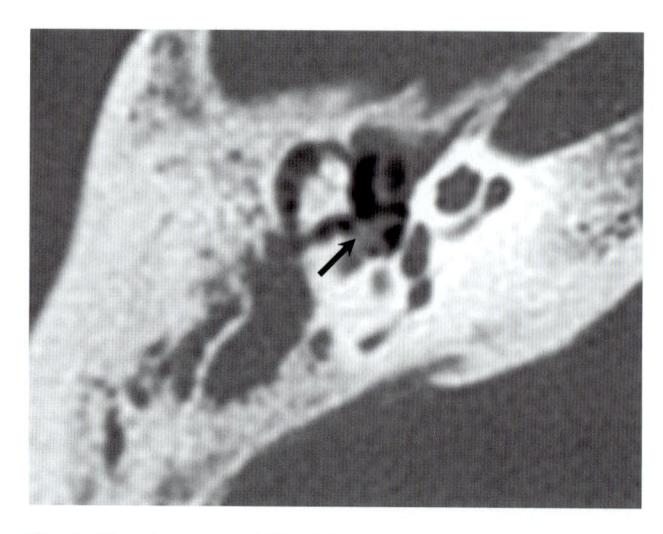

Fig. 6 Chronic otomastoiditis with ossicular chain fixation. On this axial CT scan a soft tissue-density mass is found around stapes, forming peri-stapedial tent

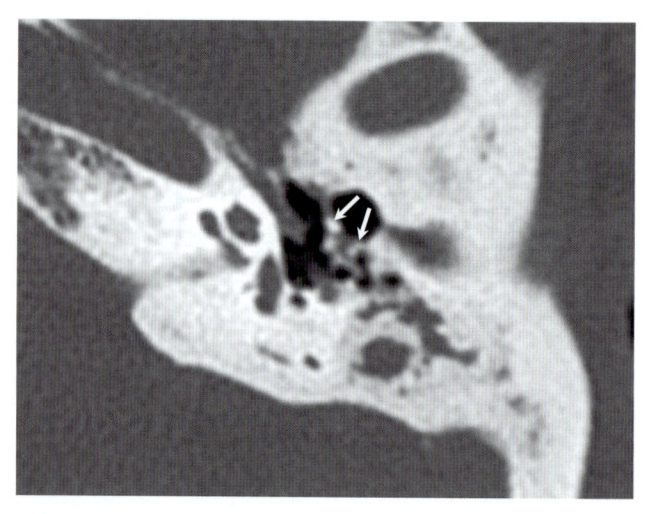

Fig. 7 This CT scan shows tympanosclerosis as post-inflammatory calcifications within epitympanum (*arrows*) in patient with chronic otitis media and hearing loss

pathologic forms (Swartz et al. 1985, Lemmerling et al. 2008, 2009):

- presence of fibrous tissue (chronic adhesive otitis media)
- hyalinization of collagen (tympanosclerosis)
- new bone formation (fibro-osseous sclerosis).

Fibrous tissue fixation appears on CT as noncalcified, soft-tissue debris encasing some or all of the ossicular chain. It is usually present in the niche of oval window, forming so called "peristapedial tent" (Fig. 6), but may also be present anywhere in meso- and epitympanum. On CT it is usually presented as a subtle mass of soft tissue density. Therefore, diagnosis of fibrous tissue fixation based on sole CT appearance should not be made, since fixation cannot be determined by imaging and the density of the mass is similar to other middle ear substances, like fluid and cholesteatoma. Diagnosis of fibrous tissue fixation can be suggested, if a soft tissue mass is seen in the setting of COM, in patient with dry ear and conductive hearing loss (Swartz et al. 1985).

Tympanosclerosis reflects deposits of hyalinized collagen in the tympanic cavity. It appears as unifocal or multifocal punctate or weblike calcifications in the middle ear cavity (Fig. 7) or on the tympanic membrane (myringosclerosis). In the tympanic cavity, it may be present in any location, visible as focal calcified densities in the middle ear cavity, along tendons, also in direct apposition to the ossicular chain. If the debris is not in a position to compromise the ossicular chain function, conductive hearing loss will not take place. On CT changes may be subtle—increased thickening of stapedial crura—or more profound (Swartz et al. 1985; Lemmerling et al. 2009). Since calcification of tendons and ligaments is a characteristic for tympanosclerosis, knowledge of normal anatomy and anatomical

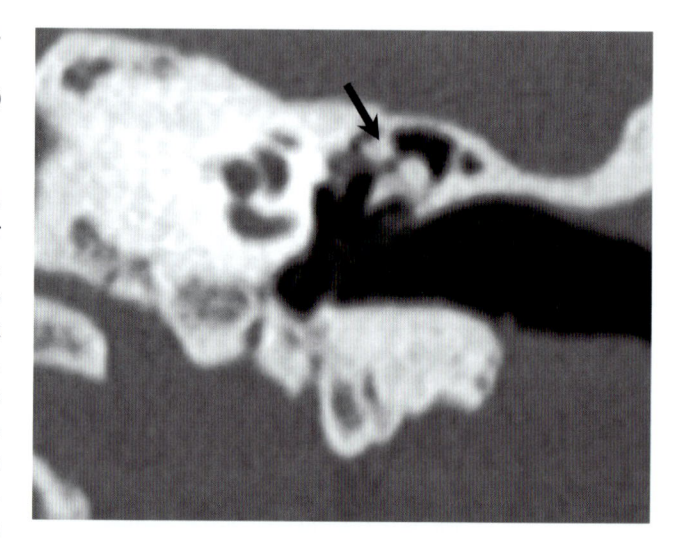

Fig. 8 This coronal temporal bone CT scan reveals large dense bone deposit (*arrow*) within epitympanum. This type of tympanosclerosis is referred to as new bone formation

variants is mandatory in order to evaluate the exact location and extent of the disease. Normal eminences, prominent bone ridges, and tendons should not be mistaken for pathological changes (Lemmerling et al. 1997; Petrus 1997).

New bone formation has been identified mostly in the epitympanum and is the least common manifestation of PIOF. It is visible as lamellar structures of high density (Fig. 8), thick bony webs, or generalized bony encasement (Lemmerling et al. 2008).

In general, CT of the temporal bone plays an important role in the evaluation of the extent of PIOF. It also enables differential diagnosis which includes other causes of

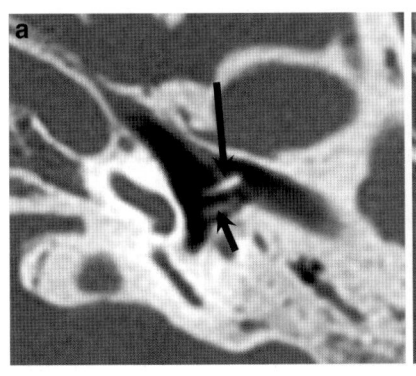

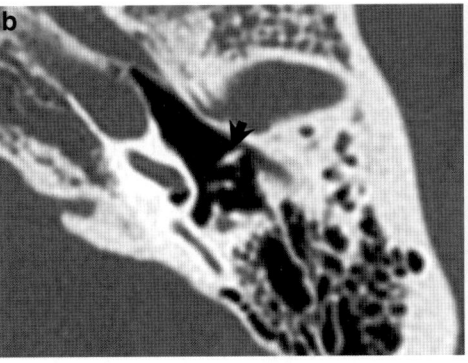

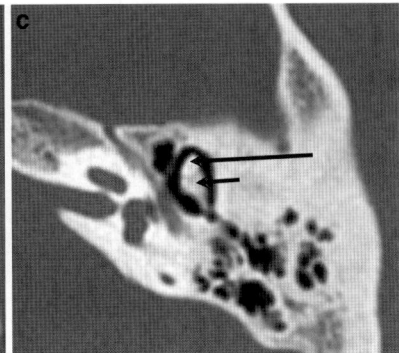

Fig. 9 Normal anatomy of the middel ear, axial CT, bone window a malleus handle (*long arrow*) and incus long process (*short arrow*) are visible, forming two parallel lines b two dots, visible posteriorly to malleus neck (*arrowhead*) represent incus lenticular process (laterally) and stapes head (medially) c malleus head (*long arrow*) and incus body (*short arrow*) with short process are visible in epitympanum, forming a so-called "ice cream cone"

conductive hearing loss, like otosclerosis, ossicular chain erosion, post-traumatic changes, developmental abnormalities. In case of suspected cholesteatoma MRI is the modality of choice (De Foer et al. 2007; Lemmerling et al. 2009).

4.4 Ossicular Chain and Tympanic Cavity Erosion

Post-inflammatory ossicular chain erosion is not very frequent in case of a non-cholesteatomatous disease, but does occur, and will affect first the incus long process and lenticular process, followed by stapes head.

For best diagnostic accuracy, images should be viewed in correct bone window setting—large window width (e.g. 4000 HU) and low window level (e.g. 0–200 HU) (Lemmerling et al. 2009).

In order to evaluate possible ossicular erosion, axial CT images should be searched for 3 distinctive signs:

"Ice cream cone" visible in epitympanum, where anterior ice cream consists of malleus head and posterior cone is made of incus body and short process (Fig. 9a).

"Two parallel lines" visible in mesotympanum, where anterior line represents tensor tympani tendon leading to malleus neck and posterior line represents incus lenticular process (Fig. 9b).

"Two dots" visible in mesotympanum, lateral dot being lenticular process and medial dot being stapes head—between them incudostapedial joint is well visible (Fig. 9c).

In cases of post-inflammatory ossicular chain erosion, any, or all of three signs will not be visualized on axial CT scans (Trojanowska et al. 2012).

It has been proven, that precise extent of bone erosion is correctly demonstrated by high resolution CT. Malleus and incus, because of their size, are well visible and effusion in the tympanic cavity does not influence their correct depiction and even more detailed evaluation. Regarding smaller structures, like stapes superstructure and incudostapedial joint, they are successfully depicted in almost 100 % of normal ears (Seeman et al. 1999). Also, high-resolution CT enables visualization of minute structures of ossicular chain in the opacified middle ear. Now it is possible to visualize routine structures like incudostapedial joint and stapes crura even with tympanic cavity filled with fluid or other soft tissue density mass (Fig. 10); inability to depict them strongly indicates abnormality (Lemmerling et al. 1997, 2008).

Post-inflammatory erosion sometimes involves walls of tympanic cavity. Based on CT examination, with the use of multiplanar images the following structures should be evaluated:
- bony cover of lateral semicircular canal
- bony cover of the second (tympanic) segment of the facial nerve
- roof of the middle ear cavity (tegmen tympani).

5 COM management—what the surgeon needs to know

Treatment depends upon the stage of the disease. Initially, efforts to control the causes of eustachian tube obstruction may prevent progression of chronic otitis media. Discharge (in exacerbation of disease) is treated with systemic antibiotics. Disease in general should be treated surgically because it cannot be definitely eradicated with conservative manners. There are four objectives of surgery for COM:
- eradication of the disease
- remodeling of the middle ear and mastoid, in order to prevent recurrence
- preservation or improvement of hearing
- prevention of complications (potentially life-threatening).

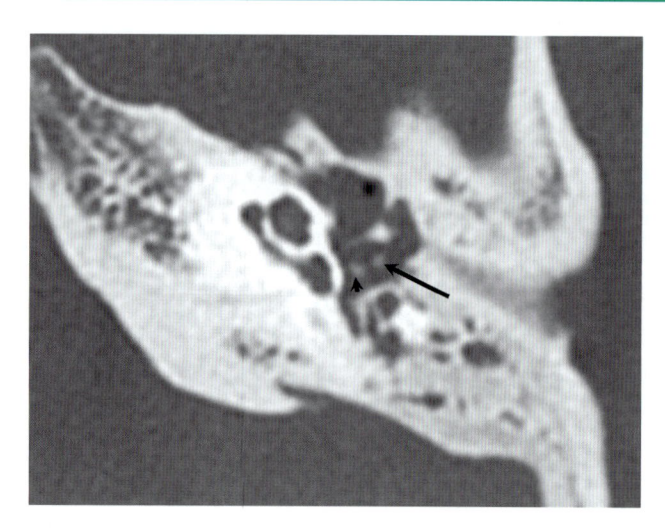

Fig. 10 Axial CT scan, chronic middle ear inflammation. Despite opacification of middle ear cavity, lenticular process (*arrow*) and head of stapes (*arrowhead*) are clearly visible. This demonstrated possibilities of CT in the visualization of minute structures, regardless of the conditions in the middle ear

Surgical procedures to achieve these objectives include tympanoplasty, mastoidectomy, or typanomastoidectomy (Applebaum 1969; Jung et al. 1999; Cruz et al. 2003).

Tympanoplasty is the surgical procedure in the middle ear and mastoid, designed to reconstruct the tympanic membrane (thus eradicating the disease if patent eustachian tube is present) and address ossicular chain destruction (to improve hearing).

There are 5 types of tympanoplasties, as described by Wullstein (Wullstein 1956).

In type I a graft is used to cover the defect in the tympanic membrane; ossicular chain is not affected. This is also called myringoplasty.

In type II tympanic membrane is repaired and ossicular chain continuity is restored by connecting head of stapes and partially eroded long process of incus (using various types of prostheses).

In type III a partial ossicular chain replacement prosthesis (PORP) is placed between tympanic membrane or malleus handle and head of stapes, or total ossicular chain replacement prosthesis (TORP) is put between tympanic membrane or malleus handle and the footplate of the stapes.

In type IV a small middle ear space is created by placing tympanic membrane graft on the promontory covering oval window (stapes footplate).

Type V is nowadays very rarely performed and consists of the preservation of reduced middle ear space and fenestration of horizontal semicircular canal.

Type III–V are accompanied by mastoidectomy.

Mastoidectomy means the removal of external mastoid cortex and exenteration of the mastoid air cells, which extends to the antrum.

Mastoidectomy can be performed in canal-wall-down (sometimes so-called simple mastoidectomy) and canal-wall-up manner.

In canal-wall-up procedure the surgeon drills between the dural plate, sigmoid sinus and supero-posterior wall of the external auditory canal, leaving the margin of the lateral epitympanic wall intact (preserving the intact external auditory canal).

In canal-wall-down procedure (also called the modified radical mastoidectomy) the mastoid bridge (the supero-posterior wall of external auditory canal) is removed. Removal of the mastoid bridge connects the mastoid cavity and external auditory canal; one common cavity is now present.

During the radical mastoidectomy (nowadays very rarely performed) remnants of the ossicles and tympanic membrane are removed.

During mastoidectomies implanted hearing aids can be applied to help restore hearing (which is beyond the scope of this chapter).

In case of disease resistant to previously described surgical treatment a subtotal petrosectomy can be performed. Procedure consists of eradication of most of temporal bone air cells and removal of ossicles, preservation of inner ear as well as Eustachian tube and external auditory canal permanent occlusion. Bone anchored hearing aids (BAHA) can be used to treat hearing impairment.

Surgical complications

Complications specific to mastoidectomy or tympanomastoidectomy usually include hearing impairment or deafness, vertigo, tinnitus, facial nerve injury, altered taste sensation, and the possible need for further surgery.

Key imaging findings for the surgeon

The radiologist should provide the following clinically valuable information (Yates et al. 2002; Watts et al. 2000):
- degree of opacification of the middle ear from the Eustachian tube to the mastoid tip
- development/sclerosis/cellularity of the mastoid and the cortex
- presence of hyalinized collagen tissue which may cause fixation of the ossicular chain (e.g., soft tissue encasing the stapes superstructure) and other signs of tympanosclerosis
- erosion of ossicular chain, especially the absence of incus long process, incudostapedial joint, or stapes superstructure
- location (relation) of dura, sigmoid sinus, and external auditory canal
- possible dehiscence of the tegmen (dura dehiscence)
- erosion of the bony labyrinth, especially lateral semicircular canal
- status of the facial nerve, its possible dehiscence or abnormal course
- alterations in anatomy with special regard to previous surgical treatment.

References

Bonafe A (1999) Imaging of conductive hearing loss. J Radiol Dec 80(12):1772–1779

Chole RA (1986) Chapter 157: Chronic ototos media, mastoiditis and petrositis. In: Cummings CE (ed) Otolaryngology head neck surgery. Mosby, St Louis, 1986:2723–2736

Cruz OL, Casse CA, Leonhart FD (2003) Efficacy of surgical treatment of chronic otitis media. Otolaryngol Head Neck Surg 128(2):263–266

De Foer B, Vercruysse JP, Bernaerts A, Maes J, Deckers F, Michiels J, Somers T, Pouillon M, Offeciers E, Casselman JW (2007) The value of single-shot turbo spin-echo diffusion-weighted MR imaging in the detection of middle ear cholesteatoma. Neuroradiology. 49(10):841–848

Jung TTK, Hanson JB (1999) Classification of otitis media and surgical principles. Otolaryngol Clin North Am 32(3):369–383

Lemmerling MM, Stambuk HE, Mancuso AA et al (1997) CT of the normal suspensory ligaments of the ossicles in the middle ear. AJNR Am J Neuroradiol 18:471–477

Lemmerling MM, De Foer B, VandeVyver V, Vercruysse JP, Verstraete KL (2008) Imaging of the opacified middle ear. Eur J Radiol 66(3):363–371

Lemmerling MM, De Foer B, Verbist BM, VandeVyver V (2009) Imaging of inflammatory and infectious diseases in the temporal bone. Neuroimaging Clin N Am 19(3):321–337

Mafee MF, Aimi K, Kahen HL, Valvassori GE, Capek V (1986) Chronicotomastoiditis: a conceptual understanding of CT findings. Radiology. 160(1):193–200

Maroldi R, Farina D, Palvarini L, Marconi A, Gadola E, Menni K, Battaglia G (2001) Computed tomography and magnetic resonance imaging of pathologic conditions of the middle ear. Eur J Radiol Nov 40(2):78–93

Meyerhoff WL, Kim CG, Paparella MM (1978) Pathology of chronic otitis media. Ann Otol Rhinol Laryngol 87(6):749–761

Pandey AK, Bapuraj JR, Gupta AK, Khandelwal N (2009) Is there a role for virtual otoscopy in the preoperative assessment of the ossicular chain in chronic suppurative otitis media? Comparison of HRCT and virtual otoscopy with surgical findings Eur Radiol 19(6):1408–1416

Petrus LV, Lo WW (1997) The anterior epitympanic recess: CT anatomy and pathology. AJNR Am J Neuroradiol 18: 1109–1114

Schuknecht HF, Applebaum EL (1969) Surgery for hearing loss. N Engl J Med 280(21):1154–1160

Seeman MD, Seeman O, Bonel H, Suckfull M, Englmeier K-H, Naumann A, Allen CM, Reiser MF (1999) Evaluation of the middle and inner ear structures: comparison of hybrid rendering, virtual endoscopy and axial 2D source images. Eur Radiol 9(9):1851–1858

Swartz JD, Wolfson RJ, Marlowe FI, Popky GL (1985) Postinflammatory ossicular chain fixation: CT analysis with surgical correlation. Radiology 154:697–700

Swartz JD, Harnsberger HR, Mukherji SK (1998) The temporal bone: contemporary diagnostic dilemmas. Radiol Clin North Am 36(5):819–853

Trojanowska A, Drop A, Trojanowski P, Rosińska-Bogusiewicz K, Klatka J, Bobek-Billewicz B (2012) External and middle ear diseases: radiological diagnosis based on clinical signs and symptoms. Insights Into Imaging. 3(1):33–48

Veillon F, Riehm S, Roedlich MN, Meriot P, Blonde E, Tongio J (2000) Imaging of middle ear pathology. Semin Roentgenol 35(1):2–11

Watts S, Flood LM, Clifford K (2000) A systematic approach to interpretation of computed tomography scans prior to surgery of middle ear cholesteatoma. J Laryngol Otol 114:248–253

Wullstein B (1956) Theory and practice of tympanoplaty. The Laryngoscope 66:1076–1093

Yates PD, Flood LM, Banerjee A, Clifford K (2002) CT scanning of middle ear cholesteatoma: what the surgeon want to know? Br J Radiol 75:847–852

Imaging of Cholesteatoma

Bert De Foer, Simon Nicolay, Jean-Philippe Vercruysse, Erwin Offeciers, Jan W. Casselman, and Marc Pouillon

Contents

1	Definition and History	69
2	Epidemiology	70
3	Classification	70
4	The Congenital Cholesteatoma	70
4.1	Introduction	70
4.2	Location	70
4.3	Clinical Signs	70
4.4	Treatment	72
4.5	Imaging	72
5	The Acquired Cholesteatoma	72
5.1	Introduction: Etiopathogenesis	72
5.2	Location	73
5.3	Clinical Signs	74
5.4	Treatment	74
5.5	Imaging	78
References		86

B. De Foer (✉) · S. Nicolay · J. W. Casselman · M. Pouillon
Department of Radiology, GZA Hospitals Sint-Augustinus,
Oosterveldlaan 24, 2610 Wilrijk, Belgium
e-mail: bert.defoer@GZA.be

J.-P. Vercruysse
Department of ENT, Heilig Hartziekenhuis,
Gasthuisstraat 1, 2400 Mol, Belgium

E. Offeciers
European Institute for ORL, GZA Hospitals Sint-Augustinus,
Oosterveldlaan 24, 2610 Wilrijk, Belgium

J. W. Casselman
Department of Radiology, AZ Sint-Jan AV, Ruddershove 10,
8000 Brugge, Belgium

J. W. Casselman
University of Ghent, Ghent, Belgium

Abstract

Whereas imaging of cholesteatoma was limited to CT scan a decade ago, MRI has become in the past few years an indispensable tool in the evaluation of the cholesteatoma patient as well as prior to first stage surgery in describing the exact location and extent of the cholesteatoma as well as prior to second stage surgery in selecting patients for second stage surgery. This chapter describes the different types of cholesteatoma as well as the different types of cholesteatoma surgery. Emphasis is put on current state-of-the art imaging of cholesteatoma as well in the non-operated patient as well as in the patient prior to second stage surgery.

1 Definition and History

Cholesteatoma is a well-demarcated non-neoplastic lesion of the temporal bone which can in fact be regarded as 'skin in the wrong place'. Cholesteatoma is gradually increasing in size due to the continuous desquamation and accumulation of keratine in the lesion.

Joseph-Guichard Du Verney, a French anatomist was the first to describe a temporal bone lesion in 1683, probably representing the first official report of a cholesteatoma (Du Verney 1683).

In 1838, this pathology was named 'cholesteatoma' by the German anatomist/pathologist Müller (1838). He described a pearly layer of fat within the ear that he thought was composed of cholesterol.

The term cholesteatoma is considered a misnomer in that it is neither a tumour, nor does it contain cholesterin or fat. 'Epidermosis', 'keratosis' of 'keratoma' are terms that are also used. However, the most commonly used expression remains the term 'cholesteatoma'.

2 Epidemiology

The annual incidence of cholesteatoma is reported to be 3 per 100,000 in children and 9.2 per 100,000 in adults with a male predominance of 1.4/1. Middle ear cholesteatomas tend to affect younger individuals, whereas external auditory canal cholesteatomas present predominantly at a higher age (40–70). Hereditary predisposition is probable. There is a high prevalence among white individuals, and cholesteatoma is rarely detected in the Asian, American Indian and Alaskan Eskimo population (Baràth et al. 2011).

3 Classification

Cholesteatoma can be classified as either congenital or acquired, though the origins are indistinguishable with histology and imaging.

The location of the lesion, the clinical history of the patient and the otologic status of the tympanic membrane may give clues to differentiate these two types of cholesteatomas (Baràth et al. 2011; De Foer et al. 2010a).

4 The Congenital Cholesteatoma

4.1 Introduction

The congenital cholesteatoma originates at the time of neural tube closure due to entrapment of ectoderm—the later skin—in the head. If the entrapment takes place inside the dura, the lesion is called epidermoid or epidermoid cyst. The most frequent location of epidermoid cyst is the cerebello-pontine angle where it is reported to be the third most frequent mass lesion after the vestibulo-cochlear schwannoma and the meningioma.

If the ectoderm gets entrapped outside the dura, but in the petrous bone, it is called a congenital cholesteatoma. Histologically, epidermoid cyst and congenital cholesteatoma are exactly the same, consisting of entrapped ectoderm or skin. As the skin is gradually exfoliating, the lesion very slowly but gradually starts to grow. Depending on its location, clinical symptoms may arise (Baràth et al. 2011; De Foer et al. 2010a).

4.2 Location

Congenital cholesteatomas can be located anywhere in the temporal bone: in the middle ear, in the mastoid, in the petrous bone apex, in the squama temporalis, within the tympanic membrane and in the external auditory canal. The location in the petrous bone apex seems to be less frequent than previously thought. Discussion still exists if a petrous bone apex cholesteatoma does not represent an acquired cholesteatoma in a pre-existing aerated petrous apex, rather than being a congenital cholesteatoma originating in the petrous bone apex.

In the petrous bone, the congenital cholesteatoma has however two predilection sites: the middle ear and the otic capsule near the geniculate ganglion.

If situated in the middle ear, it is most frequently situated in the anterior–superior part, where it can be found around the ossicular chain most frequently the malleus head and incus body (Fig. 1) (Baràth et al. 2011; De Foer et al. 2010a; Nelson et al. 2002; Darrouzet et al. 2002). From there on, it can extend towards the antrum and mastoid. It can also be situated in the mesotympanon in which it can extend to the long process of the incus, the incudostapedial joint or the crurae of the stapes, with subsequent erosion (Nelson et al. 2002; Darrouzet et al. 2002).

By definition, a congenital cholesteatoma is found behind an intact tympanic membrane without any signs of infection (Baràth et al. 2011; De Foer et al. 2010a; Nelson et al. 2002; Darrouzet et al. 2002).

Middle ear congenital cholesteatoma represent approximately 2 % of all middle ear cholesteatomas (Baràth et al. 2011). In the paediatric population, the number of congenital cholesteatomas in the overall paediatric cholesteatoma population is higher, reaching 16 % (Darrouzet et al. 2002).

Congenital cholesteatoma can also be situated in the petrous bone near the otic capsule (Fig. 2). In those cases, it is very often found near the geniculate ganglion in which it can have a component protruding in the middle ear as well as an inner ear component (De Foer et al. 2010a). The middle ear component can give rise to conductive hearing loss, the inner ear component around the geniculate ganglion can give rise to a progressive facial nerve palsy. Care should be taken that at surgery both components of the congenital cholesteatoma are resected as any residual cholesteatoma in the inner ear may continue to grow. Usually, these patients are young.

It should be noted that congenital cholesteatoma can be found anywhere around the structures of the membranous labyrinth. When situated around the structures of the inner ear, profound sensorineural hearing loss can be found.

4.3 Clinical Signs

The clinical presentation of a congenital middle ear cholesteatoma may be an asymptomatic white mass behind an intact tympanic membrane, usually discovered incidentally in the course of the evaluation of conductive hearing loss (Baràth et al. 2011; De Foer et al. 2010a; Nelson et al. 2002; Darrouzet et al. 2002). In advanced stages, congenital

Imaging of Cholesteatoma

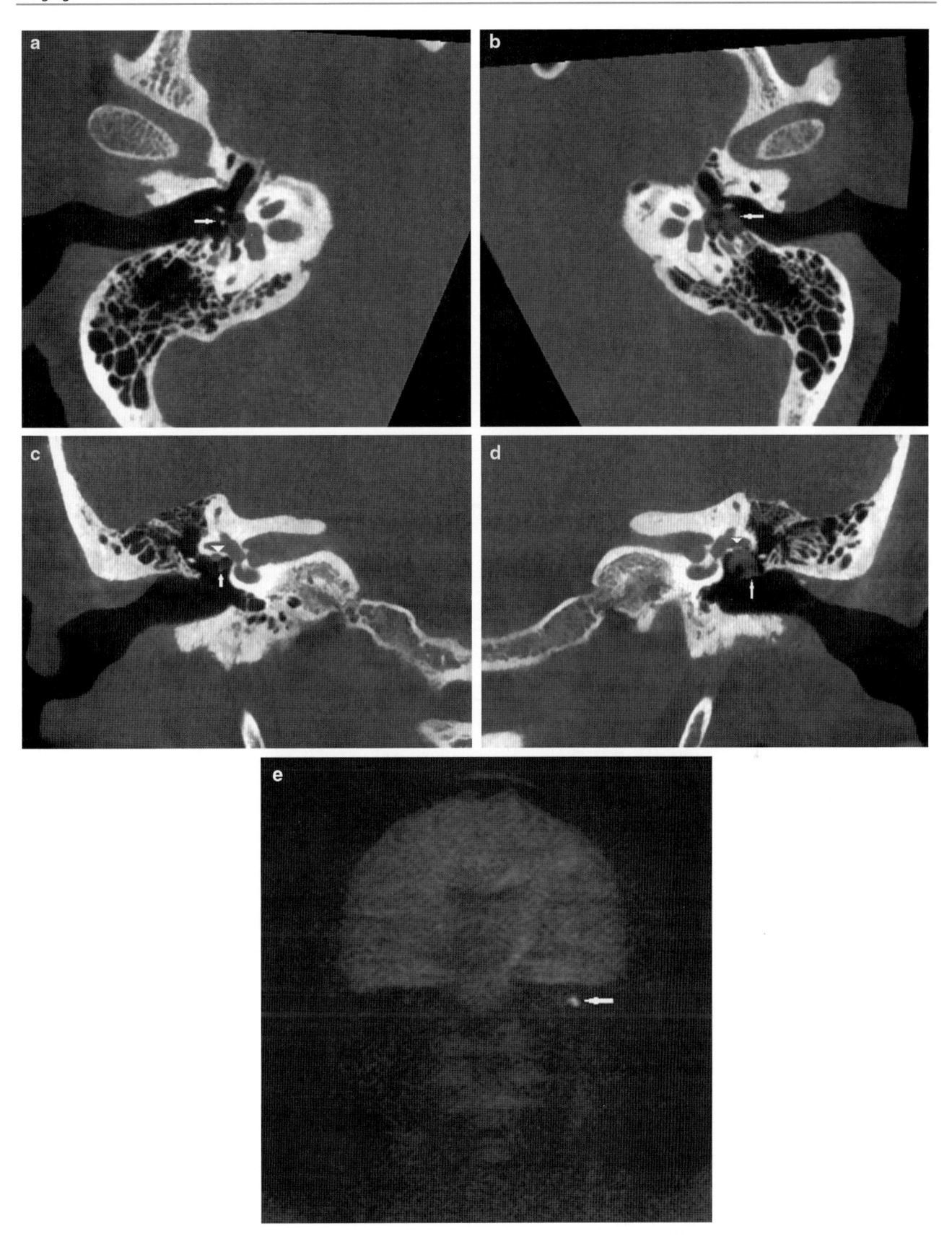

Fig. 1 A 41-year-old-female investigated for conductive hearing loss on the left side. At otoscopy, an intact tympanic membrane was found with suspicion of a whitish lesion behind it. *b*1000 HASTE diffusion-weighted sequence confirmed the presence of a congenital cholesteatoma. CBCT located the lesion and showed the erosive effect of the cholesteatoma on the ossicular chain. At surgery, the bony delineation over the second segment of the facial nerve canal was eroded. **a** Double oblique CBCT reformation through the plane of stapes and footplate on the *right side* (same level as Fig. 1b) demonstrating a normal footplate and a normal aspect and alignment of the tip of incus long process, capitellum and stapes crurae (*arrow*). **b** Double oblique CBCT reformation through the plane of stapes and footplate on the left side. There is a nodular soft tissue lesion (*arrow*) with loss of delineation of incus long process, capitellum and crurae of the stapes (compare to normal findings on the *right side* in Fig. 1a). **c** Coronal CBCT reformation at the level of the oval window (same level as Fig. 1d). In front of the oval window, the capitellum can be noted (*arrow*). Note the bony delineation over the second segment of the facial nerve running underneath the lateral semicircular canal (*arrowhead*). **d** Coronal CBCT reformation at the level of the oval window. Large semi-lunar soft tissue nodule in the mesotympanon (*arrow*). Note the loss of delineation of the capitellum (compare to the normal findings in Fig. 1c). The lesion is also abutting the second segment of the facial nerve (*arrowhead*). **e** Coronal *b*1000 HASTE diffusion-weighted image clearly demonstrates the nodular high signal intensity of the lesion, compatible with a congenital cholesteatoma (*arrow*)

cholesteatoma may cause the same symptoms as the acquired one (Baràth et al. 2011; De Foer et al. 2010a) (see below).

In case of a congenital cholesteatoma situated in or near the otic capsule, sensorineural hearing loss is usually found. Association to facial nerve palsy can be found in case of extension to the geniculate ganglion region (De Foer et al. 2010a).

4.4 Treatment

The treatment of congenital cholesteatoma is almost always surgery. Depending on its location, surgery can be extremely difficult with considerable postoperative morbidity due to temporary balance disturbances and definite sensorineural hearing loss in case of invasion of the membranous labyrinth.

In case of a middle ear location, reconstructive surgery of the ossicular chain is very often required. Most frequently, closed techniques are used (De Foer et al. 2010a; Nelson et al. 2002; Darrouzet et al. 2002) (see below).

If the congenital cholesteatoma is located near the geniculate ganglion, care should be taken to remove the entire congenital cholesteatoma as retained parts of the congenital cholesteatoma—mainly the inner ear components—may continue to grow.

4.5 Imaging

In the particular setting of a young patient presenting with conductive hearing loss and a whitish lesion at otoscopy behind an intact tympanic membrane, CT scan will nicely demonstrate the cholesteatoma as a usually rather small nodular soft tissue lesion in the anterosuperior part of the middle ear. It will also show the relationship to the ossicles and eventual ossicular erosion (Fig. 1) (Baràth et al. 2011; De Foer et al. 2010a).

Discussion still remains whether cone beam CT or CT should be used to evaluate middle ear structures and whether cone beam CT should be used to perform cholesteatoma evaluation on CT. The role of cone beam CT seems however to be increasing. It should be noted also that radiation dose in CBCT of temporal bones is substantially lower than that of CT (own unpublished data).

In case of a location in the inner ear or membranous labyrinth, the congenital cholesteatoma presents itself as a sharply delineated punched-out lesion in the temporal bone pyramid abutting or involving the structures of the membranous labyrinth. As already mentioned, the geniculate ganglion of the facial nerve is very often involved (Fig. 2).

Very often, Magnetic Resonance Imaging (MRI) is required to evaluate the involvement of the membranous labyrinth. On non-echo planar (EP) diffusion-weighted (DW) sequences, the congenital cholesteatoma will demonstrate as a clear—usually nodular—hyper-intensity on *b*1000 images (Figs. 1, 2). On ADC maps, the congenital cholesteatoma displays low signal intensity due to diffusion restriction. On T2-weighted images, the lesion shows a moderate hyper-intensity. Intensity on T1-weighted images is low, with possibly some peripheral enhancement after intravenous administration of gadolinium (Fig. 2).

Differential diagnosis should be made with other lytic temporal bone lesions. Metastatic lesions can be found anywhere in the temporal bone but usually involve a different age group of patients. These lesions are almost always ill-defined contrary to the sharply delineated punched-out lesions of the congenital cholesteatoma. The glomus jugulo-tympanicum has an entirely different clinical presentation, very often with pulsatile tinnitus. At otoscopy, a blueish lesion can be found behind an intact tympanic membrane. Moreover the lesion is invariably centred over the jugular foramen, with—contrary to the congenital cholesteatoma—ill-defined borders (De Foer et al. 2010a).

5 The Acquired Cholesteatoma

5.1 Introduction: Etiopathogenesis

There are many theories regarding the etiopathogenic mechanism of acquired cholesteatoma. The 'retraction pocket theory' is the generally most accepted one.

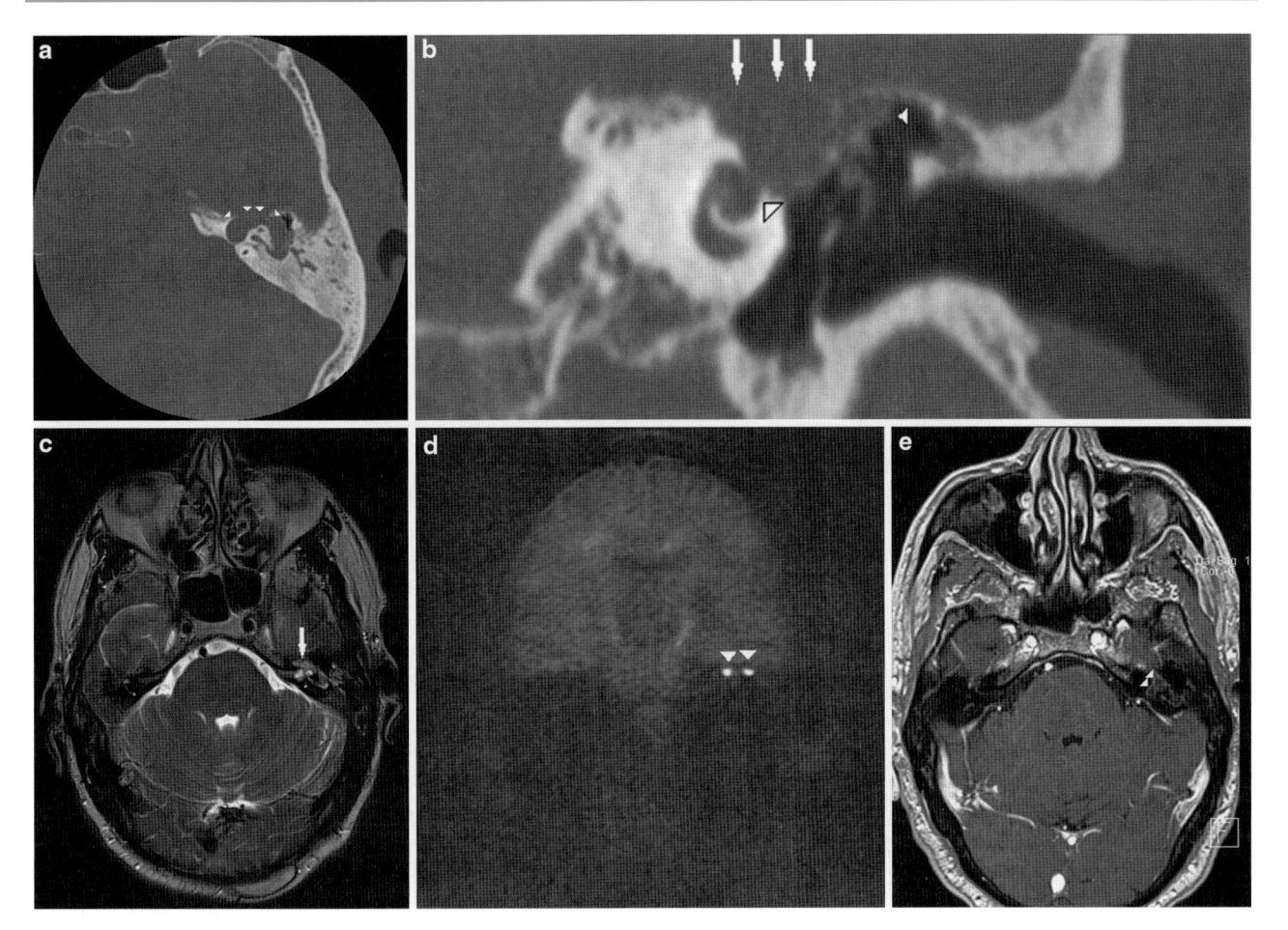

Fig. 2 A 51-year-old male with a long-standing history of mixed hearing loss on the left side and a sudden onset of facial nerve paralysis on the left side (House–Brackmann grade III). The sharply delineated punched-out lesion on CT in the left petrous bone apex, near the region of the geniculate ganglion with invasion in the membranous labyrinth, is higly suspicious of a congenital cholesteatoma. The lesion probably had a large middle ear component which was partially evacuated through the tympanic membrane into the external auditory canal. MR findings confirm the presence of a congenital cholesteatoma as the lesion displays a clear hyper-intense signal on *b*1000 diffusion-weighted images. **a** Axial CT image at the level of the superior semicircular canal on the left side. A sharply delineated semi-lunar punched-out soft tissue lesion (*arrowheads*) anteriorly located in the petrous bone apex around the anterior limb of the superior semicircular canal can be noted. **b** Coronal CT image at the level of the geniculate ganglion and cochlea. Note the large sharply delineated punched-out soft tissue lesion in the region of the geniculate ganglion (*arrows*). The lesion is abutting the cochlea (*large arrowhead*). There is a small component of soft tissues extending in the middle ear attic (*small arrowhead*). The delineation of the ossicles is lost due to erosion and subsequent partial evacuation of the middle ear component of the congenital cholesteatoma. **c** Axial TSE T2-weighted image at the level of the membranous labyrinth on the left side. There is small moderate intense nodular lesion anterior in the petrous bone apex (*arrow*). **d** Coronal *b*1000 HASTE diffusion-weighted image (same level as Fig. 2b). Bilobular hyper-intense lesion, underneath the tegmen (*arrowheads*), pathognomonic for a congenital cholesteatoma. **e** Axial T1-weighted image 45 min after intravenous administration of gadolinium-DTPA. Anterior and medial in the petrous bone apex, a bilobular peripherally enhancing low intense lesion is noted (*arrowheads*). The lesion displays signal characteristics and enhancement pattern of a cholesteatoma

In this theory, the acquired cholesteatoma is regarded as a type of chronic middle ear infection. Together with poor ventilation of the middle ear and mastoid—due to Eustachian tube dysfunction—this leads to an increased negative pressure in the tympanic cavity, resulting in retraction of the tympanic membrane with invagination of a part of it in the middle ear (Baràth et al. 2011).

5.2 Location

There are two different subtypes of cholesteatoma depending on the location of origin of the cholesteatoma, the pars flaccida cholesteatoma and the pars tensa cholesteatoma.

Most frequently, these retraction pockets are situated at the upper part of the tympanic membrane, the so-called pars flaccida (Baràth et al. 2011; De Foer et al. 2010a; Lemmerling and De Foer 2001). Pars flaccida retraction pockets expand into the lateral epitympanic recess, the so-called Prusack's space. By gradually exfoliating, the retraction pocket enlarges and will start to erode surrounding structures. It can erode the malleus head, incus body and lateral epitympanic wall (Fig. 3). If the lesion grows further, it will start to fill up the attic with possible further erosion of the tegmen of the middle ear, the bony delineation of the tympanic segment of the facial nerve and the lateral semicircular canal (Baràth et al. 2011; De Foer et al. 2010a; Lemmerling and De Foer 2001). By doing so, the cholesteatoma may invade the middle cranial fossa or the membranous labyrinth. In case of membranous labyrinth invasion, it is usually the surrounding inflammation that is invading the membranous labyrinth and not the cholesteatoma as such (Baràth et al. 2011; De Foer et al. 2010a; Lemmerling and De Foer 2001).

If the retraction pocket originates at the posterior-inferior part of the tympanic membrane—the so-called pars tensa—the cholesteatoma will expand around the long apophysis of the incus with extension medially to the ossicles (Fig. 4). This type of cholesteatoma is also called the sinus cholesteatoma. Contrary to the pars flaccida cholesteatoma, the pars tensa cholesteatoma grows from the lower part of the mesotympanon upwards and will displace the ossicles laterally. The pars tensa cholesteatoma is much less frequent than the pars flaccida cholesteatoma.

5.3 Clinical Signs

Patients with acquired cholesteatoma have a history of recurrent ear disease, Eustachian tube dysfunction, atelectasis of the middle ear and reduced pneumatisation of the mastoid. They usually have a long-standing history of chronic middle ear infection. At otoscopy, an intact or perforated tympanic membrane can be found. The cholesteatoma presents itself as a whitish, pearly soft tissue mass on or behind the tympanic membrane. Very often the clinician will be unable to exactly evaluate the extent of the cholesteatoma.

Special attention should be paid to the entity of the 'empty cholesteatoma'—also called mural cholesteatoma. In these particular cases, the content of the cholesteatoma has evacuated itself—either by auto-evacuation either by suction cleaning—via the external auditory canal. The cholesteatoma epithelium however is still adherent to the walls of the middle ear and mastoid (Fig. 5).

Middle ear cholesteatoma may present with the following clinical signs (Baràth et al. 2011; De Foer et al. 2010a; Lemmerling and De Foer 2001).

Chronic ear discharge of the ear is one of the most frequent complaints. Some form of hearing loss is found in the majority of patients, ranging from 60 to 80 %. The hearing loss can be conductive or mixed. Less frequently, sensorineural hearing loss is found. Patients may also present with a dead ear (Baràth et al. 2011; De Foer et al. 2010a; Lemmerling and De Foer 2001). Facial paralysis occurs rarely with middle ear cholesteatomas. Only in extensive cases, the bony delineation of the facial nerve canal may become eroded with subsequent paralysis. Sudden vertigo can be seen in cases with erosion of the lateral semicircular canal and membranous labyrinth invasion.

5.4 Treatment

Treatment of the acquired cholesteatoma is in most cases performed by surgery.

Different surgical approaches exist.

In the canal wall down (CWD) approach or radical mastoidectomy, the mastoid is opened, the wall of the external auditory canal is removed with total eradication of pathology. The large postoperative cavity enables a good control and inspection for the surgeon but has major drawbacks for the patient. The patient is for example no longer allowed to swim as contact of the water with the exposed lateral semicircular canal may give rise to a sudden onset of vertigo (Lemmerling and De Foer 2001).

Most frequently however, the canal wall up (CWU) procedure is used. In this type of procedure, the wall of the external auditory canal is preserved, the mastoid is opened and the pathology is eradicated. At the same time, a tympanic membrane graft and/or ossicular chain reconstruction can be performed. However, sometimes the reconstruction of the ossicular chain needs to be performed during a second-look procedure (De Foer et al. 2010a; Lemmerling and De Foer 2001; Brown 1982) (Figs. 6, 7).

One of the major drawbacks of this technique is the risk of leaving cholesteatomatous tissue behind, as the intact external auditory canal does not allow direct inspection of the antrum and mastoid (Lemmerling and De Foer 2001; Brown 1982; Shelton and Sheehy 1990) (Fig. 6). This 'residual' or left behind cholesteatoma can be found anywhere in the middle ear, antrum or mastoidectomy cavity. It is usually small and difficult to detect.

Differentiation definitely should be made with cholesteatoma recurrence (Sheehy et al. 1977). The recurrent cholesteatoma by definition always originates at the tympanic membrane or tympanic membrane graft. It usually takes more time to develop and is very often larger at time of detection (Sheehy et al. 1977).

Therefore, about 1 year after the first-stage surgery, a so-called second-look surgery is performed to evaluate the presence of a residual cholesteatoma. This second-stage is performed in a high number of patients reaching about

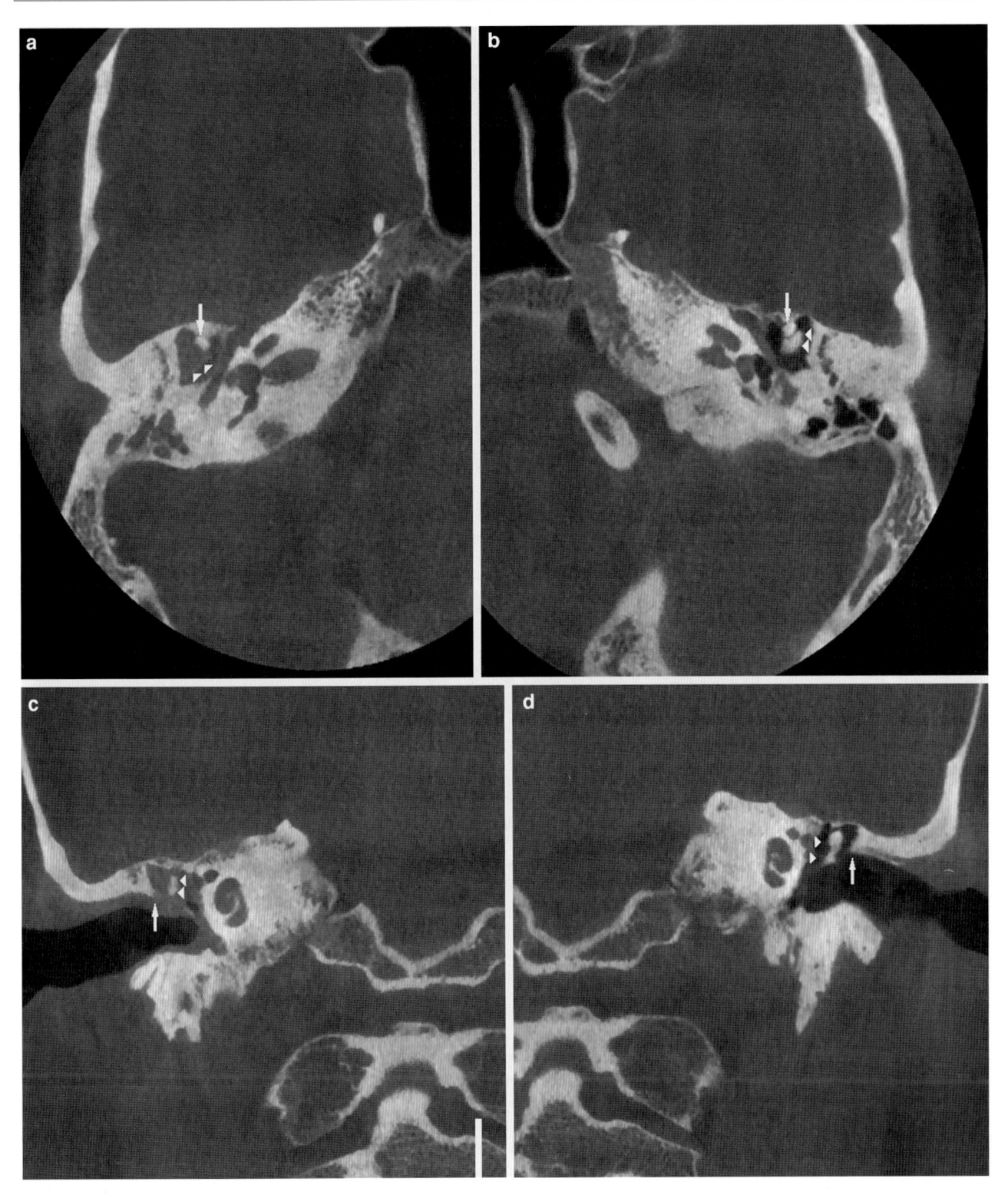

Fig. 3 A 24-year-old male with a history of chronic ear discharge on the right side and with suspicion of a retraction pocket at otoscopy. Pathognomonic image at CBCT of a pars flaccida cholesteatoma presenting itself as a soft tissue opacification in Prussak's space with clear erosion of incus body and short process. **a** Axial CBCT image on the right side at the level of the second segment of the facial nerve. Note the complete opacification of the poorly aerated middle ear. There is almost complete erosion of the incus body and short process (*arrowheads*). Note the intact appearance of the malleus head (*arrow*). Compare to the normal *left side* in Fig. 3b. **b** Axial CBCT image on the left side at the level of the second segment of the facial nerve (same level as Fig. 3a). Again, there is a poorly aerated middle ear. There is a normal delineation of the malleus head (*arrow*) and incus body (*arrowheads*). The incus short process cannot be delineated on this image due to partial volume effect. **c** Coronal CBCT image on the *right side* at the level of the cochlea. Note the opacification of the meso- and epitympanon with erosion of the scutum (*arrow*). The complex of malleus head and incus body—compare to the normal side in Fig. 3d—looks thinned and eroded (*arrowheads*). **d** Coronal CBCT image on the left side at the level of the cochlea (same level as Fig. 3c). There is a complete aeration of the middle ear with completely intact delineation of the complex malleus and incus body (*arrowheads*). Note the intact delineation of the scutum (*arrow*) and the aerated Prussak's space

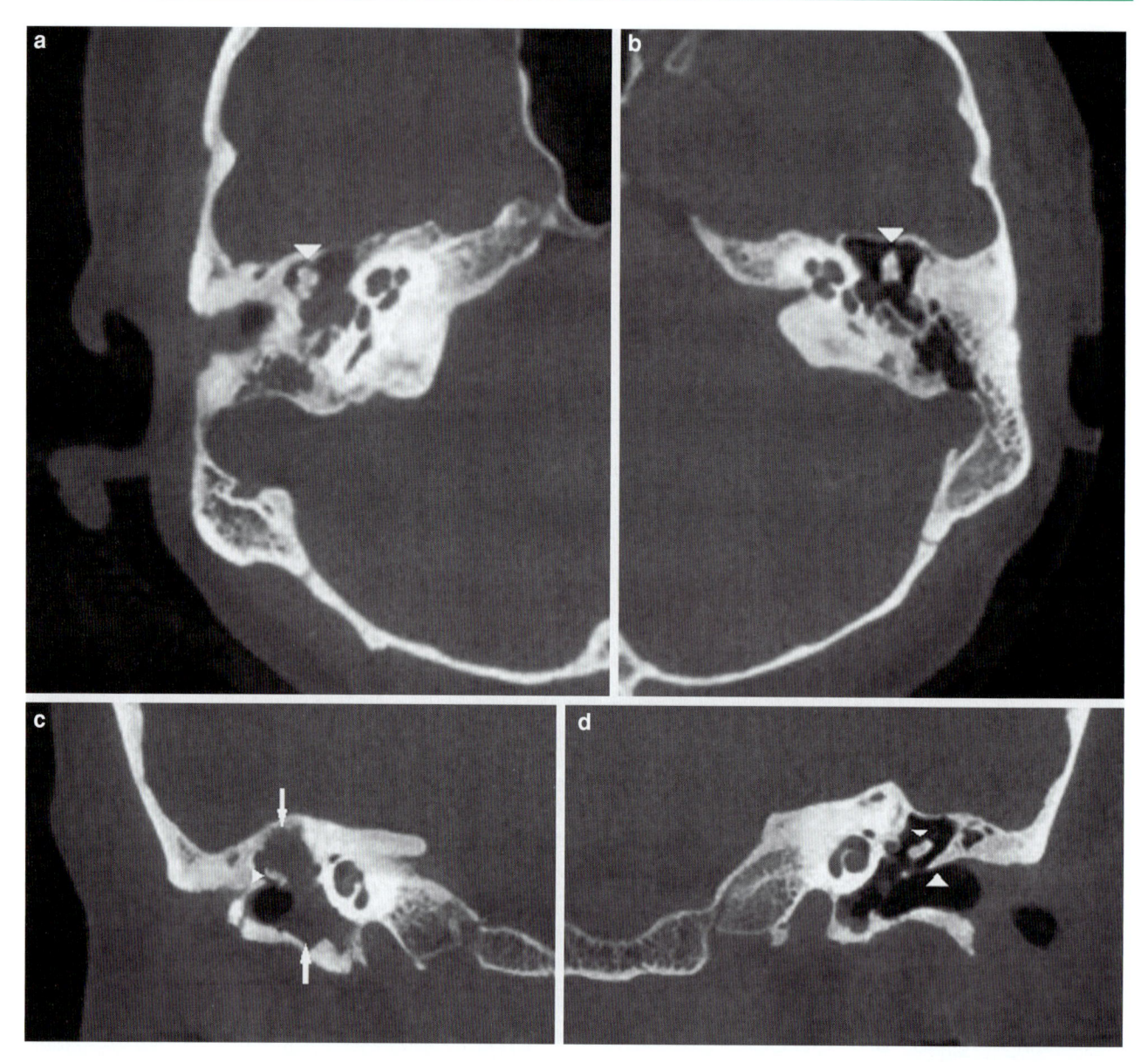

Fig. 4 An 18-year-old woman with a conductive hearing loss on the right side and a whitish lesion behind the pars tensa of an intact tympanic membrane. Findings on this CBCT examination are typical for a pars tensa cholesteatoma with ossicular erosion and lateral displacement of the ossicles. **a** Axial CBCT image at the level of the oval window. There is complete opacification of the middle ear with an intact delineation of the malleus and incus (*arrowhead*). Malleus and incus look displaced laterally (compare to the normal side, Fig. 4b). **b** Axial CBCT image at the level of the oval window (same level as Fig. 4a). The middle ear is completely aerated with a normal delineation of the ossicular chain (*arrowhead*). **c** Coronal CBCT image at the level of the cochlea. There is complete opacification of the middle ear, antrum and mastoid (*arrows*). The incus corpus seems to be slightly eroded (*small arrowhead*) with lateral displacement of the ossicles (compare to the normal situation on the *left side* in Fig. 4d). **d** Coronal CBCT image at the level of the cochlea. The middle ear and mastoid are completely aerated. There is a normal delineation of the ossicular chain (*small arrowhead*) and scutum (*large arrowhead*). Compare to Fig. 4c to evaluate the position of the ossicles

60–65 %. This percentage is even higher in children reaching about 80 %. The percentage of residual cholesteatoma found at second-look surgery is about 10–15 % (Schilder et al. 1997). Reported numbers in literature can however be higher in children, varying between 23 and 44 % (Schilder et al. 1997; Darrouzet et al. 2000).

In order to lower the residual and recurrence rate of cholesteatoma, a third technique is used, the so-called primary bony obliteration technique (PBOT—also called Mercke technique). This technique can be used during primary cholesteatoma surgery in order to treat middle ear and mastoid cholesteatoma but can also be assessed in

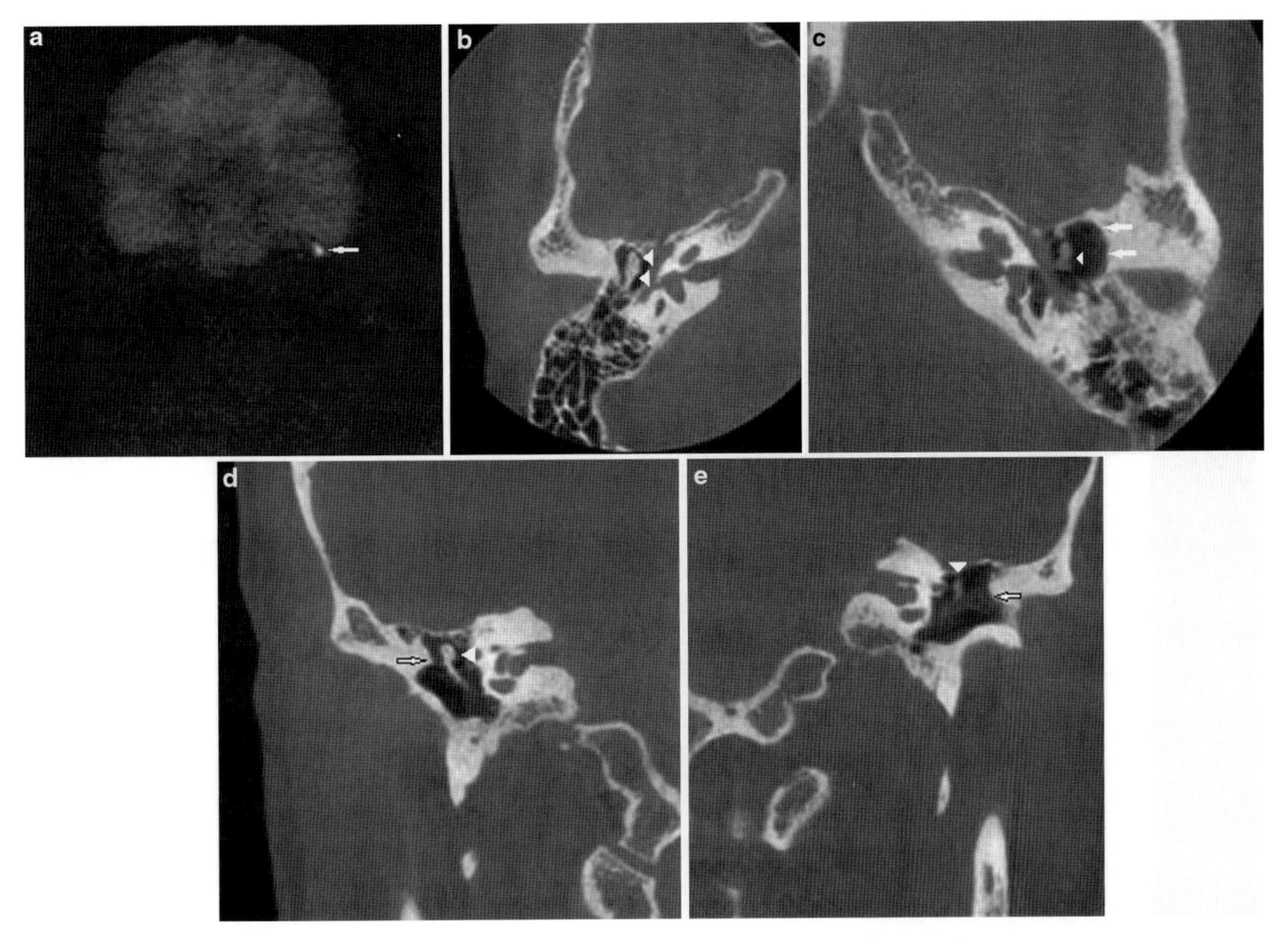

Fig. 5 A 42-year-old male with a clinically and otoscopically known middle ear cholesteatoma on the left side. HASTE diffusion-weighted image clearly demonstrates a high signal intensity on the left side, pathognomic for a middle ear cholesteatoma. However, CBCT performed 4 months later—prior to surgery—shows no clear soft tissue density in the left middle ear and/or mastoid. However, the indirect signs of cholesteatoma—e.g. ossicular erosion—are still present. It was concluded that the cholesteatoma had been evacuated in the time period elapsed between the MRI and CBCT examination probably due to auto evacuation of the cholesteatoma. The content of the cholesteatoma sac was evacuated but the cholesteatoma matrix is still adherent to the walls of the middle ear. **a** Coronal b1000 HASTE diffusion-weighted sequence clearly demonstrates a nodular hyper-intensity on the left side pathognomonic of middle ear cholesteatoma (*arrow*). **b** Axial CBCT image at the level of the second segment of the facial nerve on the right side. There is a normal delineation of the ossicular chain (*arrowheads*) without any associated soft tissues. Note the higher density of the ossicles when compared with the demineralised aspect of the ossicles on the left side (see Fig. 5c). **c** Axial CBCT image at the level of the second segment of the facial nerve on the left side. Compared to the normal side in Fig. 5b, the lateral epitympanic wall seems to be eroded (*arrows*) and the incus body also seems to be eroded (*arrowhead*). Note that the residual ossicular chain looks also demineralised compared to the *normal right side* in Fig. 5b. Clear nodular soft tissues cannot be found. **d** Coronal CBCT image at the level of the internal auditory canal on the right side. There is a normal delineation of the ossicular chain (*arrowhead*) without any associated soft tissues. Note that Prussak's space is free and that the scutum is sharp (*arrow*). **e** Coronal CBCT image at the level of the internal auditory canal on the left side. There are no clear associated soft tissues. The scutum looks amputated (*arrow*), with an eroded ossicular chain (*arrowhead*) looking also demineralised. Compare to the *normal side* in Fig. 5d

revision cases of recurrent cholesteatoma. In this technique, the CWU tympanoplasty is subsequently filled up with a mixture of bone and bone pâté in order to diminish the number of recurrences through new retractions of the tympanic membrane (Fig. 8) (Offeciers et al. 2008; Vercruysse et al. 2008). A functional ossicular chain reconstruction is performed either in the same stage either in a second stage.

The number of residual cholesteatoma after using this technique is reported to be lower than in the CWU technique with a recurrence rate of about 2 %. It should be pointed out that—in our experience—eventual residual and recurrent cholesteatoma in this technique is only found at the periphery of the obliterated cavity of the middle ear, but never in the obliterated cavity as such (Offeciers et al. 2008; Vercruysse et al. 2008).

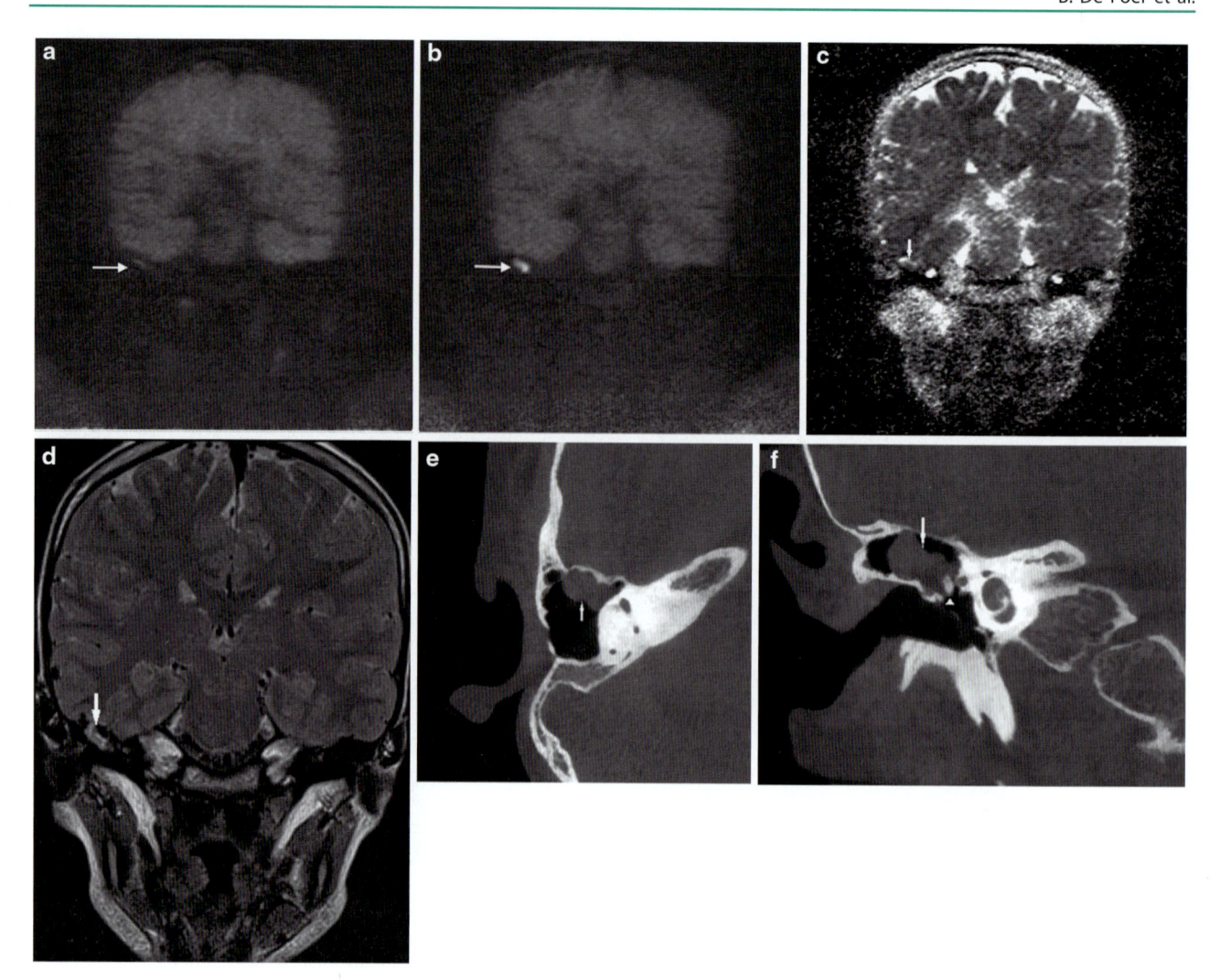

Fig. 6 An 8-year-old girl with a prior history of surgery for an attical cholesteatoma on the right side, treated by CWU tympanoplasty. This case illustrates the current state-of-the-art way of working in cholesteatoma follow-up. The first MRI follow-up examination displayed a doubtful high signal intensity on b1000 HASTE diffusion-weighted images which became a clear nodular high signal intensity on MRI follow-up. CT scan—in this case CBCT, resulting in a substantially lower radiation dose—is reserved for the pre-operative setting. **a** Coronal b1000 HASTE diffusion-weighted image 1 year after first-stage surgery demonstrates a doubtful high signal intensity (*arrow*) in the right temporal bone, underneath the tegmen. Based upon this image, diagnosis of a cholesteatoma cannot be confirmed. MRI follow-up examination after 1 year was advised. **b** Coronal b1000 HASTE diffusion-weighted image acquired 1 year after Fig. 1a showing a clear bilobular nodular high signal intensity (*arrow*) compatible with a large residual cholesteatoma. **c** Corresponding ADC map, same level as Fig. 6a and b. The cholesteatoma corresponds to a nodular zone of clear signal drop (*arrow*). **d** Corresponding coronal TSE T2-weighted image, same level as Fig. 6a, b and c. The cholesteatoma corresponds to a bilobular nodular moderate intense lesion under the tegmen on the right side (*arrow*). **e** Axial CBCT image—performed in a preoperative setting—through the superior semicircular canal. The cholesteatoma is seen as a bilobular nodular soft tissue lesion (*arrow*), located anterior in the mastoidectomy cavity. **f** Coronal CBCT image—performed in a preoperative setting—at the level of the cochlea. Large nodular soft tissue lesion, anterior in the canal-wall-up tympanoplasty cavity (*arrow*), partially situated around the malleus head (*arrowhead*): residual cholesteatoma. Note the persistent delineation of the external auditory canal typical for a CWU tympanoplasty

5.5 Imaging

5.5.1 Prior to First Stage Surgery

In most cases of an acquired cholesteatoma—which is the most common type of cholesteatoma encountered in the routine daily practice—imaging evaluation prior to first stage surgery is performed using high resolution CT. CT will be able to demonstrate the soft tissue of the cholesteatoma and its most characteristic features: signs of erosion of the ossicular chain, the scutum and the lateral epitympanic wall (Fig. 3) (Lemmerling et al. 2008).

In case of a pars flaccida cholesteatoma, erosion is most often situated at the lateral side of the malleus head and incus body. The short process of the incus can also be

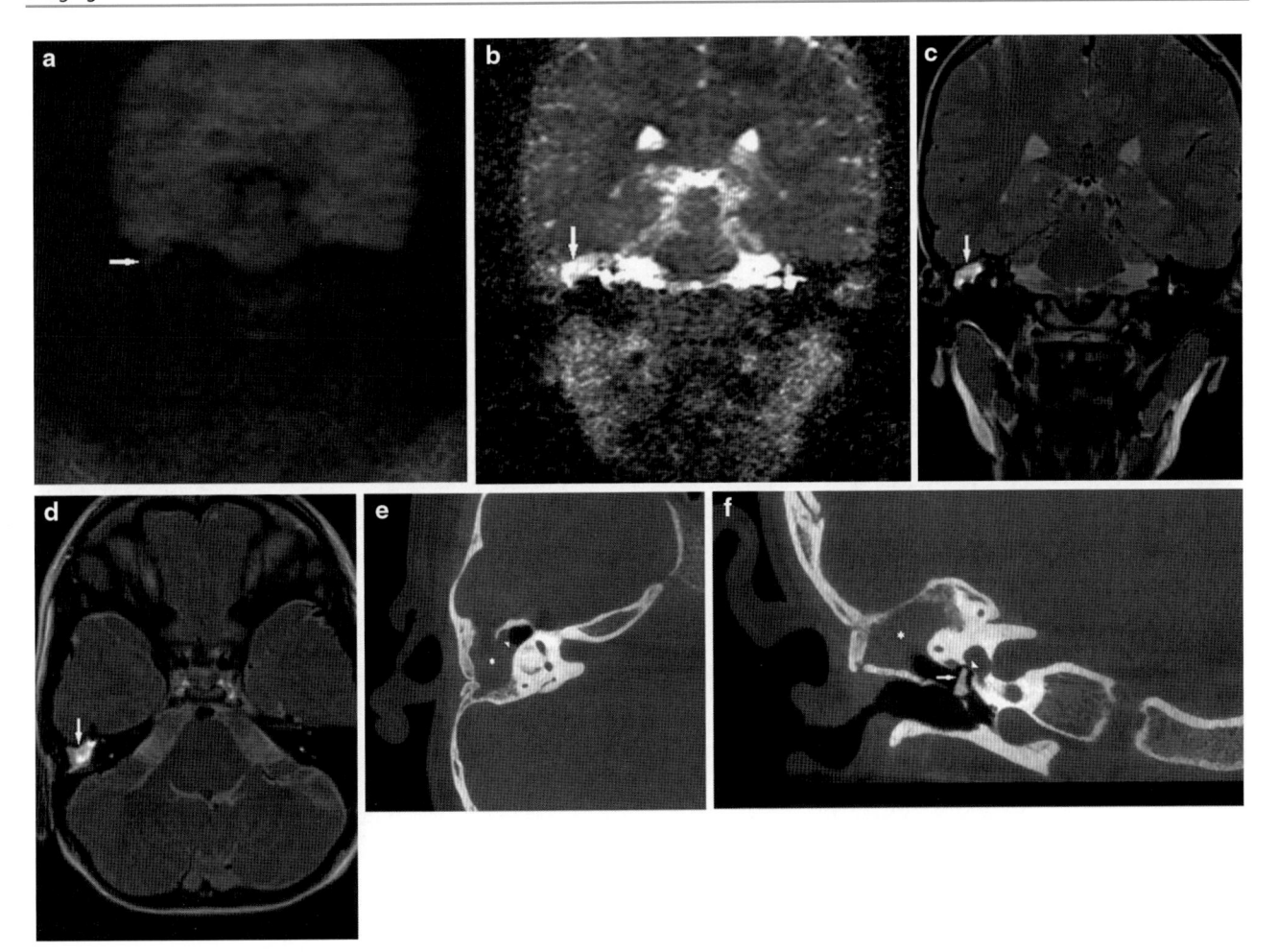

Fig. 7 A 6-year-old boy with a history of cholesteatoma surgery 1 year prior on the right side. The shortened MRI protocol (*b*0, *b*1000 HASTE diffusion, coronal and axial TSE T2-weighted images) excludes the presence of a cholesteatoma. CBCT was performed prior to surgery in order to correct the malpositioned ossicular reconstruction. **a** Coronal *b*1000 HASTE diffusion-weighted image. On the right side, there is an isointense lesion underneath the tegmen (*arrow*). The low signal intensity excludes the presence of a cholesteatoma. **b** Corresponding ADC map (same level as Fig. 7a). On the right side, there is a persisting hyper-intense signal on ADC map, confirming the absence of cholesteatoma (*arrow*). **c** Coronal TSE T2-weighted image at the level of the cochlea (same level as Fig. 7a and b). There is a clear hyper-intensity on the right side (*arrow*). Signal intensity is by far too high to be compatible with a cholesteatoma. The resection cavity is filled with post-operative tissue. **d** Axial TSE T2-weighted image at the level of the superior semicircular canal. Again a clear hyper-intensity on the right side is noted (*arrow*). Signal intensity is again too high to be compatible with a cholesteatoma. **e** Axial CBCT image on the right side at the level of the superior semicircular canal. There is a subtotal opacification (*asterisk*) of the resection cavity with a posterior convex delineation (*arrowhead*). The subtotal opacification on CBCT cannot be differentiated. **f** Coronal CBCT image on the right side at the level of the oval window. Note again the homogeneous opacification (*asterisk*) of the resection cavity. Again the soft tissue opacification cannot be differentiated. There is an ossicular reconstruction based on a remodelled incus (*arrow*). The remodelled incus is not abutting the oval window (*arrowhead*). Surgical reintervention is hence mandatory. Note again the intact delineation of the roof of the external auditory canal compatible with a CWU tympanoplasty technique

eroded. This type of erosion is never seen in case of chronic middle ear infection and can be regarded as a pathognomonic sign of cholesteatoma (Fig. 3).

Sometimes, clinical and otoscopical differentiation between chronic middle ear infection and cholesteatoma can be present simultaneously (Fig. 9).

The lateral epitympanic wall can be eroded as well and the soft tissue of the cholesteatoma will displace the ossicles medially.

CT is also able to evaluate the integrity of the bony delineation of the lateral semicircular canal. On coronal reconstructions, it will also allow evaluation of the delineation of the roof of the tegmen of the middle ear cavity (Lemmerling and De Foer 2001; Lemmerling et al. 2008).

In case of a pars tensa cholesteatoma, soft tissues are mainly located in the lower part of the middle ear, the so called hypotympanon. Ossicular erosion is most often situated at the incus long process and stapes. However, erosion of the incus

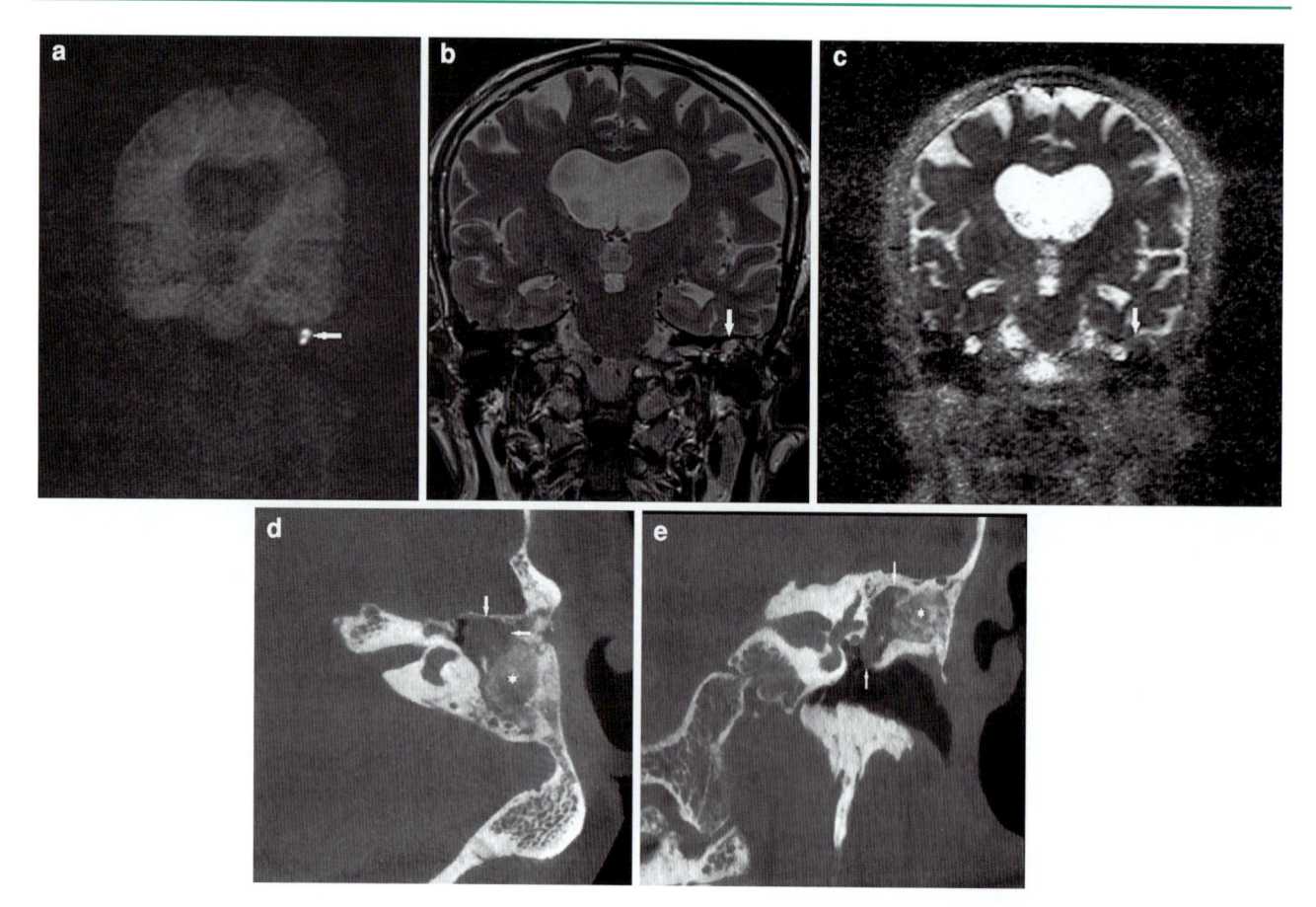

Fig. 8 A 77-year-old-male with a history of cholesteatoma surgery, 3 years prior on the left side. A CWU tympanoplasty was performed at that time in combination with a bony obliteration of the tympanoplasty cavity (PBOT). Clinically and otoscopically there was suspicion of a cholesteatoma. MRI—and especially the HASTE diffusion-weighted sequence—cleary demonstrates the cholesteatoma. CBCT was performed in a pre-operative setting, showing the partial erosion of the obliterated cavity by the cholesteatoma. **a** Coronal *b*1000 HASTE diffusion-weighted image demonstrates a large left-sided nodular high signal intensity, compatible with a large recurrent cholesteatoma (*arrow*). Note that it is impossible to exactly locate the lesion in the middle ear, due to the absence of any clear anatomical reference. **b** Coronal TSE T2-weighted image showing the cholesteatoma as a nodular moderately intense lesion in the antrum (*arrow*) at the level of the vestibule and lateral semicircular canal. **c** Coronal ADC map (same level as Fig. 8a and b). The cholesteatoma displays a clear drop in signal (*arrow*). **d** Axial CBCT image at the level of the vestibule. Note the homogeneous hyper-dense aspect of the posterior part of the mastoid (*asterisk*) compatible with the obliterated cavity. A small nodular soft tissue lesion is situated anteriorly (*arrows*) and is compatible with the recurrent cholesteatoma. **e** Coronal CBCT image at the level of the vestibule and lateral semicircular canal (same level as Fig. 8a, b and c). The lateral part of the mastoidectomy cavity is filled with a mixture of bone and bone pâté resulting in a homogeneously dense filled mastoidectomy cavity (*asterisk*). At the medial side, the cholesteatoma is seen as a nodular soft tissue density (*arrows*)

long process can also be seen in chronic middle ear infection so differentiation can sometimes be very difficult.

In case of a pars tensa cholesteatoma, the soft tissues of the cholesteatoma displace the ossicles lateral contrary to the medial displacement by a pars flaccida cholesteatoma (Fig. 4) (Lemmerling and De Foer 2001; Lemmerling et al. 2008). Erosion of incus long process can be seen in cholesteatoma as well as chronic middle ear infection, so sometimes differentiation can be difficult.

Chronic middle ear infection and cholesteatoma can be present simultaneously (Fig. 10).

One of the main goals of CT is also to demonstrate important anatomical landmarks for the surgeon and possible anatomical variants, prior to surgery.

However, in case of associated infection and/or inflammation and possible complications such as fistulisation to the lateral semicircular canal, CT will be unable to differentiate the cholesteatoma from the surrounding inflammation (Baràth

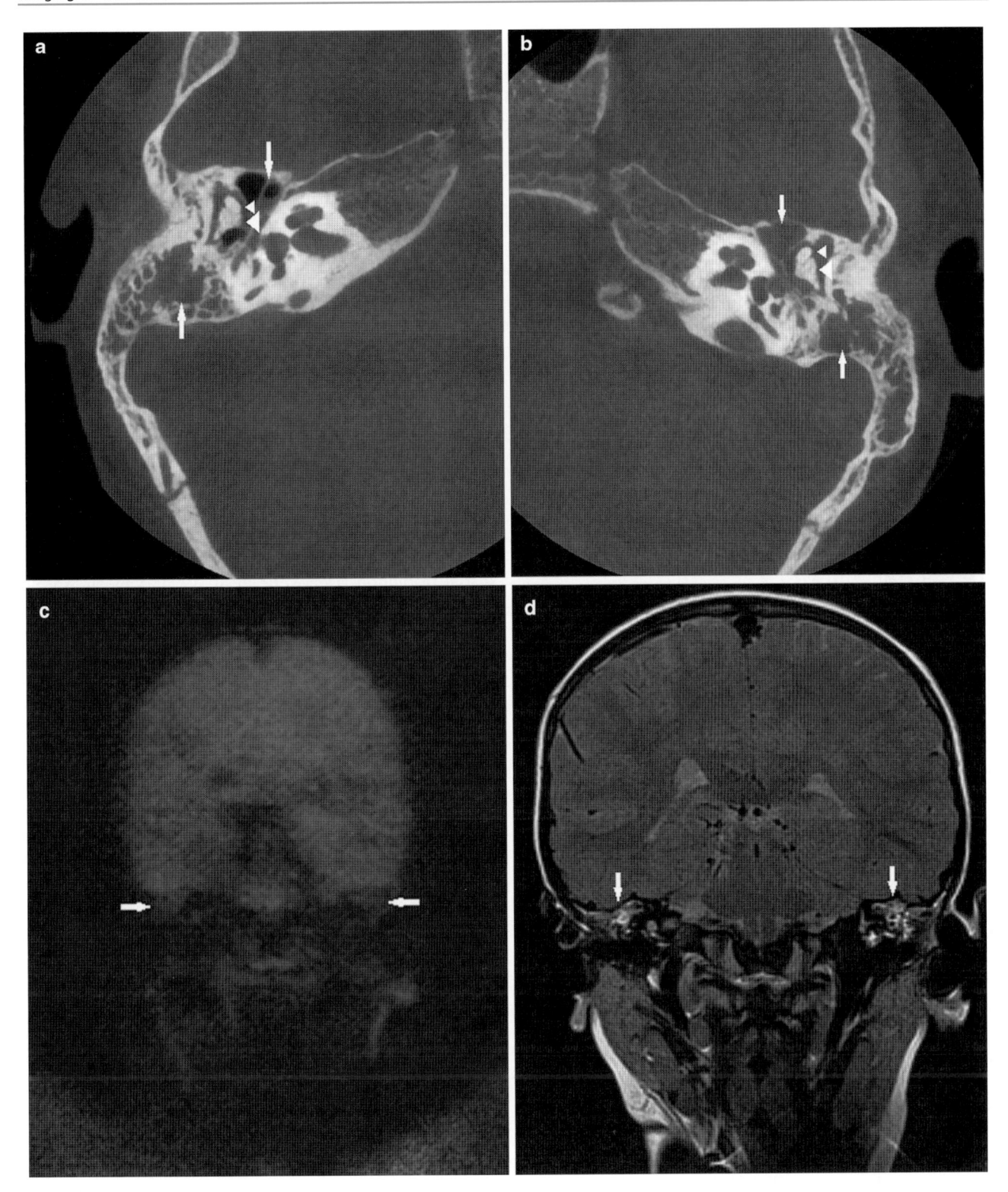

Imaging of Cholesteatoma

Fig. 9 A 5-year-old girl with conductive hearing loss on the left side. Otoscopically, a retraction pocket on the left side is seen with suspicion of an underlying cholesteatoma. The findings on CBCT could not demonstrate any erosion making the diagnosis on CBCT of a cholesteatoma highly unlikely. The absence of a cholesteatoma was confirmed on MRI by the absence of high signal on b1000 HASTE diffusion-weighted images. Based upon CBCT and MRI, it was concluded that both ears had chronic inflammatory changes but no cholesteatoma. **a** Axial CBCT image on the right side at the level of the oval window. On this side there is subtotal opacification of the middle ear and mastoid (*arrows*). There is an intact delineation of the malleus head (*small arrowhead*) and incus body and short process (*large arrowhead*). The absence of ossicular erosion makes the diagnosis of a cholesteatoma highly unlikely. **b** Axial CBCT image on the left side at the level of the oval window. There is complete opacification of the middle ear and mastoid (*arrow*). There is an intact delineation of the malleus head (*small arrowhead*) and incus body and short process (*large arrowhead*). The absence of ossicular erosion makes the diagnosis of a cholesteatoma highly unlikely. **c** Coronal b1000 HASTE diffusion-weighted image. On both sides, a low signal intensity lesion is found, almost completely filling up both middle ears (*arrows*). The absence of a clear hyper-intense signal excludes the presence of a cholesteatoma. The ADC map (not shown) also demonstrated a high signal intensity compatible with chronic inflammatory changes. **d** Coronal TSE T2-weighted image at the level of the vestibule on both sides. Both middle ears are completely filled with mixed to moderate to high intensity signals on both sides (*arrows*). Based upon this sequence alone, the presence of cholesteatoma cannot be confirmed nor can it be excluded

et al. 2011; De Foer et al. 2010a; Lemmerling and De Foer 2001; Lemmerling et al. 2008). CT is very limited in demonstrating the exact degree of involvement of the membranous labyrinth and the possible extension into the middle cranial fossa.

In these cases, MRI plays an important role in the exact delineation of the cholesteatoma and in the description of extension of the cholesteatoma in the membranous labyrinth (De Foer et al. 2010a).

5.5.2 Prior to Second-Look Surgery

In CWU patients prior to second-stage surgery, CT will only be able to exclude cholesteatoma in case of a well-aerated middle ear and mastoidectomy cavity, without any associated soft tissue. Only in case of a nodular soft tissue lesion, CT will be able to make the positive diagnosis of a residual cholesteatoma (Lemmerling et al. 2008; Williams et al. 2003).

Unfortunately, most post-cholesteatoma surgery temporal bones do not present with well-aerated middle ear and mastoidectomy cavities or with a well-circumscribed nodular soft tissue lesion. The vast majority of post-operative CWU mastoidectomy patients present with subtotal/total soft tissue opacification of the middle ear and mastoid. Unfortunately, CT is unable to differentiate these soft tissue opacifications (Figs. 6, 7) (Tierney et al. 1999; Blaney et al. 2001).

However—in spite of these important limitations—CT is still worldwide used in patients evaluated prior to second-stage surgery. It is however known that CT is an increasing source of radiation exposure and that its use should be rationalised (Brenner and Hall 2007).

It was already noted in early papers that MR imaging using gadolinium-enhanced T1-weighted sequences was able to make the differential diagnosis between cholesteatoma and chronic inflammation (Martin et al. 1990). This is based on the fact that chronic inflammation will enhance on gadolinium-enhanced T1-weighted images in contrast to the lack of enhancement of the avascular cholesteatoma (Martin et al. 1990).

Several papers have however evaluated the use of standard MR imaging sequences including T2-weighted and gadolinium-enhanced T1-weighted images in the detection of residual cholesteatoma prior to second-look. It was concluded that standard sequences alone were unable to replace second-look surgery, due to poor contrast and spatial resolution (Denoyelle et al. 1994; Vanden Abeele et al. 1999; Kimitsuki et al. 2001).

Several reports suggested the improvement of other MR imaging techniques in diagnosing middle ear cholesteatoma—as well as prior to first-stage and second-stage surgery—using delayed contrast-enhanced T1-weighted imaging (Williams et al. 2003; Ayache et al. 2005) and DW MR imaging (Aikele et al. 2003; Maheshwari and Mukherji 2002; Stasolla et al. 2004).

Williams et al. used delayed gadolinium-enhanced T1-weighted sequences to detect residual cholesteatoma after CWU tympanoplasty. Patients were pre-selected based on CT scan. The rationale behind this technique was that the postoperative scar tissue takes time to enhance and that early scanning will result in false-positive results. Using delayed gadolinium-enhanced T1-weighted images, they achieved a sensitivity, specificity, PPV and inter-observer agreement of 85.2, 92.6, 92.6 %, respectively, and a kappa of 0.78. The conclusion was that delayed contrast-enhanced T1-weighted MR imaging was reliable for the detection of residual cholesteatoma in patients having undergone CWU tympanoplasty. Residual cholesteatoma as small as 3 mm could be detected (Williams et al. 2003; Ayache et al. 2005).

The mechanism of DW MR imaging is based upon the Brownian motion of water molecules in tissue and, more importantly, on the hindrances/facilitations of water molecule movements in various types of tissue. In order to make an MR imaging sequence sensitive to diffusion of water molecules, the sequence is expanded with a diffusion-sensitizing gradient scheme, usually a very fast, single-shot gradient-echo data collecting sequence (EP imaging).

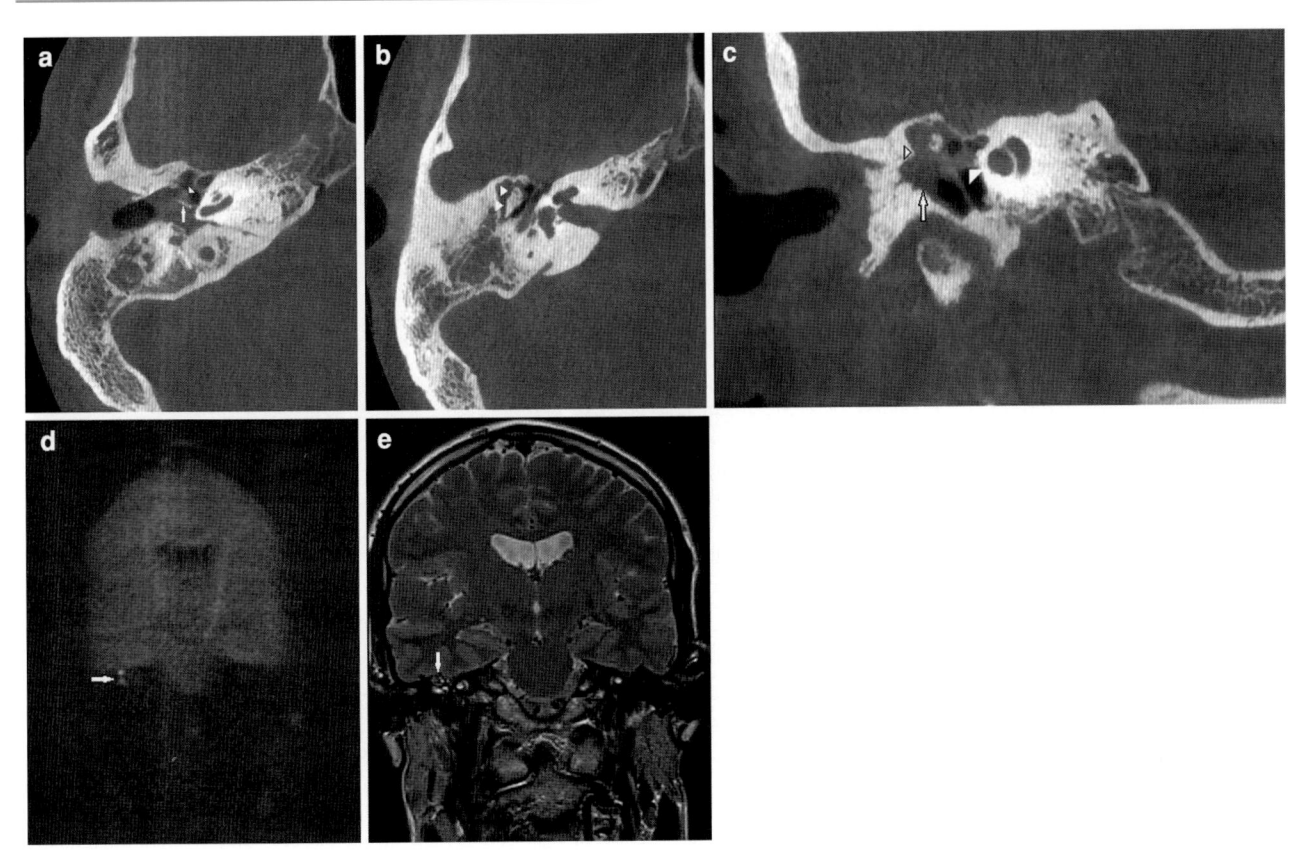

Fig. 10 A 24-year-old man with a history of chronic ear infection, severe conductive hearing loss and a suspicion of cholesteatoma at otoscopy on the right side. CBCT demonstrates signs of a specific form of chronic middle ear infection: tympanosclerosis. Apart from an amputation of the scutum, no direct signs of cholesteatoma can be found. MRI however clearly demonstrates the co-existence of a cholesteatoma by demonstrating a high signal intensity on b1000 HASTE diffusion-weighted images, with corresponding low signal intensity on ADC map. In this particular case, there is a co-existence of a cholesteatoma and tympanosclerosis. This case was surgically confirmed. **a** Axial CBCT image at the level of the basal turn of the cochlea on the right side. There is a subtotal opacification of the hypotympanon. Note that there are subtle calcifications (*arrowhead*) anterior to the malleus handle (*arrow*). These subtle calcifications are the handmark of a subtype of chronic middle ear infection called tympanosclerosis. **b** Axial CBCT image at the level of the second segment of the facial nerve. There is opacification of the middle ear and mastoid. There is no evident erosion of the ossicular chain (*arrowheads*). **c** Coronal CBCT image at the level of the cochlea. There is opacification of the lateral epitympanic recess (Prussak's space) (*arrow*) with amputation of the scutum (*small arrowhead*). Note again the subtle calcifications of the soft tissues anterior and medial to the malleus (*large arrowhead*). **d** Coronal HASTE diffusion weighted image (same level as Fig. 10c). There is a bilobular clear hyper-intensity underneath the tegmen on the right side (*arrow*). The lesion also demonstrates a clear signal drop on ADC map (not shown). This image is pathognomonic of a middle ear and epitympanic cholesteatoma. **e** Coronal TSE T2-weighted image (same level as Fig. 10c and d) demonstrating mixed moderate and high signal intensities underneath the tegmen (*arrow*). Because of the mixed signal intensities, diagnosis of a cholesteatoma cannot be made based upon this sequence alone

The amount of diffusion-sensitizing gradient applied is usually indicated by the *b*-value. In routine clinical practice, images are generally acquired with a *b*-value of 0 and 1.000 s/mm^2.

ADC images are calculated from DW images with at least two different *b*-values (typically, $b = 0$ and $b = 1.000$ s/mm^2). The contrast corresponds to the spatially distributed (apparent) diffusion coefficient of the acquired tissues and does not contain T1 or T2* parts. The lower the grey value of a pixel in the ADC image, the more diffusion is restricted in this pixel (Vercruysse et al. 2006).

However, numerous artefacts can be generated during acquisition of EP DW MR imaging such as eddy current artefacts, susceptibility artefacts, chemical shift and motion artefacts. With the use of higher magnetic fields, these artefacts and image distortions on EP DW imaging are even more pronounced (De Foer et al. 2006). In the temporal bone region, the interface between air, bone and the temporal lobe is in particular prone to susceptibility artefacts.

Other acquisition sequences that are less sensitive to susceptibility artefacts such as multi-shot EP DW imaging sequences or non-EP DW imaging sequences can be used.

These non-EP DW imaging sequences are turbo SE or fast SE-based DW sequences, have a higher spatial resolution, generate thinner slices (down to 2 mm) and do not suffer at all from susceptibility artefacts. The most frequently used

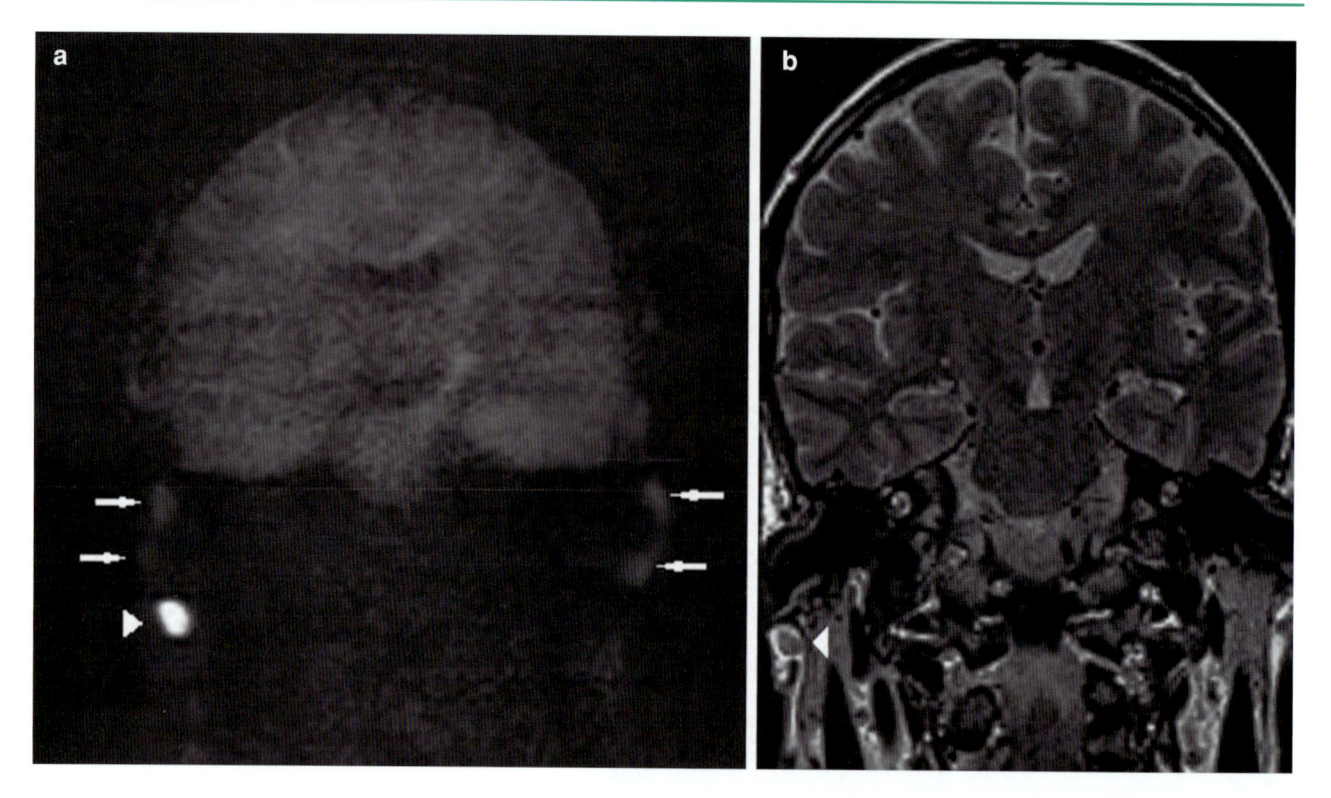

Fig. 11 A 43-year-old male investigated for conductive hearing loss on the left side. Otoscopically, a small retraction pocket was suspected. The large nodular high signal intensity on the right side displays all signs of a cholesteatoma. However, the lesion is situated by far too lateral and inferior to be located in the middle ear. Theoretically, this can be a congenital cholesteatoma in the mastoid but correlation to the T2-weighted sequences demonstrates that the lesion is situated outside the temporal bone. The lesion is located behind the right ear. Clinical inspection clearly shows the presence of a large sebum cyst behind the right ear. The content of a sebum cyst is exactly the same as the content of a cholesteatoma: both contain exfoliated skin. **a** Coronal *b*1000 HASTE diffusion-weighted image shows no high signal intensity on the left side. There is a clear nodular high signal intensity on the right side (*arrowhead*). Note the semi-lunar intensities at the lateral side of both signal voids of the temporal bone on both sides (*arrows*), caused by the external ear. Note that the nodular high signal intensity on the right side is located rather low and lateral to the temporal bone, almost near the right external ear. Corresponding ADC map (not shown) clearly shows a drop in signal intensity. **b** Coronal TSE T2-weighted image (same level as Fig. 11a) at the level of the cochlea. The lesion as demonstrated on the *b*1000 HASTE diffusion-weighted image corresponds to a nodular moderate intense lesion located behind the right ear, superficially to the parotid gland (*arrowhead*). Clinical inspection shows the presence of a large sebum cyst behind the right ear

non-EP DW imaging sequence in the literature is the half-Fourier acquisition single-shot turbo spin-echo (HASTE) DW sequence (De Foer et al. 2006, 2007, 2008, 2010a; Jeunen et al. 2008; Dhepnorrarat et al. 2009) followed by the periodically rotated overlapping parallel lines with enhanced reconstruction (PROPELLER) DW MR sequence (De Foer et al. 2006; Lehmann et al. 2009; Fitzek et al. 2002).

At the onset, studies were mainly focused on the use of EP DW imaging sequences and/or in combination with immediate gadolinium enhanced T1-weighted sequences (Aikele et al. 2003; Maheshwari and Mukherji 2002; Stasolla et al. 2004; Vercruysse et al. 2006). Fitzek was one of the first to evaluate cholesteatoma opposed to chronic middle ear infection on DW imaging, especially on *b*1000 EP DW images. The hyper-intense aspect of cholesteatoma was completely different from the complete lack of hyper-intensity of middle ear inflammatory changes on *b*1000 EP DW images (Fitzek et al. 2002).

Reports on the use of EP DW images at first seemed to be very promising. Aikele et al. reported a sensitivity of 77 %, a specificity of 100 % and PPV and NPV of 100 and 75 %, respectively, using the combination of DW MR imaging and standard MR sequences. The minimum size of cholesteatoma detection was 5 mm using this technique (Fitzek et al. 2002). Stasolla et al. reported a sensitivity of 86 %, a specificity of 100 % and PPV and NPV of 100 and 92 %, respectively, in diagnosing relapsing/residual cholesteatoma after CWU tympanoplasty (Stasolla et al. 2004).

Vercruysse et al. however reported on the use of EP DW sequences in combination with immediate gadolinium-enhanced T1-weighted sequences with a sensitivity of 12.5 %, a specificity of 100 % and a PPV and NPV of 100 and

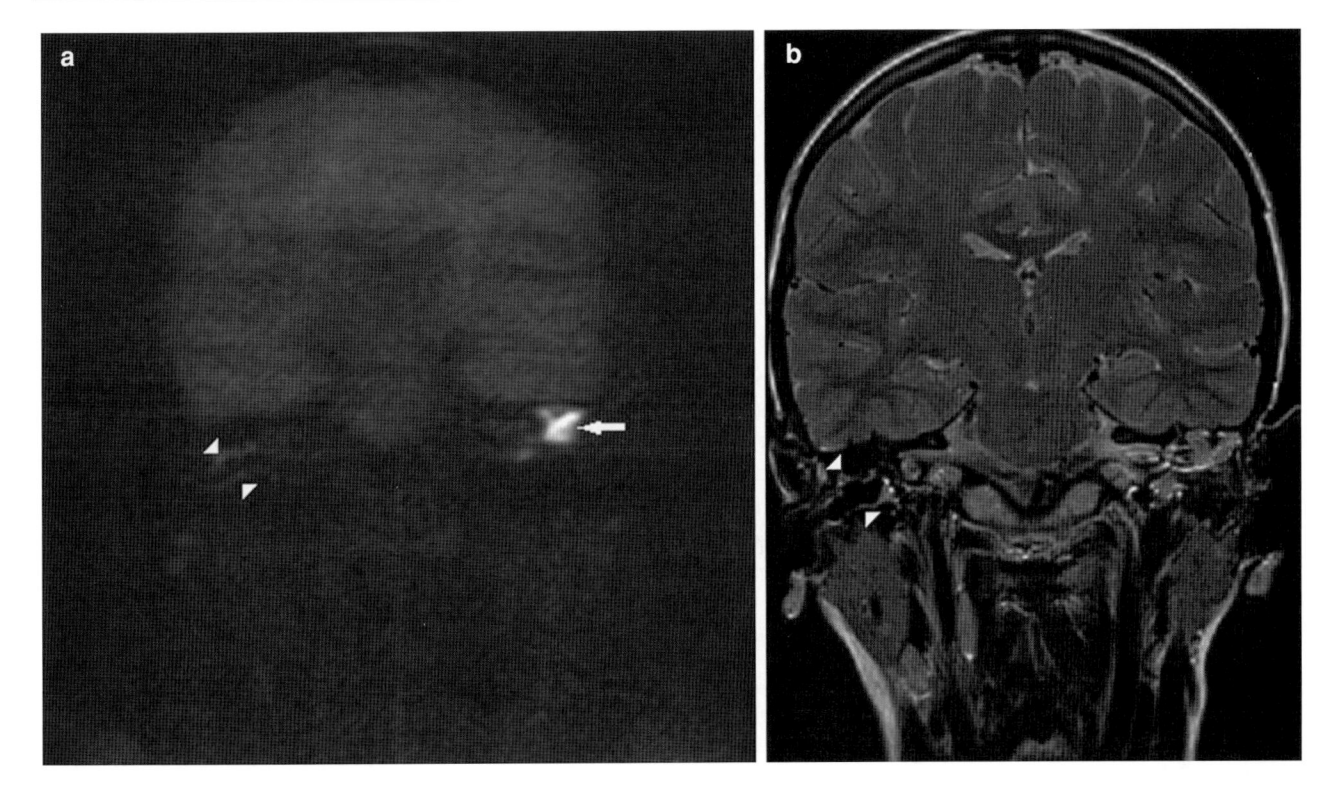

Fig. 12 A 14-year-old boy with a history of prior surgery for cholesteatoma on the left side. Clinical and otoscopical, there is evidence of a large recurrent cholesteatoma. MRI was performed in a pre-operative setting. **a** Coronal *b*1000 HASTE diffusion-weighted image demonstrates a large nodular hyper-intensity nearly completely filling up the left middle ear, compatible with a large recurrent cholesteatoma (*arrow*). On the right side, two linear hyper-intensities (*arrowheads*) are seen rather low in the middle ear. **b** Coronal TSE T2-weighted image (same level as Fig. 12a). The linear hyper-intensities correspond to moderate intense soft tissues along the course of the external auditory canal (*arrowheads*). Clinical inspection shows the presence of sebum along the walls of the external auditory canal

84 %, respectively, in patients prior to second-look surgery. With this high PPV, it was concluded that a nodular hyper-intensity on EP DW sequence equalled cholesteatoma provided that artefacts were not misinterpreted as cholesteatoma (Vercruysse et al. 2006). However, this very low sensitivity tempered the initial enthusiasm over EP DW sequences.

This low sensitivity could be explained by the fact that in this last study patients were not preselected based upon CT. Moreover, only residual cholesteatoma were included.

The studies by Aikele et al. (Aikele et al. 2003) and Stassola et al. (Maheshwari and Mukherji 2002) both incorporated a combination of residual and recurrent cholesteatoma finally resulting in a patient population with cholesteatoma of a larger size. One of the most imported conclusions of the paper of Vercruysse et al. was that EP DW sequences are unable to detect cholesteatoma smaller than 5 mm and that its sensitivity can be augmented by using the combination with standard sequences (Vercruysse et al. 2006). Numerous papers have in the mean time confirmed this size limit of 5 mm using EP DW sequences (Jeunen et al. 2008; Venail et al. 2008; Toyama et al. 2008; Emonot et al. 2008). It was concluded that EP DW sequences were unable to replace second-look surgery.

By using the combination of non-EP DW sequences and delayed gadolinium enhanced T1-weighted images, De Foer et al. reported a size limit for detection of cholesteatoma of 2 mm as well as prior to first stage surgery (De Foer et al. 2007) as well as prior to second stage surgery (De Foer et al. 2008). Reported sensitivity in patients prior to second-look surgery was 90 % with a specificity of 100 %. PPV was 100 % with an NPV of 96 %. It was concluded that the combination of delayed gadolinium-enhanced T1-weighted sequences with non-EP DW sequences could replace second-look surgery avoiding unnecessary surgical interventions. The superiority of non-EP DW sequences over EP DW sequences has been reported in several other papers (Dhepnorrarat et al. 2009; Rajan et al. 2010; Huins et al. 2010; Khemani et al. 2011; Dremmen et al. 2012).

In three meta-analyses of the recent literature it was concluded that non-EP DW sequences such as half-Fourier acquisition single-shot turbo spin echo sequences are more reliable in identifying residual or recurrent cholesteatoma compared to EP DW sequences (Aarts et al. 2010; Jindal et al. 2011; Li 2013).

In another paper, De Foer et al. concluded that non-EP DW sequences can be used as a stand-alone sequence for the diagnosis of middle ear cholesteatoma and that the use of added, delayed and gadolinium-enhanced T1-weighted sequences does not yield a higher sensitivity, specificity, PPV or NPV (De Foer et al. 2010b, c).

A state-of the art MRI protocol for cholesteatoma detection currently comprises a $b0$ and $b1000$ non-EP DW sequence with ADC map and an axial and coronal T2-weighted sequence in order to localise any suspected hyper-intensities on the DW sequence (Fig. 6) (Li 2013; De Foer et al. 2010b, c).

It is nowadays also considered the routine practice to select patients for second-look surgery using the above-mentioned non-EP DW MRI. In these cases, CT scanning is preserved for the immediate preoperative setting (Figs. 6, 7). By doing so, the number of useless operated patients will drop significantly as well as the number of useless irradiated patients prior to second-look surgery (De Foer et al. 2010b, c).

5.5.3 The Issue of False Positives and False Negatives

There are two major causes of false negative examinations.

Motion artefacts can cause false negative examinations and are most frequently reported in children. The high signal intensity of small lesions will be dispersed by motion over multiple pixels causing a lack of high signal intensity (De Foer et al. 2008).

The other—most important cause—is the emptying of the cholesteatoma sack. The high signal intensity of the cholesteatoma is caused by the exfoliated keratin in the cholesteatoma sack (De Foer et al. 2008). Sebum cysts—which are also filled with keratin—can be located in the skin around the external ear, and can present with a nodular high signal intensity (Fig. 11). However, these sebum cysts are clearly located outside the temporal bone pyramid. In incidental cases the external auditory canal can be seen as linear hyper-intensities on $b1000$ non-EP DW sequences due to adherent sebum and keratine along the external auditory canal (Fig. 12).

A cholesteatoma sack can empty through the external auditory canal, either by itself either by suction cleaning by the ENT surgeon. In both cases, the nodular high signal intensity will no longer be visible (Fig. 5). In the literature, this type of cholesteatoma is also called mural cholesteatoma (Baràth et al. 2011). It should be noted that in these cases, the cholesteatoma epithelium or matrix is still adherent to the walls of the middle ear or mastoid. Theoretically, one should be able to see this matrix or cholesteatoma epithelium on T1-weighted images due to its enhancement but delineation of the enhancing epithelium is sometimes very difficult due to the surrounding inflammation.

However, in most cases, the ENT surgeon will suspect these so-called empty cholesteatoma sac at otoscopy.

The few false-positive cases with DWI described in the literature turned out to be acute otitis media, bone powder, scar tissue, a silastic sheet, granulation tissue, cholesterol granuloma and endocrine adenoma (Baràth et al. 2011). In clinical practice, cholesterol granuloma is the most frequent entity displaying a possible high intensity on $b1000$ DW images probably due to T2-shine through effect.

Most of these entities display a hyper-intensity on un-enhanced T1-weighted images contrary to the low intensity of cholesteatoma.

Correlation to ADC maps will show a clear drop in signal in case of cholesteatoma contrary to the persistent high signal of inflammation and/or cholesterol granuloma.

Correlation to ADC maps is hence obligatory (Mas-Estelles et al. 2012; Lingam et al. 2013).

References

Aarts MC, Rovers MM, Van Der Veen EL et al (2010) The diagnostic value of diffusion-weighted magnetic resonance imaging in detecting a residual cholesteatoma. Otolaryngol Head Neck Surg 143:12–16

Aikele P, Kittner T, Offergeld C et al (2003) Diffusion-weighted MR imaging of cholesteatoma in pediatric and adult patients who have undergone middle ear surgery. Am J Roentgenol 181:261–265

Ayache D, Williams MT, Lejeune D et al (2005) Usefullness of delayed postcontrast magnetic resonance imaging in the detection of residual cholesteatoma after canal wall-up tympanoplasty. Laryngoscope 115:607–610

Baràth K, Huber AM, Stämpfli P et al (2011) Neuroradiology of cholesteatomas. AJNR Am J Neuroradiol 32:221–229 Epub 2010 Apr 1

Blaney SP, Tierney P, Oyarazabal M, Bowdler DA (2001) CT scanning in "second look" combined approach tympanoplasty. Rev Laryngol Otol Rhinol (Bord) 121:79–81

Brenner DJ, Hall EJ (2007) Computed Tomography—an increasing source of radiation exposure. N Engl J Med 357:2277–2284

Brown JS (1982) A ten year statistical follow-up of 1142 consecutive cases of cholesteatoma: the closed versus the open technique. Laryngoscope 92:390–396

Darrouzet V, Duclos JY, Portmann D et al (2000) Preference for the closed technique in management of cholesteatoma of the middle ear in children: a retrospective study of 215 consecutive patients treated over 10 years. Am J Otol 21:474–481

Darrouzet V, Duclos JY, Portmann D et al (2002) Congenital middle ear cholesteatoma in children: our experience in 34 cases. Otolaryngol Head Neck Surg 126:34–40

De Foer B, Vercruysse JP, Pilet B et al (2006) Single-shot, turbo spin-echo, diffusion-weighted imaging versus spin-echo-planar, diffusion-weighted imaging in the detection of acquired middle ear cholesteatoma. Am J Neuroradiol 27:1480–1482

De Foer B, Vercruysse JP, Bernaerts A et al (2007) The value of single-shot turbo spin-echo difusion-weighted MR imaging in the detection of middle ear cholesteatoma. Neuroradiology 28:230–234

De Foer B, Vercruysse JP, Bernaert A et al (2008) Detection of postoperative residual cholesteatoma with non-echo-planar diffusion-weighted magnetic resonance imaging. Otol Neurotol 29: 513–517

De Foer B, Vercruysse JP, Spaepen M et al (2010a) Diffusion-weighted magnetic resonance imaging of the temporal bone. Neuroradiology 52:785–807 Epub 2010 Jul 15

De Foer B, Vercruysse JP, Bernaert A et al (2010b) Middle ear cholesteatoma: non-echo-planar diffusion-weighted MRI imaging versus delayed gadolinium-enhanced T1-weighted MR imaging: value in detection. Radiology 255:866–872

De Foer B, Vercruysse JP, Spaepen M et al (2010c) Diffusion-weighted magnetic resonance imaging of the temporal bone. Neuroradiology 52:785–807

Denoyelle F, Silberman B, Garabedian EN (1994) Value of magnetic resonance imaging associated with X-ray computed tomography in the screening of residual cholesteatoma after primary surgery. Ann Otolaryngol Chir Cervicofac 111:85–88

Dhepnorrarat RC, Wood B, Rajan GP (2009) Postoperative non-echo-planar diffusion-weighted magnetic resonance imaging after cholesteatoma surgery: implications for cholesteatoma screening. Otol Neurotol 30:54–58

Dremmen MH, Hofman PA, Hof JR (2012) The diagnostic accuray of non-echo-planar diffusion-weighted imaging in the detection of residual and/or recurrent cholesteatoma of the temporal bone. Am J Neuroradiol 33:439–444

Du Verney JG (1683) Traité de l'Organe de l'Ouie. Paris: E. Michaillet

Emonot G, Veyret C, Dumollard JM et al (2008) Apport de l'imagerie aud diagnostic de cholesteatome residuel. Fr ORL 94:366–374

Fitzek C, Mewes T, Fitzek S et al (2002) Diffusion-weighted MRI of cholesteatoma of the petrous bone. J Magn Reson Imaging 15:636–641

Huins CT, Singh A, Lingam RK et al (2010) Detecting cholesteatoma with non-echo planar (HASTE) diffusion-weighted magnetic resonance imaging. Otolaryngol Head Neck Surg 143:141–148

Jeunen G, Desloovere C, Hermans R (2008) The value of magnetic resonance imaging in the diagnosis of residual or recurrent acquired cholesteatoma after canal wall-up tympanoplasty. Otol Neurotol 29:16–18

Jindal M, Riskalla A, Jiang D et al (2011) A systematic review of diffusion-weighted magnetic resonance imaging in the assessment of postoperative cholesteatoma. Otol Neurotol 32:1243–1249

Khemani S, Lingam RK, Kalan A et al (2011) The value of non-echo planar HASTE diffusion-weighted MR imaging in the detection, localisation and prediction of extent of postoperative cholesteatoma. Clin Otolaryngol 36:306–312

Kimitsuki T, Suda Y, Kawano H et al (2001) Correlation between MRI findings and second-look operation in cholesteatoma surgery. ORL J Otorhinolaryngol Relat Spec 63:291–293

Lehmann P, Saliou G, Brocart C et al (2009) 3 T MR imaging of postoperative recurrent middle ear cholesteatoma: value of periodically rotated overlapping parallel lines with enhanced reconstruction diffusion-weighted MR imaging. Am J Neuroradiol 30:423–427

Lemmerling M, De Foer B (2001) Imaging of cholesteatomatous and non-cholesteatomatous middle ear disease. In: Lemmerling M, Kollias SS (eds) Radiology of the petrous bone. Springer, New York, pp 31–47

Lemmerling MM, De Foer B, Vandevyver V et al (2008) Imaging of the opacified middle ear. Eur J Radiol 66:363–371

Li PM, Linos E, Gurgel RK et al (2013) Evaluating the utility of non-echo-planar diffusion-weighted imaging in the preoperative evaluation of cholesteatoma: a meta-analysis. Laryngoscope 123:1247–1250

Lingam RK, Khatri P, Hughes J et al (2013). Apparent diffusion coefficients for detection of postoperative middle ear cholesteatoma on non-echo-planar diffusion-weighted images. Radiol 269:504–510

Maheshwari S, Mukherji SK (2002) Diffusion-weighted imaging for differentiating recurrent cholesteatoma from granulation tissue after mastoidectomy: case report. Am J Neuroradiol 23:847–849

Martin N, Sterkers O, Nahum H (1990) Chronic inflammatory disease of the middle ear cavities: Gd-DTPA-enhanced imaging. Radiology 176:399–405

Mas-Estelles F, Mateos-Fernandez M, Carrascosa-Bisquert B et al (2012) Contemporary non-echo-planar diffusion-weighted imaging of middle ear cholesteatomas. Radiographics 32:1197–1213

Müller J (1838) Ueber den feineren Bau und die formen der krankhaften Geschwülste. G. Reimer, Berlin

Nelson M, Roger G, Koltai PJ et al (2002) Congenital cholesteatoma: classification, management, and outcome. Arch Otolaryngol Head Neck Surg 128:810–814

Offeciers E, Vercruysse JP, De Foer B et al (2008) Mastoid and epitympanic obliteration. The obliteration technique. In: Ars B (ed) Chronic Otitis Media. Pathogenesis Oriented Therapeutic Treatment. Kugler, Amsterdam, pp 299-327

Rajan GP, Ambett R, Wun L et al (2010) Preliminary outcomes of cholesteatoma screening in children using non-echo-planar diffusion-weighted magnetic resonance imaging. Int J Pediatric Otorhinolaryngol 74:297–301

Schilder AG, Govaerts PJ, Somers T et al (1997) Tympano-ossicular allografts for cholesteatoma in children. Int J Pediatr Otorhinolaryngol 42:31–40

Sheehy JL, Brackmann DE, Graham MD (1977) Cholesteatoma surgery: residual and recurrent disease. A review of 1,024 cases. Ann Otol Rhinol Laryngol 86:451–462

Shelton C, Sheehy JL (1990) Tympanoplasty: review of 400 staged cases. Laryngoscope 100:679–681

Stasolla A, Magliulo G, Parrott D et al (2004) Detection of postoperative relapsing/residual cholesteatomas with diffusion-weighted echo-planar magnetic resonance imaging. Otol Neurotol 25:679–684

Tierney PA, Pracy P, Blaney SP et al (1999) An assessment of the value of the preoperative computed tomography scans prior to otoendoscopic 'second look' in intact canal wall mastoid surgery. Clin Otolaryngol Allied Sci 24:274–276

Toyama C, Leite Cda C, Barauna Filho IS et al (2008) The role of magnetic resonance imaging in the postoperative management of cholesteatomas. Braz J Otorhinolaryngol 74:693–696

Vanden Abeele D, Coen E, Parizel PM et al (1999) Can MRI replace a second look operation in cholesteatoma surgery. Acta Otolaryngol 119:555–561

Venail F, Bonafe A, Poirrier V et al (2008) Comparison of echo-planar diffusion-weighted imaging and delayed postcontrast T1-weighted MR imaging for the detection of residual cholesteatoma Am. J Neuroradiol 29:1363–1368

Vercruysse JP, De Foer B, Pouillon M et al (2006) The value of diffusion-weighted MR imaging in the diagnosis of primary acquired and residual cholesteatoma: a surgical verified study of 100 patients. Eur Radiol 16:1461–1467

Vercruysse JP, De Foer B, Somers T et al (2008) Mastoid and epitympanic bony obliteration in pediatric cholesteatoma. Otol Neurotol 829:953–960

Williams MT, Ayache D, Alberti C et al (2003) Detection of postoperative residual cholesteatoma with delayed contrast-enhanced MR-imaging: initial findings. Eur Radiol 13:169–174

Otosclerosis

Marc Lemmerling

Contents

1 Etiology and Categories 89
2 CT/CBCT and MRI Appearance 93
3 Differential Diagnosis 94
4 The Cochlear Cleft: Potential Imaging Pitfall in Children 95
References 95

Abstract

Otosclerosis is a disorder of the bony labyrinth with usual onset in the third decade. The disease is bilateral in a majority of cases and such patients have conductive hearing loss. In case of fenestral otosclerosis hypodense foci are seen on CT/CBCT just anterior to the oval window, at the so-called fissula ante fenestram region. In case of retrofenestral otosclerosis additional foci are seen in the otic capsule around the cochlea.

1 Etiology and Categories

Otosclerosis is a disorder of the bony labyrinth and exclusively affects human beings. In otosclerosis, the ivory-like enchondral bone of the otic capsule is replaced by immature and spongy new bone, and this process of remodeling occurs continuously. The process can become quiescent at any time or may become reactivated, in a way that otosclerotic foci commonly contain both active and inactive regions (Schuknecht 1993a). Unilateral involvement is only seen in about 10–15 % of the cases and there is a 2:1 female predominance. The risk to an affected person of having a child who will eventually develop otosclerosis is 1 in 4 (Donnell and Alfi 1980; Shin et al. 2001a). In comparison with patients with a sporadic form of otosclerosis, the radiologic lesions are more often detectable, bilateral, and severe in the familial forms (Shin et al. 2001a).

Otosclerosis usually has its clinical onset in the third decade, with symptoms of conductive hearing loss due to the impaired movement of the stapes by invasion of the stapediovestibular articulation. Under the age of 18 years old the diagnosis is rarely made (Lescanne et al. 2008). Fixation of the stapes by foci located anterior to the oval window—in the so-called region of the fissula ante fenestram—is found in 96 % of ears from persons with clinical otosclerosis. In 49 % of the cases, otosclerotic foci are also present in other locations, of which the most frequent ones are the oval window

M. Lemmerling (✉)
Department of Radiology, AZ St.-Lucas Hospital, Groenebriel 1, 9000 Gent, Belgium
e-mail: marc.lemmerling@azstlucas.be

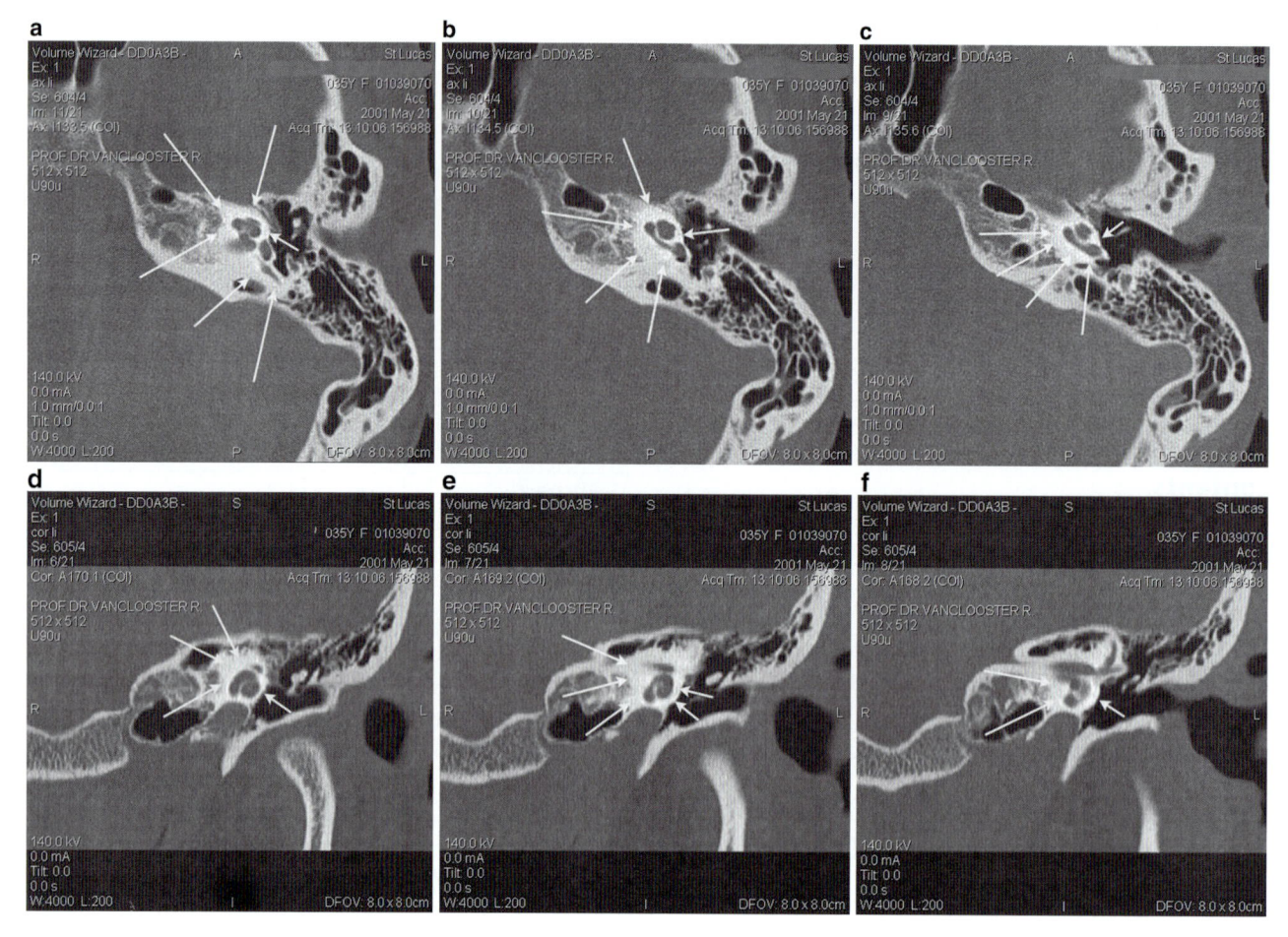

Fig. 1 Three consecutive axial (**a**–**c**) and coronal (**d**–**f**) CT images are shown in a nonotospongiotic ear to insist on the careful inspection of the dense appearance of the normal bone in many regions. It is very important to systematically inspect the region of the fissula ante fenestram on the axial image set, situated just anterior to the oval window and anterior stapes crus, in order to be sure that fenestral otosclerosis is excluded (*small arrows* on images **a**–**c**). The same region can be inspected on the coronal images too (*small arrows* on images **d**–**f**). An intensely high density must be present in the otic capsule region surrounding the cochlea, in order to be sure that cochlear otosclerosis is excluded (*large arrows* on images **a**–**f**)

Fig. 2 The axial CT image at oval window level shows a hypodense region of otosclerotic origin in the footplate itself, and anterior to the oval window (*arrows*). Note that the footplate is thickened

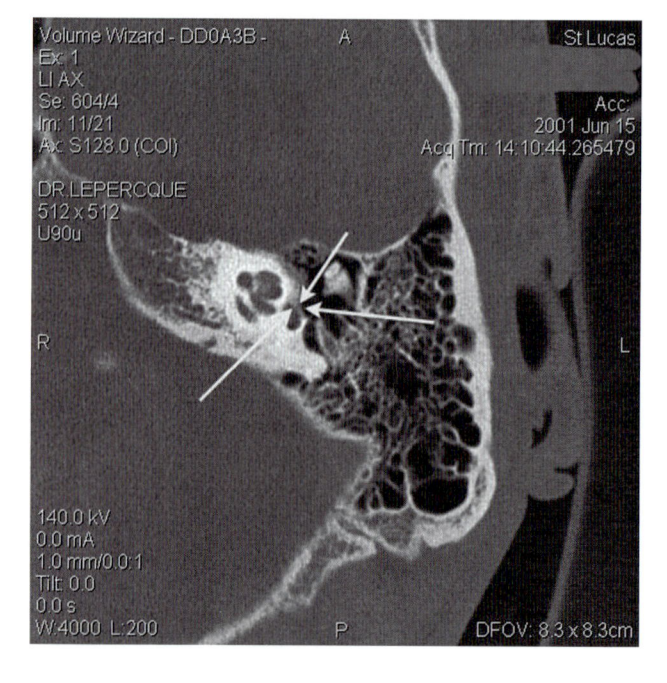

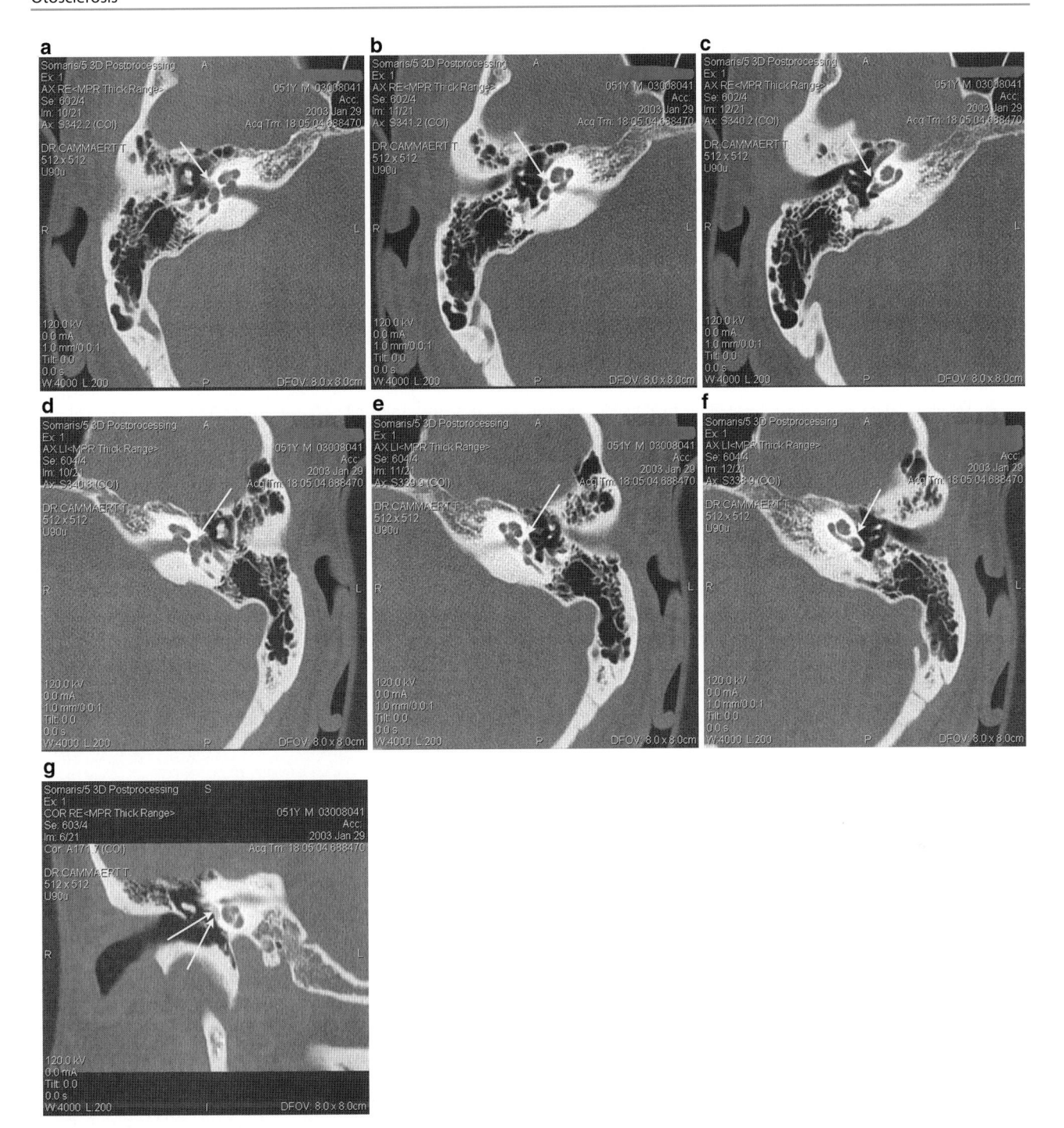

Fig. 3 In the right ear three consecutive CT images (**a–c**) show a lucent area just anterior to and extending to the oval window: fenestral otosclerosis (*arrow*). In the same patient, the normal contralateral ear is shown. Note the normal high density anterior to the footplate (**d–f**). In this same patient, a coronal reconstruction (**g**) obviously depicts the otospongiotic focus in the region of the promontory (*arrows*)

niche (30 %), the cochlear apex (12 %), and posterior to the oval window (12 %). Round window obliteration is seen in 7 % of ears with clinical otosclerosis. Other even rarer sites of involvement are the walls of the internal auditory canal, around the cochlear aqueduct, around the semicircular canals, and within the footplate (Schuknecht and Barber 1985). Incus and malleus invasion each have been reported once, and the internal auditory canal itself is never invaded. Invasion of the labyrinthine spaces rarely occurs (Schuknecht 1993a). The extension of otosclerosis as seen on CT/CBCT scans seems to generally correlate with the preoperative and postoperative hearing loss (Marx et al. 2011).

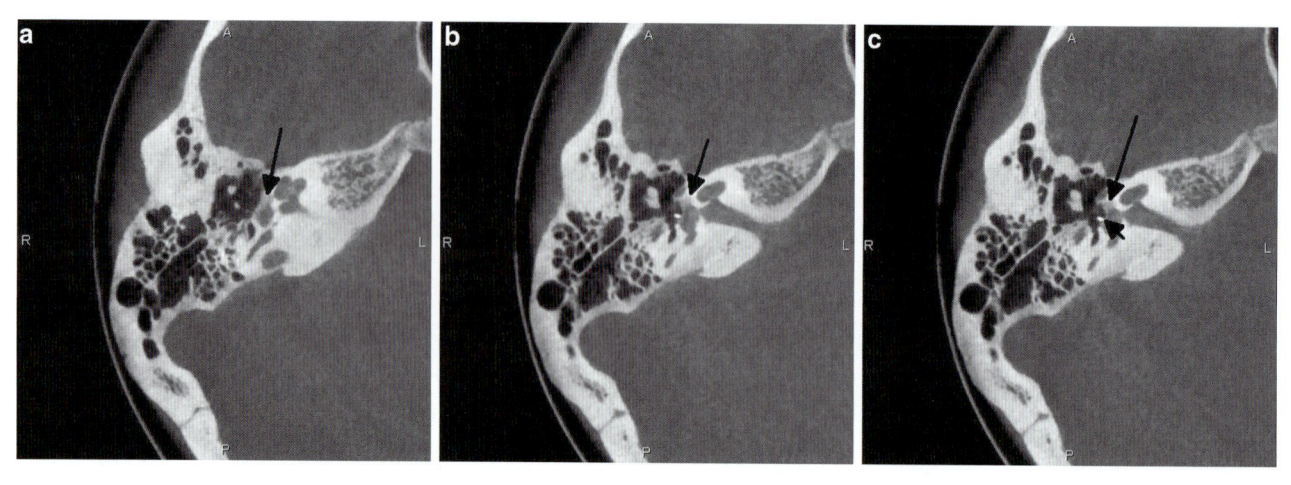

Fig. 4 On these axial CBCT images (**a–c**) of the right middle ear, a hypodense focus of otosclerosis is nicely depicted in the region just anterior to the oval window (*large arrow*). The patient is treated with a stapes prosthesis (*small arrow*)

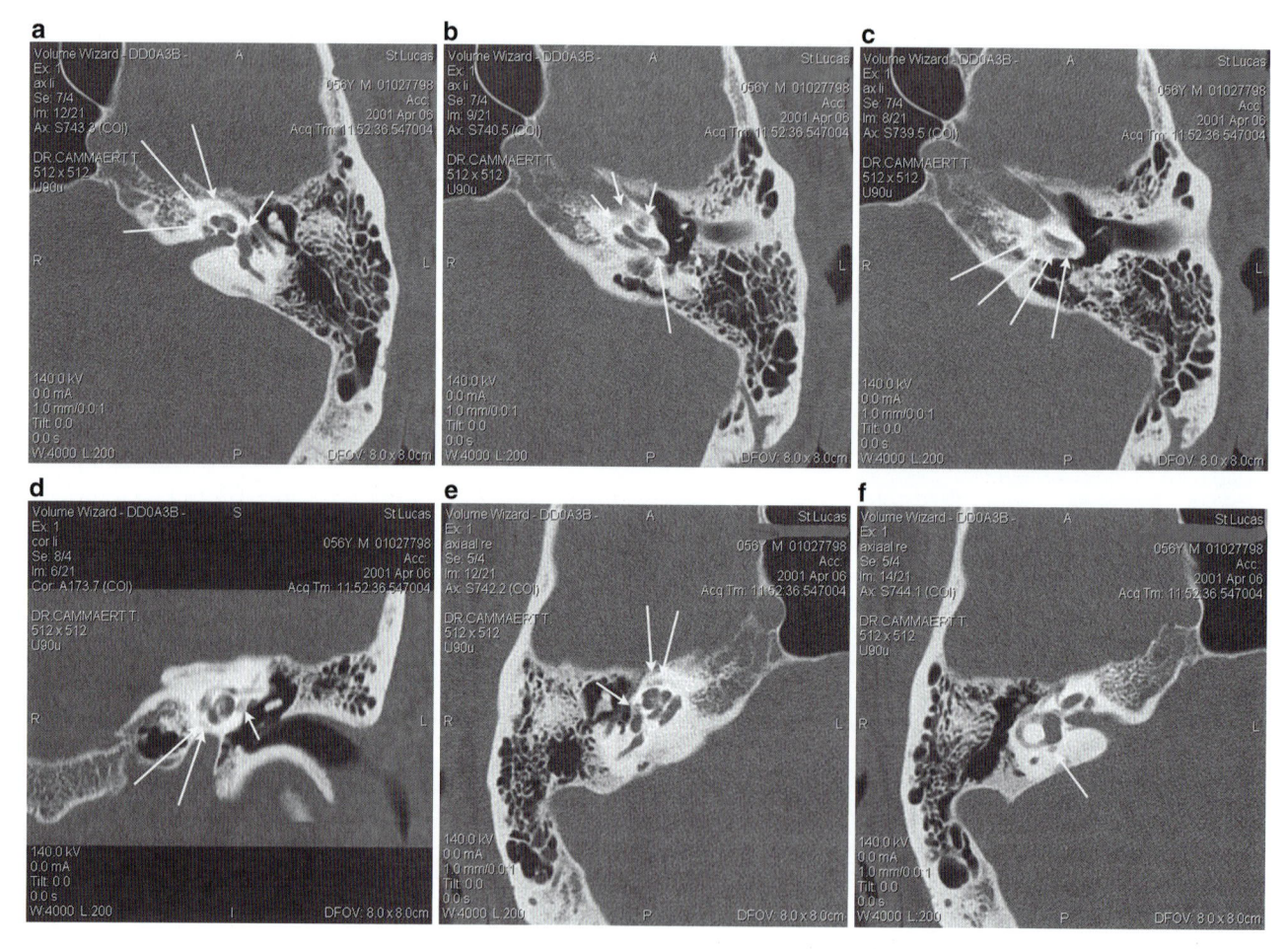

Fig. 5 Multiple CT images are shown from a patient with bilateral fenestral and retrofenestral otosclerosis. On the most cranial axial image on the left side (**a**) lucencies of otosclerotic origin are seen around the cochlea (*large arrows*) and anterior to the oval window (*small arrow*). On the image below (**b**) cochlear otosclerosis is seen medial to the apical and middle cochlear turns (*small arrows*), but also around the basal cochlear turn, and in the round window region (*large arrows*). On the slice more caudally (**c**) more otosclerotic foci are obviously present around the basal turn of the cochlea. The coronal image from the same left ear confirms the presence of fenestral (*small arrow*) and retrofenestral (*large arrows*) foci of otosclerosis (**d**). In the contralateral right ear, the axial image performed at footplate level (**e**) shows more otosclerotic lucencies at the fissula ante fenestram (*small arrow*) and in the pericochlear otic capsule (*large arrows*). On the slice performed 2 mm more caudally (**f**) otosclerosis is seen posterior to the vestibule (*arrow*)

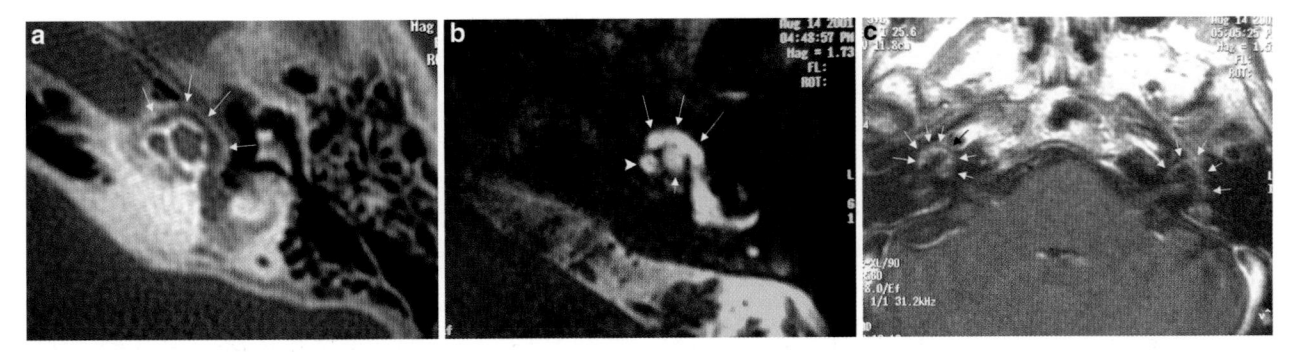

Fig. 6 The axial CT image at the level of the middle and apical turns of the left cochlea (**a**) shows otosclerotic changes around the cochlea: the so-called fourth ring of Valvassori is seen (*arrows*). The axial 3D FSE T2-weighted image at the same level (**b**) again demonstrates the fourth ring of Valvassori (*large arrows*), now seen as a semicircular hyperintensity around the middle (*arrowhead*) and apical (*small arrow*) turns of the cochlea. On the axial contrast-enhanced T1-weighted image through both inner ears (**c**) diffuse semicircular enhancement is noted around the cochlea bilaterally: the diagnosis of bilateral severe retrofenestral otosclerosis in the active phase can be made (Courtesy by Dr. B. Defoer, Antwerp, Belgium)

Sensorineural hearing loss can be seen in patients with otosclerosis, and is believed to be caused by the accumulation in the inner ear of products liberated by the growth of the otosclerotic foci that are present in the pericochlear region (Schuknecht 1993a). In patients with pericochlear otosclerotic foci, sensorineural hearing loss is present with a higher degree (Guneri et al. 1996).

Many authors have used CT grading systems of otosclerosis in their studies. Some authors grade on the basis of disease site and progression (Valvassori 1993), or on the basis of disease site with subdivision of these different sites (Shin et al. 2001b), whereas others categorize the presence of otosclerosis on the basis of the location and appearance of the disease (Marshall et al. 2005). We use a simple system with two categories of otosclerosis described on the basis of where the anomalies are seen: fenestral and retrofenestral otosclerosis. As the name suggests (fenestra is the latin word for window) fenestral otosclerosis affects the lateral labyrinthine wall, including the promontory, facial nerve canal, and both the oval and round window niche (Swartz and Harnsberger 1992). Retrofenestral otosclerosis involves the pericochlear otic capsule and is almost always present together with fenestral otosclerosis. For this latter reason it is better to use the term retrofenestral otosclerosis than cochlear otosclerosis, another term also in use.

2 CT/CBCT and MRI Appearance

CT or CBCT is the tool of choice to investigate for the eventual presence of otosclerotic lesions (Weissman 1996), and its sensitivity to make the diagnosis was recently estimated as high as about 90–95 % (Lagleyre et al. 2009). Both axial and coronal images are performed in order to give a detailed description of the extent and location of the lesions. During the reading of the CT/CBCT images, inspection for contralateral otosclerotic foci is always mandatory, even in case of unilateral clinical findings. CBCT allows to make images with a higher spatial resolution than does CT, and this is achieved with a much lower radiation dose.

In normal circumstances, the bone of the otic capsule is homogeneously dense (Fig. 1). The otosclerotic foci contain spongy new bone, which appears lucent on CT/CBCT (Valvassori and Dobben 1985; Miura et al. 1996). These are seen in the medial wall of the labyrinth in case of fenestral otosclerosis (Mafee et al. 1985a). It is important to inspect the region of the fissula ante fenestram very carefully, since otosclerotic foci can be very small. Especially, the axial images will be helpful to do so. In some cases, footplate thickening is noted (Veillon et al. 2001) (Figs. 2, 3, and 4). Additional foci of retrofenestral otosclerosis can be seen in the otic capsule around the cochlea (Mafee et al. 1985b) (Fig. 5). It is important to notice round window localizations, since these can obliterate the window and cause problems to insert a cochlear implant. In extensive cases of retrofenestral otosclerosis, a so-called 'fourth ring of Valvassori' is described (Figs. 6 and 7).

MRI is sporadically used in case of otosclerosis. Otosclerosis very often leads to severe hearing loss in a chronic progressive manner. Initially an otospongiotic phase takes place and causes an inflammatory osteolytic process in the otic capsule. During this 'active' phase, the otospongiotic foci will enhance on T1-weighted SE MRI images performed after IV injection of gadolinium (Ziyeh et al. 1997; Stimmer et al. 2002). On the T1-weighted images before gadolinium injection, a ring of intermediate signal can be present in the pericochlear and perilabyrinthine regions, and an increased signal may also be seen on the T2-weighted images (Goh et al. 2002) (Fig. 6). MRI has also proven its usefulness in the investigation of complications of stapes surgery performed for otosclerosis. Some of these complications, such as reparative intravestibular

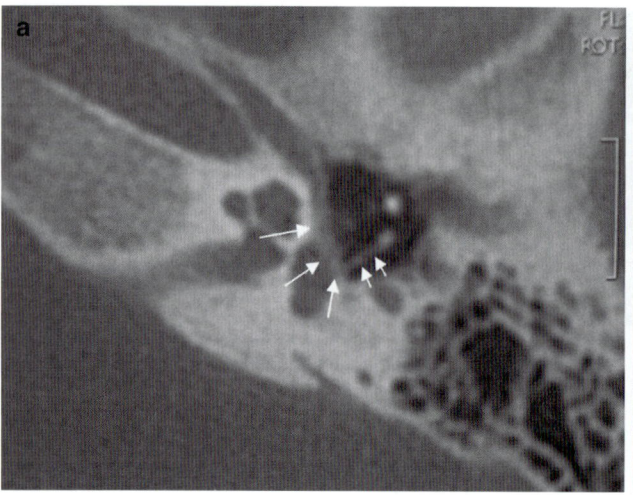

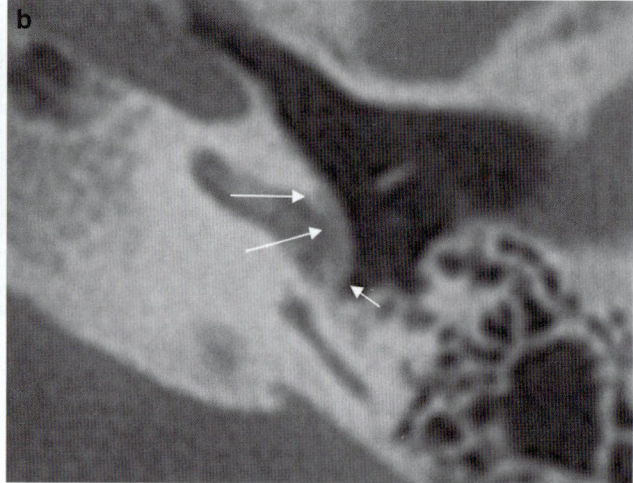

Fig. 7 The axial CT image at the level of the oval window (**a**) shows an otosclerosis focus at the fissula ante fenestram extending over the oval window, and with diffuse and severe thickening of the footplate (*large arrows*). Note the postoperative status with stapedectomie and replacement by a piston, posteriorly displaced (*small arrows*). The axial CT image at the level of the basal cochlear turn and round window (**b**) demonstrates the extension of the otosclerotic changes over the promontory toward the round window niche (*large arrows*). There is extension of the otosclerotic changes to the round window with total obliteration of the access to the round window (*small arrow*), thus making a later cochlear implantation virtually impossible (Courtesy by Dr. B. Defoer, Antwerp, Belgium)

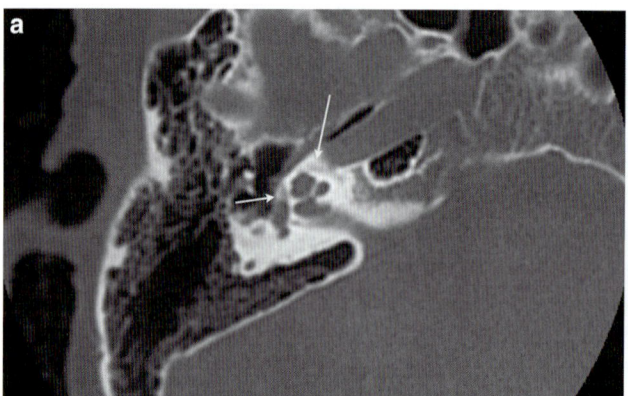

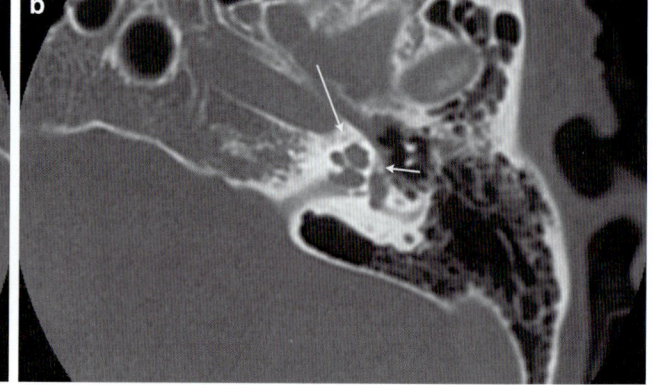

Fig. 8 The axial CT images at footplate level are shown in both temporal bones from a patient with proved osteogenesis imperfecta. Note that the bone in the region of the fissula ante fenestram (*small arrow*) and in the pericochlear region (*large arrow*) has become lucent. The CT findings do not differ from those seen in patients with combined fenestral and retrofenestral otosclerosis (Courtesy by Dr. B Defoer, Antwerp, Belgium)

granuloma formation, intralabyrinthine hemorrhage, and bacterial labyrinthitis are detectable with MRI, while they pass unrecognized on CT/CBCT examinations (Rangheard et al. 2001).

3 Differential Diagnosis

Osteogenesis imperfecta is a rare disease and is often associated with hearing loss. It is an inherited generalized disorder of type-I collagen synthesis (Zajtchuk and Lindsay 1975; Berghstrom 1981; Berger et al. 1985; Schuknecht 1993b). The classic triad of blue sclerae, spontaneous fractures, and hearing loss is known as the Van der Hoeve and De Kleyn syndrome (Schuknecht 1993b; Czerny and Temmel 1999). The CT/CBCT appearance can be undistinguishable from otosclerosis, with lucent bone anterior to the oval window and in the pericochlear otic capsule (Fig. 8). On MRI similar findings have been described as those seen in the active phase of otosclerosis: pericochlear soft tissue signal intensities and enhancement after contrast injection (Ziyeh et al. 2000).

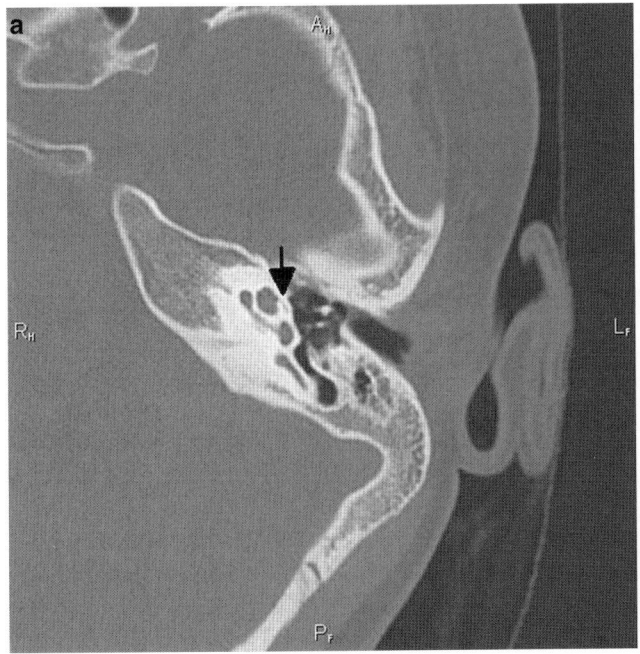

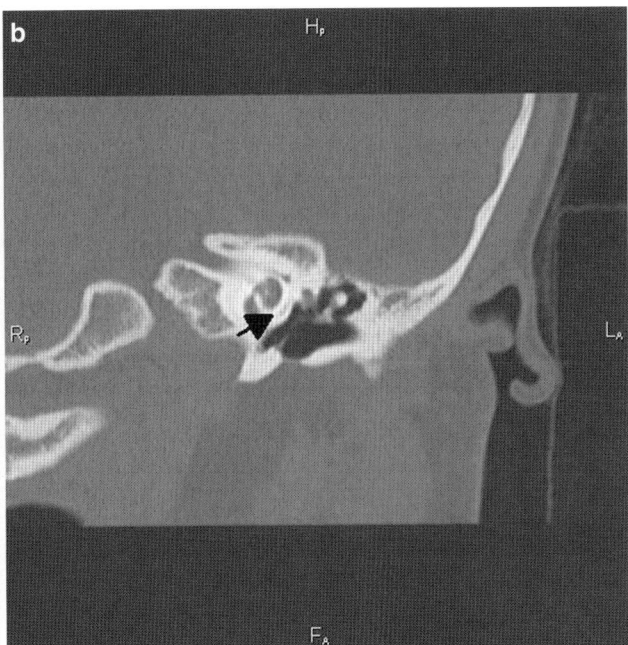

Fig. 9 On the axial CT image (**a**) in a 10-year-old child performed in the region of the fissula ante fenestram, the hypointense C-shaped cochlear cleft is noted in the otic capsule. On the corresponding coronal image (**b**) the cochlear cleft often has a more linear shape

Paget disease is another condition to be excluded if a decreased attenuation is seen in the otic capsule (Mafee et al. 1985b).

4   The Cochlear Cleft: Potential Imaging Pitfall in Children

The so-called 'cochlear cleft' is a hypodense cleft in the cochlear otic capsule seen on CT/CBCT examinations in the region anterior to the oval window. It is particularly seen in children with an average incidence of about 40 % (age group from 0.5 to 19.3 years old) (Chadwell et al. 2004). Another group of investigators noted an incidence of 32 % in a pediatric population aged between 0 and 9 years old (Pekkola et al. 2004). Its incidence decreases with age. The finding is believed to be a space in the interface between the endosteal and outer layers of the otic capsule or that it is related to the fissula ante fenestram (Fig. 9). The finding does not have any pathological implication in the absence of a clinical evidence for otosclerosis or osteogenesis imperfecta.

References

Berger G, Hawke M, Johnson A, Proops D (1985) Histopathology of the temporal bone in osteogenesis imperfecta congenita: a report of 5 cases. Laryngoscope 95(2):193–199

Bergstrom L (1981) Fragile bones and fragile ears. Clin Orthop 159:58–63

Chadwell JB, Halsted MJ, Choo DI, Greinwald JH, Benton C (2004) The cochlear cleft. AJNR Am J Neuroradiol 25:21–24

Czerny C, Temmel AF (1999) Osteogenesis imperfecta tarda with association of the inner ear also called Van Hoeve-Klein-syndrome. Eur J Radiol 30(2):162–164

Donnell GN, Alfi OS (1980) Medical genetics for the otorhinolaryngologist. Laryngoscope 90:40–46

Ea Guneri, Ada E, Ceryan K, Guneri A (1996) High-resolution computed tomographic evaluation of the cochlear capsule in otosclerosis: relationscihp between densitometry and sensorineural hearing loss. Ann Otol Rhinol Laryngol 105(8):659–664

Goh JP, Chan LL, Tan TY (2002) MRI of cochlear otosclerosis. Br J Radiol 75(894):502–505

Lagleyre S, Sorrentino T, Calmels MN, Shin YJ, Escudé B, Deguine O, Fraysse B (2009) Reliability of high-resolution CT scan in diagnosis of otosclerosis. Otol neurotol 30(8):1152–1159

Lescanne E, Bakhos D, Metais JP, Robier A, Moriniere S (2008) Otosclerosis in children and adolescents: a clinical and CT-scan survey with review of the literature. Int J Pediatr Otorhinolaryngol 72(2):147–152

Mafee MF, Henrikson GC, Deitch RL, Norouzi P, Kumar A, Kriz R, Valvassori GE (1985a) Use of CT in stapedial otosclerosis. Radiology 156(3):709–714

Mafee MF, Valvassori GE, Deitch RL, Norouzi P, Henrikson GC, Capek V, Applebaum EL (1985b) Use of CT in the evaluation of cochlear otosclerosis. Radiology 156(3):703–708

Marshall AH, Fanning N, Symons S, Shipp D, Chen JM, Nedzelski JM (2005) Cochlear implantation in cochlear otosclerosis. Laryngoscope 115:1728–1733

Marx M, Lagleyre S, Escudé B, Demeslay J, Elhadi T, Deguine O, Fraysse B (2011) Correlations between CT scan findings and hearing thresholds in otosclerosis. Acta Otolaryngol 131(4):351–357

Miura M, Naito Y, Takahashi H, Honjo I (1996) Computed tomographic image analysis of ears with otosclerosis. ORL J Otorhinolaryngol Relat Spec 58(4):200–203

Pekkola J, Pitkäranta A, Jappel A, Czerny C, Baumgartner WD, Heliövaara M, Robinson S (2004) Localized pericochlear hypoattenuating foci at temporal-bone thin-section CT in pediatric patients: nonpathologic differential diagnostic entity. Radiology 230:88–92

Rangheard AS, Marsot-Dupuch K, Mark AS, Meyer B, Tubiana JM (2001) Postoperative complications in otospongiosis: usefulness of MR imaging. AJNR Am J Neuroradiol 22(6):1171–1178

Schuknecht HF (1993a) Disorders of bone. In: Bussy RK (ed) Pathology of the ear, 2nd edn. Lea and Febiger, Philadelphia, pp 365–379

Schuknecht HF (1993b) Disorders of bone. In: Bussy RK (ed) Pathology of the ear, 2nd edn. Lea and Febiger, Philadelphia, pp 390–392

Schuknecht HF, Barber W (1985) Histologic variants in otosclerosis. Laryngoscope 95:1307–1317

Shin YJ, Calvas P, Deguine O, Charlet JP, Cognard C, Fraysse B (2001a) Correlations between computed tomography findings and family history in otosclerotic patients. Otol Neurotol 22(4):461–464

Shin YJ, Fraysse B, Deguine O, Cognard C, Charlet JP, Sévely A (2001b) Sensorineural hearing loss and otosclerosis: a clinical and radiological survey of 437 cases. Acta Otolaryngol 121:200–204

Stimmer H, Arnold W, Schwaiger M, Laubenacher C (2002) Magnetic resonance imaging and high-resolution computed tomography in the otospongiotic phase of otosclerosis. ORL J Otorhinolaryngol Relat Spec 64(6):451–453

Swartz JD, Harnsberger HR (1992) The otic capsule and otodystrophies. In: Imaging of the temporal bone, 2nd edn. Thieme Medical Publishers, New York, pp 227–242

Valvassori GE (1993) Imaging of otosclerosis. Otolaryngol Clin North Am 26:359–371

Valvassori GE, Dobben GD (1985) CT densitometry of the cochlear capsule in otosclerosis. AJNR Am J Neuroradiol 6(5):661–667

Veillon F, Riehm S, Emachescu B, Haba D, Roedlich MN, Greget M, Tongio J (2001) Imaging of the windows of the temporal bone. Semin Ultrasound CT MR 22(3):271–280

Weissman JL (1996) Hearing loss. Radiology 199(3):593–611

Zajtchuk JT, Lindsay JR (1975) Osteogenisis imperfecta congenital and tarda: a temporal bone report. Ann Otol Rhinol Laryngol 84(3 Pt 1):350–358

Ziyeh S, Berlis A, Ross UH, Reinhardt MJ, Schumacher M (1997) MRI of active otosclerosis. Neuroradiology 39(6):453–457

Ziyeh S, Berger R, Reisner K (2000) MRI-visible pericochlear lesions in osteogenesis imperfecta type I. Eur Radiol 10(10):1675–1677

Temporal Bone Trauma

Sabrina Kösling and A. Noll

Contents

1 Imaging Techniques 98
2 Fracture Classification 98
2.1 Longitudinal Fractures 98
2.2 Transversal Fractures 100
2.3 Mixed Fractures 103
3 Ossicular Injuries 103
4 Contusio Labyrinthi 104
References 104

Abstract

In this chapter, radiological relevant injuries of the temporal bone are described and illustrated by selected images: fractures including nowadays used classifications, ossicular injuries and labyrinthine contusion. At the beginning, possibilities and limits of single radiological methods in the diagnostics of the temporal bone trauma are explained. Thereby, CT is still the imaging method of choice.

Compared to the rest of the body, the temporal bone is rarely affected in traumatic injuries. However, fractures of the temporal bone have been described as common (about 10 %) in patients with head trauma (Exadaktylos et al. 2003). Fractures of the temporal bone, which are also called laterobasal fractures, can occur without or with brain injuries. They result from blunt head injuries, which are caused by motor vehicle accidents (45 %), falls (31 %) and assaults (11 %) in the majority of cases (Saraiya and Aygun 2009).

On one side, not each temporal bone fracture presents with clinical symptoms (Turetschek et al. 1997), on the other side, the diagnosis is not uncommonly delayed in polytrauma because life-threatening injuries have priority and limit the clinical evaluation for signs of temporal bone trauma. Apart from the fractured bone, further structures may be more or less often injured in temporal bone trauma: tympanic cavity or labyrinth (hemotympanum, contusio labyrinthi), rupture of the drum, dural laceration, injuries of ossicles, the facial nerve and rarely great arterial or venous vessels.

Most of the temporal bone injuries do not require a surgical intervention. Only in the immediate facial nerve palsy an indication for rapid surgical management is given. Indications for operations in the interval are dislocations of ossicles, perilymphatic fistulas and cerebrospinal fluid (CSF) leaks that persist longer than 2 weeks. Patients with severe sensorineural hearing loss might be considered for a

S. Kösling (✉) · A. Noll
Martin Luther Universität Halle-Wittenberg,
Universitätsklinik für Diagnostische Radiologie,
E-Grube-Str. 40, 06097 Halle, Germany
e-mail: sabrina.koesling@medizin.uni-halle.de

cochlear implant (Gladwell and Viozzi 2008; Turetschek et al. 1997).

Nowadays, CT is the modality of choice for the detection or exclusion of temporal bone fractures and associated complications. MRI is rarely applied for special questions.

In soft tissue injuries of the external ear, acute or chronic noise damage, imaging of the temporal bone plays a less important role.

1 Imaging Techniques

Basically, the imaging technique of temporal bone trauma does not differ from the technique described in Chap.2.

For subtle details, as for instance an injury of the ossicular chain, it is important to achieve a spatial resolution as best as possible in **CT**. This means a small slice thickness, small collimation in Multi-detector CT and high zoom (low field of view). According to one's CT device these requirements cannot be exactly accomplished in polytrauma. Usually, injuries of the temporal bone are not life threatening. Temporal bone reconstructions are of secondary importance. The maximum slice thickness for optimal findings should not exceed more than one millimetre. Thin-sliced maximum intensity projections can be helpful in cases with difficult delineation of fracture lines.

Recently, **Conebeam CT** is achieved in otolaryngology too. Due to its high special resolution and low radiation exposure it is a valuable option for the isolated temporal bone trauma, but only for cases in which a soft tissue window and intravenous application of contrast medium is not needed.

In radiological studies **MRI** has been described as helpful in the assessment of an injured facial nerve, especially in the pre-operative localisation of the site of facial nerve injury if CT cannot provide this information (Kinoshita et al. 2001; Sartoretti-Schefer et al. 1997). Possible causes of facial nerve injury include oedema, intraneural haematoma, transsection, and bony impingement on the nerve (Gladwell and Viozzi 2008). Requirements for visualisation on MRI are thin-sliced high resolution T2-w, non-contrast and contrast enhanced T1-w sequences. From the clinician's point of view the benefit of MRI in facial nerve injuries is challenged: often found oedema and enhancement of the entire course of facial nerve can obscure the exact location of the injury; the proof of a nerve transsection is hardly successful (Saraiya and Aygun 2009). Clinical findings of severity of facial nerve paralysis and timing of the palsy are considered as more helpful in determining treatment than MRI (Saraiya and Aygun 2009).

Although the verification of an intra-labyrinthine bleeding does not have a therapeutic consequence it can be required in legal actions. Bleedings are best seen as hyperintensity on thin-sliced non-contrast T1-w or FLAIR images in the methaemoglobin phase between the fourth day and the first month after the trauma.

2 Fracture Classification

Optimal classifications deliver a statement about the pathomechanisms, the extent and severity as well as the prognosis of a disease. They help in therapeutic decisions and facilitate the comparability of scientific studies. A classification fulfilling all these criteria does not exist for temporal bone fractures.

The so-called traditional classification distinguishes according to the course of the fracture in relation to the long axis of the petrous bone between longitudinal, transversal and mixed or complex fractures. This classification allows a conclusion about causative forces and certain clinical signs (Jäger et al. 1997; Kösling and Neumann 2010; Schuknecht and Graetz 2005; Turetschek et al. 1997). However, the association with complications (conductive or sensorineural hearing loss, facial nerve weakness, CSF leak) and prediction of prognosis has been described as poor (Ishman and Friedlan 2004). Distinguishing petrous from non-petrous involvement should demonstrate a better correlation with the occurrence of serious sequelae (Ishman and Friedlan 2004). A similar approach with comparable conclusions has been reported on a third classification dividing otic capsule-sparing and otic capsule-violating fractures (Little and Kesser 2006). Nonetheless, not all authors confirm the superiority of the newer classification (Rafferty et al. 2006).

In the clinical situation, the traditional classification is still the most commonly used classification of temporal bone fractures. With an extended interpretation of fracture lines all temporal bone fractures can be adequately classified. In the following the incidence, clinical and radiological appearance of these fractures as well as their typical complications will be described.

2.1 Longitudinal Fractures

With about 70 % longitudinal fractures are the most common fractures of the temporal bone. They result from laterally directed forces. The fracture runs more or less parallel to the long axis of the petrous bone (Figs. 1, 2). Not uncommonly, the middle ear is involved in this type. Longitudinal fractures can be further differentiated into an anterior and posterior subtype.

Compared to transverse fractures facial nerve palsy occurs more seldom (10–20 %). Mostly, it is delayed, incomplete and transitory, caused by pressure of an extraneural haematoma on the nerve. Dural lacerations with a

Fig. 1 Longitudinal fracture of the anterior subtype. Fall on the head, after 3 days an incomplete peripheral facial nerve palsy has developed. Fracture lines through the anterior squamous portion of the temporal bone (*white arrows*) and opacifications (stars) in the mastoid and tympanic cavity especially at the fossa geniculi as expression of bleedings. **a, b** CT axial; **c, d** CT coronal

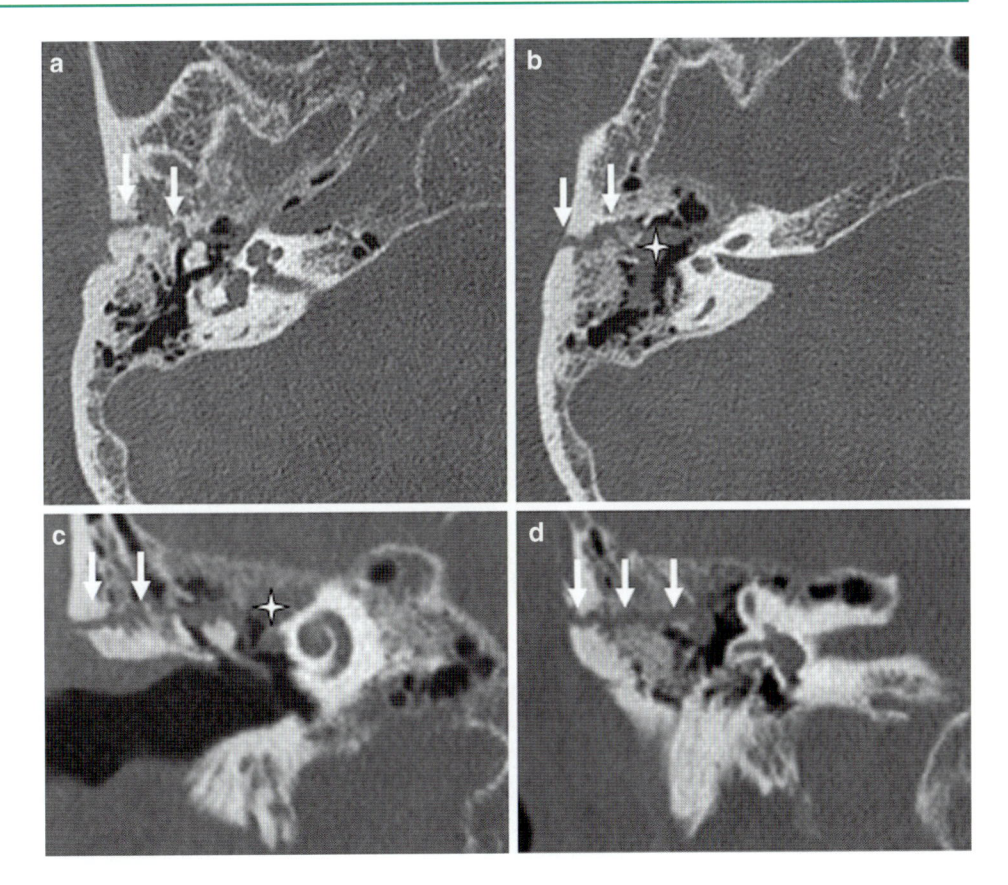

CSF leak may occur, but most leaks close spontaneously. As late complication the development of a cholesteatoma is observed. (Gladwell and Viozzi 2008; Jäger et al. 1997; Kösling and Neumann 2010; Rafferty et al. 2006; Schuknecht and Graetz 2005; Turetschek et al. 1997).

Clinical findings:
- Palpable step in the external auditory canal
- Perforation of the drum
- Haemtotympanum
- Conductive hearing loss
- Otoliquorrhea; in intact drum 'false rhinoliquorrhea' (drainage via the tuba auditiva)
- Peripheral facial nerve palsy.

Radiological findings:
- *Anterior subtype* (more common): fracture line(s) through the anterior and/or middle squamous portion of the temporal bone, the anterior wall of the external auditory canal, the tegmen tympani, toward the geniculate ganglion and possibly along the anterior border of the petrous portion or through the tuba auditiva (Fig. 1), rarely extend into the central skull base
- *Posterior subtype* (less common): fracture line(s) through the posterior squamous portion of the temporal bone or through the mastoid process, the posterior wall of the external auditory canal, the second knee of the facial nerve or its mastoid portion and may extend to the surrounding of the foramen lacerum and seldom into the jugular foramen (Fig. 2)
- *Attendant signs in both subtypes*: opacifications of the mastoid, cavum tympani and external auditory canal—sometimes with fluid levels as expression of bleedings (Figs. 1, 2); injuries of ossicles (see below); occasionally involvement of the carotid canal; rarely intracranial air as a sign for an open skull base fracture (Fig. 2b).

Differential diagnosis:

Small canals, fine sutures (pseudofractures) (Fig. 2c)—comparison with the contralateral side (when it is unaffected) helps in the differentiation.

Important points:
- Knowledge of the clinical findings supports the radiological assessment
- Analyze the roof of the middle ear and mastoid carefully on coronal reconstructions; traumatic gaps may occur with CSF leaks and can lead to cephaloceles and/or meningitis (Fig. 3)
- The canal of the ICA and facial nerve has to be analysed carefully, but not each fracture line is linked with an injury of the vessel and nerve, respectively
- Dislocated fragments of the carotid canal should implicate a non-invasive imaging of cerebral arteries or DSA (depending on the available technique, no unique recommendations)

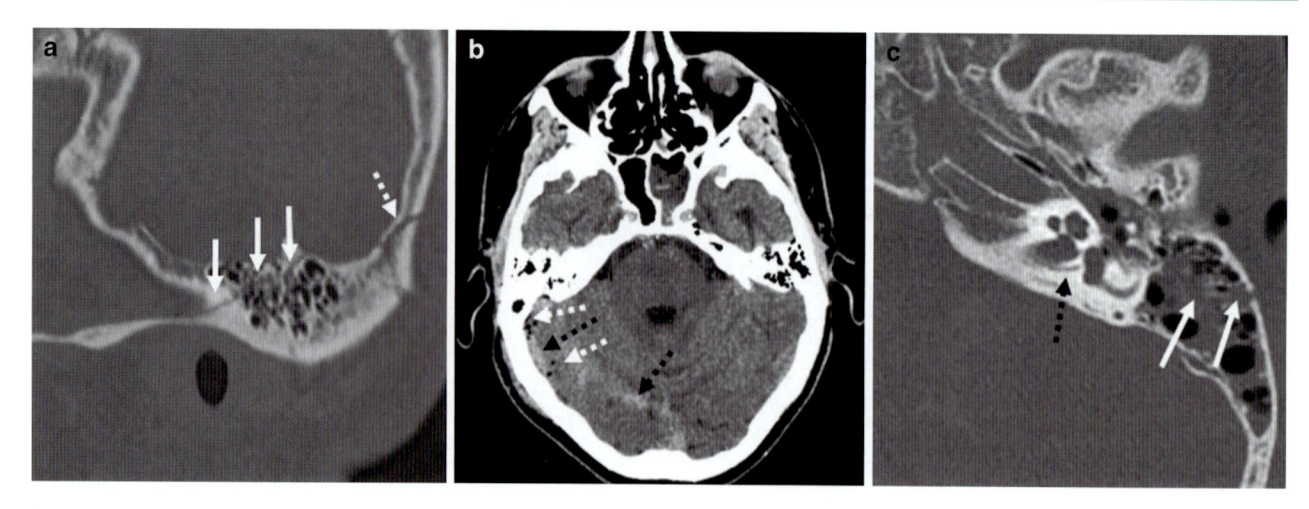

Fig. 2 Longitudinal fractures of the posterior subtype. Fall in alcoholised condition (**a**, **b**). A cupboard fell on the head (**c**). Fracture lines through the mastoid (*white arrows* in **a** and **c**) and occipital bone (*dotted arrow* in **a**), intracranial air (*white dotted arrows* in **b**) and infratentorial subdural haematoma (*black dotted arrows* in **b**). The prominent singular canal (*black dotted arrow* in **c**) should not be confused with a fracture. **a** CT sagittal; **b** brain CT axial; **c** CT axial

Fig. 3 Post-traumatic meningoencephalocele. Head trauma many years ago. On CT a broad gap in the roof of the mastoid is visible (*arrow* in **a**). MRI demonstrates the prolapse of brain into the mastoid (*star*). **a** CT coronal; **b** MRI T2-w coronal. (**b** with permission from Kösling and Neumann (2010))

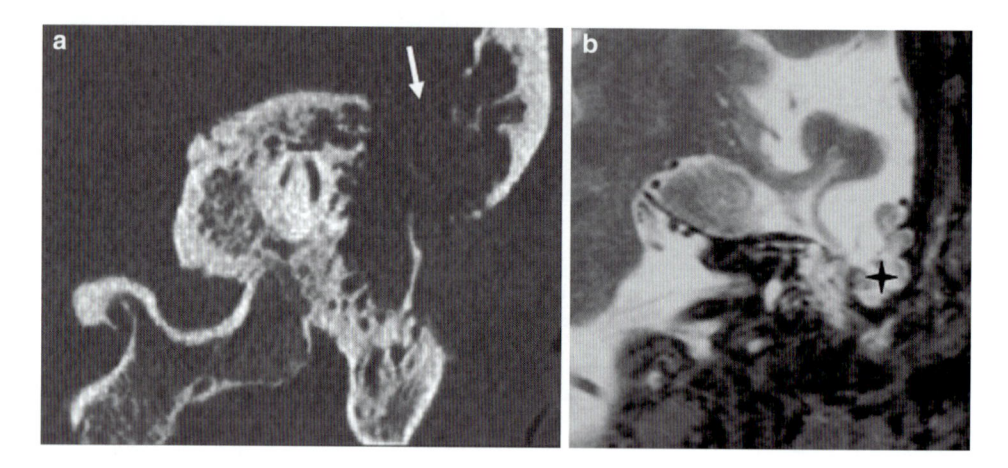

- Fracture lines through the jugular foramen are extremely rarely accompanied by venous complications (Saraiya and Aygun 2009).

2.2 Transversal Fractures

Transversal fractures arise from frontal or occipital directed forces. They are less common (about 20 % of all temporal bone fractures). Fractures pass off perpendicular to the long axis of the petrous bone and can be linked with a damage of the inner ear (Figs. 4, 5). Transversal fractures can be further differentiated into a lateral and medial subtype.

A mostly immediate and complete facial nerve palsy, which is caused by a direct damage of the nerve, is found in about half of cases. From the lateral subtype, labyrinthine fistulas may result. Fibrosing and ossification of the labyrinth are possible serious sequelae (Fig. 6) (Gladwell and Viozzi 2008; Jäger et al. 1997; Kösling and Neumann 2010; Rafferty et al. 2006; Schuknecht and Graetz 2005; Turetschek et al. 1997).

Clinical findings:
- Sensorineural hearing loss or deafness
- Damage of the vestibular organ (vertigo, vomiting and spontaneous nystagmus to the contralateral side)
- Peripheral facial nerve palsy.

Radiological findings:
- *Lateral subtype* (more common): fracture line(s) laterally of the internal auditory canal through petrous bone often with involvement of the labyrinth, the medial wall of the tympanic cavity (windows may be affected) and the facial nerve (predominately the fossa geniculi or labyrinthine segment, rarely the tympanic segment) (Figs. 4, 5).
  Attendant signs: pneumolabyrinth (Fig. 4a–c) and fluid level in the sinus tympani as an indirect sign of a labyrinthine fistula; opacifications of tympanic cavity and mastoid according to haemorrhage (Fig. 4a–c); intracranial

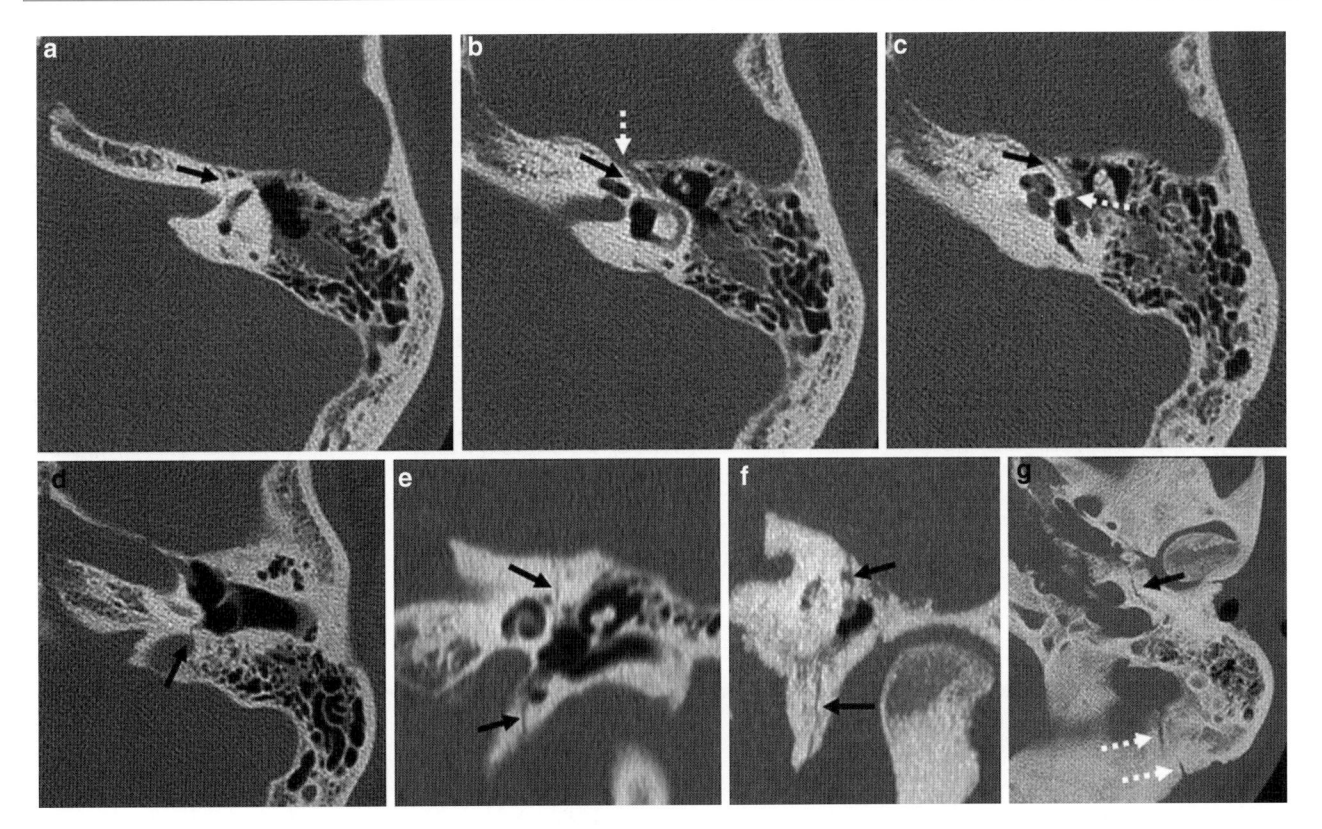

Fig. 4 Transversal fracture of the lateral subtype. Traumatic brain injury of first degree. Fracture lines (*black arrows*) through the otic capsule with involvement of the labyrinth, the fossa geniculi (*white dotted arrow* in **b**), the oval window (*white dotted arrow* in **c**), the jugular fossa (*arrow* in **d**) as well as a described opacification in the antrum. The occipitomastoid suture (*white dotted arrows* in **g**) should not be confused with a fracture. **a–d** CT axial; **e** CT coronal; **f** CT coronal thin-sliced maximum intensity projection; **g** CT axial thin-sliced maximum intensity projection

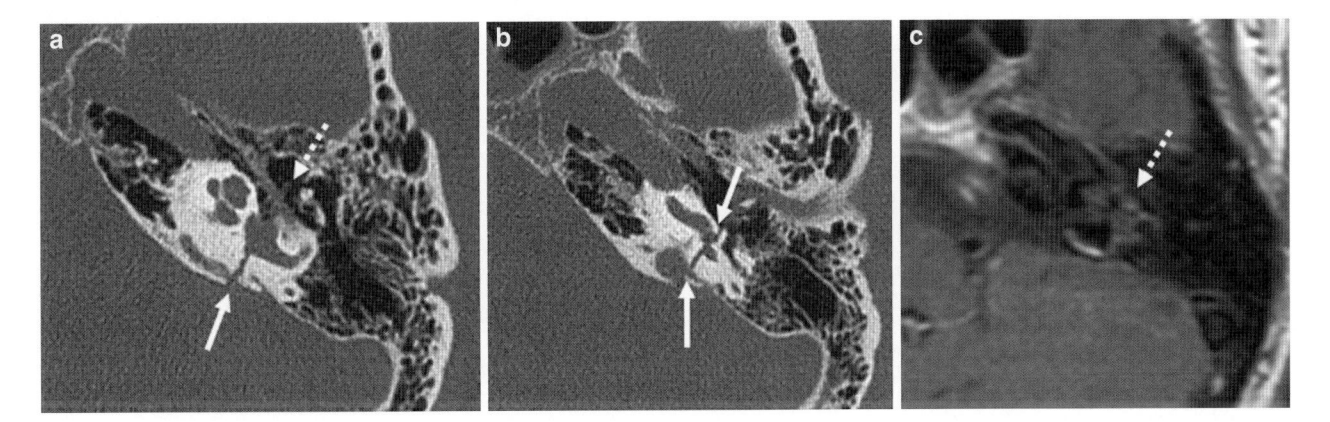

Fig. 5 Transversal fracture of the lateral subtype. Motor vehicle accident, immediate peripheral facial nerve palsy. On CT fracture lines (*white arrows*) through the labyrinth including the jugular foramen and subtle opacifications around the tympanic segment of the facial nerve (*dotted white arrow* in **a**). On MRI an enhancement of the tympanic segment of the facial nerve is visible (*dotted white arrow* in **c**). **a, b** CT axial; **c** MRI T1-w with contrast medium, axial. (**a, c** with permission from Kösling and Neumann (2010))

air; rarely injuries of ossicles; inclusion of jugular foramen (Fig. 4d)
- *Medial subtype* (rare): fracture line from the posterior cranial fossa through the internal auditory canal to the middle cranial fossa (foramen spinosum and ovale may be included), in severe injuries to the anterior skull base and midface
- *Attendant signs in both subtypes*: possibly inclusion of the carotid canal.

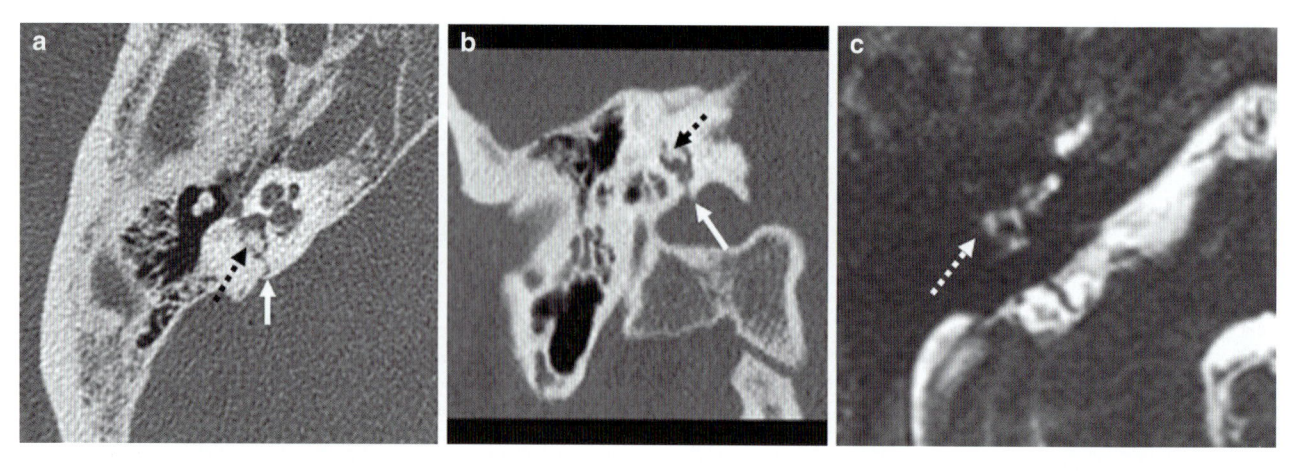

Fig. 6 Sequelae of transversal fracture. Deafness after accident at work. On CT fracture lines (*white arrows*) and partial ossification of the labyrinth (*dotted black arrows*) are visible—on MRI there is a partial signal loss in the labyrinth (white dotted arrow). **a** CT axial; **b** CT coronal; **c** MRI T2*-w axial

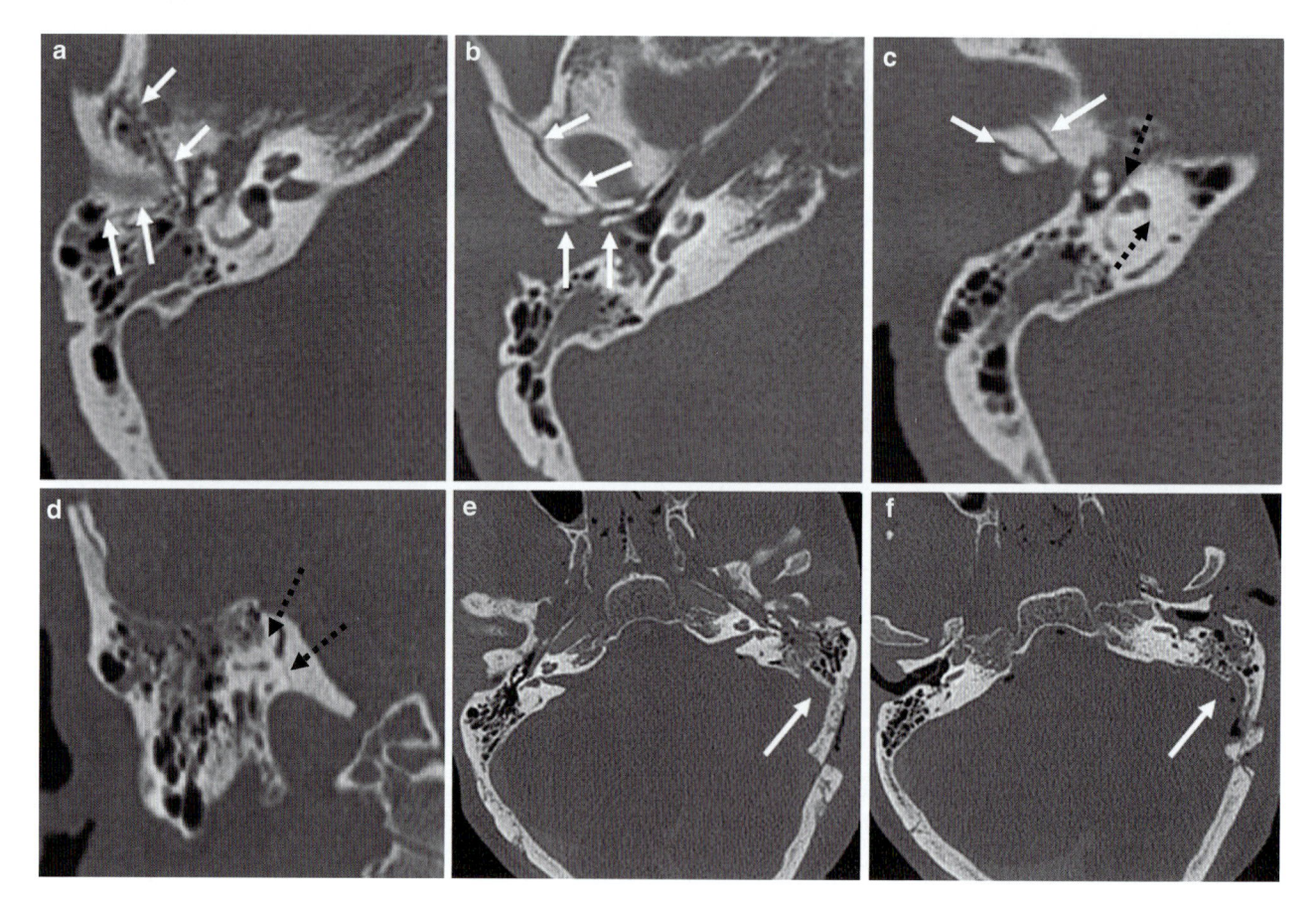

Fig. 7 Complex fractures. Open traumatic brain injury after fall (**a–d**). Polytrauma (**e, f**). In the first case (**a–d**) longitudinal (*white arrows*) and transversal (*dotted black arrows*) fracture lines can be recognised. In the second case (**e, f**) there is an impression fracture (*white arrows*). **a–c, e, f** CT axial; **d** CT coronal

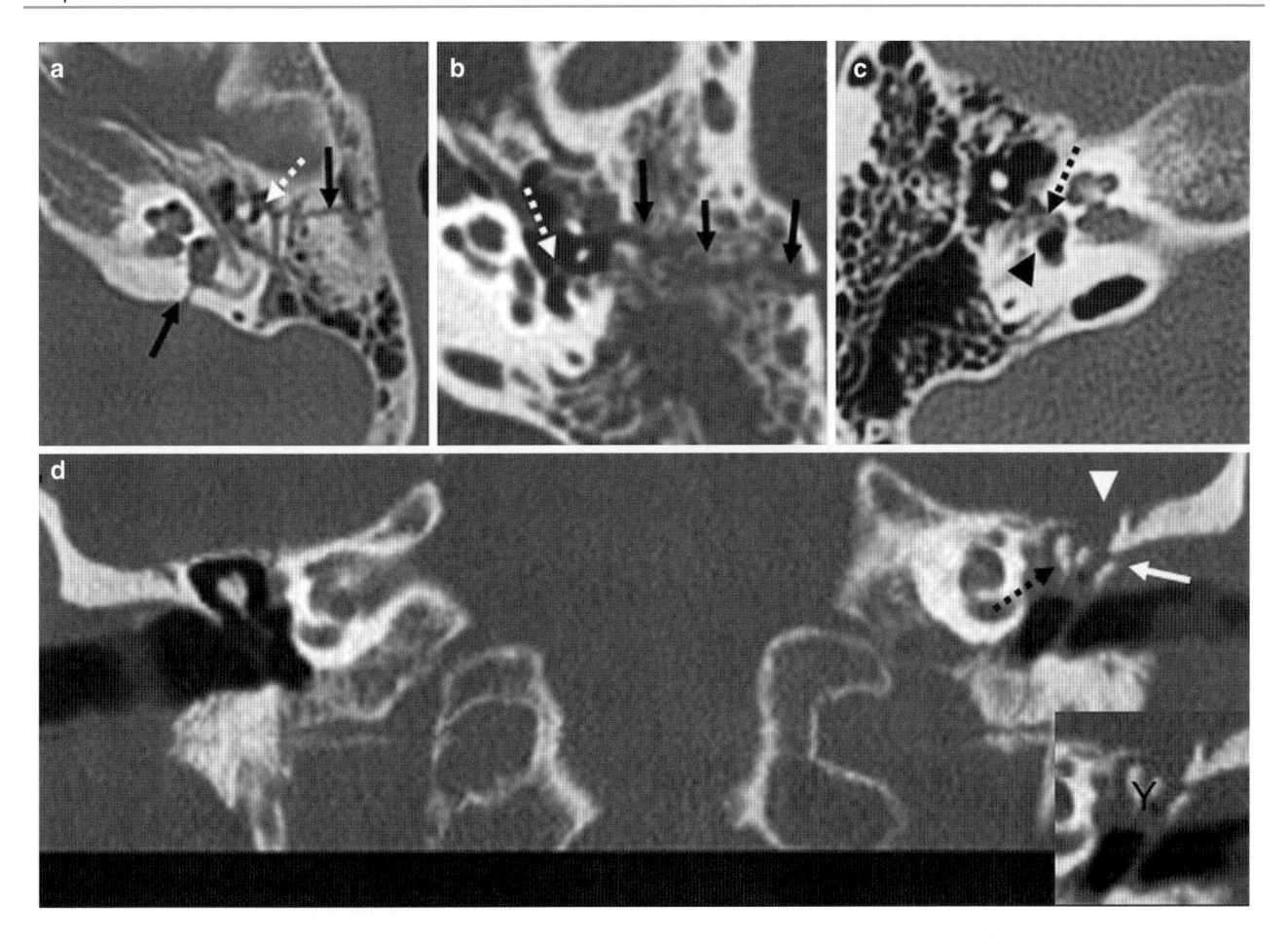

Fig. 8 Ossicular injuries. **a** Incudomalleolar joint separation (*white dotted arrow*) and complex temporal bone fracture (black arrows). **b** Incudostadpedial joint separation (*white dotted arrow*) and longitudinal temporal bone fracture (*black arrows*). **c** Stapediovestibular dislocation (*black dotted arrow*) and pneumolabyrinth (*arrowhead*). **d** Dislocation of the incus with y-sign, fracture of malleus (*black dotted arrow*) and longitudinal temporal bone fracture (*white arrow*) causing a gap in the roof of tympanic cavity. The comparison with the contralateral side is helpful. **a–c** CT axial; **d** CT coronal. (**b, c** with permission from Kösling and Neumann (2010))

Differential diagnosis:

Small canals, fine sutures (pseudofractures) (Fig. 4g)—comparison with the contralateral side (when it is unaffected) helps in the differentiation.

Important points:

- Knowledge of the clinical findings supports the radiological assessment
- The canal of the ICA and facial nerve has to be analysed carefully, but not each fracture line is linked with an injury of the vessel and nerve, respectively
- Dislocated fragments of the carotid canal should implicate a non-invasive imaging of cerebral arteries or DSA (depending on the available technique, no uniform recommendations)
- Fracture lines through the jugular foramen are extremely rarely accompanied by venous complications (Saraiya and Aygun 2009)
- MRI can provide additional information regarding a facial nerve injury (see Sect. 1) (Fig. 5c)
- Persistent severe sensorineural hearing loss after trauma may be an indication for cochlear implant.

2.3 Mixed Fractures

Mixed or complex fractures show characteristics of longitudinal as well as transversal fractures (Fig. 7). They are seen more frequently in severe head injuries and can be combined with considerable dislocation or impression of fragments. (Kösling and Neumann 2010; Rafferty et al. 2006; Turetschek et al. 1997).

3 Ossicular Injuries

Blows to the temporal, occipital or parietal region are the main mechanisms of ossicular injuries. Often, the ossicular chain is damaged in longitudinal or mixed fractures of the temporal bone (Fig. 8). Other causes as transverse fractures,

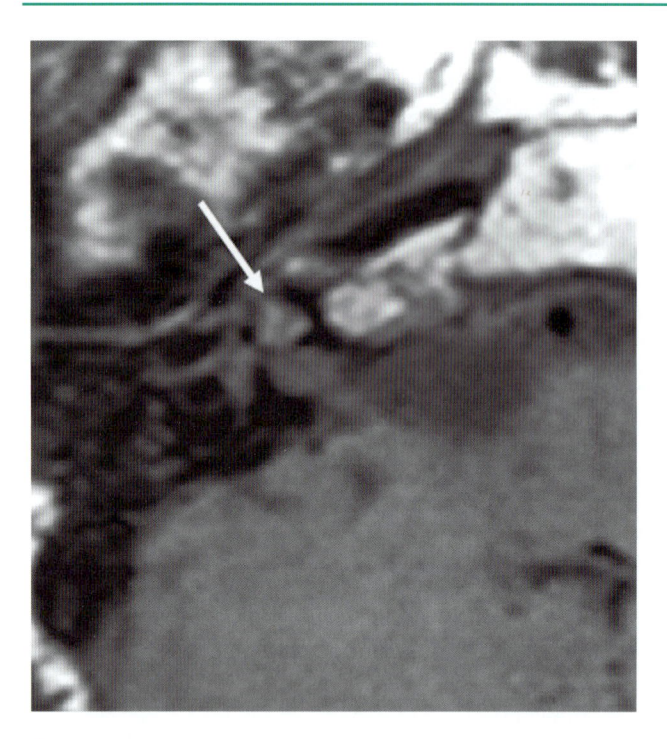

Fig. 9 Contusio labyrinthi. Deafness after accident at work, 4 weeks after trauma. Increased signal intensity of the cochlea (*arrow*). MRI T1-w without contrast medium, axial. (with permission from Kösling and Neumann (2010))

explosion trauma and direct mechanical impairment are uncommon.

Mainly ossicular injuries occur as dislocations; fractures are rarely found. Due to a diverse ligamentary attachment and orientation the single ossicles are affected with different frequency. (Kösling and Neumann 2010; Lourenco et al. 1995; Meriot et al. 1997).

Clinical findings:
– Persistent conductive (or rarely mixed) hearing loss after trauma
– Rarely vertigo and/or tinnitus
– Rarely rupture of tympanic membrane.

Radiological findings:
– Incudomalleolar joint separation (common): gap between the body of incus and head of malleus, best seen on axial images (Fig. 8a)
– Incudostapedial joint separation (common): widening of the distance between the head of the stapes and the lenticular process of the incus, best seen on axial images (Fig. 8b)
– Dislocation of the incus (due to weak ligamentary attachment more common than a dislocation of malleus): Y-sign (Lourenco et al. 1995) of the incudomalleolar complex on coronal images (Fig. 8d)
– Dislocation of the incudomalleolar complex: in intact incudomalleolar joint the incus and malleus may dislocate together in different direction, partly there is a consecutive rupture of the incudostapedial joint
– Stapediovestibular dislocation (rare): dislocation of the stapes into vestibulum, often accompanied by a perilymphatic fistula (Fig. 8c)
– Fractures of single ossicles (very rare): especially fractures of the stapes are hardly detectable on CT (Fig. 8d).

Differential diagnosis:
– Normal finding (for avoidance best spatial resolution is needed)
– Malformation (other clinical situation).

Important points:
– In haemtotympanum the assessment of the stapes may be aggravated
– Comparison with the contralateral side (when it is unaffected) helps in the detection of an incorrect position of ossicles
– The oval window region has to be analysed carefully
– Air in the labyrinth is an indirect sign of a perilymphatic fistula (Fig. 8c)
– Tympanoscopy is the golden standard for the assessment of the ossicular chain; with optimised CT technique or Conebeam CT most, but not all ossicular injuries can be diagnosed non-invasively.

4 Contusio Labyrinthi

The contusio labyrinthi is a traumatic lesion of the inner ear of different degree without a temporal bone fracture. On the basis of CT the diagnosis can be made only indirectly if CT is negative regarding fractures and the patient has typical clinical findings of a disturbed inner ear function. Opacifications of pneumatised areas can be seen occasionally.

A direct verification is enabled through MRI by demonstration of an intra-labyrinthine bleeding (see Sect. 1) (Fig. 9). Less common as in transverse fractures, fibrosing and ossification of the labyrinth can develop (Jäger et al. 1997; Kösling and Neumann 2010).

References

Exadaktylos AK, Sclabas GM, Nuyens M et al (2003) The clinical correlation of temporal bone fractures and spiral computed tomographic scan: a prospective and consecutive study at a level I trauma center. J Trauma 55:704–706

Gladwell M, Viozzi C (2008) Temporal bone fractures: a review for the oral and maxillofacial surgeon. J Oral Maxillofac Surg 66:513–522

Ishman SL, Friedlan DR (2004) Temporal bone fractures: traditional classification and clinical relevance. Laryngoscope 114:1734–1741

Jäger L, Strupp M, Brandt T et al (1997) Imaging of labyrinth and vestibular nerve. Nervenarzt 86:443–458

Kinoshita T, Ishii K, Okitsu T et al (2001) Facial nerve palsy: evaluation by contrast-enhanced MR imaging. Clin Radiol 56:926–932

Kösling S, Neumann K (2010) Schläfenbein und hintere Schädelbasis. Traumatisch bedingte Erkrankungen. In: Kösling S, Bootz F (eds) Bildgebung HNO-Heilkunde. Springer, Berlin, pp 59–69

Little SC, Kesser BW (2006) Radiographic classification of temporal bone fractures. Arch Otolaryngol Head Neck Surg 132:1300–1304

Lourenco MTC, Yeakley JW, Ghorayeb BY (1995) The "Y" sign of lateral dislocation of the incus. Am J Otol 16:387–392

Meriot P, Veillon F, Garcia JF et al (1997) CT appearances of ossicular injuries. RadioGraphics 17:1445–1454

Rafferty MA, Mc Conn Walsh R, Walsh MA (2006) A comparison of temporal bone fracture classification systems. Clin Otolaryngol 31:287–291

Saraiya PV, Aygun N (2009) Temporal bone fractures. Emerg Radiol 16:255–265

Sartoretti-Schefer S, Scherler M, Wichmann W et al (1997) Contrast enhanced MR of the facial nerve in patients with posttraumatic peripheral facial nerve palsy. Am J Neuroradiol 18:1115–1125

Schuknecht B, Graetz K (2005) Radiologic assessment of maxillofacial, mandibular, and skull base trauma. Eur Radiol 15:560–568

Turetschek K, Czerny C, Wunderbaldinger et al (1997) Temporal bone trauma and imaging. Radiologe 37:977–982

Temporal Bone Tumours

Cheng K. Ong, Eric Ting, and Vincent F. H. Chong

Contents

1	Introduction	107
2	Imaging Anatomy	107
3	Pathologic Anatomy	108
4	External Auditory Canal	108
4.1	Carcinoma of the External Auditory Canal	108
5	Middle Ear-Mastoid Complex	108
5.1	Glomus Tympanicum Paraganglioma	109
5.2	Middle Ear Schwannoma	109
5.3	Other Middle Ear Tumours	109
6	Inner Ear and Internal Auditory Canal	110
6.1	Schwannoma	111
6.2	Endolymphatic Sac Tumour	113
7	Petrous Apex	114
7.1	Pseudolesions	114
7.2	Benign Lesions	114
7.3	Malignant Tumours	115
	References	117

Abstract

Temporal bone tumours are rare entities and when encountered on cross sectional imaging, can be diagnostically challenging. Imaging plays a key role in diagnosis, treatment planning and follow-up of these tumours. Imaging evaluation of temporal bone tumours requires careful assessment of location, imaging characteristics and tumour extent. This chapter provides an overview of the most common tumours of the temporal bone with respect to anatomical location, typical imaging appearances and patterns of spread.

1 Introduction

Malignant tumours of the temporal bone are rare, with an estimated incidence between one and six cases per 1 million population per year (Barrs 2001). Management of these tumours is challenging as the accumulated experience of any particular individual or institution is often rather limited. The problem is further compounded by the absence of a universally accepted tumour staging system, rendering treatment outcome comparison difficult.

2 Imaging Anatomy

The temporal bone straddles the middle and posterior cranial fossae, with the petrous ridge (to which the tentorium cerebelli attaches) as the dividing line between the central and posterior skull base.

The temporal bone consists of five bony parts: squamous, tympanic, styloid, mastoid and petrous. It constitutes the external auditory canal (EAC), middle ear-mastoid complex, inner ear and internal auditory canal (IAC), and petrous apex. The facial nerve and petrous internal carotid artery course through the temporal bone to exit the stylomastoid foramen and petrous apex respectively.

C. K. Ong (✉) · E. Ting · V. F. H. Chong
Department of Diagnostic Radiology,
National University Hospital,
5 Lower Kent Ridge Road, Singapore 119074, Singapore
e-mail: cheng_kang_ong@nuhs.edu.sg; ongck22@hotmail.com

C. K. Ong · E. Ting · V. F. H. Chong
Yong Loo Lin School of Medicine, National University of Singapore,
5 Lower Kent Ridge Road, Singapore 119074, Singapore

Fig. 1 **a** Axial contrast-enhanced T1-weighted MR image shows an enhancing squamous cell carcinoma along the right EAC (*arrow*). **b** Axial and **c** coronal CT images show underlying osseous destruction of the right EAC (*arrow*). **d** Axial contrast-enhanced CT image shows an enlarged right parotid node (*arrow*), the first echelon node of EAC carcinoma

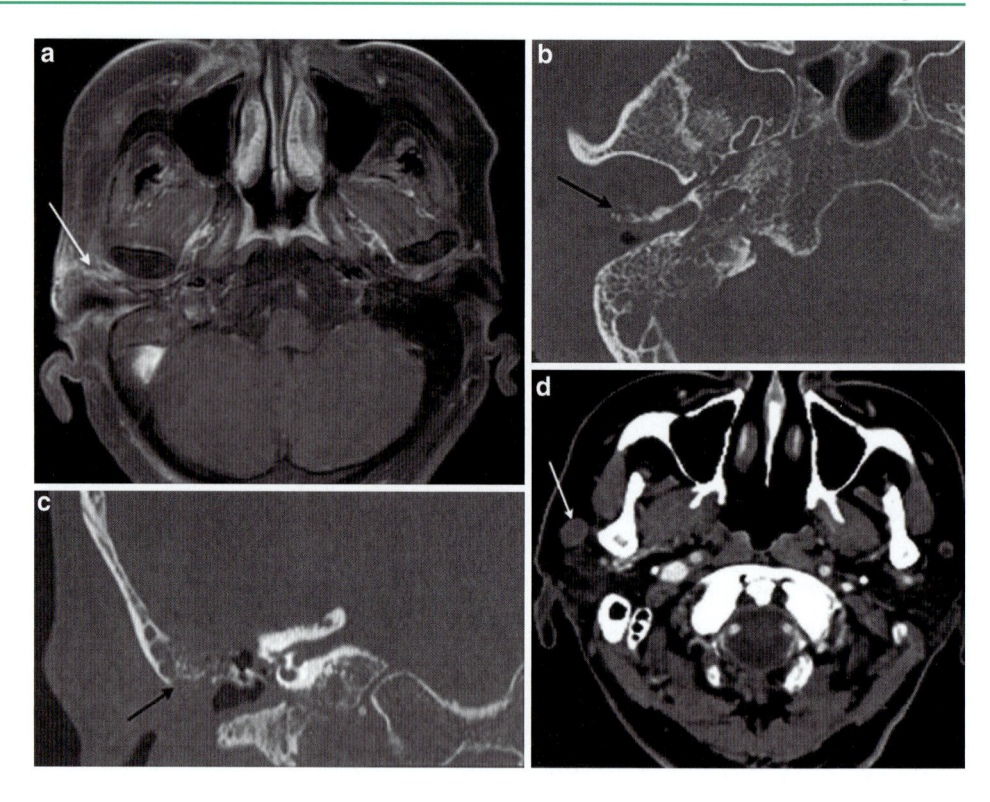

3 Pathologic Anatomy

A temporal bone tumour may be categorised into one of the following compartments: EAC, middle ear-mastoid complex, inner ear or petrous apex. A differential diagnosis may then be formulated based on the location of the lesion.

4 External Auditory Canal

The EAC comprises a fibrocartilaginous portion in the lateral third and a bony portion (the tympanic bone) in the medial two-thirds. The canal is lined by a thin layer of stratified squamous epithelium.

4.1 Carcinoma of the External Auditory Canal

Carcinomas of the EAC are usually disease of the elderly, often diagnosed in their 60s or 70s. Squamous cell carcinoma (SCC) is the most common malignancy of the EAC, approximately four times more common than basal cell carcinoma (Lobo et al. 2008). These tumours have been associated with chronic infection or inflammation of the EAC, and previous radiotherapy for other head and neck neoplasms (Lim et al. 2000).

On imaging, an early carcinoma is usually seen as a soft tissue mass in the EAC. As the disease progresses, underlying bony destructive changes become evident and the tumour infiltrates into the surrounding soft tissues (Ong et al. 2008). Carcinoma of the EAC most commonly spreads inferiorly through the fissures of Santorini along the floor of the cartilaginous EAC. The parotid nodes are the first echelon nodes (Choi et al. 2003) (Fig. 1). Malignant pre- and post-auricular lymphadenopathy is also commonly seen. Cervical nodal metastasis and the presence of facial palsy at presentation are the most important unfavourable prognostic factors (Moffat et al. 2005; Yin et al. 2006).

Diagnosis EAC carcinoma may be delayed as the initial presenting symptoms of otorrhoea and otalgia often mimic otitis externa. In addition, even the histological samples may sometimes be confused with pseudoepitheliomatous hyperplasia (Gacek et al. 1998). Essentially, any EAC lesion associated with bony destruction should be considered malignant until proven otherwise.

5 Middle Ear-Mastoid Complex

The middle ear is connected to the mastoid via the aditus ad antrum. Tumours of the middle ear may grow freely through the air spaces of the middle ear and mastoid. They can spread to other parts of the temporal bone via the oval and round windows as well as through the tympanic membrane. Other potential pathways beyond the middle ear-mastoid complex include the eustachian tube and along neurovascular structures into the nasopharynx, infratemporal fossa or

Fig. 2 A 49 year-old female with pulsatile tinnitus and a *red* retrotympanic mass. **a** Axial temporal bone CT image shows a soft tissue tympanic mass over the cochlear promontory (*arrow*). **b** Coronal temporal bone CT image shows the tumour in the meso- and hypotympanum bulging against the lower tympanic membrane (*arrow*). The clinical and imaging features are consistent with a glomus tympanicum paraganglioma

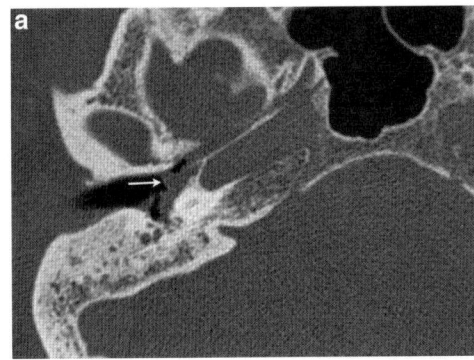

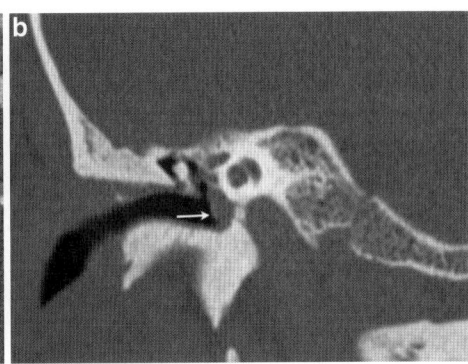

neck. Aggressive tumours may erode directly through bone, particularly through the thin tegmen tympani or sigmoid plate into the middle or posterior cranial fossa and sigmoid sinus.

5.1 Glomus Tympanicum Paraganglioma

The most common benign tumour of the middle ear and mastoid is the glomus tympanicum paraganglioma (O'Leary et al. 1991). Paragangliomas are neuroendocrine tumours, originating from chromaffin cells in paraganglia or chromaffin-negative glomus cells derived from the embryonic neural crest. In the middle ear, these cells are found anywhere along the course of Jacobson's nerve (the tympanic branch of the glossopharyngeal nerve) which enters the middle ear through the tympanic canaliculus and forms the tympanic plexus, which ramifies on the surface of the cochlear promontory and medial wall of the middle ear. The term glomus jugulotympanicum refers to paragangliomas that involve both the jugular foramen and middle ear. These tumours usually arise from glomus cells derived either from Jacobson's nerve or Arnold's nerve (the mastoid or auricular branch of the vagus nerve). Peak incidence is in the fifth and sixth decades and there is a clear female predominance (3:1).

The most common presenting symptom is pulsatile tinnitus. If the tumour is large, it may cause conductive hearing loss. Facial nerve palsy, sensorineural hearing loss or vertigo may result if the facial nerve or inner ear becomes involved. Other cranial nerve palsies may result from extension to the jugular foramen or hypoglossal canal. Occasionally, they may be asymptomatic. On clinical examination, a vascular retrotympanic mass is seen. The symptoms and clinical findings of a glomus tympanicum tumour may be indistinguishable from glomus jugulotympanicum, aberrant internal carotid artery or a dehiscent, high-riding jugular bulb and imaging is required to differentiate these entities. On high resolution CT, a nodular soft tissue mass is typically seen in the hypotympanum near the cochlear promontory (Fig. 2). The mass may fill the middle ear cavity but generally spares the ossicles. Bone erosion is usually not a feature, even in large tumours. Tumours may fill the epitympanum, attic and antrum, resulting in fluid retention in the mastoid. On MRI, the mass is seen as a strongly enhancing lesion within the signal void of the middle ear-mastoid complex, on T1-weighted post-contrast sequences, with variable T2-weighted signal. Larger tumours may exhibit the characteristic 'salt and pepper' appearance on T1-weighted sequences, with the 'pepper' representing hypointense signal flow voids caused by the large feeding arteries and the 'salt' representing subacute haemorrhage within the tumour.

5.2 Middle Ear Schwannoma

The next most common tumour involving the middle ear is the schwannoma. The most common schwannoma of the middle ear arises from the facial nerve, though it may arise from any nerve of the middle ear, including Jacobson's nerve and Arnold's nerve (Aydin et al. 2000; Wiet et al. 1985). On clinical examination, schwannomas may appear as a fleshy-white mass behind an intact tympanic membrane. On imaging, a well-circumscribed lobulated mass may be seen arising from the tympanic or mastoid segments of the facial nerve (Fig. 3) or lying separate from the facial nerve canal when the facial nerve is not involved. Post-contrast T1-weighted MRI shows enhancement of the mass.

5.3 Other Middle Ear Tumours

Congenital cholesteatomas are the next most common differential for a middle ear mass. Congenital cholesteatomas typically present with a whitish mass seen behind an intact tympanic membrane, as opposed to acquired cholesteatomas, which arise from a perforation or retraction pocket in the tympanic membrane and are associated with a history of chronic otorrhoea and recurrent middle ear infection.

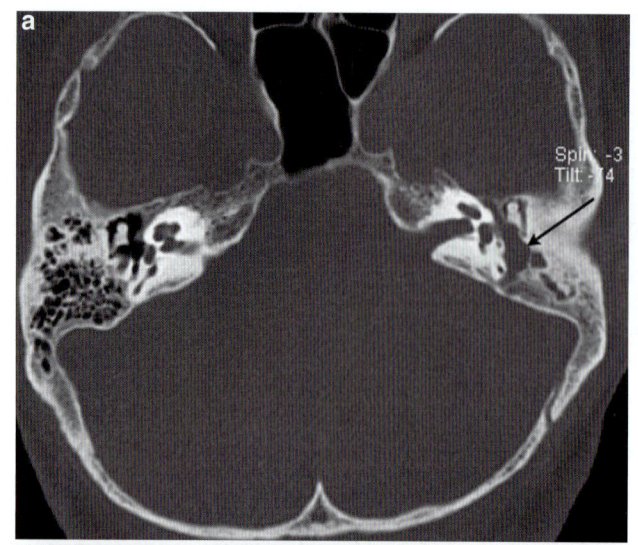

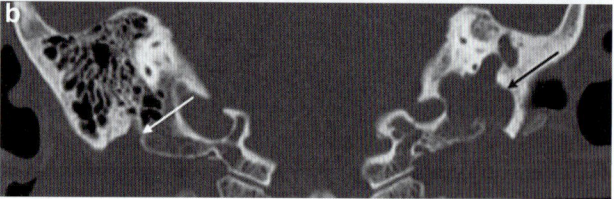

Fig. 3 Facial nerve schwannoma. **a** Axial temporal bone CT image shows a facial nerve schwannoma enlarging the posterior tympanic segment of the left facial nerve canal (*arrow*). **b** Coronal temporal bone CT image shows the schwannoma extending along the mastoid segment of the left facial nerve canal (*black arrow*). Note the normal right mastoid facial nerve canal, which opens through the stylomastoid foramen (*white arrow*)

Congenital cholesteatomas arise when there is aberrant migration of external canal ectoderm beyond the tympanic ring. As a result, the tympanic membrane is intact. Both congenital and acquired cholesteatomas form as a result of the accumulation of exfoliated keratinous material in a sac lined by squamous epithelial cells. On CT, congenital cholesteatomas appear as a nodular soft tissue mass in the hypo- or mesotympanum, with or without ossicular erosion. Prussak's space and the scutum are typically normal. On MRI, congenital cholesteatomas demonstrate intermediate signal intensity on T2-weighted and hypointense signal intensity on T1-weighted sequences without any enhancement post contrast. Rim enhancement is occasionally seen due to surrounding granulation tissue. Diffusion weighted MRI (DWI) may be used to differentiate congenital cholesteatoma from other middle ear masses, as cholesteatomas appear hyperintense on B1000 DWI sequences. Non-echoplanar sequences are preferred, as they allow for thinner sections and are less sensitive to susceptibility artefacts at the brain-bone interface (De Foer et al. 2006; Schwartz et al. 2011).

The middle ear adenoma is a rare tumour of the middle ear, considered by some to encompass a spectrum of histological types ranging from adenoma to carcinoid, depending on the degree of glandular or neuroendocrine differentiation (Torske et al. 2002). Middle ear adenomas most commonly present with conductive hearing loss and a soft tissue mass behind an intact tympanic membrane. On CT, they appear as a soft tissue mass engulfing the ossicles, indistinguishable from the far more common congenital cholesteatoma. Larger tumours may cause ossicular erosion. On MRI, they appear as an enhancing mass not confined to the cochlear promontory and may mimic glomus tympanicum (Zan et al. 2009).

Malignant tumours of the middle ear are rare. The most common malignant middle ear tumour is SCC, which is thought to arise secondary to squamous metaplasia, mainly in the setting of chronic otitis media (Fig. 4). A high prevalence of human papilloma virus (HPV) has also been reported in middle ear SCC associated with chronic otitis media (Jin et al. 1997).

Rhabdomyosarcomas are the most common paediatric soft tissue sarcoma and most common middle ear malignancy in children, although the temporal bone is an uncommon site of involvement (Adrassy 1997). Initially, the tumour may present as chronic otitis media, unresponsive to antibiotics. Cranial nerve dysfunction is common, particularly facial nerve palsy. CT may demonstrate a soft tissue mass with extensive bony destruction. MRI is useful to delineate the extent of the tumour, the intracranial extent and to differentiate tumour from fluid, although findings are non-specific. Rhabdomyosarcomas are typically isointense to muscle on T1-weighted, iso- to slightly hyperintense to muscle on T2-weighted and diffusely enhancing on contrast enhanced T1-weighted sequences. Langerhans cell histiocytosis (LCH) is the main differential for a soft tissue mass with aggressive bony destruction in a child. LCH may indistinguishable from rhabdomyosarcoma on imaging and biopsy is often necessary. Acute coalescent otomastoiditis may also be associated with soft tissue density in the middle ear and bony destruction, however patients are usually acutely ill and respond to antibiotics.

6 Inner Ear and Internal Auditory Canal

The inner ear comprises the membranous labyrinth bathed in perilymph within the bony labyrinth. The membranous labyrinth is a closed system of endolymph-filled tubes and chambers, which includes the vestibule (utricle and saccule), the semicircular ducts, the cochlear duct (scala media of cochlea), the endolymphatic duct and sac. The endolymphatic duct arises from the utriculosaccular duct (which connects the utricle and the saccule), and passes within the bony vestibular aqueduct to the endolymphatic sac which is lodged at the fovea of the vestibular aqueduct along the posterior wall of the temporal bone.

Fig. 4 Carcinoma of the middle ear. **a** Axial contrast-enhanced T1-weighted MR image shows a heterogeneously enhancing tumour arising from the left middle ear (*white arrow*), invading the petrous apex and surrounding the left petrous internal carotid artery (*black arrow*). **b** Coronal contrast-enhanced T1-weighted MR image shows superior spread with intracranial tumour extension (*arrow*)

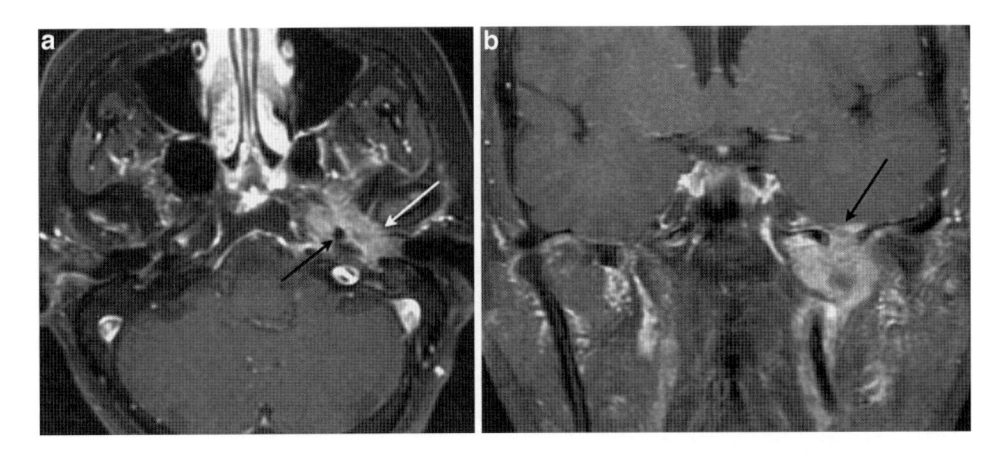

Fig. 5 **a** Axial high-resolution heavily T2-weighted MR image shows a cylindrical right intracanalicular vestibular schwannoma, and an "ice cream on cone" left CPA-IAC vestibular schwannoma. **b** Axial contrast-enhanced fat-saturated T1-weighted MR image shows avid enhancement in both schwannomas, with intramural cystic changes in the larger left-sided lesion. Bilateral vestibular schwannomas are hallmark of type 2 neurofibromatosis

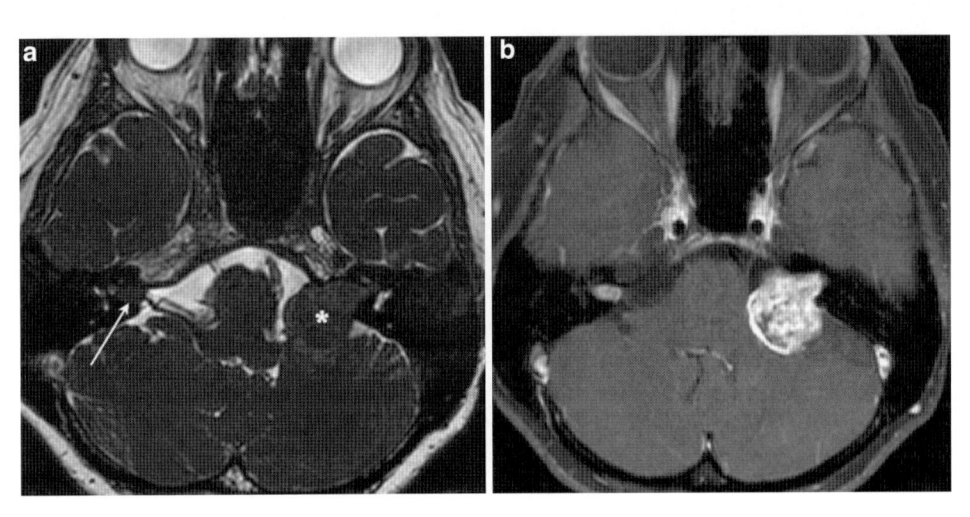

The IAC is approximately 10 mm long and transmits the facial and vestibulocochlear nerves between the posterior cranial fossa and the inner ear. The canal is divided by a horizontal crest of bone, the crista falciformis into an upper compartment (which houses the facial nerve anteriorly and the superior vestibular nerve posteriorly) and a lower compartment (which contains the cochlear nerve anteriorly and the inferior vestibular nerve posteriorly). The facial and superior vestibular nerves are further divided by a vertical Bill bar, although this small bony structure is not visible on imaging.

6.1 Schwannoma

Schwannomas are benign encapsulated tumours arising from the Schwann cells that wrap around cranial nerves. Histologically, they comprise of differentiated Schwann cells forming Antoni A (areas of compact spindle cells) and B patterns (areas of loosely arranged matrix with lipid-laden cells and cysts). Malignant schwannomas are very rare but have been reported (Balasubramaniam 1999).

6.1.1 Intracanalicular Schwannoma

It is postulated that schwannomas in the IAC most commonly arise from the vestibular division of the vestibulocochlear nerve (CN8) at the glial-Schwann cell junction, which is usually near the porous acousticus and hence their common presentation as a combined cerebellopontine angle (CPA)-IAC mass. However, there are also lesions that are entirely intracanalicular and it has been hypothesised that some of these tumours may have originated from the Scarpa's ganglion on the vestibular nerve near the fundus of the IAC (De Foer et al. 2010).

The peak age for vestibular schwannomas is between 40 and 60 years old. Patients most often complain of unilateral progressive sensorineural hearing loss, sometimes with tinnitus and vertigo. On MR imaging, this tumour appears as an avidly enhancing cylindrical (intracanalicular schwannoma) or "ice cream on cone" (CPA-IAC schwannoma) mass (Fig. 5). Although intramural cysts are not uncommon in larger schwannomas (up to 25 %), they are hardly seen in the smaller intracanalicular lesions. Haemorrhagic schwannomas are rare (0.5 %). On imaging, it is important to look for any negative prognostic features for

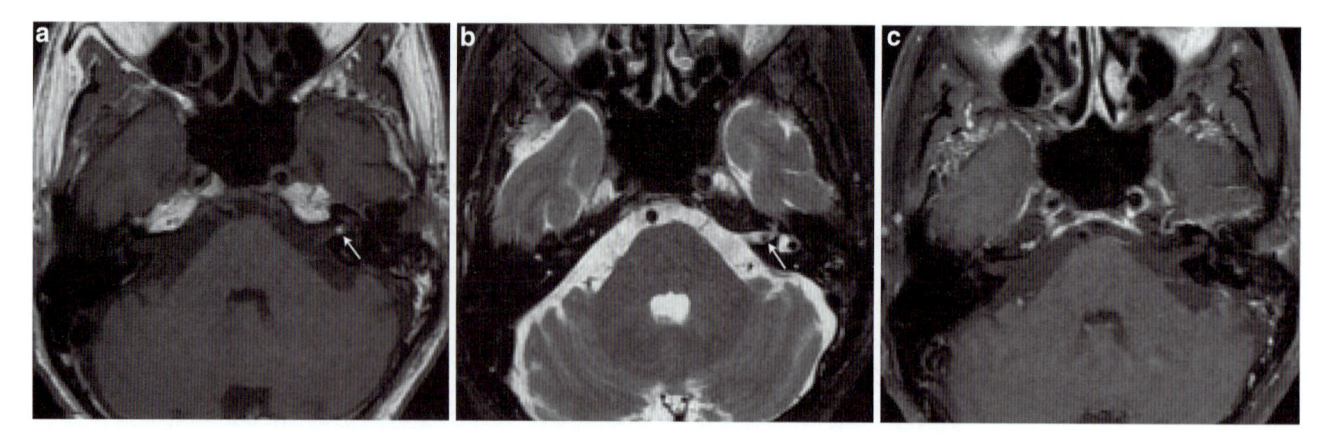

Fig. 6 Internal auditory canal lipoma. **a** Axial T1-weighted MR image shows a small hyperintense left intracanalicular lesion (*arrow*). **b** Axial T2-weighted fat-saturated MR image shows signal suppression of the lesion, which appears as a "filling defect" in the left IAC surrounded by the high signal cerebrospinal fluid (*arrow*). **c** Axial contrast-enhanced fat-saturated T1-weighted MR image shows no enhancement of the lesion, in keeping with a lipoma

hearing preservation following surgery, which include a tumour size larger than 2 cm and tumour involvement of the IAC fundus or cochlear aperture (Somers et al. 2001).

Although a well-circumscribed IAC lesion should be considered a vestibular schwannoma unless proven otherwise, a few differential diagnoses exist.

An IAC *facial nerve schwannoma* may mimic a vestibular schwannoma clinically, although facial nerve (CN7) palsy is more common in the former (up to 73 %) (Ulku et al. 2004). If the tumour is confined within the IAC, it is indistinguishable from a vestibular schwannoma on imaging. An imaging diagnosis of facial nerve schwannoma is achieved when the tumour is seen extending into the labyrinthine segment of the facial nerve, giving rise to a "labyrinthine tail" detected on contrast-enhanced MRI.

While CPA-IAC meningiomas account for 5–8 % of all intracranial meningiomas, meningiomas arising from and confined to the IAC are rare with only a handful of case reports in the literature (Bohrer and Chole 1996; Langman et al. 1990). The clinical presentations of *intracanalicular meningiomas* are similar to those of vestibular schwannomas (up to 80 % with unilateral progressive sensorineural hearing loss and 50 % with tinnitus), although they tend to become symptomatic earlier (Laudadio et al. 2004). The imaging features often associated with other intracranial meningiomas, such as intramural calcification, dural tail and bone hyperostosis have never been described in all the intracanalicular meningiomas documented in the literature. As a result, they appear identical to IAC vestibular schwannomas on imaging and the definitive diagnosis requires histological confirmation.

Intracanalicular lipomas are rare congenital lesions believed to arise from maldifferentiation of meningeal precursor tissue (meninx primitiva). They are seen as non-enhancing IAC lesions with homogeneous hyperintense signal on T1-weighted MR imaging, which is clearly suppressed on fat-saturated sequence (Bonneville et al. 2007) (Fig. 6). A concurrent intravestibular lipoma may be present. Most of the IAC lipomas are discovered incidentally on MR imaging of the temporal bones (Swartz 2008). They usually incorporate CN7 and CN8 with dense adhesion, and should be considered "leave me alone" lesions as any surgical interventions might do more harm than good (De Foer et al. 2010).

6.1.2 Intralabyrinthine Schwannoma

Intralabyrinthine schwannomas originate from the perineural Schwann cells of the intralabyrinthine branches of the CN8. Approximately 80 % of these tumours are confined to the cochlea, often located anteriorly between the basal and second turns (Tieleman et al. 2008). Intralabyrinthine schwannomas may grow from the cochlea into the vestibule, and vice versa. They may also extend from the cochlea (transmodiolar) or vestibule (transmacular) into the fundus of the IAC.

The main presenting symptom is slowly progressive unilateral sensorineural hearing loss, often associated with tinnitus and vertigo.

Intralabyrinthine schwannomas are mildly more hyperintense than its surrounding endolymph and perilymph on T1-weighted MR imaging, and show avid enhancement following intravenous contrast administration. They appear as sharply circumscribed hypointense intralabyrinthine lesions on high-resolution heavily T2-weighted 3D sequences (Tieleman et al. 2008) (Fig. 7).

When intralabyrinthine enhancement is detected, the most important differential diagnosis to consider is *labyrinthitis*, which usually has an acute clinical onset. In labyrinthitis, the enhancement tends to involve most or all of the membranous labyrinth and on high-resolution T2-

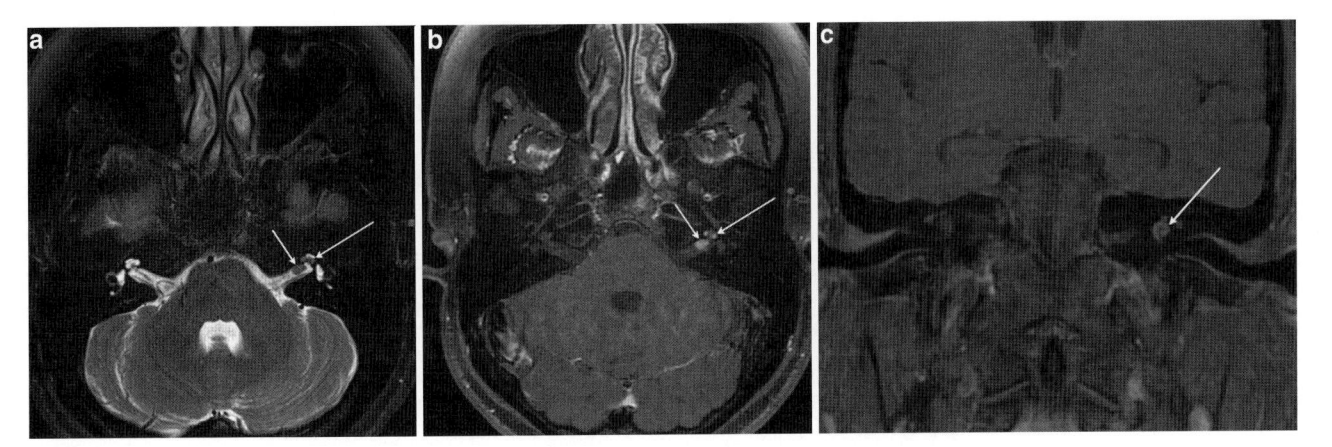

Fig. 7 Cochlear schwannoma. **a** Axial fat-saturated T2-weighted MR image shows an intracanalicular cochlear schwannoma in the antero-inferior aspect of the left IAC (*short arrow*) and an intralabyrinthine schwannoma occupying the basal turn of the left cochlea (*long arrow*). **b** Axial contrast-enhanced T1-weighted MR image with fat-saturation shows enhancement of both intracanalicular (*short arrow*) and intralabyrinthine (*long arrow*) cochlear schwannomas. **c** Coronal contrast-enhanced T1-weighted MR image with fat-saturation shows the enhancing schwannoma filling the basal turn of the left cochlea (*arrow*)

weighted sequence, no discrete hypointense mass is seen replacing the high signal inner ear fluid.

On the other hand, *ossifying labyrinthitis*, a sequelae of suppurative membranous labyrinthitis, may present as focal low signal lesion within the high signal intralabyrinthine fluid on high-resolution T2-weighted MR imaging. However, there is usually minimal or no post-contrast enhancement. High-resolution, 1 mm thick bone algorithm CT would show focal bony encroachment on the membranous labyrinth. The membranous labyrinth may be obliterated by bone in severe ossifying labyrinthitis (Fig. 8).

6.2 Endolymphatic Sac Tumour

Endolymphatic sac tumours are low grade papillary adenocarcinoma, often centred in the fovea of endolymphatic sac along the posterior surface of the petrous temporal bone. Most authors nowadays accept the hypothesis proposed by Heffner that these tumours originate from the endolymphatic sac, which is lined by a neuroectodermally derived epithelium (Heffner 1989). Most endolymphatic sac tumours are sporadic but some (especially bilateral tumours) are associated with von Hippel–Lindau disease. These tumours generally affect adults with the peak incidence in the third and fourth decades (Devaney et al. 2003). The most common presenting symptoms include sensorineural deafness, vertigo and tinnitus.

A notable feature of this tumour is the discrepancy between its low-grade histological appearance and its aggressively infiltrative behaviour (Devaney et al. 2005). CT shows a destructive soft tissue mass with intratumoural residual bone spicules arising from the retrolabyrinthine petrous temporal bone (Mukherji et al. 1997; Stendel et al. 1998). On MRI, hyperintense foci are frequently seen within the tumour on T1-weighted sequence, which may represent subacute haemorrhage (extracellular methaemoglobin) or intramural cysts with high protein content (Ho et al. 1996). Flow voids may been seen in the larger tumours, as they are hypervascular. Heterogeneous enhancement is also demonstrated following intravenous contrast (Fig. 9). These tumours are usually fairly large at presentation, extending into the CPA cistern and jugular foramen or permeating through the middle ear.

An important differential diagnosis is the more commonly encountered *glomus jugulare paraganglioma*. This tumour is also particularly vascular and may show hyperintense foci and high velocity flow voids on T1-weighted MR imaging (the "salt and pepper" appearance), mimicking the endolymphatic sac tumours and vice versa (Roncaroli et al. 1997). However, glomus jugulare paragangliomas arise from the jugular foramen and spread along the path of least resistance, usually through the jugular plate superolaterally into the middle ear (so-called "glomus jugulotympanicum paraganglioma") and rarely involve the dense retrolabyrinthine temporal bone (Ong and Chong 2009).

Metastasis from papillary thyroid carcinoma may resemble endolymphatic sac tumours on imaging and histological examinations, although fortunately they usually stain positive for thyroglobulin (Heffner 1989). Middle ear adenomas may also bear significant histological similarity with endolymphatic sac tumours. However, they are indolent tumours, which do not destroy the adjacent temporal bone (Devaney et al. 2005).

Fig. 8 Severe ossifying labyrinthitis. **a** Axial temporal bone CT image at the level of the semicircular canals shows complete replacement of the left semicircular canals with bone (*arrow*). **b** Axial and **c** coronal temporal bone CT images through the cochlea reveal almost complete obliteration of the left cochlea (*arrow*)

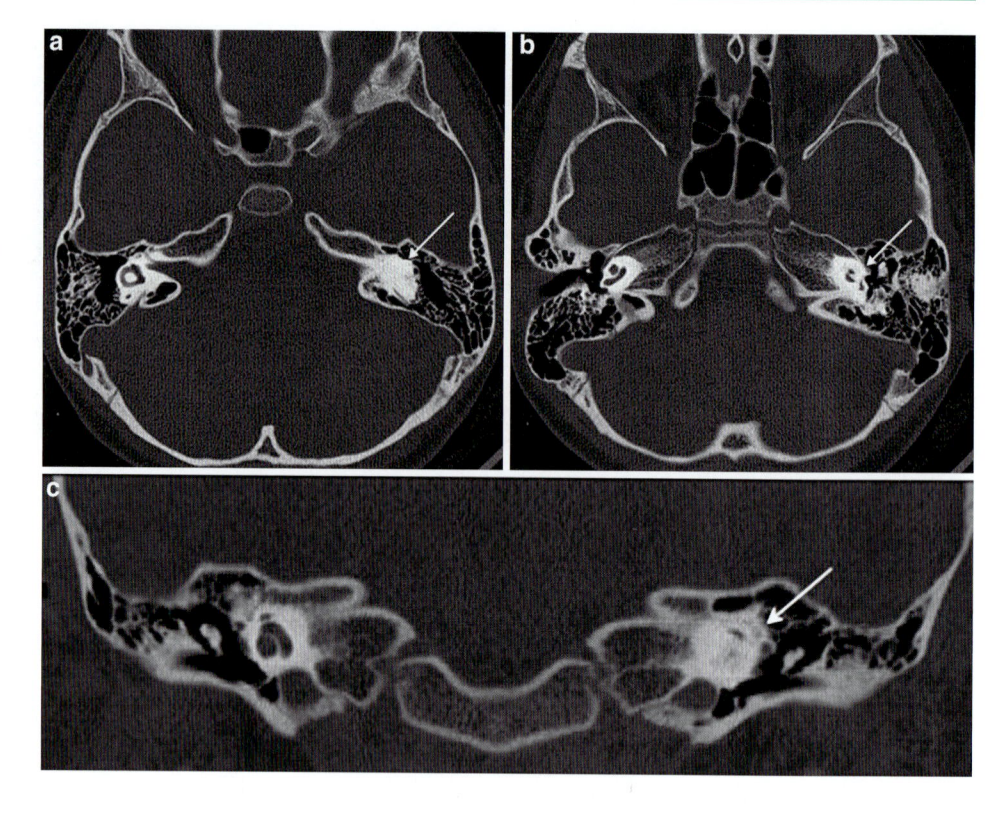

7 Petrous Apex

The petrous apex is defined as the petrous temporal bone anteromedial to the inner ear. It contains the horizontal segment of the petrous internal carotid artery (ICA). The abducens nerve (CN6) arches over the medial aspect of the petrous apex within the Dorello canal, and the trigeminal nerve (CN5) courses immediately superomedial to the petrous apex. Approximately 33 % of people have pneumatised petrous apices, the extent of which often correlates with the degree of mastoid pneumatisation (Virapongse et al. 1985). Apart from malignant neoplasms, many abnormalities of the petrous apex are related to the presence of pneumatisation (Moore et al. 1998).

7.1 Pseudolesions

Asymmetrical fatty marrow, trapped fluid of the petrous apex and petrous apex cephalocoele are three "leave me alone" lesions, which are often detected during unrelated MR imaging of the brain. Diploic fatty marrow in an asymmetrically non-pneumatised or less pneumatised petrous apex may be seen in 5–10 % of individuals. This marrow is characterised by high signal intensity on T1-weighted images and intermediate to high signal intensity on T2-weighted images, following signals of the orbital fat (Leonetti et al. 2001). The diagnosis is confirmed when the signal is suppressed on the fat-saturated sequence.

Trapped fluid in a pneumatised petrous apex is identified in approximately 1 % of MR imaging. It occurs when the interconnecting tracks between the middle ear-mastoid complex and the petrous apex are obstructed following a bout of otomastoiditis, trapping sterile fluid within the petrous apex air-cells. High T2-weighted signal is demonstrated with variable T1-weighted signal, depending on the protein content of the fluid. CT shows no bone expansion, cortical erosion or trabecular disruption (Moore et al. 1998).

Petrous apex cephalocoele is rare, and represents congenital or acquired herniation of the posterolateral wall of Meckel cave into the petrous apex. CT and MR imaging show a lesion of cerebrospinal fluid density and intensity, which communicates with the Meckel cave. Smooth excavation or expansion of the petrous apex may be detected on bone algorithm CT (Fig. 10). This lesion usually shows no enhancement, unless part of the trigeminal ganglion and its periganglionic venous plexus protrude into the cephalocoele (Moore et al. 2001).

7.2 Benign Lesions

These lesions are characterised by the CT appearance of a well-demarcated expansile mass with smooth margins (Connor et al. 2008).

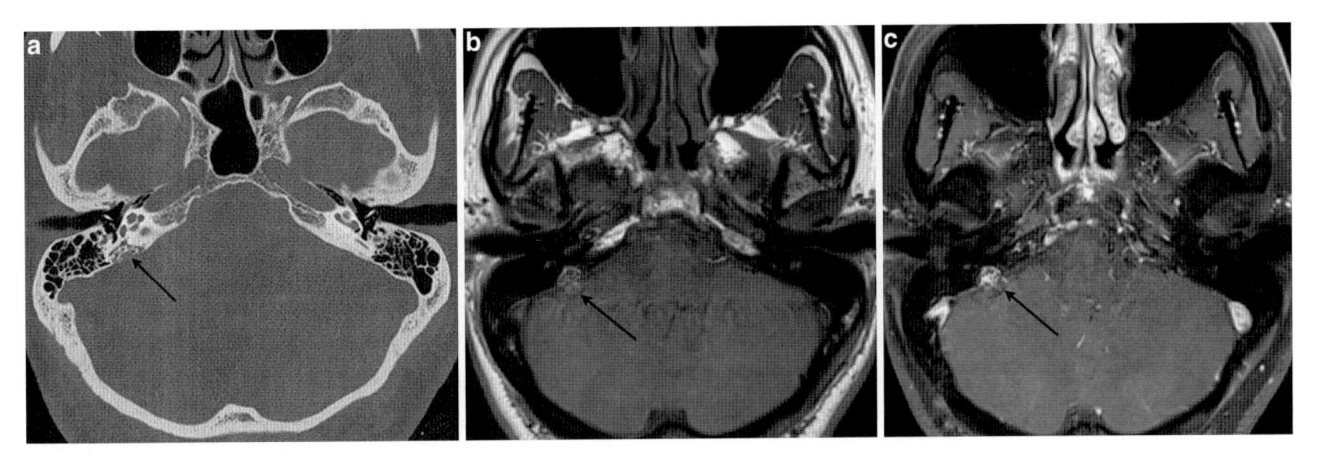

Fig. 9 Endolymphatic sac tumour **a** Axial temporal bone CT image shows typical permeative bone changes in the retrolabyrinthine right petrous temporal bone (*arrow*). **b** Axial T1-weighted MR image shows the tumour with characteristic intramural high signal foci (*arrow*). **c** Axial fat-saturated contrast-enhanced T1-weighted image shows heterogeneous enhancement of the lesion (*arrow*)

Fig. 10 Bilateral petrous apex cephalocoeles. **a** Axial high-resolution T2-weighted MR image shows bilateral CSF intensity petrous apex cephalocoeles, with direct communication with the Meckel caves (*arrows*). **b** Axial temporal bone CT image shows smooth, non-aggressive excavation of the petrous apices (*arrows*)

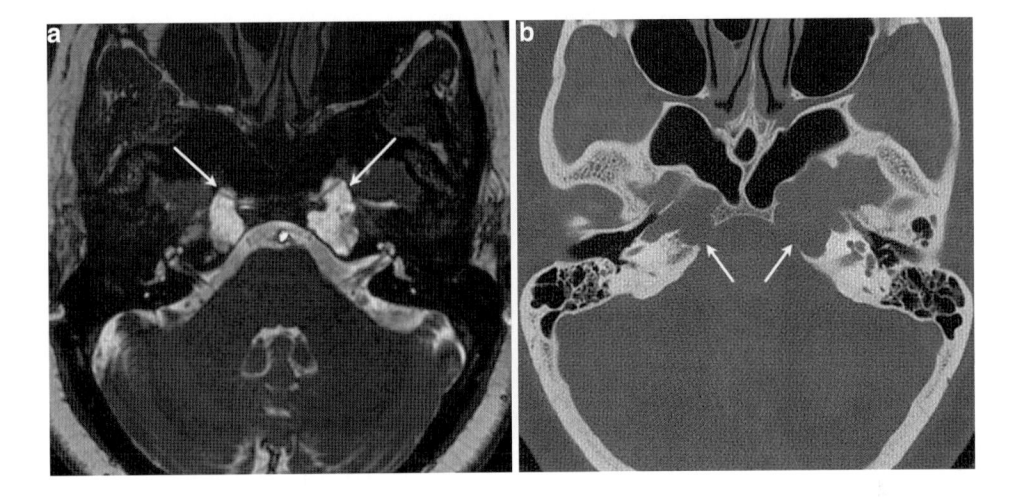

Cholesterol granuloma is the most common surgical lesion of the petrous apex (Greenberg et al. 1988). It results from an inflammatory response to the presence of cholesterol crystals, a degradation product of microhaemorrhages within the petrous apex air-cells (Jackler and Cho 2003). It is characterised by an expansile mass of high T1 and T2-weighted signals, with a hypointense rim (due to haemosiderin deposition) and no enhancement.

Mucocoele of the petrous apex is a rare lesion, which results from continuous mucous secretion into obstructed air-cells. The MR signals of this expansile lesion vary according to the degree of hydration or inspissation of the contents (Larson and Wong 1992). This lesion shows no enhancement, the presence of which should raise the suspicion of superimposed infection or underlying tumours.

Petrous apex cholesteatomas are very rare, accounting for less than 1 % of all detected petrous apex lesions. This cholesteatoma may develop from aberrant epithelial rests of embryonal origin within the petrous apex air-cells or less commonly, extension of an acquired middle ear cholesteatoma (Profant and Steno 2000).

7.3 Malignant Tumours

The imaging features of malignant lesions of the petrous apex are frequently non-specific. CT reveals lytic or permeative bone destruction, while MR imaging shows variable T1 and T2-weighted signal intensities with post-contrast enhancement (Connor et al. 2008).

In elderly patients, *metastasis* (most commonly from breast or lung cancer) and *plasmacytoma* or *multiple myeloma* are the principal differential diagnoses (Fig. 11). The petrous apex is the most common site for metastatic deposit in the temporal bone, and marrow-filled petrous apices may predispose to metastases (Gloria-Cruz et al. 2000).

In the paediatric population, *rhabdomyosarcoma* and *Langerhans cell histiocytosis* are the key considerations.

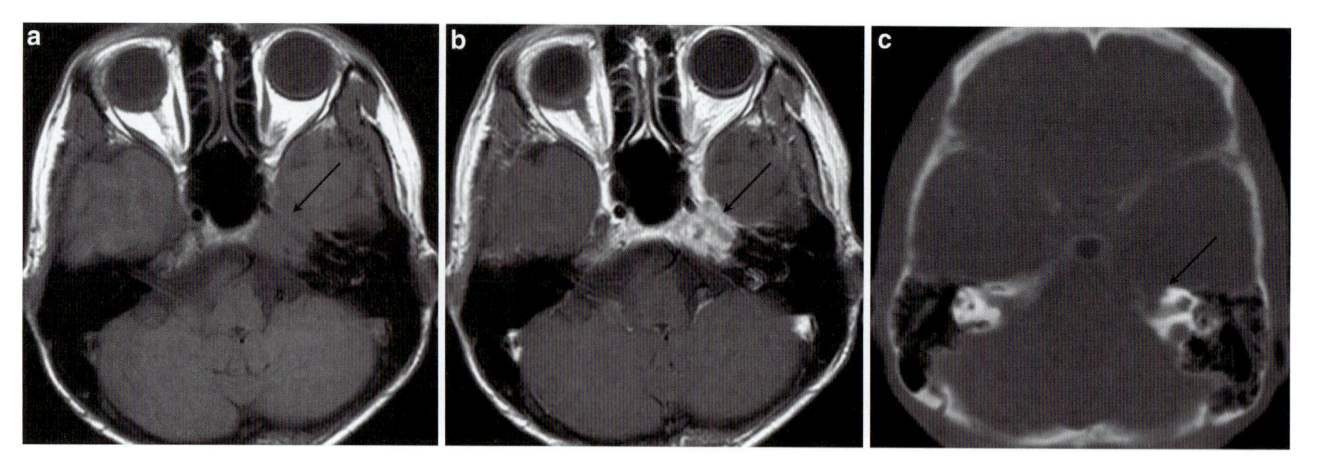

Fig. 11 Petrous apex metastasis from breast cancer. **a** Axial T1-weighted MR image shows soft tissue replacement of the left petrous apex (*arrow*), surrounding the petrous ICA. **b** Axial contrast-enhanced T1-weighted MR image shows avid enhancement of the lesion (*arrow*). **c** Axial bone algorithm CT image shows bony destruction of the left petrous apex (*arrow*)

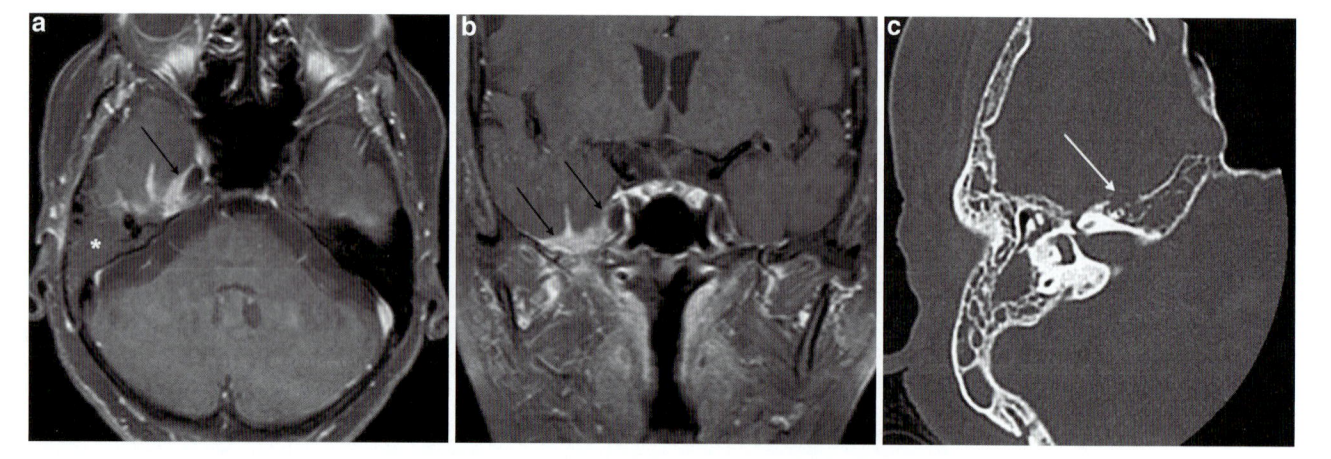

Fig. 12 Apical petrositis in a 47-year-old female with fever, right otorrhoea and deep-seated facial pain. **a** Axial fat-saturated contrast-enhanced T1-weighted MR image shows enhancement of the right petrous apex, and meningeal enhancement over the adjacent Meckel cave (*arrow*). Right mastoiditis is evident (*asterisk*) **b** Coronal fat-saturated contrast-enhanced T1-weighted MR image shows marked meningeal thickening with avid enhancement over the floor of the right middle cranial fossa and cavernous sinus (*arrows*). **c** Axial right temporal bone CT image shows petrous apex opacification with trabecular disruption and cortical erosion (*arrow*)

Although approximately 30 % of all paediatric rhabdomyosarcomas occur in the head and neck, the temporal bone is an uncommon site of involvement (Adrassy 1997). The diagnosis is often delayed as the presentation may mimic chronic otitis media. Chronic ear discharge unresponsive to antibiotics in paediatric patients should prompt further investigations, especially if associated with any periauricular mass, lymphadenopathy or cranial neuropathy (Durve et al. 2004). Langerhans cell histiocytosis may involve the petrous apex, although it most commonly arise from the mastoid air-cells.

The petrous apex may also be involved by *chondrosarcoma* and *chordoma*, which typically originate from adjacent structures. The skull base develops by endochondral ossification. Skull base chondrosarcomas arise de novo from remnants of embryonic cartilage, most commonly in the petro-occipital fissure (Neff et al. 2002). CT shows a lytic bone lesion with sharp transition margin, and chondroid calcification is seen in up to 50 % of the cases. They are hypointense to isointense on T1-weighted images and hyperintense on T2-weighted images, with heterogeneous post-contrast enhancement (Schmidinger et al. 2002). Chordomas, which originate from the embronic notochord, shares similar imaging findings with chondrosarcomas. The key differentiating feature from chondrosarcomas is their midline clival origin. Rarely, chordomas may develop from ectopic notochordal remnants in the petrous apex, when they are virtually indistinguishable from chondrosarcomas (Lowenheim et al. 2006).

Apical petrositis is an important differential diagnosis when aggressive cortical erosion and trabecular breakdown are seen in the petrous apex. This infection of the petrous apices (most of which are pneumatised) usually results from middle ear infection spreading through interconnecting air-cell tracts (Connor et al. 2008). Otorrhoea is the most common symptom. Gradenigo syndrome, which consists of the clinical triad of otomastoiditis, deep facial pain (trigeminal neuropathy) and lateral rectus palsy (abducens neuropathy), is a rare but classis presentation. Contrast enhanced MR imaging may show a peripherally enhancing fluid-filled petrous apex (similar to an abscess collection) with adjacent meningeal thickening and enhancement (Fig. 12).

References

Adrassy R (1997) Rhabdomyosarcoma. J Semin Pediatr Surg 6:17–23

Aydin K, Maya MM, Lo WWM, et al (2000) Jacobson's nerve schwannoma presenting as middle ear mass. AJNR Am J Neuroradiol 21:1331–1333

Balasubramaniam C (1999) A case of malignant tumor of jugular foramen in a young infant. Childs Nerv Syst 15:347–350

Barrs DM (2001) Temporal bone carcinoma. Otolaryngol Clin North Am 34:1197–1218

Bohrer PS, Chole RA (1996) Unusual lesions of the internal auditory canal. Am J Otol 17:143–149

Bonneville F, Savatovsky J, Chiras J (2007) Imaging of cerebello-pontine angle lesions: an update. Part 2: intra-axial lesions, skull base lesions that may invade CPA region, and non-enhancing extra-axial lesions. Eur Radiol 17:2908–2920

Choi JY, Choi EC, Lee HK et al (2003) Mode of parotid involvement in external auditory canal carcinoma. J Laryngol Otol 117:951–954

Connor SEJ, Leung R, Natas S (2008) Imaging of the petrous apex: a pictorial review. Br J Radiol 81:427–435

De Foer B, Vercruysse J-P, Pilet B et al (2006) Single-shot, turbo spin-echo, diffusion-weighted imaging versus spinecho-planar, diffusion-weighted imaging in the detection of acquired middle ear cholesteatoma. AJNR Am J Neuroradiol 27:1480–1482

De Foer B, Kenis C, Van Melkebeke D et al (2010) Pathology of the vestibulocochlear nerve. Eur J Radiol 74:349–358

Devaney KO, Ferlito A, Rinaldo A (2003) Endolymphatic sac tumor (low-grade papillary adenocarcinoma) of the temporal bone. Acta Otolaryngol 123:1022–1026

Devaney KO, Boschman CR, Willard SC et al (2005) Tumours of the external ear and temporal bone. Lancet Oncol 6:411–420

Durve DV, Kanegaonkar RG, Albert D et al (2004) Paediatric rhabdomyosarcoma of the ear and temporal bone. Clin Otolaryngol 29:32–37

Gacek MR, Gacek RR, Gantz B et al (1998) Pseudoepitheliomatous hyperplasia versus squamous cell carcinoma of the external auditory canal. Laryngoscope 108:620–623

Gloria-Cruz TI, Schachern PA, Paparella MM et al (2000) Metastases to temporal bones from primary nonsystemic malignant neoplasms. Arch Otolaryngol Head Neck Surg 126:209–214

Greenberg JJ, Oot RF, Wismer GL et al (1988) Cholesterol granuloma of the petrous apex: MR and CT evaluation. Am J Neuroradiol 9:1205–1214

Heffner DK (1989) Low-grade adenocarcinoma of probable endolymphatic sac origin. A clinicopathologic study of 20 cases. Cancer 64:2292–2302

Ho VT, Rao VM, Doan HT (1996) Low-grade adenocarcinoma of probable endolymphatic sac orign: CT and MR appearance. AJNR Am J Neuroradiol 17:168–170

Jackler RK, Cho M (2003) A new theory to explain the genesis of petrous apex cholesterol granuloma. Otol Neurotol 24:96–106

Jin YT, Tsai ST, Li C, et al (1997) Prevalence of human papillomavirus in middle ear carcinoma associated with chronic otitis media. Am J of Pathology 150:1327–1333

Langman AW, Jackler RK, Althaus SR (1990) Meningioma of the internal auditory canal. Am J Otol 11:201–204

Larson TL, Wong ML (1992) Primary mucocele of the petrous apex: MR appearance. Am J Neuroradiol 13:203–204

Laudadio P, Berni Canani F, Cunsolo E (2004) Meningioma of the internal auditory canal. Acta Otolaryngol 124:1231–1234

Leonetti JP, Shownkeen H, Marzo SJ (2001) Incidental petrous apex findings on magnetic resonance imaging. Ear Nose Throat J 80(200–202):205–206

Lim LHY, Goh YH, Chan YM et al (2000) Malignancy of the temporal bone and external auditory canal. Otolaryngol Head Neck Surg 122:882–886

Lobo D, Llorente JL, Suarez C (2008) Squamous cell carcinoma of the external auditory canal. Skull Base 18:167–172

Lowenheim H, Koerbel A, Ebner FH et al (2006) Differentiating imaging findings in primary and secondary tumors of the jugular foramen. Neurosurg Rev 29:1–11

Moffat DA, Wagstaff SA, Hardy DG (2005) The outcome of radical surgery and postoperative radiotherapy for squamous cell carcinoma of the temporal bone. Laryngoscope 115:341–347

Moore KR, Harnsberger HR, Shelton C et al (1998) "Leave me alone" lesions of the petrous apex. Am J Neuroradiol 19:733–738

Moore KR, Fischbein NJ, Harnsberger HR et al (2001) Petrous apex cephaloceles. Am J Neuroradiol 22:1867–1871

Mukherji SK, Albernaz VS, Lo WW et al (1997) Papillary endolymphatic sca tumors; CT, MR imaging, and angiographic findings in 20 patients. Radiology 202:801–808

Neff B, Sataloff RT, Storey L et al (2002) Chondrosarcoma of the skull base. Laryngoscope 112:134–139

O'Leary MJ, Shelton C, Giddings NA et al (1991) Glomus tympanicum tumors: a clinical perspective. Laryngoscope 101:1038–1043

Ong CK, Chong VF (2009) Imaging of jugular foramen. Neuroimaging Clin N Am 19:469–482

Ong CK, Pua U, Chong VF (2008) Imaging of carcinoma of the external auditory canal: a pictorial essay. ICIS Cancer Imaging 20:191–198

Profant M, Steno J (2000) Petrous apex cholesteatoma. Acta Otolaryngol 120:164–167

Roncaroli F, Giangaspero F, Piana S et al (1997) Low-grade adenocarcinoma of endolymphatic sac mimicking jugular paraganglioma at clinical and neuroradiological examination. Clin Neuropathol 16:243–246

Schmidinger A, Rosahl SK, Vorkapic P et al (2002) Natural history of chondroid skull base lesions: case report and review. Neuroradiology 44:268–271

Schwartz KM, Lane JI, Bolster BD Jr et al (2011) The utility of diffusion-weighted imaging for cholesteatoma evaluation. AJNR Am J Neuroradiol 32:430–436

Somers T, Casselman J, de Ceuler G et al (2001) Prognostic value of magnetic resonance imaging findings in hearing preservation surgery for vestibular schwannoma. Otol Neurotol 22:1368–1376

Stendel R, Suess O, Prosene N et al (1998) Neoplasm of endolymphatic sac origin: clinical, radiological and pathological features. Acta Neurochir (Wien) 140:1083–1087

Swartz JD (2008) Pathology of the vestibulocochlear nerve. Neuroimaging Clin N Am 18:321–346

Tieleman A, Casselman JW, Somers T et al (2008) Imaging of intralabyrinthine schwannomas: a retrospective study of 52 cases with emphasis on lesion growth. Am J Neuroradiol 29:898–905

Torske KR, Thompsom L (2002) Adenoma versus carcinoid tumor of the middle ear: a study of 48 cases and review of the literature. Mod Pathol 15:543–555

Ulku CH, Uyar Y, Acar O et al (2004) Facial nerve schwanommas: a report of four cases and a review of the literature. Am J Otolaryngol 25:426–431

Virapongse C, Sarwwar M, Bhimani S et al (1985) Computed tomography of temporal bone pneumatization, 1: normal pattern and morphology. Am J Roentgenol 145:473–481

Wiet RJ, Lotan AN, Brackmann DE (1985) Neurilemmoma of the chorda tympani nerve. Otolaryngol Head Neck Surg 93:119–121

Yin M, Ishikawa K, Honda K et al (2006) Analysis of 95 cases of squamous cell carcinoma of the external and middle ear. Auris Nasus Larynx 33:251–257

Zan E, Limb CJ, Koehler JF et al (2009) Middle ear adenoma: a challenging diagnosis. AJNR Am J Neuroadiol 30:1602–1603

Congenital Malformations of the Temporal Bone

J. W. Casselman, J. Delanote, R. Kuhweide, J. van Dinther,
B. De Foer, and E. F. Offeciers

Contents

1 Imaging Techniques 120
2 Congenital Malformations of the External Auditory Canal, Tympanic Membrane and Ring 121
2.1 Embryology 121
2.2 Stenosis and Atresia of the External Auditory Canal 122
3 Congenital Malformations of the Middle Ear 127
3.1 Embryology 127
3.2 Middle Ear Malformations Associated with External Auditory Canal Deformities 127
3.3 Middle Ear Malformations in the Absence of EAC Stenosis and EAC Atresia 127
4 Congenital Malformations of the Inner Ear 133
4.1 Embryology 133
4.2 Classifications and Malformations of the Labyrinth 134

References 152

J. W. Casselman (✉) · J. Delanote
Department of Radiology and Medical Imaging,
AZ St-Jan Brugge-Oostende, Bruges, Belgium
e-mail: jan.casselman@azsintjan.be

J. W. Casselman · B. De Foer
Department of Radiology, AZ St-Augustinus,
Antwerp, Belgium

J. W. Casselman
Ghent University, Ghent, Belgium

R. Kuhweide
Department of ENT, AZ St-Jan Brugge-Oostende,
Bruges, Belgium

J. van Dinther · E. F. Offeciers
Department of ENT, AZ St-Augustinus, Antwerp, Belgium

J. van Dinther · E. F. Offeciers
European Institute for ENT- Head and Neck Surgery,
AZ St-Augustinus, Antwerp, Belgium

Abstract

Computed tomography is the technique of choice to study the malformations of the auricle, external auditory canal (EAC) and middle ear. The best image quality with the lowest radiation dose can be achieved when high-end Cone Beam CT scanners are used. The 125 μm spatial resolution images they provide are crucial in the detection of subtle ossicular and oval/round window malformations. Knowledge of the embryology helps to understand which malformations can be found and atresia and stenosis of the EAC are the most frequently found malformations of the outer ear. First Branchial Cleft Anomalies are rare and are best studied using MR. Middle ear malformations can develop in association with or in the absence of EAC deformities. Anomalies of the ossicles, facial nerve, oval window, round window, etc., can all be studied in detail with CT. However, MR is needed for the detection of congenital middle ear cholesteatomas and for cholesteatomas which are caused by congenital middle ear malformations and their resulting bad middle ear aeration. Inner ear malformations normally are not associated with middle and outer ear anomalies and high-resolution MR is the best adapted technique to detect vestibular, cochlear and cochleovestibular nerve malformations. New classifications of the labyrinthine malformations and VIIIth nerve malformations are used and their goal is to warn the surgeon for potential hazards during surgery and especially when cochlear implantation is considered. Finally the outer, middle and inner ear can be involved together in syndromes and therefore both MR and CT are often required in these patients. In this chapter the embryology and most frequent malformations of the outer, middle and inner ear will be discussed as well as the contemporary imaging techniques that should be used.

1 Imaging Techniques

Congenital malformations of the outer ear (auricle and the external auditory canal (EAC)), middle ear, inner ear and auditory pathways can be very complex (e.g. syndromes). On the other hand sometimes only very subtle isolated malformations are present. Therefore, imaging with the highest possible spatial and/or contrast resolution is needed.

Malformations of the auricle, microtia, severe dysplasia of the auricle and anotia can be diagnosed clinically. However, they are often associated with external, middle and less frequently inner ear malformations and therefore detailed imaging is required in these patients as well.

Computed tomography (CT) is the method of choice to study EAC and middle ear malformations (Romo et al. 2011; Veillon et al. 2014; Verbist et al. 2011). Today, MultiDetector CT (MDCT) systems using a spiral acquisition technique are widely available and provide submillimetric 0.625–0.5 mm thick CT images and high-end MDCT systems produce even thinner images. The in-plane resolution of these images is similar and the high-end systems even have an in-plane resolution between 0.2 and 0.25 mm. But even with such a high spatial resolution, it remains necessary to reconstruct these images every 0.1 mm (or at least every 0.2 mm) and to recalculate images of the left and right ear separately with a smaller field of view (6 × 6 or 8 × 8 cm) using a bone window setting. Many of these patients are neonates, children and young adults and hence the radiation should be kept as low as possible. New high-end systems with iterative reconstruction and fast scan possibilities allow scanning with a considerable dose reduction. However, a minimum of radiation dose is needed to guarantee high-quality CT imaging of the temporal bone. The images will no longer be diagnostic if one is tempted to reduce the dose too much and this will often result in a re-scan in another institution with at the end an overall higher radiation dose. For the same reason, coronal images should be reformatted from the original axial 0.1 or 0.2 mm thick recalculated images in order to keep the radiation dose low. Scanning in both the axial and coronal plane can no longer be justified. Finally, the axial images through the temporal bone must be angled, so that they pass below the lens. Even higher resolution is today possible with the latest generation Cone Beam CTs (CBCT). These systems provide isotropic images with a spatial resolution of 0.075–0.125 mm instead of the routine 0.5 mm images of most of the MDCTs and axial, coronal and sagittal reformatted images have the same quality (Casselman et al. 2014b; Dahmani-Causse et al. 2011; Penninger et al. 2011). Moreover, CBCT also allows further radiation dose reduction. But there is one disadvantage. The total CBCT scan time is 40 s, resulting in movement artefacts in neonates and young children and less cooperative patients. Ossicular and especially stapedial and footplate or oval window malformations can be very subtle. They are often only discernable on double-oblique reformatted images. These images correct the 15–25° posterior (with regard to the coronal plane) and 20–30° superior (with regard to the axial plane) angulation of the stapes and its footplate, revealing the most detailed anatomy and/or malformations of these very small structures. It is often impossible to exclude stapedial or oval window malformations in the absence of double-oblique reformatted images (Fig. 1).

Magnetic resonance (MR) imaging has become the primary imaging technique for screening of congenital inner ear malformations. The imaging quality increased with the advent of better phased-array coils, a higher main magnetic field and stronger gradients. Three-dimensional (3D) heavily T2-weighted images provide excellent contrast between the high-signal intensity of cerebrospinal fluid (CSF), endolymphatic and perilymphatic fluid and the low-signal intensity surrounding osseous structures of the temporal bone. Similar images allow separate visualization of the three branches of the VIIIth nerve and the facial nerve inside the internal auditory canal (IAC). At 3.0 Tesla, the signal-to-noise is good enough to acquire submillimetric (isotropic 0.3^3–0.4^3 mm) images with enough contrast resolution and anatomic detail, even when a routine phased-array head coil is used. At 1.5 Tesla, phased-array surface coils are often needed to compensate for the lower signal-to-noise ratio (Schmalbrock et al. 1995). Three-dimensional Fourier transform constructive interference in steady state (3DFT-CISS), 3D turbo spin-echo (3D-TSE), 3D fast imaging employing steady-state acquisition (3D-FIESTA) and 3D driven equilibrium radio frequency reset pulse (3D-DRIVE) are some of the best known heavily T2-weighted sequences used to study the inner ear (Brogan et al. 1991; Casselman et al. 1993a, b, 1996; Schmalbrock et al. 1993; Tien et al. 1993). Even small anatomic structures like the utricular macula and the ganglion of Scarpa can be depicted on these high-quality images. Subtle congenital inner ear malformations like modiolar anomalies, incomplete partition anomalies of the cochlea and hypoplasia or aplasia of the cochleovestibular nerve or its cochlear branch can all be recognised on these images. They can also be used to produce 3D-maximum intensity projections (3D-MIP) and 3D-virtual reality (VR) surface rendered images. They are very helpful in the analysis of complex malformations which are difficult to evaluate on routine orthogonal images. T1-weighted images lack this good contrast between bone, nerves and fluid. Nevertheless, gadolinium-enhanced T1-weighted images remain the most sensitive images if one wants to exclude concomitant tumoral and inflammatory changes in adult patients with congenital sensorineural hearing loss (SNHL). The diagnosis of a congenital cholesteatoma can be made on CT when the middle ear is normally aerated. However, it can be very difficult to depict a congenital cholesteatoma on CT when a middle ear effusion is present. In these cases, non-echo-planar diffusion-weighted imaging (non-EPI DWI) with a b-value of 1,000 (b = 1,000 s/mm^2) can be used to distinguish the cholesteatoma from the middle ear effusion (De Foer et al. 2010).

2 Congenital Malformations of the External Auditory Canal, Tympanic Membrane and Ring

2.1 Embryology

By about 4–5 weeks of fetal age, the first branchial groove deepens to become the primitive external auditory meatus. The first pharyngeal pouch which arises from endoderm of the primitive foregut grows outward and upward and will lead to the development of the primitive eustachian tube. For a short time, the epithelium of the first branchial groove and the endoderm of the first pharyngeal pouch will be in contact at the site where the future tympanic membrane will develop. During the next 20 fetal weeks, the first branchial groove contributes to the development of the mature external auditory canal, the outer layer of the tympanic membrane and the tympanic ring. The eustachian tube and middle ear cavity and its epithelial lining develop from the first pharyngeal pouch.

At 8 weeks, inward extension of the first branchial groove in the direction of the middle ear creates a primitive canal between the first and second branchial arches. At 9 weeks, the "meatal plug", a solid cord of ectoderm grows from the fundus of the primitive EAC towards the middle ear. Ingrowth of mesoderm between the meatal plug and the middle ear forms the central fibrous portion of the tympanic membrane and explains why the mature tympanic membrane has an outer ectodermal (squamous epithelium), middle mesodermal (fibrous) and inner endodermal (respiratory epithelium) layer. At the same time, the first ossification centre of the bony tympanic ring appears. Disintegration and canalization of the meatal plug, which starts in the deepest part of the meatal plug near the tympanic membrane, will result in the formation of the bony part of the EAC. Failure of development of the first branchial groove resulting in non-formation of the primitive auditory canal or incomplete or absent canalization of the meatal plug will result in a spectrum of EAC, tympanic membrane and the tympanic ring malformations ranging from minor EAC stenosis to severe EAC atresia. Normal growth of the temporomandibular joint (TMJ) and middle ear also depends on the presence of a normal meatus and tympanic ring development. Congenital middle ear cholesteatomas can also develop when

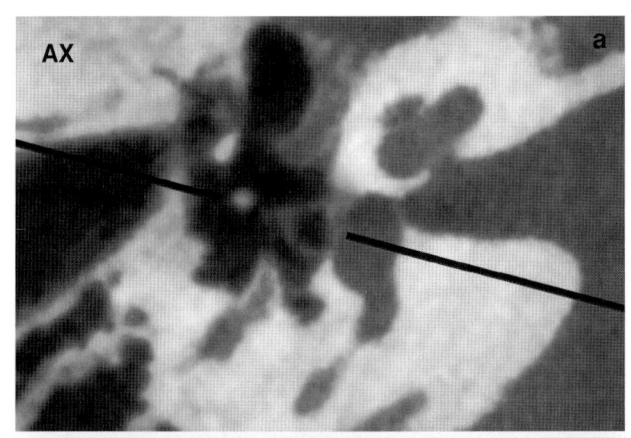

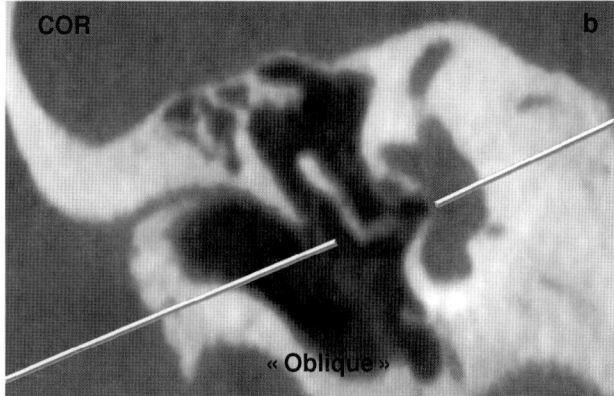

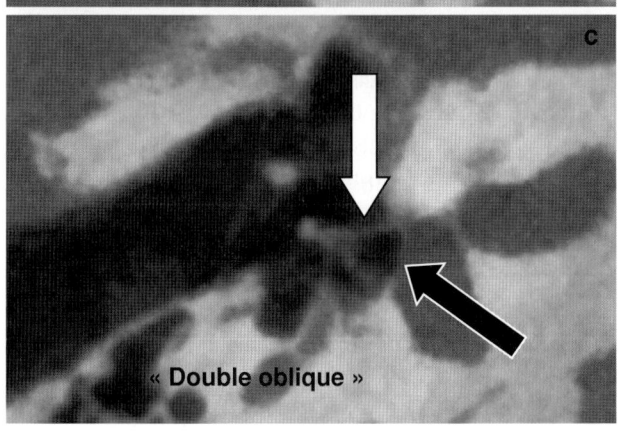

Fig. 1 Cone-Beam CT—double-oblique reformatted images. **a** On axial images, the incudostapedial axis is angulated 15–25° posteriorly with regard to the coronal plane. Images must be reformatted along this line, passing through the joint and between the two crurae of the stapes (*black line*). Note the false appearance of a *thickened* footplate seen as high density between the grey fluid in the labyrinth and the black air in the middle ear. **b** On the oblique reformatted image (made along the *black line* in a), the incudostapedial joint is now angulated 20–30° superiorly with regard to the axial plane. Images must be reformatted along this line, passing through the joint and the centre of the oval window (*white line*). Note that the footplate no longer seems to be thickened. **c** On this double-oblique reformatted image (made along the *black line* in a and *white line* in b) one can see the joint, the crurae (*white arrow*) and the footplate (*black arrow*) in one plane. The footplate is normal and the fluid is in contact with the air without any bone density in between. Compare with "**a**" where this was not the case and the density between the fluid and air represented partial volume through the bone around the oval window/footplate

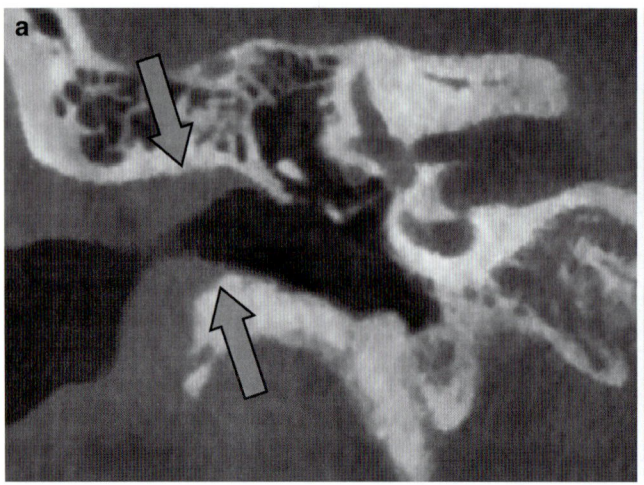

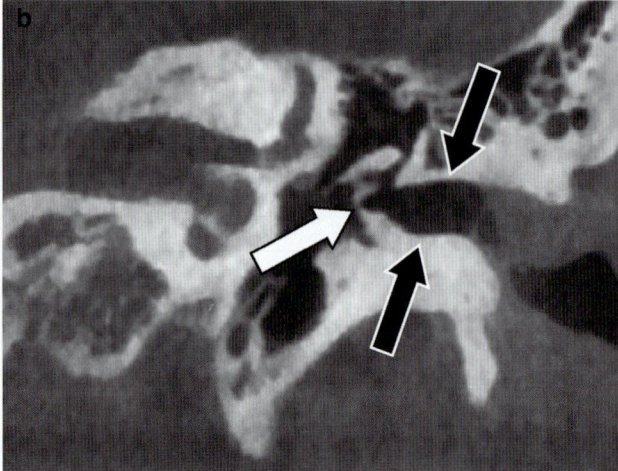

Fig. 2 Stenosis of the external auditory canal. **a** Coronal CBCT image on the *right side* with normal size of the external auditory canal (*grey arrows*). **b** Coronal CBCT image on the *left side* stenosis of the bony part of the external auditory canal (*black arrows*). Fixation of the malleus to the tympanic ring (*white arrow*). There was no fibrous or bony atresia in this patient

ectodermal tissue rests remain in the middle ear during fetal gestation.

The cartilaginous and osseous portions of the EAC develop from the first branchial arch mesoderm. The cartilages from the first and second branchial arch also form the ossicles as well as the mandible and midface. Hence ossicular anomalies, especially ossicular fusion, and more severe facial and mandibular deformities can occur together with EAC atresia. Unlike the rest of the ossicles, the anterior process of the malleus differentiates from the primitive tympanic ring. This explains why the malleus is frequently fixed to the atretic plate at this site (Dayal 1973; Bellucci 1981; Schuknecht 1989; Curtin et al. 2011).

2.2 Stenosis and Atresia of the External Auditory Canal

Stenosis or atresia of the EAC occurs once per 10,000–20,000 births and is most frequently unilateral. (Jafek et al. 1975). Its occurrence is sporadic due to spontaneous chromosomal abnormalities, which can be caused by infections or toxicity during gestation. However, genetic transmission explains the association of EAC atresia and many syndromes: hemifacial microsomia, Treacher Collins syndrome, Branchio-Oto-Renal syndrome (BOR), Crouzon or Alport syndrome, Klippel-Feil anomaly etc. (Romo et al. 2011). These patients present with conductive hearing loss.

2.2.1 Stenosis of the External Auditory Canal

The cartilaginous portion of the EAC can be stenotic, short or its course can be abnormal. The bony external auditory canal is considered stenotic when its diameter is smaller than 4 mm. Stenosis can also be associated with middle ear and ossicular abnormalities, but this association is more frequently seen in case of atresia (Fig. 2). Epithelial debris gets entrapped in the medial part of the EAC once the diameter of the EAC is smaller than 2–3 mm. These patients are prone to the development of an acquired EAC cholesteatoma (Cole and Jarsdoerfer 1990; Benton and Bellet 2000).

2.2.2 Atresia of the External Auditory Canal

Atresia of the EAC can be membranous or bony. In "membranous atresia", the bony EAC is usually stenotic and a soft tissue mass is occupying the region where the tympanic membrane normally is located. Associated malformations of the ossicles and middle ear are less frequent in case of membranous atresia (Fig. 3).

In "bony atresia" of the EAC, the tympanic membrane is replaced by a bony plate of variable thickness, extending in the EAC, however, this bony atresia can also be incomplete (Fig. 4).

In "complete bony atresia", the EAC is absent and a bony atresia plate seals the lateral wall of the middle ear cavity. The surrounding skull base structures show a centripetal shift towards the area where the EAC should have been (Benton and Bellet 2000). Complete bony atresia is often associated with:

- A higher and posterior displaced condylar fossa
- An anterior displaced mastoid process
- A shift of the condyle towards the mastoid process and localization lateral to the middle ear cavity
- Absence of the ascending ramus of the mandible
- A high jugular bulb and low tegmen
- A dehiscent and/or inferior displaced tympanic segment of the facial nerve
- An anterior and lateral displacement of the mastoid segment of the facial nerve (Figs. 4 and 6).

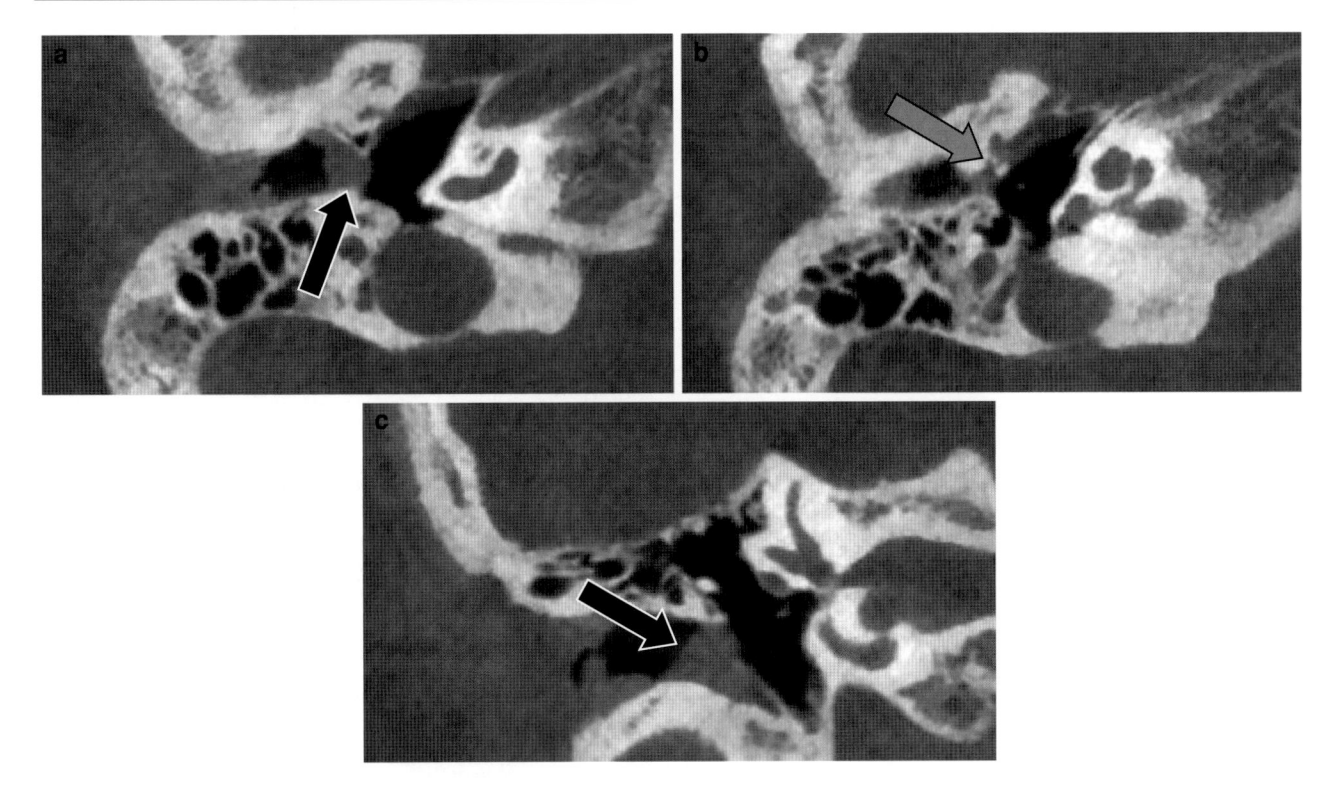

Fig. 3 Membranous atresia of the external auditory canal—Jahrsdoerfer Type B. **a** Axial CBCT image through the EAC shows a soft tissue mass at the site where the tympanic membrane is normally situated (*black arrow*). **b** Axial CBCT image made more cranial than image a. The anterior process of the malleus, which differentiates unlike the rest of the ossicles from the primitive tympanic ring, is fixed to the tympanic ring (*grey arrow*). **c** Coronal CBCT image through the EAC. Membranous atresia with soft tissues at the site of the tympanic membrane (*black arrow*)

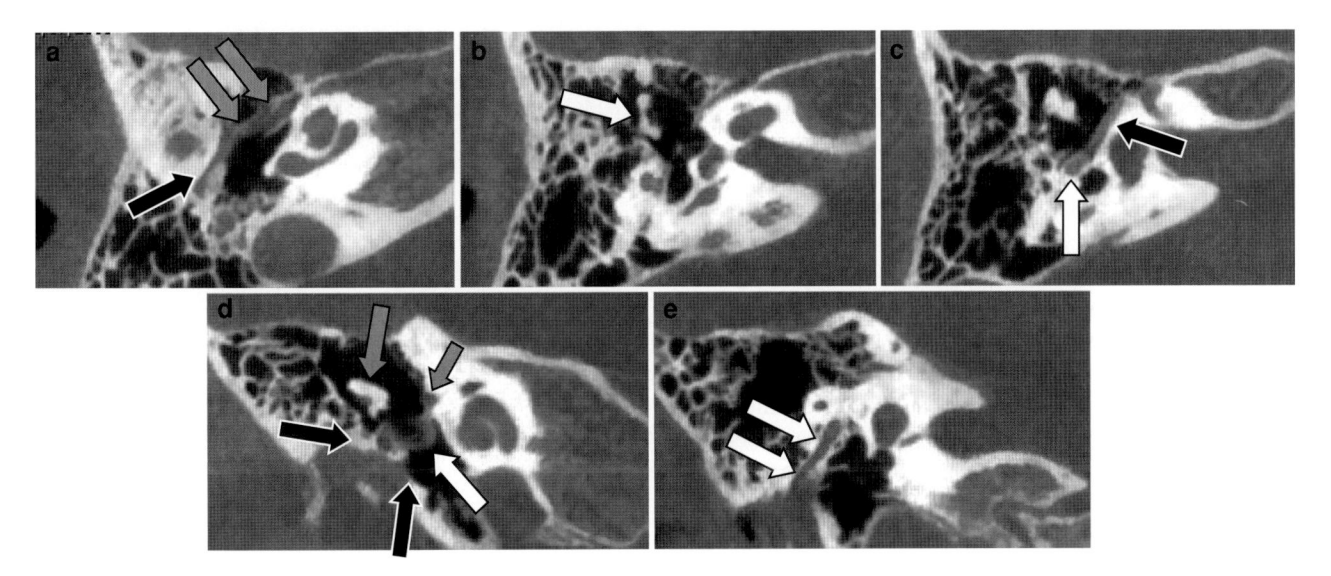

Fig. 4 Incomplete bony atresia of the EAC with abnormal course of the facial nerve and tensor tympani muscle. **a** Axial CBCT image at the level of the tensor tympani muscle shows how this muscles follows an abnormal course through the middle ear cavity (*grey arrows*) and ends at the bony atresia plate (*black arrow*). **b** Axial CBCT image at the level of the oval window shows a normal position and development of the stapes but the malleus and incus are malformed and fused (*arrow*). **c** Axial CBCT image at the level of the tympanic segment of the facial nerve canal (*black arrow*). The posterior genu and mastoid segment of the facial nerve are showing a slightly anterolateral displacement (*white arrow*). Notice that the articulation of the malleus and incus has an abnormal mediolateral orientation. **d** Coronal CBCT image through the anterior part of the middle ear shows the incomplete bony atresia (*black arrows*), the fused malleus and incus (*grey arrow*) and the abnormal course of the thickened tensor tympani muscle (*white arrow*). Tympanic segment of the facial nerve canal (*small arrow*). **e** Coronal CBCT image through the posterior part of the middle ear cavity showing the abnormal oblique lateral shift of the mastoid segment of the facial nerve canal (*white arrows*)

A simple and useful classification of EAC stenosis and atresia was proposed by Schuknecht and was modified by Benton and Jahrsdoerfer (Schuknecht 1989; Benton and Bellet 2000; Yeakley and Jahrsdoerfer 1996). It facilitates the communication between radiologists and otological surgeons and further helps to make the choice between surgery and placement of an osteo-integrated bone-conduction device (BAHA system) (Evans and Kazahaya 2007).

- Type A or meatal atresia: The lateral fibrocartilaginous part of the canal is stenotic
- Type B or partial atresia: The fibrocartilaginous and bony parts of the canal are narrowed and sometimes tortuous. The tympanic membrane is small. The manubrium of the malleus is frequently short and curved and the malleus may be fixed to the epitympanum or tympanic ring (Fig. 3)
- Type C or total atresia: There is absence of the external auditory canal, a partial or complete atresia plate and a well-developed middle ear cavity are present. The malleus and incus are deformed and fused, the malleus neck is fused to the atretic plate (Fig. 5)
- Type D or hypopneumatic total atresia. Similar to Type C but the middle ear cavity is underdeveloped and there is little or no mastoid pneumatization. The facial nerve is often aberrant (Fig. 7).

This classification already helps the radiologist to look carefully at the structures which could jeopardize surgical repair. The following findings make repair of the EAC and ossicular chain more difficult or impossible:

- Mandibular condyle lateral to the middle ear cavity—difficult to reconstruct the EAC
- Small middle ear cavity (distance promontory—atretic plate of less than 3 mm)
- Closed or stenotic oval and/or round window
- Abnormal course of the facial nerve interfering with the surgical approach
- Absence of normal malleus-incus complex (severe deformity or dissociation), absence of the incudostapedial articulation, absence of the stapes suprastructure.

Finally, in severe aural atresia inner ear malformations can be present, although the inner ear develops completely separately from the EAC and middle ear. Hence, inner ear imaging is needed to exclude inner ear malformations in these patients.

2.2.3 First Branchial Cleft Anomalies

First branchial cleft anomalies occur when there is incomplete obliteration of the first branchial apparatus. Remnants of the first branchial cleft can then give rise to a first branchial cleft cyst, fistula or sinus and the majority of first branchial cleft remnants are cysts. In "Type I" first branchial cleft cysts (first BCC), which are of ectodermal origin, a soft and painless well-circumscribed cyst is found just anterior, inferior or posterior to the EAC and they can run parallel with the EAC and are often only related to the membranous EAC. However, the cyst can beak towards the bony-cartilaginous junction of the EAC in both Type I and Type II first BCCs. ""Type II"" first BCCs are of ectodermal and mesodermal origin and can extend from the EAC to the angle of the mandible (Fig. 8) and can even reach the posterior submandibular space. They are found deep to—and even in the parapharyngeal space (Fig. 9), in or superficial to the anterior part of the parotid gland, anterior to the sternocleidomastoid muscle, superior to the

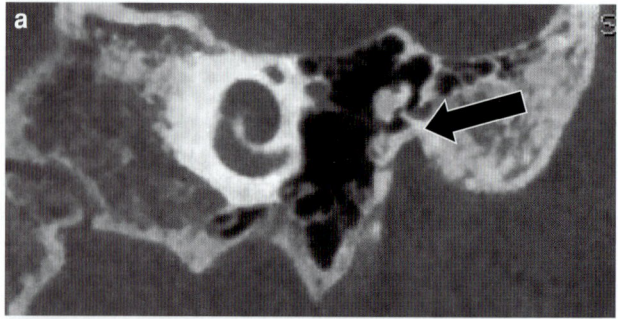

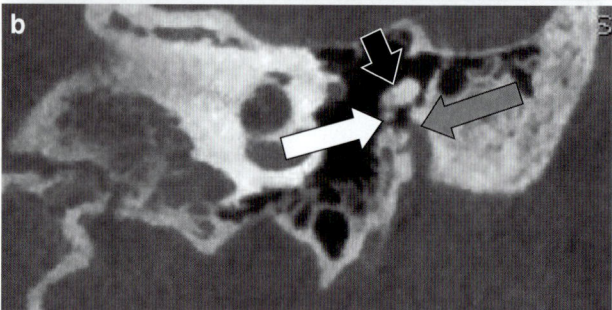

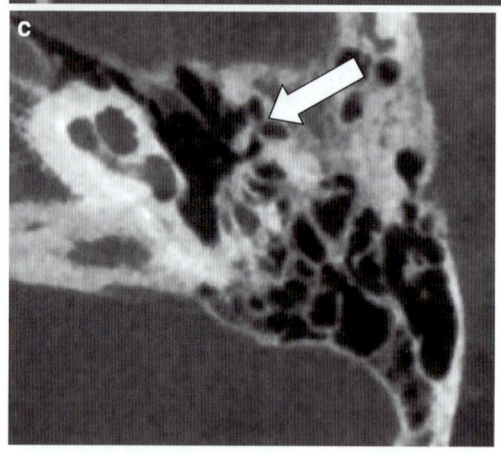

Fig. 5 Bony atresia—Jahrsdoerfer Type C. **a** Coronal CBCT image through the anterior part of the middle ear cavity. The tympanic membrane is replaced by a bony plate (*black arrow*). **b** Coronal CBCT image posterior to "**a**". The bony atresia is not complete. There is still some membranous atresia and a very stenotic EAC filled with soft tissue can be seen (*grey arrow*). Notice the fixation of the anterior process of the malleus to the tympanic bony atresia plate (*white arrow*). The head of the malleus and body of the incus are fused (*short arrow*). **c** Axial CBCT image showing the fixation of the anterior process of the malleus to the bony atresia plate (*white arrow*)

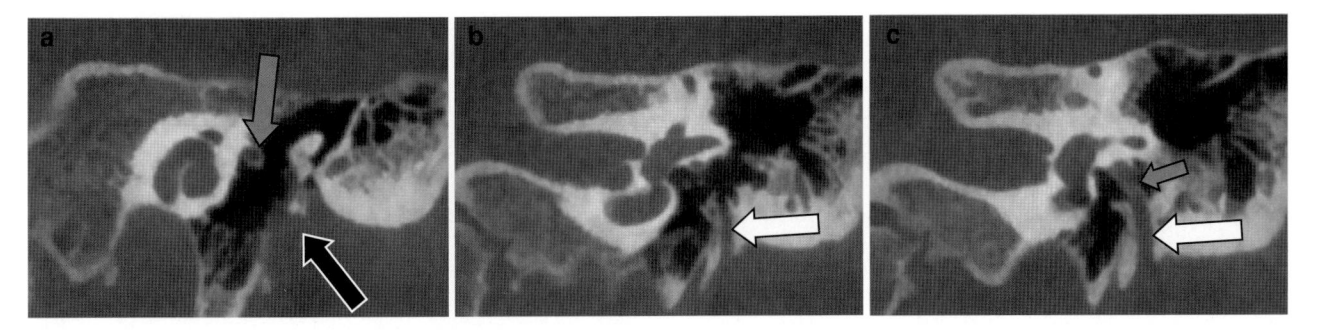

Fig. 6 Membranous atresia, abnormal course of the mastoid segment of the facial nerve. **a** Coronal CBCT image through the anterior part of the middle ear cavity showing the membranous atresia of the external auditory canal (*black arrow*) and the normal position of the tympanic segment of the facial nerve canal (*grey arrow*). **b** Coronal CBCT image posterior to (**a**) showing the anterolateral displacement of the mastoid segment of the facial nerve canal (*white arrow*). **c** Coronal CBCT image at the level of the round window showing the anterolateral displaced dehiscent mastoid segment of the facial nerve running through the middle ear cavity (*short arrow*) and through its anterolateral displaced canal (*white arrow*)

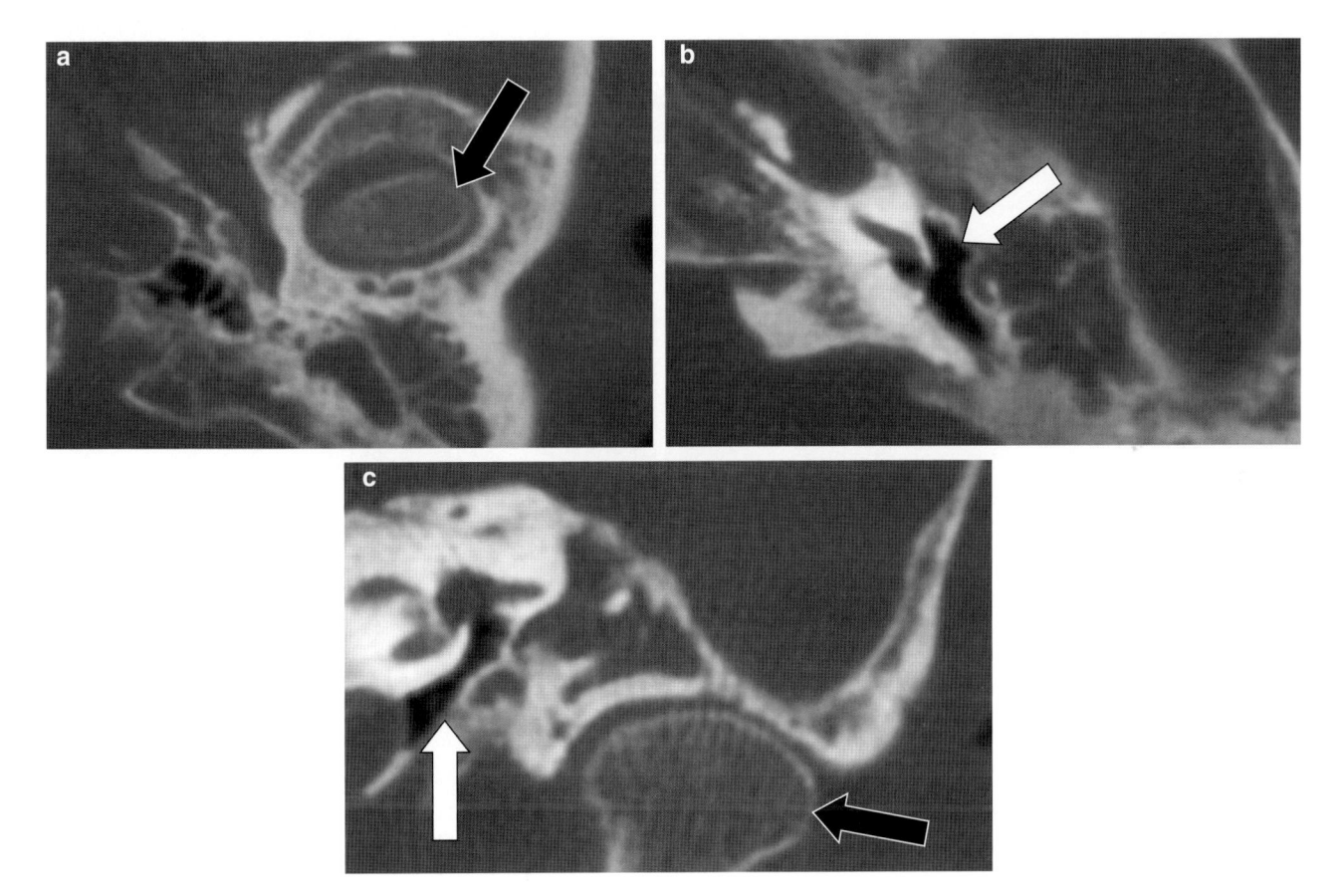

Fig. 7 Bony atresia with hypoplasia of the middle ear cavity—Jahrsdoerfer Type D. **a** Axial MDCT image through the mastoid showing the protrusion of the TMJ in the skull base (*black arrow*). **b** Axial MDCT image at the level of the round window: atresia of the EAC and extreme hypoplastic middle ear cavity (*white arrow*). **c** Coronal MDCT image through the TMJ showing the cranial displacement of the TMJ (*black arrow*) which is now situated lateral to the hypoplastic middle ear cavity (*white arrow*). Notice the absence of the ossicles

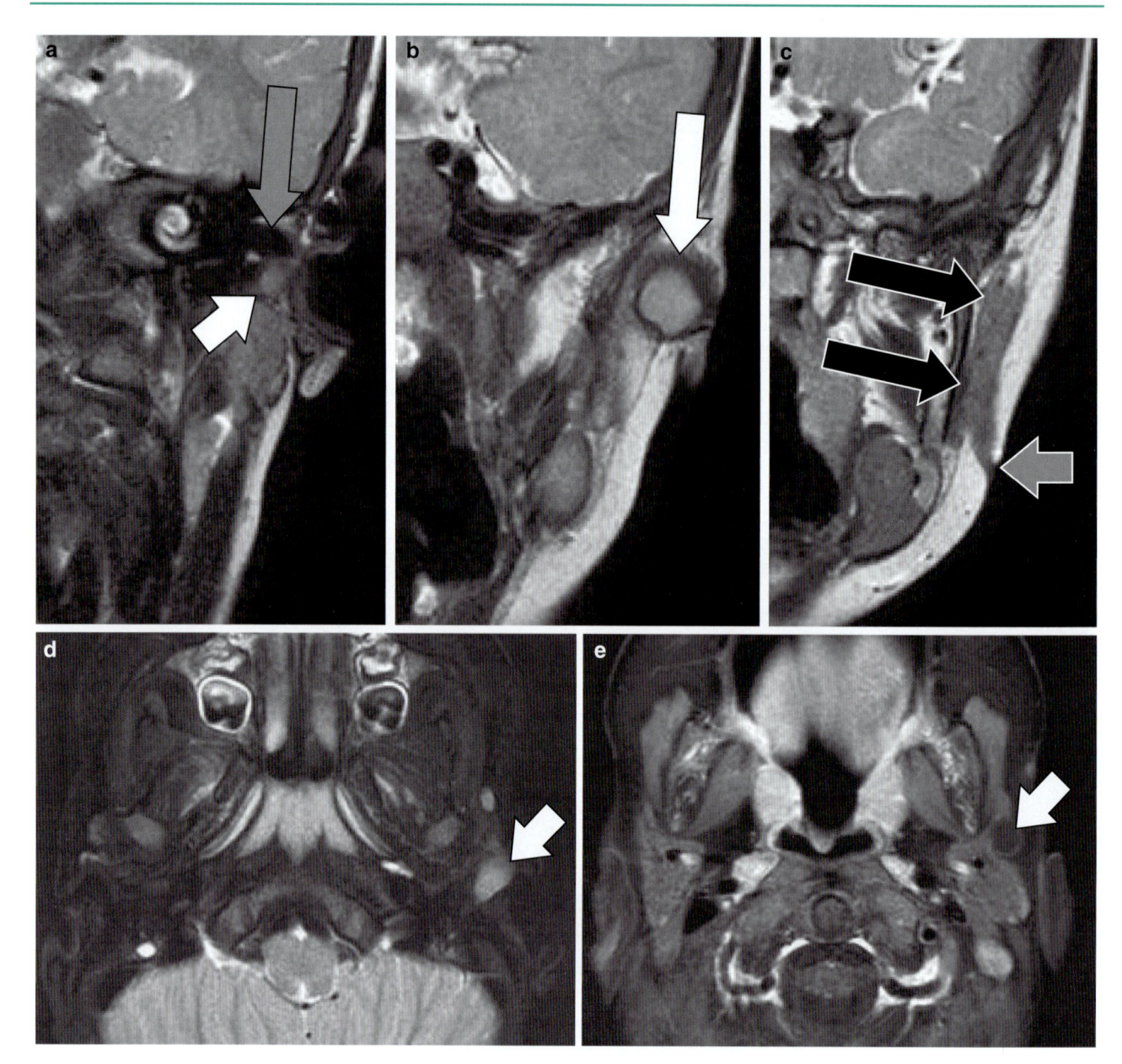

Fig. 8 Type II cyst and fistula of the first branchial cleft. **a–c** Coronal T2-weighted turbo spin-echo images through the external auditory canal (EAC) (**a**), the retromandibular region (**b**) and ascending ramus of the mandible (**c**). A cyst can be followed to the bony-cartilaginous junction of the floor of the EAC (*small white arrow*) and becomes larger in the region anterior to the EAC (*large white arrow*). A large fistula (*black arrows*) can be followed downward to the mandibular angle where the cutaneous opening of the fistula is seen (*small grey arrow*). Roof of the EAC (*large grey arrow*). **d** Axial T2-weighted image with fat suppression at the level of the floor of the EAC showing the high-signal intensity in the branchial cleft cyst (*arrow*). **e** Axial gadolinium-enhanced T1-weighted image with fat suppression at the level of the parotid gland demonstrating the first branchial cleft fistula along the anterolateral border of the parotid gland with subtle enhancement of the wall of the fistula (*arrow*)

hyoid bone and end at the bony-cartilaginous junction of the EAC. Typically, the wall of the cyst is not enhancing, enhancement of a thickened wall is only seen when the first BCC is infected. Complete surgical resection is needed to treat the associated recurrent periauricular abscess formation or chronic otorrhea caused by the sinus tract drainage. Good facial nerve exposure is needed during surgery because of the often close relation of the first BCC with the facial nerve (Lambert and Dodson 1996; Mukherji et al. 1993; Triglia et al. 1998; Work and Proctor 1963).

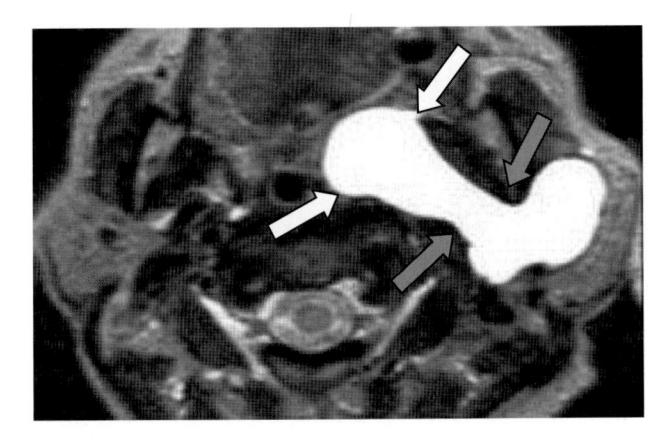

Fig. 9 Type II cyst of the first branchial cleft with extension in the prestyloid parapharyngeal space. Axial T2-weighted image through the parotid glands showing a very rare extension of a first branchial cleft cyst deep to the left parotid gland, through the stylomandibular tunnel (*grey arrows*) into the prestyloid parapharyngeal space (*white arrows*)

3 Congenital Malformations of the Middle Ear

3.1 Embryology

At the third gestational week, an outpouching of the endoderm-lined first pharyngeal pouch, will form the tympanic cavity and auditory tube. This outpouching of the foregut, the tubotympanic recess, grows dorsally between the otic capsule and primitive external auditory canal. Progressive resorption of the mesenchyma surrounding the primary middle ear cavity will lead by the end of the eight gestational week to cavitation and expansion of the tympanic cavity. Remnants of the mesenchyma eventually form the ligaments which will support the middle ear ossicles. The mesoderm of the first and second branchial arch forms the remaining middle ear structures being the ossicles, muscles and tendons. Meckel's cartilage, the cartilage anlage of the first branchial arch, forms the head and neck of the malleus, the malleal ligaments, the body and short process of the incus and the tensor tympani muscle. The tensor tympani muscle is innervated by the mandibular nerve, the nerve of the first branchial arch. Reichert's cartilage, the cartilage anlage of the second branchial arch, forms the manubrium of the malleus, the long process of the incus, the capitulum, crura and the larger central part of the footplate (Thompson et al. 2012) and the stapedius muscle which is innervated by the facial nerve, the nerve of the second branchial arch. As already mentioned, the anterior process of the malleus differentiates from the primitive tympanic ring unlike the rest of the ossicles. During the 5th–6th week of gestation, the stapes, derived from the second branchial arch, develops around the stapedial artery, explaining the ring-like configuration of the stapes. The stapedial ring will further enlarge and the mesenchymal tissue will differentiate into cartilage. The stapes will reach the otic capsule at the region of the future oval window by 4 months and the area of fusion is the dense fibrous tissue of the oval window that forms at the end of the fissure between primordial otic and basioccipital ossification centers (Thompson et al. 2012, Clack 2002) and will become the medial vestibular surface of the footplate. (Arey and Real 1974; Anson et al. 1991; Williams 1992).

3.2 Middle Ear Malformations Associated with External Auditory Canal Deformities

These malformations were described and discussed above (see "Atresia of the External Auditory Canal").

3.3 Middle Ear Malformations in the Absence of EAC Stenosis and EAC Atresia

3.3.1 Isolated Ossicular Deformities

Isolated ossicular deformities occur in 38 % of the congenital malformations of the external and/or middle ear and are bilateral in half of the cases (Anson and Donaldson 1981; Swartz and Faerber 1985; Sando et al. 1988; Nager 1993). Anomalies of the middle ear and ossicles without EAC stenosis and EAC atresia are much less common than outer ear anomalies. The stapes and the incus are the most frequently affected ossicles. These ossicular anomalies can be inherited but association with syndromes, especially with Goldenhar's and Treacher Collins syndromes, is known. Isolated maldevelopment of the first branchial arch (Meckel's cartilage) will cause anomalies of the neck and head of the malleus, and of the body and short process of the incus. The mandible is also formed by Meckel's cartilage and hence mandibular and first branchial arch ossicular malformations are often associated. Maldevelopment of the second branchial arch (Reichert's cartilage) will cause anomalies of the manubrium of the malleus, long process of the incus, stapes superstructure and lateral surface of the footplate of the stapes, styloid process and facial nerve canal. Maldevelopment of both the first and second branchial arch can of course result in complete absence of one or more of the ossicles. The stapes is the most frequently involved ossicle and a broad spectrum of anomalies can be found: footplate fixation, hypoplasia of the stapes, subtle abnormalities of the crura, monopodal stapes and in the worst case absence of the complete stapes (Fig. 10). Subtle anomalies of the footplate were only rarely reported in the past, but with the advent of high-resolution CT and CBCT and the use of double-oblique reconstructions, these

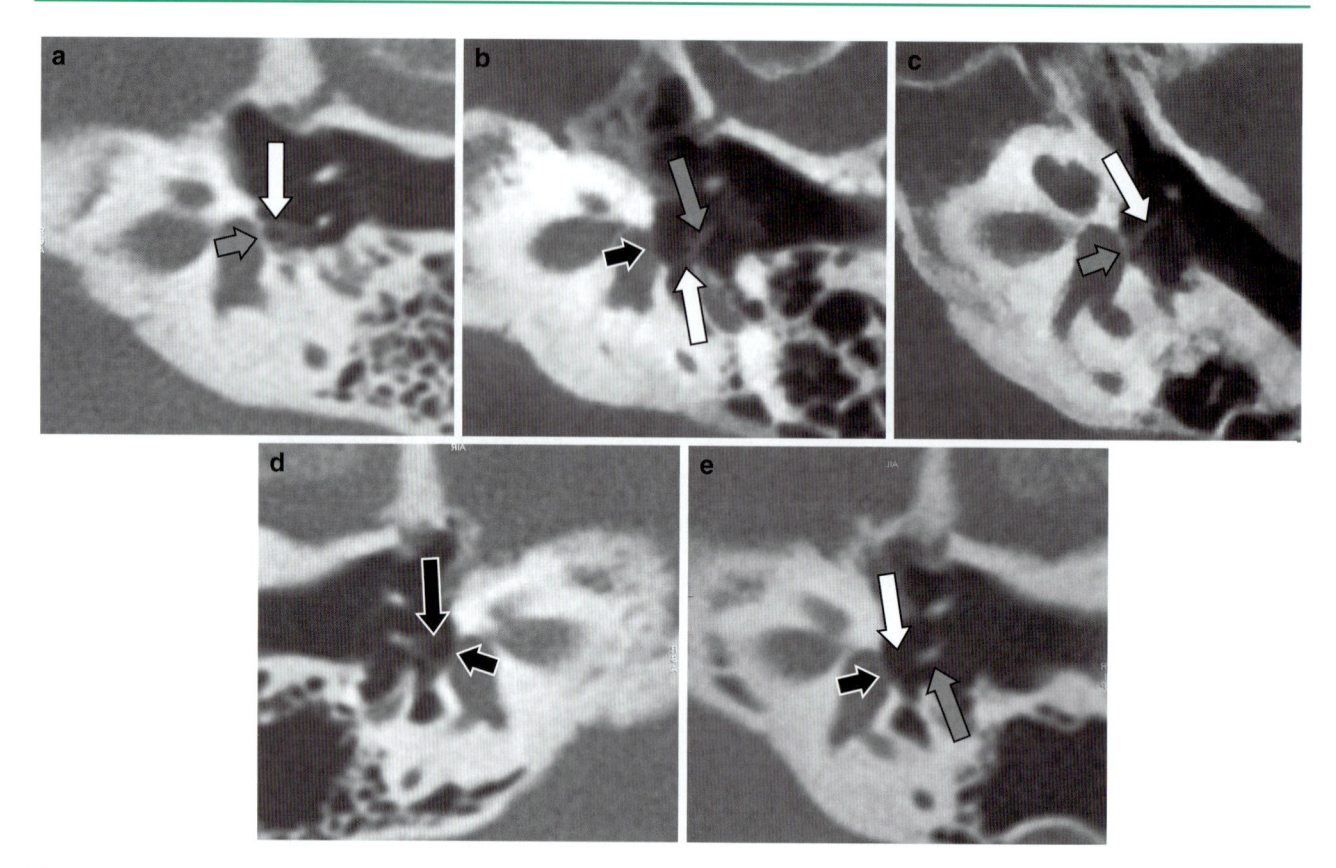

Fig. 10 Isolated congenital stapes deformities. **a** Double-oblique reformatted MDCT image of the left middle ear in a patient with a hypoplastic stapes (*white arrow*), compare with a normal-size stapes in Figs. 1c and 10d. Abnormal footplate (*grey arrow*). **b** Double-oblique reformatted CBCT image of the left middle ear in a patient with a stapes with only a posterior crus (*white arrow*), the anterior crus was absent. Capitulum of the stapes (*grey arrow*), normal footplate without any calcification located between the fluid in the vestibule and air in the middle ear (*black arrow*). **c** Double-oblique reformatted CBCT image of the left middle ear in a patient with a monopodal stapes (*white arrow*) fixed on the centre of a thickened and calcified footplate (*grey arrow*). This deformity was present on both sides in this patient. **d–e** Double-oblique reformatted MDCT image of the right (**d**) and left (**e**) middle ear in a patient with aplasia of the left stapes (*white arrow*). Normal stapes on the right side (*black arrow*), lenticular process of the incus on the left side (*grey arrow*), normal footplate (*small black arrows*)

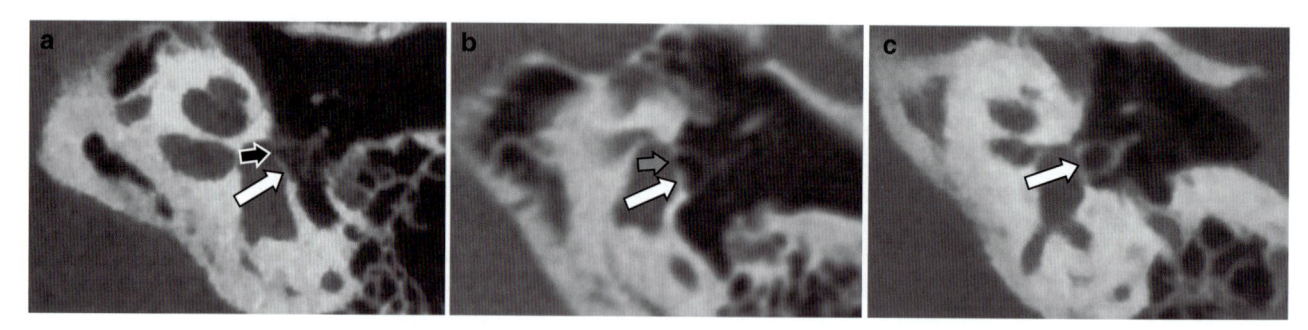

Fig. 11 Congenital footplate thickening/oval window closure in patients with a normal stapes suprastructure and normal course of the facial nerve and who presented with congenital conductive hearing loss. **a** Double-oblique reformatted CBCT image in a patient with an almost completely calcified and closed footplate/oval window (*white arrow*) and a remaining subtle opening at the anterior border of the footplate (*black arrow*). Non-ossified hypodense stapes suprastructure. **b** Double-oblique reformatted MDCT image in a patient with a remaining central opening in the footplate/oval window (*grey arrow*) located between a smaller anterior and larger posterior (*white arrow*) calcified footplate plaque. Non-ossified hypodense stapes suprastructure. **c** Double-oblique reformatted CBCT image in a patient with a completely closed and calcified footplate/oval window (*white arrow*). Ossified hyperdense stapes suprastructure

anomalies are more frequently reported (Fig. 11). Incus aplasia, long process malformations, absent incudostapedial joint or fibrous appearance of this joint are some of the most frequent anomalies of the incus (Figs. 12 and 13). Anomalies of the malleus are: aplasia, disappearance of the joint with the incus and fusion with the incus (Fig. 14), fusion of the

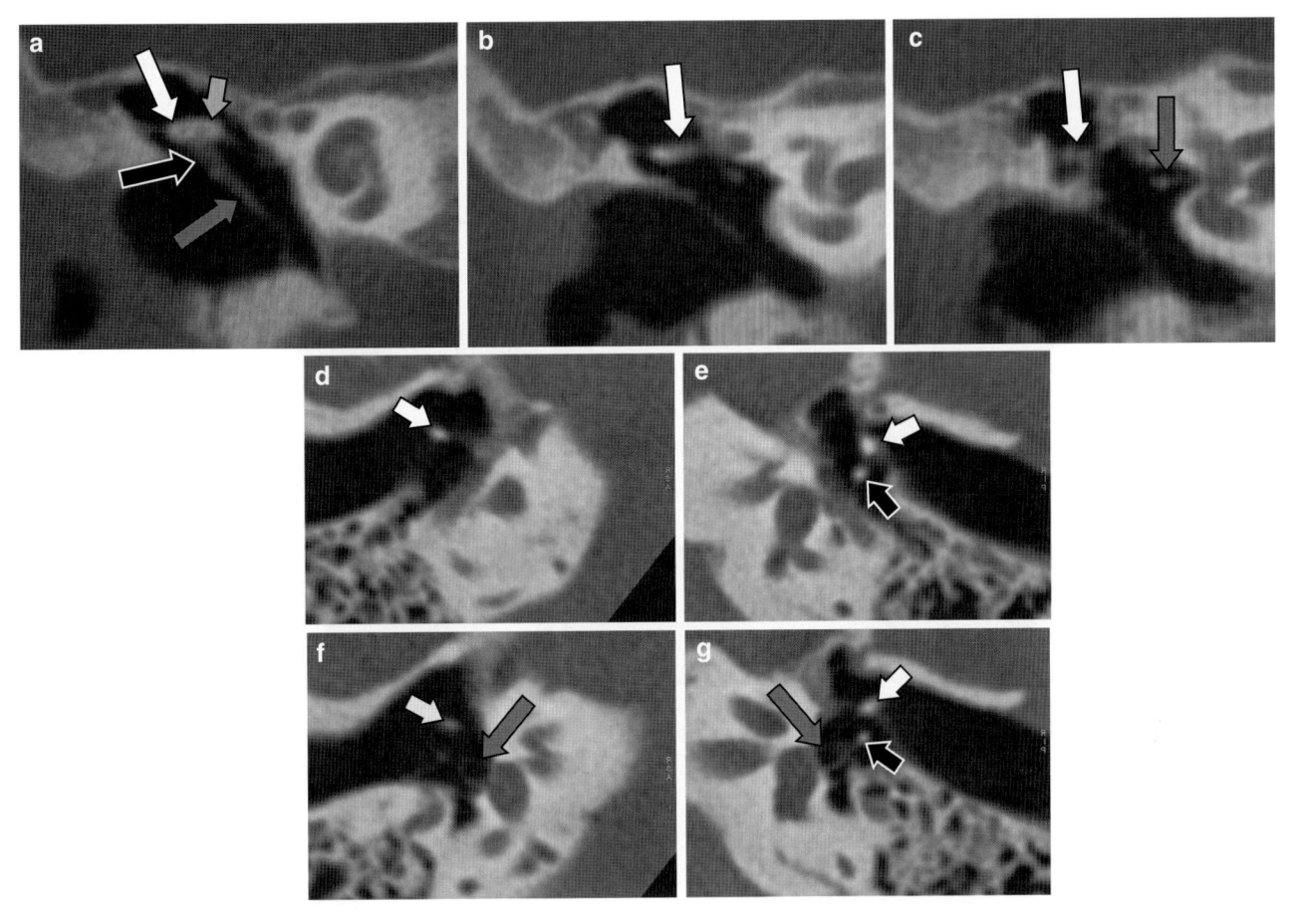

Fig. 12 Aplasia of the long process of the incus. a Coronal MDCT image through the normal malleus: malleus head (*small white arrow*), neck of the malleus (*black arrow*), handle of the malleus (*grey arrow*) and corpus of the incus (*large white arrow*). b Coronal MDCT image through the incus: incus body (*white arrow*). c Coronal MDCT image through the stapes: short process of the incus (*white arrow*), stapes (*grey arrow*). d–g Axial MDCT images at the level of the long process of the incus (d, e) and incudostapedial joint (f, g). The long process of the incus can be seen on the left side (*black arrows*) but is absent on the right side, aplasia. Neck and handle of the malleus (*white arrows*), normal stapes (*grey arrows*)

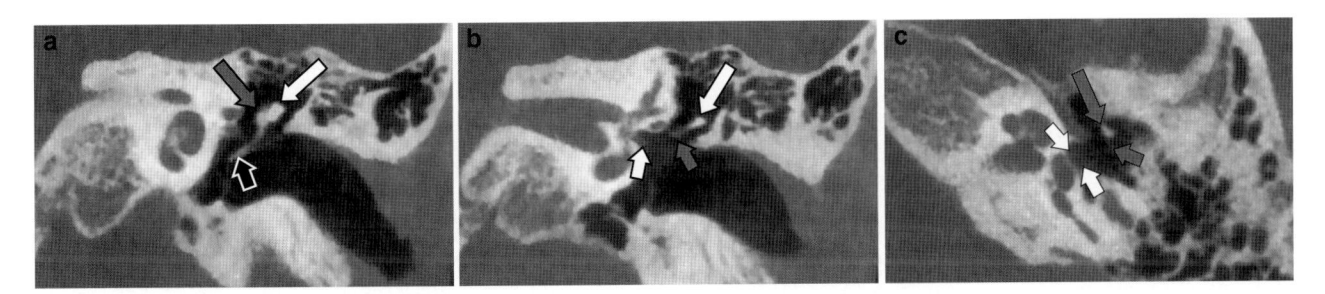

Fig. 13 Aplasia (bilateral) of the long process of the incus in a patient with Treacher Collins syndrome. a Coronal CBCT image through the malleus. Normal head of the malleus (*grey arrow*), handle of the malleus (*black arrow*) and body of the incus (*white arrow*). b Coronal CBCT image through the body of the incus (*white arrow*). The long process of the incus is absent and is partially replaced by a fibrous structure (*grey arrow*). Normal stapes in the oval window niche (*small white arrow*). c Axial CBCT image through the stapes (*white arrows*). The normal ossified neck of the malleus can be seen (*large grey arrow*), the long process of the incus is absent and is replaced by a hardly visible fibrous structure (*small grey arrow*)

manubrium with the long process of the incus and the capitulum of the stapes and fixation of the head of the malleus to the epitympanic wall with a "malleus bar" (Fig. 15).

Detailed imaging of the facial nerve, oval window and middle ear cavity itself is required whenever surgical reconstruction of the malformed ossicular chain is considered.

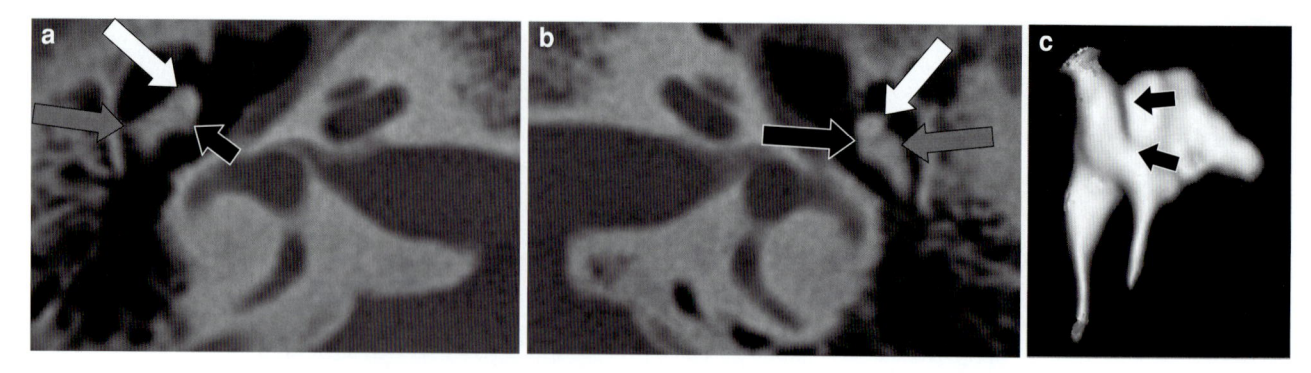

Fig. 14 Incudomallear fusion. **a–b** Axial MDCT images through the right (**a**) and left (**b**) middle ear. Head of the malleus (*white arrows*), corpus of the incus (*grey arrows*) with a slightly malformed body of the incus on the right side. Normal incudomallear joint on the left side (*black arrow*), absent joint on the right side as the head of the malleus and the corpus of the incus are fused (*small black arrow*). **c** 3D surface rendering of the right malleus and incus: absence of the joint between the head of the malleus and the corpus of the incus (*black arrows*)

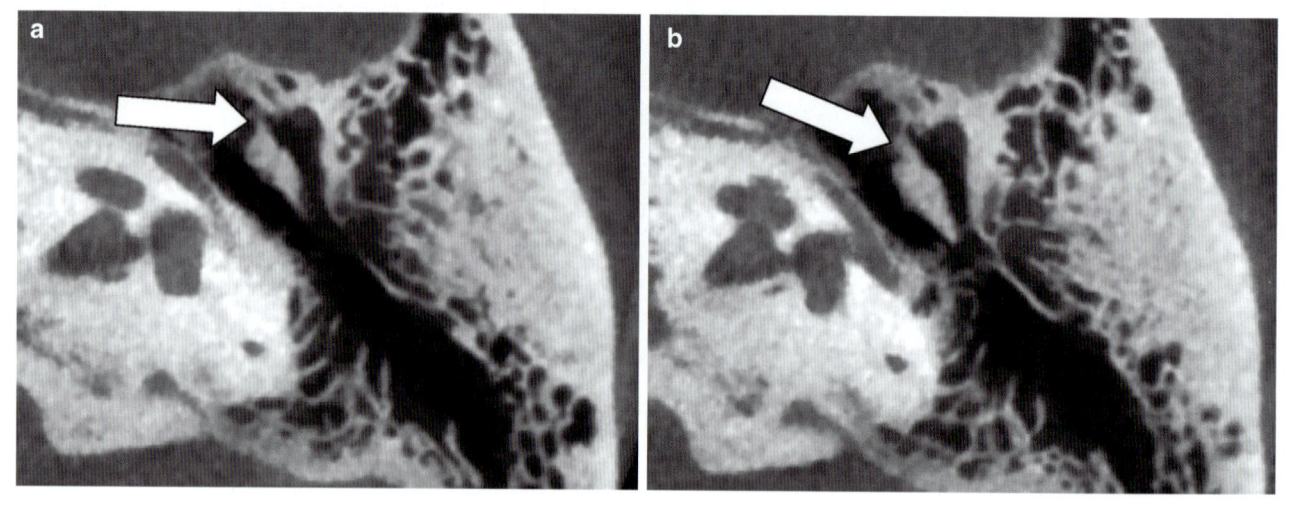

Fig. 15 Congenital fixation of the head of the malleus to the anterior wall of the middle ear cavity—mallear bar. **a–b** Axial MDCT images through the upper and lower part of the head of the malleus on the left side. A calcified bridge (*white arrows*) is seen between the head of the malleus and the anterior wall of the middle ear cavity, reducing the mobility of the incus: mallear bar

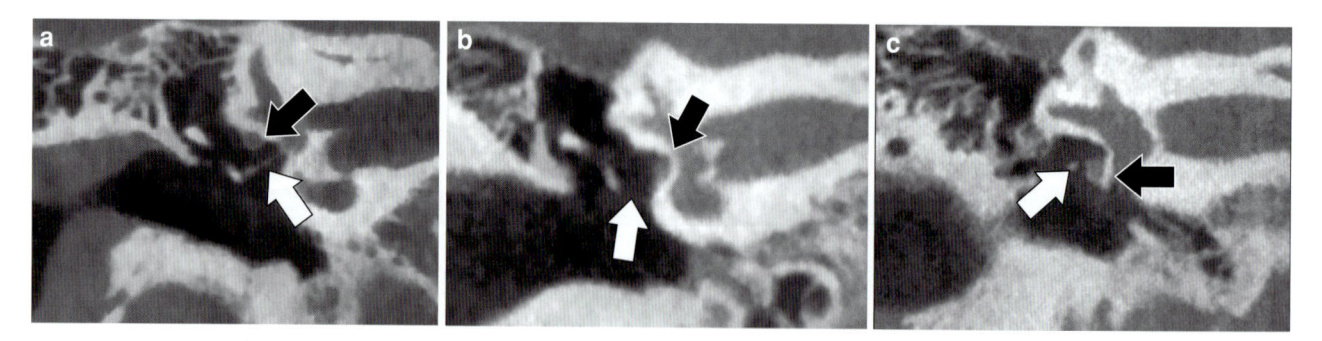

Fig. 16 Abnormal course of the tympanic segment of the facial nerve. **a** Coronal CBCT image through a normal right middle ear illustrating the normal position of the tympanic segment of the facial nerve canal under the lateral semicircular canal (*black arrow*) and above the stapes (*white arrow*). Notice the normal thickness of the footplate. **b** Coronal CBCT of the right middle ear. The facial nerve (*black arrow*) is lying on the surface of the closed/not developed oval window. The stapes cannot be depicted: aplasia of the stapes (*white arrow*). **c** Coronal CBCT of the right middle ear. The facial nerve (*black arrow*) is lying on the promontory below the oval window niche and the stapes (*white arrow*) can be seen above the facial nerve but below the completely closed or not formed oval window

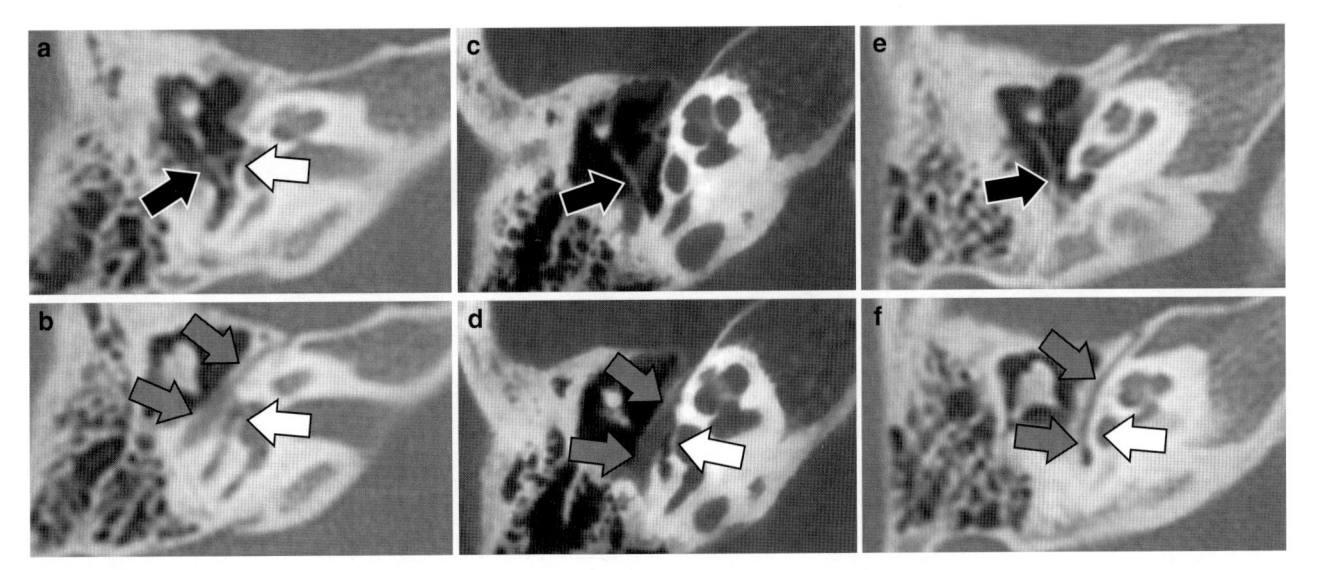

Fig. 17 Congenital absence or hypoplasia of the oval window. Axial MDCT (**a, b, e, f**) and CBCT (**c, d**) images at the level of the inferiorly displaced stapes (**a, c, e**) and at the level of the tympanic segment of the facial nerve canal and aplastic or hypoplastic oval window (**b, d, f**). **a, b** The stapes is displaced inferiorly and slightly posteriorly and is not longer exactly centred on the oval window area (*black arrow*). The oval window is extremely hypoplastic and only a small opening can be seen (*white arrow*). The tympanic segment of the facial nerve canal is positioned lateral to the hypoplastic oval window (*grey arrows*). **c, d** The stapes completely missed its contact with the oval window and is displaced inferoposteriorly in the sinus tympani (*black arrow*). The oval window is absent (*white arrow*) and the tympanic segment of the facial nerve canal (*grey arrows*) passes just lateral of the place where the oval window should have been formed. **e, f** The stapes again completely missed the contact with the oval window area and is displaced inferoposteriorly in the sinus tympani (*black arrow*). The oval window is not formed (*white arrow*) and the tympanic segment of the facial nerve is lying on the surface of the labyrinth at the site where the oval window should have developed (*grey arrows*). Images 17 **c, d** *Courtesy* Dr. Sebastien Janssens de Varebeke, ENT Department, Virga Jesse Hospital, Hasselt, Belgium

3.3.2 Facial Nerve, Oval Window and Round Window Anomalies

Both the facial nerve and part of the ossicles develop from the second branchial arch. This explains why the facial nerve often has an anomalous course in the presence of ossicular malformations. In patients with congenital middle ear malformations and a normal EAC, the tympanic segment of the facial nerve can run over the oval window, can be found below the stapes under the oval window and sometimes lies on the stapes (Fig. 16). An abnormally wide Obtuse angle of the first or anterior genu of the facial nerve canal can also be present.

Congenital malformation of the oval window is an associated finding in patients with a congenital abnormal course of the facial nerve. The hypothesis is that the abnormal position of the facial nerve prevents the stapes to make contact with the developing otic capsule at the site of the future oval window. Consequently, the development of the oval window is not induced. More subtle oval window anomalies like hypoplasia or partial absence of the oval window or thickening of the footplate could be caused by less important facial nerve hinderance (Fig. 17). These more subtle oval window anomalies and the abnormal course of the facial nerve can today be detected on high-resolution CT/CBCT images. However, the footplate of the stapes can only be evaluated in a reliable way when double-oblique reconstructions are made, otherwise subtle stapes and especially footplate anomalies may remain undetected (Jahrsdoerfer 1981; 1988; Zeifer et al. 2000; Miura et al. 2003; Vercruysse et al. 2006).

Absence of the round window is rare and is bilateral in nearly 50 % of the cases (Fig. 18), and is most frequently not associated with oval window anomalies. Stenosis of the round window and/or round window recess is more frequently found and the diagnosis is made when the round window or round window recess measures less than 1.5 mm. This is best measured in the sagittal plane (Veillon et al. 2014).

3.3.3 Other Middle Ear Anomalies and Congenital Middle Ear Cholesteatoma

The middle ear cavity can be hypoplastic (Fig. 7) which can also jeopardize surgical reconstruction. Absence of the stapedius muscle and/or tendon, absence or elongation of the pyramid eminence, abnormal course of the tensor tympani tendon (Figs. 4 and 19), absence of a normal cochleariform process, etc. are some of the other congenital anomalies which can be found in the middle ear. Congenital cholesteatomas account for 2 % of all middle ear cholesteatomas and can also be found in the middle ear cavity in the absence of EAC stenosis and EAC atresia. They are

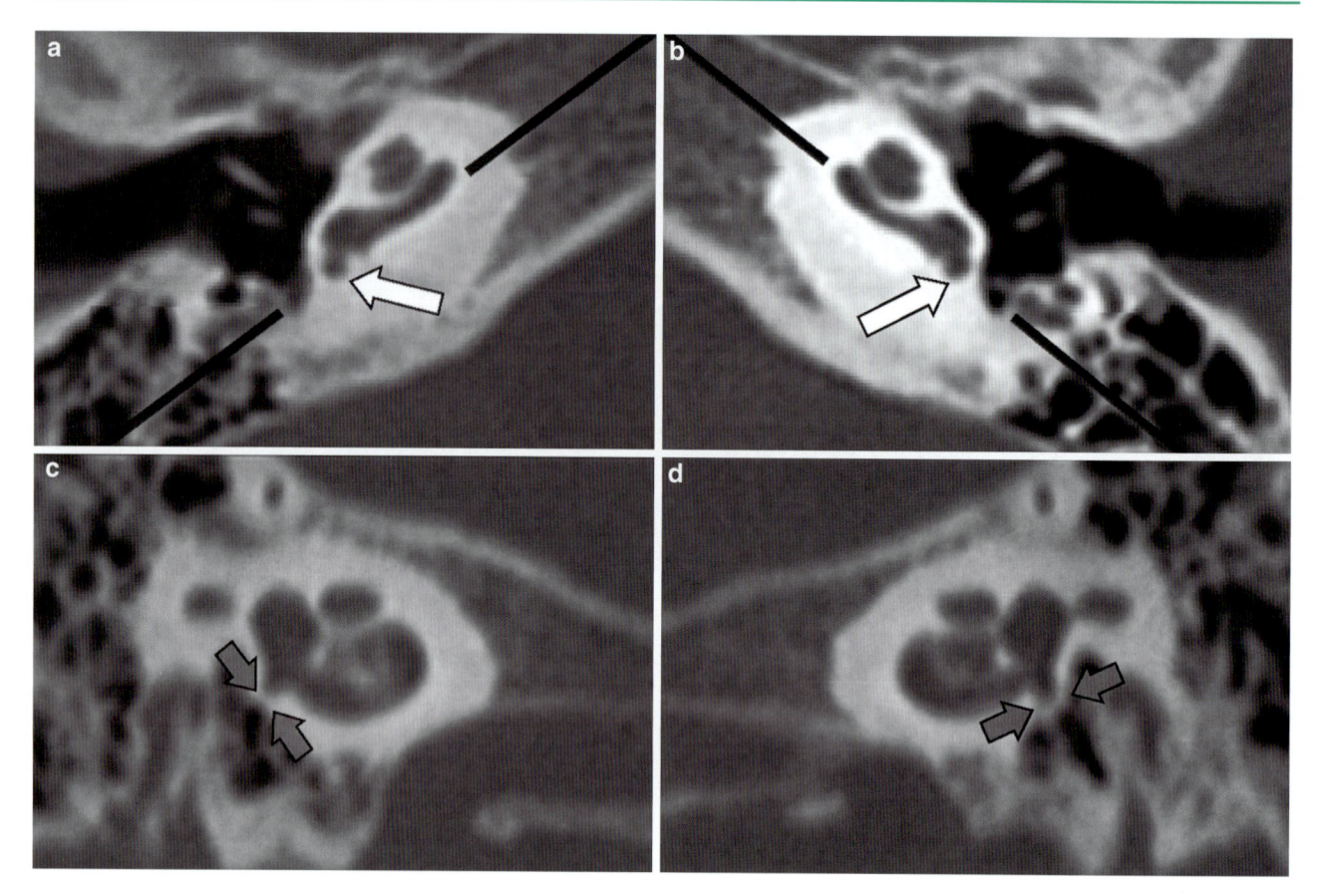

Fig. 18 Bilateral absence of the round window. Images of the right (a, c) and left (b, d) round window made in the axial (a, b) and parasagittal plane (c, d), the latter made along the black lines on the axial images. a, b The round window and round window recess are completely closed (*white arrows*). c, d The complete absence of the round window and round window recess is confirmed on the parasagittal images (*grey arrows*)

the result of misplaced embryonic rests of squamous cell epithelium (ectoderm) in the middle ear cavity (endoderm) during the development of the middle ear. In these cases, the tympanic membrane is completely normal and often there are no other signs of middle ear inflammation. These congenital cholesteatomas are most frequently located in the vicinity of the tensor tympani muscle canal and medial to the ossicles while acquired cholesteatomas are most often found lateral to the ossicles (Fig. 20). These congenital cholesteatomas have a convex shape. They are detected at the age of 4–5 years and are more frequent in boys (Levenson et al. 1989; Mc Gill et al. 1999).

3.3.4 Congenital Dermoids

Congenital dermoids of the temporal bone can be considered as benign developmental anomalies. During the fourth week of gestation, there is a short contact between the endoderm lining of the first pharyngeal pouch and the ectoderm of the first branchial groove (see "Embryology".). Inclusion of ectoderm into the endoderm at the time of this short contact probably causes the development of these temporal bone dermoids (Kollias et al. 1995). These dermoids can be found in the petrous apex, middle ear cavity, mastoid air cells and Eustachian tube (Fig. 21). In the latter case, the Eustachian tube is blocked and the patients present with chronic otitis media and ear drainage resistant to therapy. Dermoids have an ectodermal and mesodermal origin which allows histological differentiation from cholesteatoma (only ectodermal origin) and teratomas (ectodermal, mesodermal and endodermal origin). On imaging, these congenital dermoids are well circumscribed, non-enhancing and contain fat and have a smooth capsule. Complete surgical removal is the treatment and therefore detailed preoperative imaging is required.

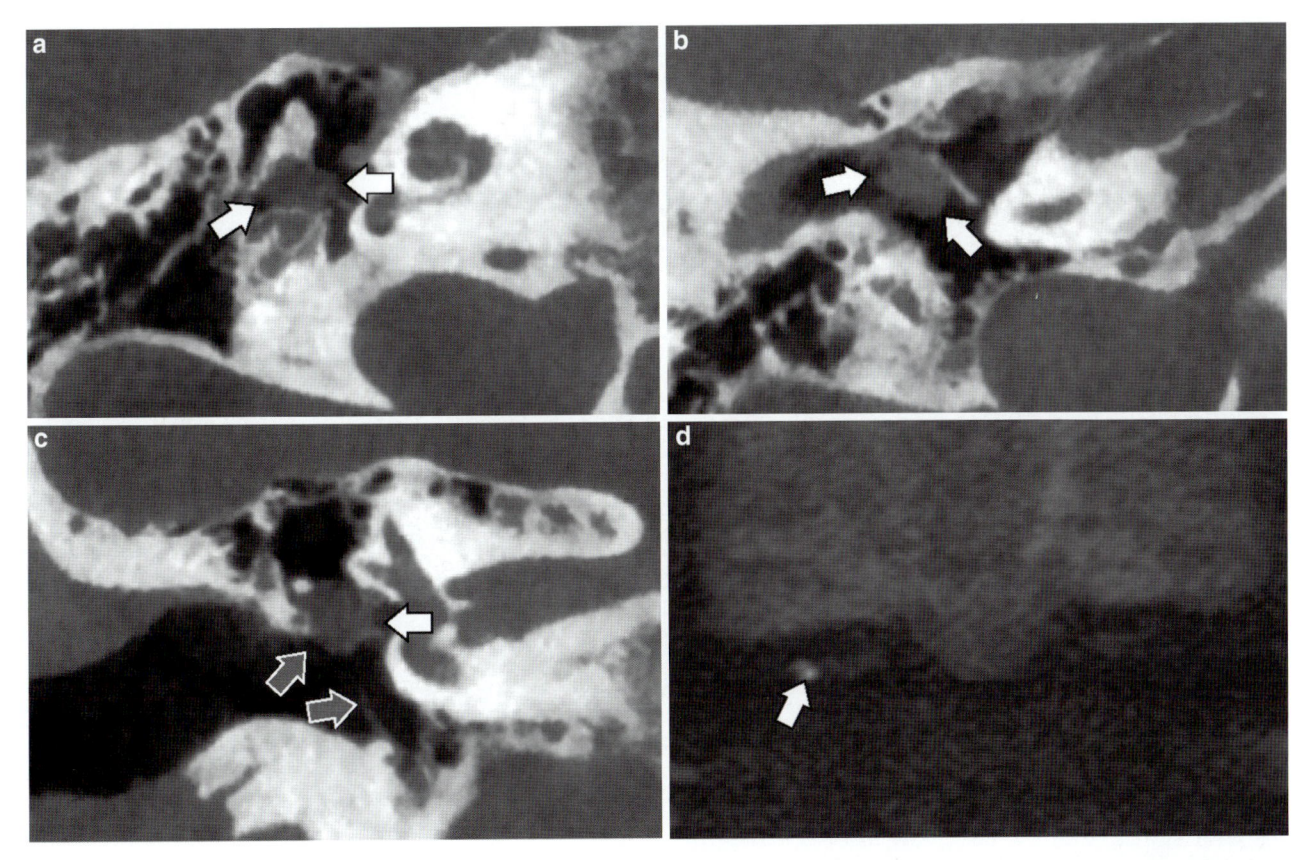

Fig. 19 Congenital cholesteatoma in a normal middle ear. **a–b** Axial CBCT images at the level of the right incus body (**a**) and malleus handle (**b**) showing a convex soft tissue lesion medial to the ossicles and posterior to the malleus handle (*white arrows*). There is a normal aeration of the rest of the middle ear, antrum and mastoid. **c** Coronal CBCT image through the lesion in the right middle ear confirms the location of the lesion medial to the ossicles near the incudostapedial junction (*white arrowhead*). Notice the normal appearance of the tympanic membrane (*grey arrows*). **d** Coronal B-1,000 non-EPI DWI image through the middle ears detects a high-signal intensity lesion and therefore confirms the presence of a cholesteatoma on the right side (*white arrow*). The MR findings together with the location of the lesion in a normal aerated ear with a normal drum confirm the diagnosis of a congenital cholesteatoma

4 Congenital Malformations of the Inner Ear

4.1 Embryology

The membranous labyrinth derives from surface ectoderm near the rhombencephalon and begins as the otic pit. During the fourth gestational week, it becomes the primitive otocyst. The mesenchyma which surrounds the otic vesicle increases in cell density and becomes precartilage which will form the primitive otic capsule. During the fifth week of gestation, the otic vesicle elongates and three projections become visible. The saccule and cochlear duct develop from the ventromedial projection, the utricle and semicircular ducts develop from the dorsal projection and the endolymphatic duct and sac develop from the dorsomedial projection. The development of the cochlea is complete at 9 weeks at the time when the appearance of the neural epithelium also has started. The formation of the saccule, utricle and endolymphatic duct is complete at 11 weeks, hence formation of the membranous labyrinth is complete between the 10 and 12 week of gestation. The semicircular canals appear during the sixth week of gestation, but are only completed between the 20th and 22nd week, the lateral semicircular canal is the last one to be completed. The perilymph, occupying the space between the inner periosteal layer of the otic capsule and the membranous labyrinth arises from the mesoderm surrounding the membranous labyrinth. This mesodermal tissue regresses and changes into precartilage and further into loose vascular reticulum. Finally, vacuolization results in the formation of an uninterrupted space which will become the perilymphatic space (Bast and Anson 1949; Gulya 2003, 2007; Curtin et al. 2011).

Neuroblasts of the cochlear ganglion separate from the otic neural epithelium and fibers from these ganglion cell bodies start to grow peripherally back into the otic epithelium and centrally into the brain stem at 9–10 weeks of gestation. Although it has been thought that the cochlear development

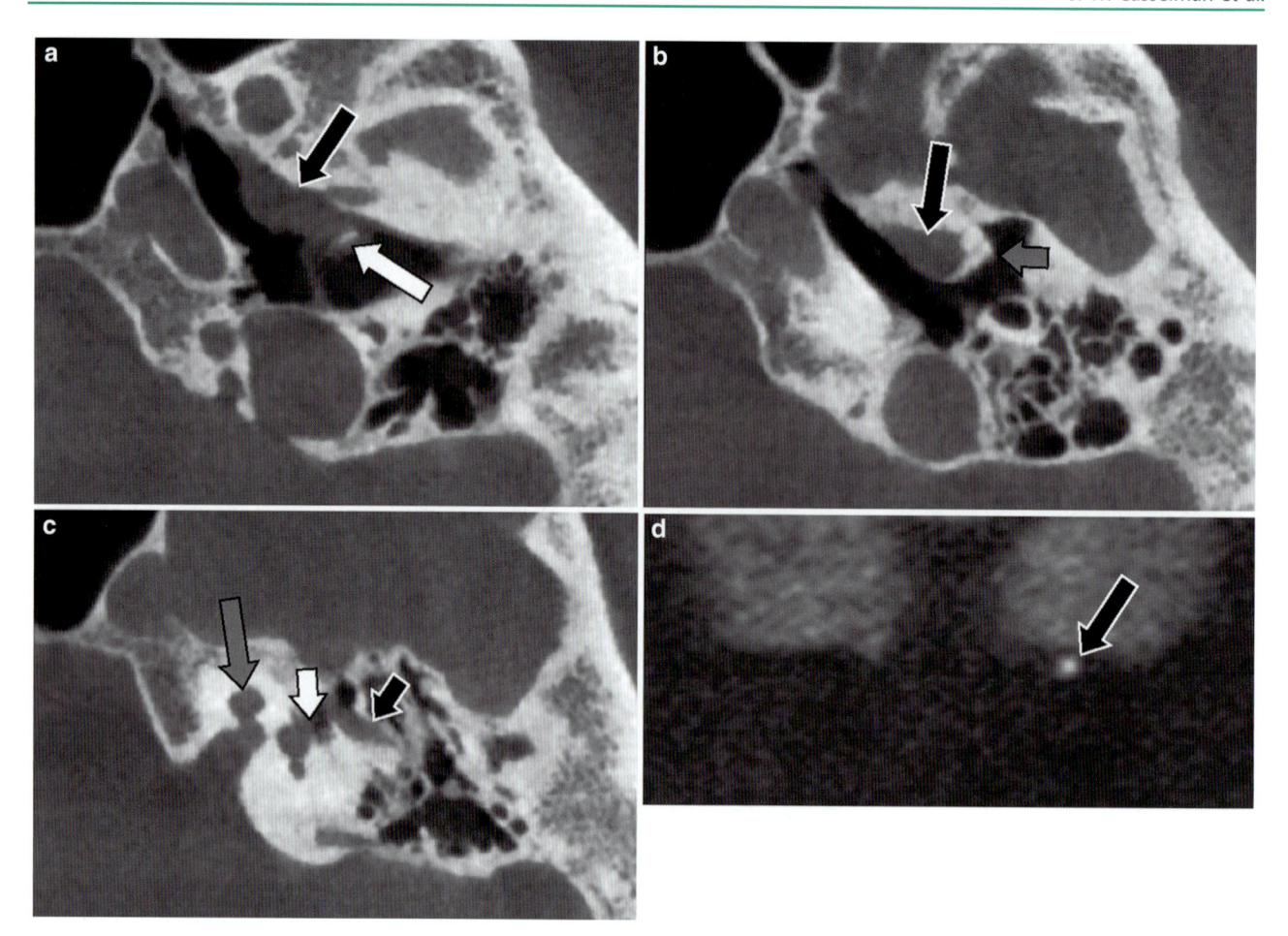

Fig. 20 Congenital cholesteatoma in a patient with middle and inner ear malformations. **a–c** Axial CBCT images of the left middle ear at the level of the hypotympanum (**a**), the incudomallear joint (**b**) and the cochlea (**c**). The tensor tympani muscle can be followed along the lateral wall of the hypotympanum and appears too thick for a normal tensor tympani muscle (*black arrows*). The lesion can be seen anterior to the handle of the malleus (*white arrow*) and the malformed incudomallear joint (*small grey arrow*). A cystic apical and second turn of the cochlea (Sennaroglu type IP-II malformation) (*grey arrow*), an aplasia of the stapes (*small white arrow*) and abnormal course of the tympanic segment of the facial nerve canal (*small black arrow*) can be seen higher up in the middle ear cavity. A cochleariform process could not be found: aplasia. **d** A coronal B-1,000 non-EPI DWI image through the middle ears demonstrates a high-signal intensity lesion on the left side and hence confirms the presence of a cholesteatoma on the left side (*black arrow*), situated between the tensor tympani muscle tendon and the anterolateral wall of the hypotympanum. The young age and history of the patient, the normal aeration of the rest of the middle ear and the normal appearance of the drum together with the above-described imaging findings confirm the presence of a congenital cholesteatoma

or differentiation depends on the innervation, this has been proved not to be the case and implies that the inner ear development is not dependant on any neuronal trigger or stimulus or trophic effect. This explains why the cochlea can be completely normal in case of vestibulocochlear nerve aplasia (Hemond and Delanty 1991; Van De Water 1976).

4.2 Classifications and Malformations of the Labyrinth

21 % of congenital SNHL is caused by Inner Ear malformations. Initially, these inner ear malformations got the name of the scientists who first described them, e.g. Bing-Siebenmann, Scheibe, Mondini, Alexander, Michel, etc. This was replaced by the classification of Robert Jackler in 1987 which was based on the hypothesis that various inner ear anomalies result from an arrest of maturation during different stages of inner ear embryogenesis (Jackler et al. 1987). Hence, the most severe malformations like complete aplasia of the labyrinth aplasia and a common cavity were the result of a problem occurring during the early development of the otic pit and cyst. The lateral semicircular canal is the last inner ear structure to be completed explaining why it is the most frequently involved inner ear structure with less important clinical consequences. Nevertheless, it became obvious that the majority of the inner ear malformations were a result of genetic

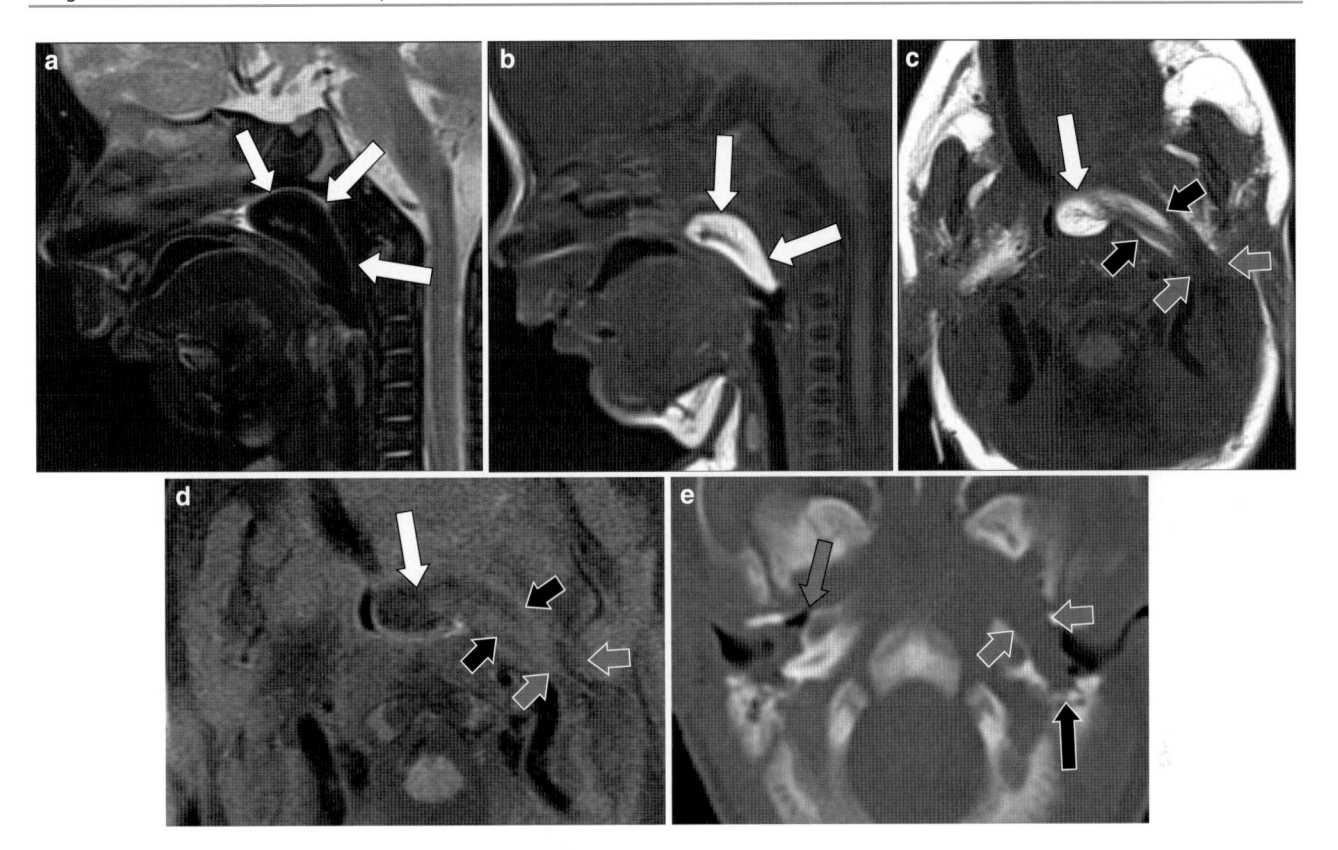

Fig. 21 Congenital dermoid with extension through the Eustachian tube into the nasopharynx. **a–b** Sagittal T2-weighted image with fat suppression (**a**) and unenhanced T1-weighted image without fat suppression through the nasopharynx (**b**). A crescent-shaped lesion (*white arrows*) can be seen in the nasopharynx above the soft palate with a high-signal intensity on T1 and a low-signal intensity on the fat suppressed T2-weigthed image. These signal intensities suggest that the lesion contains fat and is a dermoid. **c–d** Axial unenhanced T1-weighted image without (**c**) and with fat suppression (**d**) through the nasopharynx. The fat in the nasopharynx is confirmed as the high-signal intensity disappears on the fat suppressed image (*white arrows*). The fat containing lesion can be followed in the left Eustachian tube (*black arrows*) and ends in an abnormally wide opening in the anteroinferior wall of the middle ear cavity (*grey arrows*). **e** Axial CT image through the nasopharynx and hypotympamun. The abnormal wide defect in the anteroinferior wall of the middle ear cavity is confirmed (*grey arrows*) and the dysfunction of the Eustachian tube causes complete opacification of the left middle ear and mastoid (*black arrow*). Notice the normal ostium of the Eustachian tube in the right pro-hypotympanum (*large grey arrow*). *Courtesy* Prof. Dr. H. Vermeersch, department of Head & Neck and Maxillo-Facial surgery, Ghent University, Belgium

etiology and not embryologic arrest. In this context, Levent Sennaroglu introduced a more practical classification of "cochlear malformations" in 2002, which helps the surgeon to find out whether cochlear or brainstem implantation is possible and warns him for potential problems like a CSF gusher, risk to get meningitis, abnormal course of the facial nerve, etc. (Sennaroglu and Saatci 2002).

4.2.1 Semicircular Canals

The most frequently malformed canal is the lateral semicircular canal as it is the last one to be formed. This also explains why isolated posterior and superior canal malformations in combination with a normal lateral semicircular canal are rare. The malformations can be subtle and frequently only a short and wide canal, narrow canal, canal with a more angular shape and/or enlarged ampulla and even partially fused canals can be seen, often without any clinical manifestation. It is, however, important to recognize and report these subtle malformations as they can herald underlying invisible inner ear malformations. This can alert the surgeon that he is dealing with a "fragile" ear with a higher potential risk of deafness following surgery. The lateral semicircular canal is considered enlarged once its posteromedial part is wider than 1.8 mm (Veillon et al. 2014) (Fig. 22). A frequently seen malformation is a single cavity which is formed by the vestibule and lateral semicircular canal. This malformation is called a "Lateral Semicircular Canal Vestibule Dysplasia—LCVD" when it occurs in the absence of any other inner ear malformation (Fig. 23) and it remains then clinically most often unnoticed. It can be bilateral and may be associated with other inner ear malformations, in the latter case, it is no longer called "LCVD". Partial or complete semicircular canal or duct aplasia (Fig. 24) is less frequent and can or cannot be associated with cochlear malformations. Absence

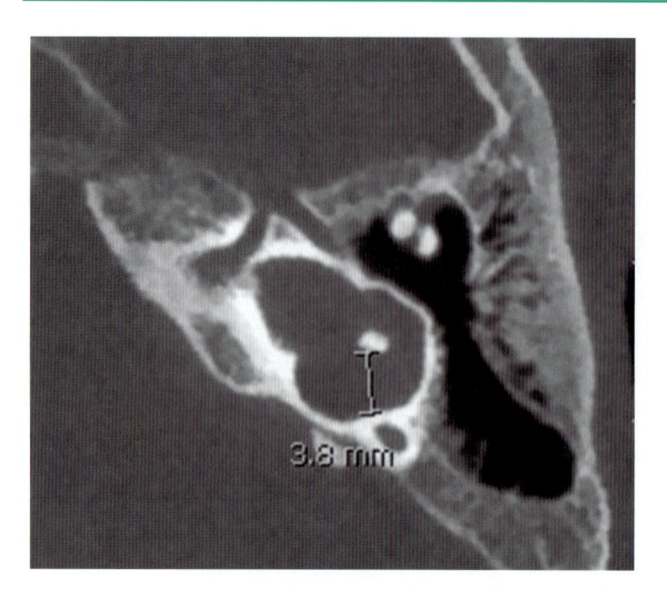

Fig. 22 Enlarged lateral semicircular canal. Axial CBCT through the left enlarged lateral semicircular canal and/or enlarged vestibule. The lateral semicircular canal is considered enlarged once its posteromedial part is wider than 1.8 mm, 3.8 mm in this patient

of a semicircular canal on heavily T2-weighted MR images must always be checked on CT as fibrous obliteration or ossification of the canal can mimic aplasia on MR. Absence of all semicircular canals with a normal cochlea is almost pathognomonic for a "CHARGE" association or syndrome (Coloboma, Heart disease, Atresia choanae, Retarded growth and development, Genital hypoplasia, Ear abnormalities) (Fig. 25). Most cases result from new mutations in the CHD7 gene (chromosome 8) but it can also be inherited in an autosomal dominant pattern (Vissers et al. 2004). Isolated aplasia of the superior semicircular duct has been described in patients with Alagille's and Waardenburg's syndrome while isolated aplasia of the posterior semicircular canal has been reported in patients with thalidomide toxicity. Superior semicircular canal dehiscence is considered as a developmental abnormality, although abnormally thin bone overlying the superior canal in approximately 1–2 % of the population (Carey et al. 2000) predisposes its development. Continuous pressure by the temporal lobe and CSF flow and/or trauma can disrupt this thin layer and this also explains why the mean age at the time of diagnosis is around 45 years. This creates a third mobile window allowing some of the sound energy, which is normally only travelling between the moving stapes in the oval window and the round window where the pressure is dissipated back to the middle ear, to be transmitted in the vestibular labyrinth. There the sound energy stimulates the hair cells where it eventually causes sound-induced vertigo and/or nystagmus, called the Tullio's phenomenon (Minor et al. 1998). A deep sulcus for the superior petrosal sinus is another more rare cause of the dehiscence (Dubrulle et al. 2009). The diagnosis can be made on CT and state of the art imaging requires reformatted images parallel and perpendicular to the superior semicircular canal. However, standard MDCT images have a spatial resolution of only 0.625–0.500 mm and the quality even decreases when reformatted images are made parallel or perpendicular to the superior semicircular canal. This explains why Cone-Beam CT became the imaging technique of choice to detect these dehiscences. It offers a much better spatial resolution between 0.1 and 0.15 mm and images can be reconstructed in any plane without loss of quality. Moreover, this can be done at a lower radiation dose. The result is that many of the MDCT made diagnoses of a "dehiscent superior semicircular canal" are corrected by CBCT as a "normal bony covered canal" (Fig. 26).

4.2.2 Vestibular Malformations

Most frequently anomalies of the vestibule and utriculosaccular structures present in association with other inner ear malformations (Lagundoye et al. 1975). Isolated deformation or enlargement of the vestibule occurs less frequent. When enlarged, the posterior part of the vestibule extends further posterior than the most posterior delineation of the lateral semicircular canal. The lateral semicircular canal becomes shorter as the vestibule becomes larger and starts to assimilate it into the vestibule. Frequently, there is an associated dilatation of the lateral semicircular canal. The vestibule can be considered enlarged once CT shows that the surface of the bone island surrounded by the lateral semicircular canal drops below 6 mm^2 (Veillon et al. 2014) (Fig. 27). Enlargement of the vestibule without assimilation of the lateral semicircular canal has been described in patients with thalidomide-induced deafness (Lagundoye et al. 1975).

4.2.3 Cochlear Malformations: Sennaroglu Classification

4.2.3.1 Labyrinthine Aplasia

This is the most severe inner ear malformation and it is also known as Michel's deformity. In these very rare cases the cochlea, vestibule and semicircular canals, vestibular aqueduct and cochlear aqueduct are absent (Schuknecht 1993) (Fig. 28). The labyrinthine aplasia can be associated with petrous bone aplasia and in these patients, the internal auditory canal is absent. When the internal auditory canal is present, it only contains a facial nerve. The VIIIth nerve is absent in patients with labyrinthine aplasia and hence cochlear implantation is not possible.

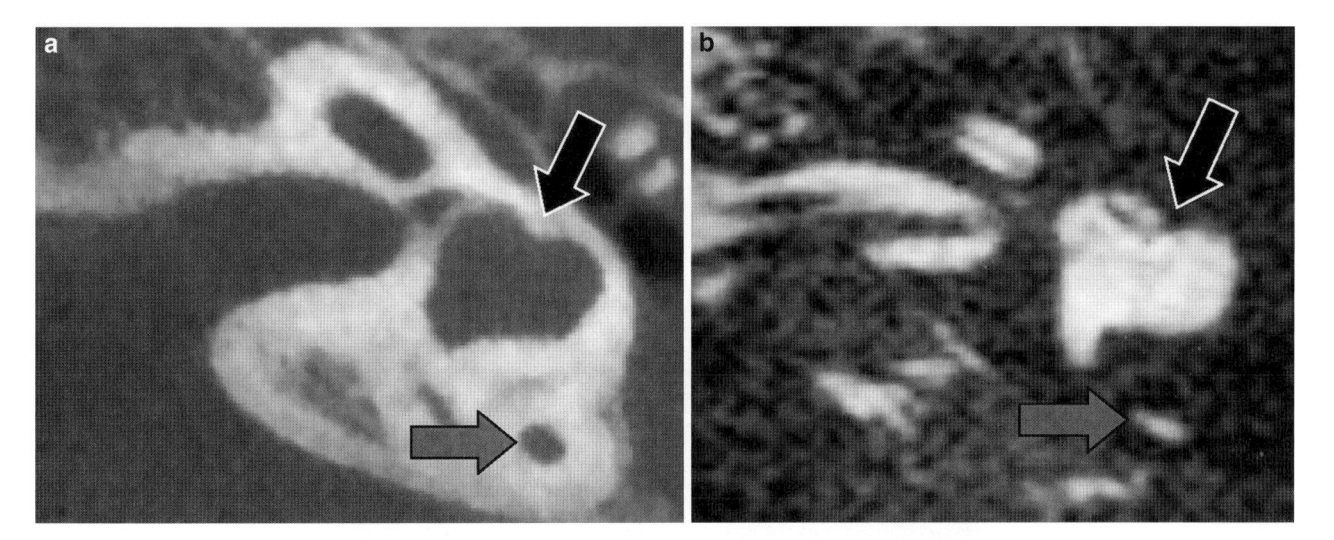

Fig. 23 Lateral semicircular Canal—Vestibule Dysplasia (LCVD). **a** Axial CBCT image. There is a cystic appearance of the left lateral semicircular canal (*black arrow*). This malformation is called an LCVD in the absence of other inner ear malformations. Normal posterior semicircular canal (*grey arrow*). **b** Axial Driven Equilibrium image showing the fluid-filled cystic lateral semicircular duct (*black arrow*). Normal fluid-filled posterior semicircular duct (*grey arrow*)

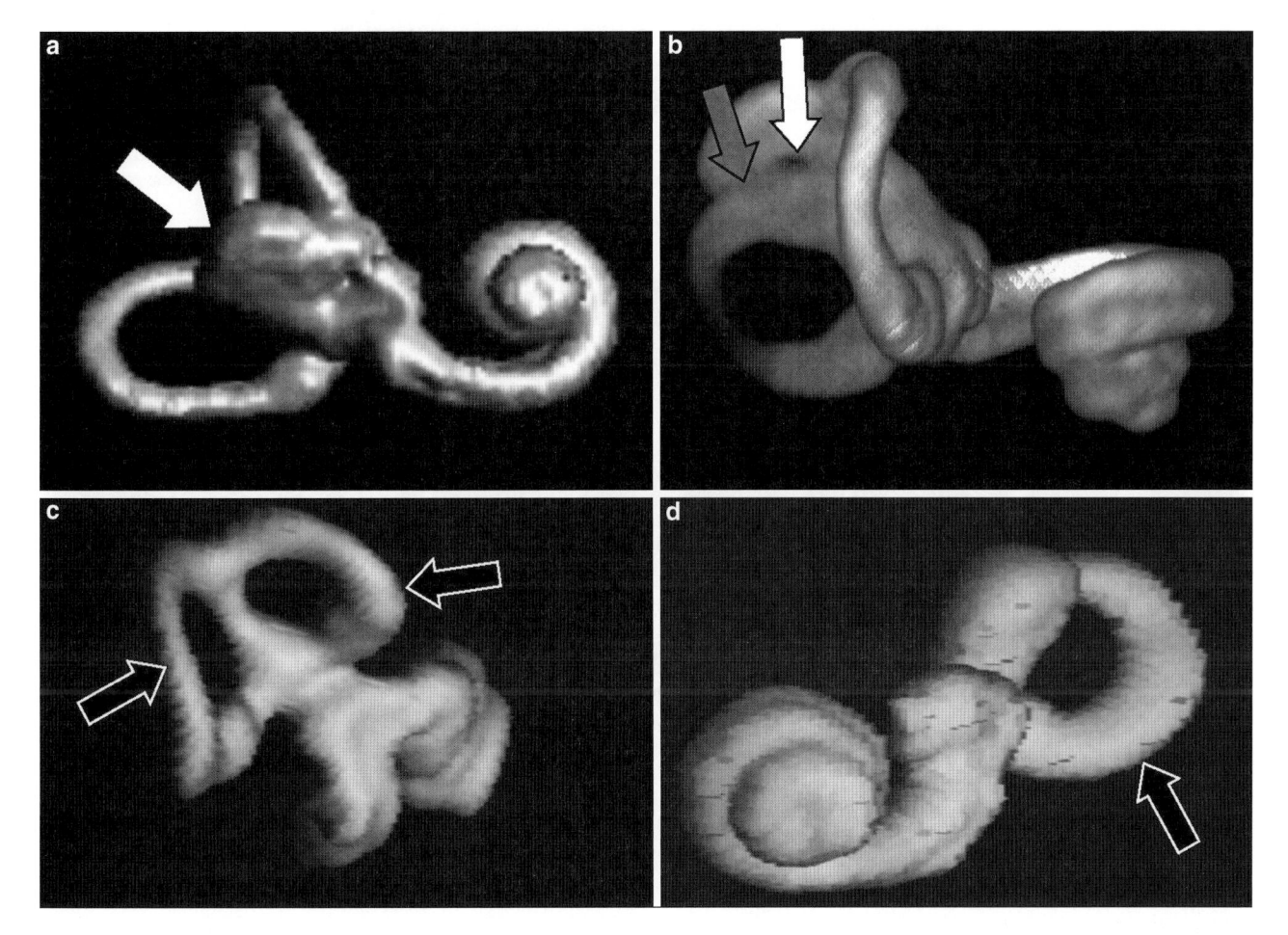

Fig. 24 T2-weighted MR Virtual Reality surface renderings of semicircular canal/duct malformations. **a** 3D surface rendering of a lateral semicircular canal—vestibule dysplasia (LCVD) (*white arrow*). **b** 3D surface rendering of a partially fused posterior and lateral semicircular duct (*grey arrow*). The posterior semicircular duct almost became cystic and the remaining central bony island (*white arrow*) is very small, <6 mm². **c** 3D surface rendering of a patient with aplasia of the lateral semicircular canal, the two remaining canals have an aberrant orientation (*black arrows*). **d** 3D surface rendering of a more severe inner ear anomaly, only one semicircular duct developed (*black arrow*)

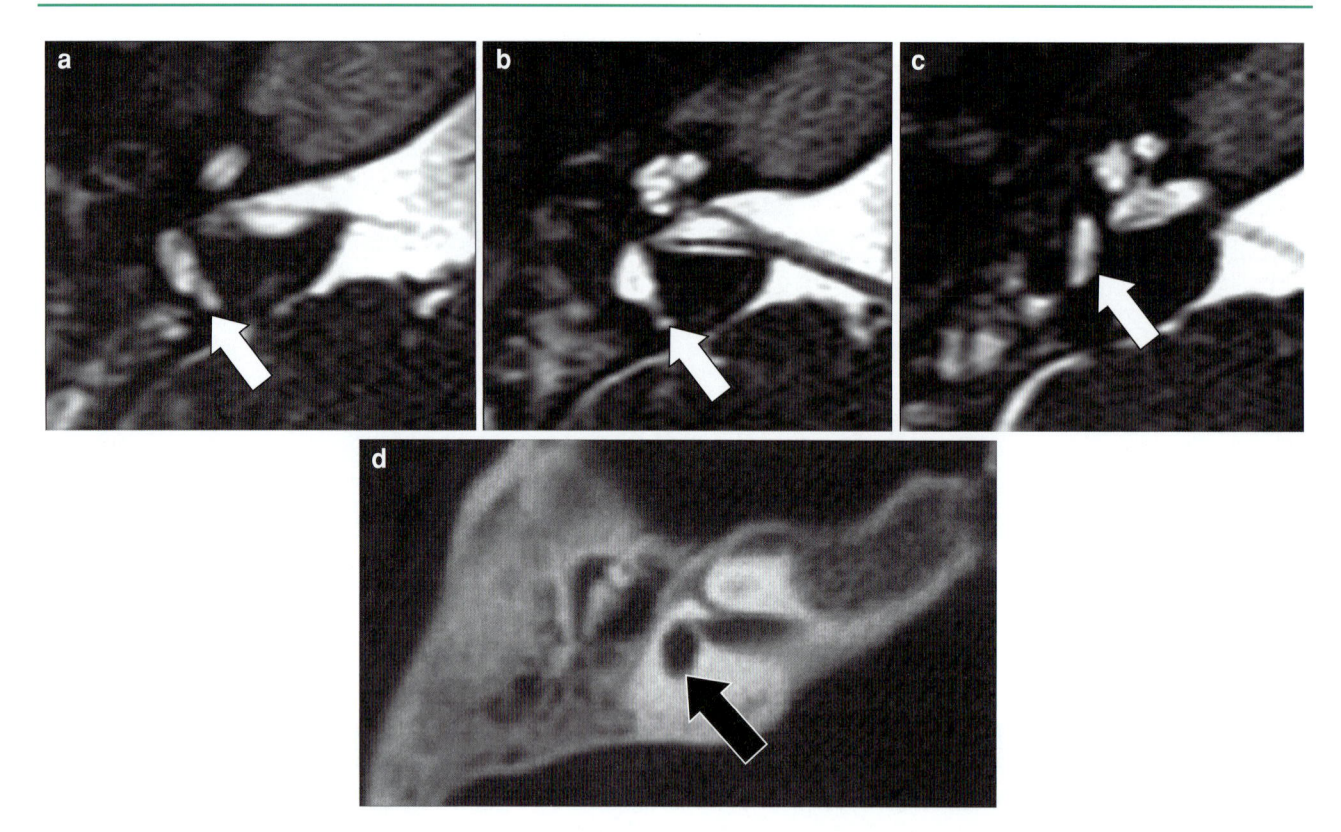

Fig. 25 CHARGE association/syndrome. **a–c** Axial T2-weighted driven equilibrium (DRIVE) images through the upper (**a**), middle (**b**) and lower (**c**) part of the vestibule showing the presence of high-signal intensity fluid in the vestibule (*white arrows*) and also confirming the absence of semicircular ducts. **d** Axial MDCT image through the inner ear confirming the absence of the semicircular canals, only the vestibule can be seen (*black arrow*)

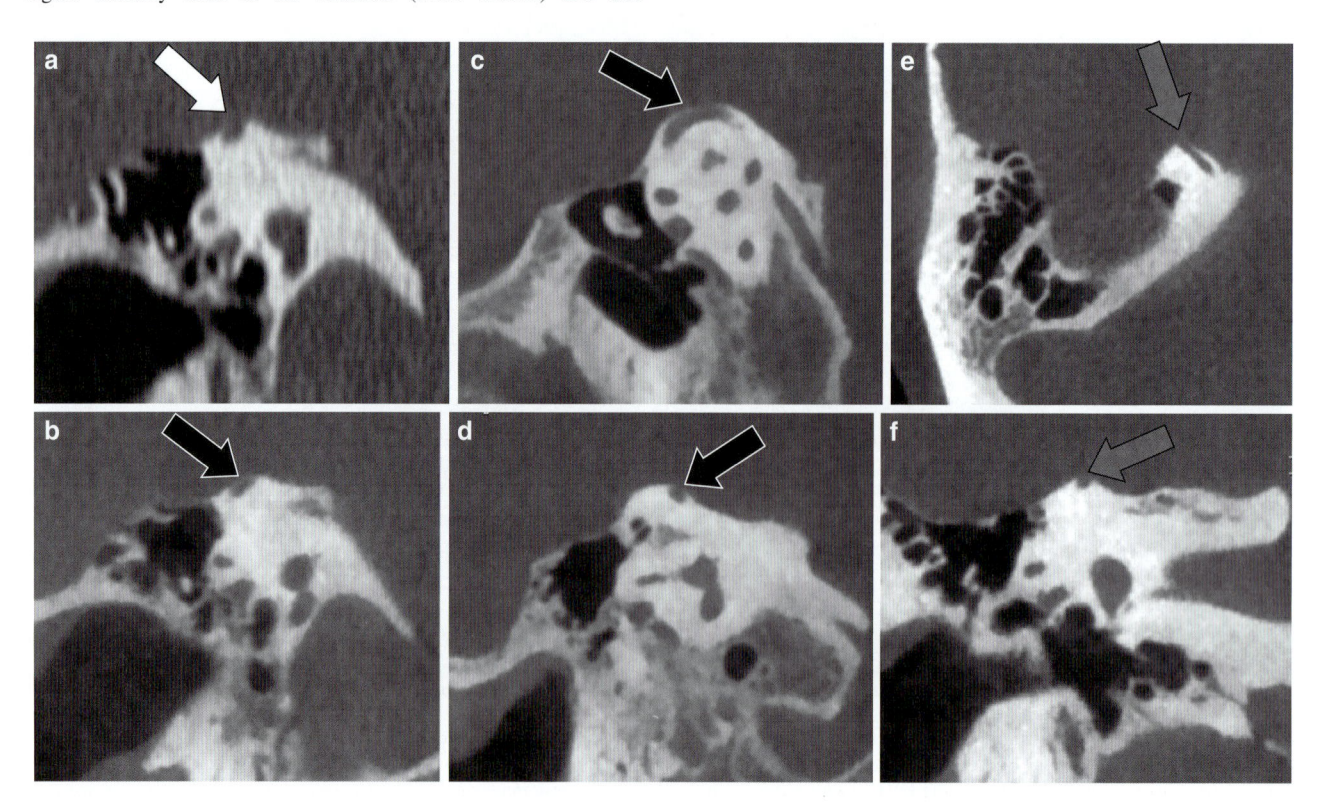

Fig. 26 False and true Dehiscent Superior Semicircular Canal—value of CBCT. **a–b** Coronal MDCT (**a**) and CBCT (**b**) through the right superior semicircular canal (SSC). The MDCT image shows a dehiscent SSC (*white arrow*). This is corrected on the CBCT where a thin bony wall of the SSC can be seen, hence CBCT is thanks to its much higher spatial resolution correcting MDCT. **c–d** The findings were checked on paracoronal (**c**) and parasagittal (**d**) reformatted CBCT images, confirming an intact bony wall of the SSC (*black arrows*). **e–f** Axial and coronal CBCT through the right SSC in another patient showing a true dehiscence of the SSC in both planes (*grey arrows*)

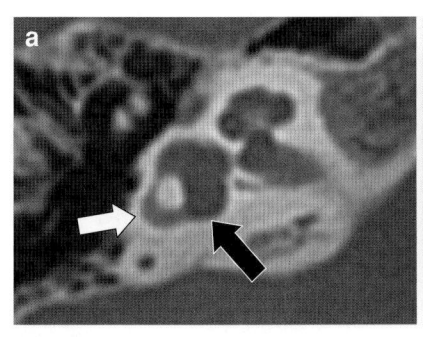

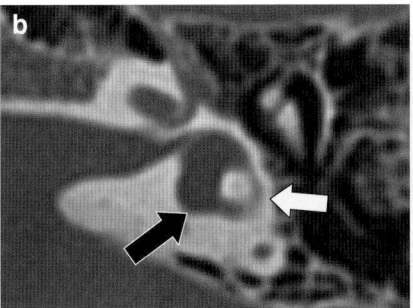

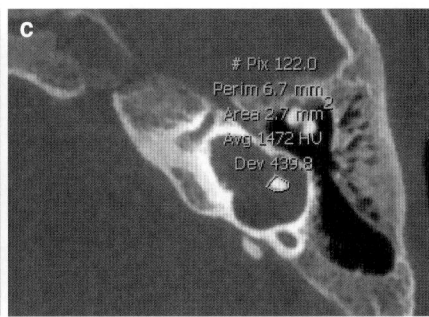

Fig. 27 Enlarged vestibule. **a–b** Axial MDCT image through the right (**a**) and left (**b**) vestibule. The vestibule is enlarged and extends further posterior than the most posterior delineation of the lateral semicircular canal (*black arrows*). The vestibule starts to assimilate the lateral semicircular canal which therefore appears shorter (*white arrows*). **c** Axial CBCT image through the left enlarged vestibule (in a different patient). The vestibule can be considered enlarged once CT shows that the surface of the bone island surrounded by the lateral semicircular canal drops below 6 mm², in this patient the remaining bone island measures 2,7 mm²

Fig. 28 Labyrinthine aplasia. **a–b** Labyrinthine aplasia in a patient with a developed petrous apex (**a**) and in a patient with petrous apex aplasia (**b**). **a** The petrous apex (*white arrows*) is present on both sides but the cochlea and vestibular structures are absent. Notice the normal development of the middle ear and mastoid and the presence of a canal for the facial nerve on the left side. **b** There is not only absence of the inner ear structures but also of the petrous bone/petrous apex (*black arrows*). *Courtesy* Prof. M. Profant, Bratislava, Slovakia

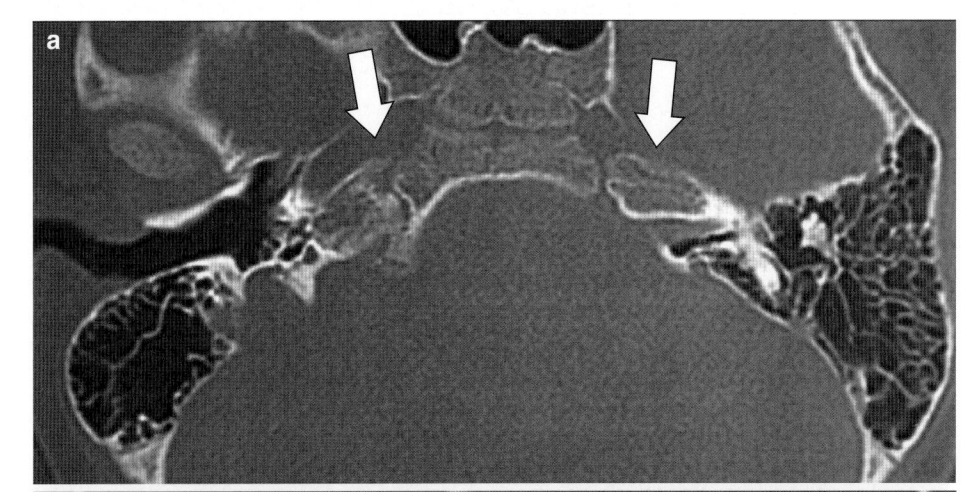

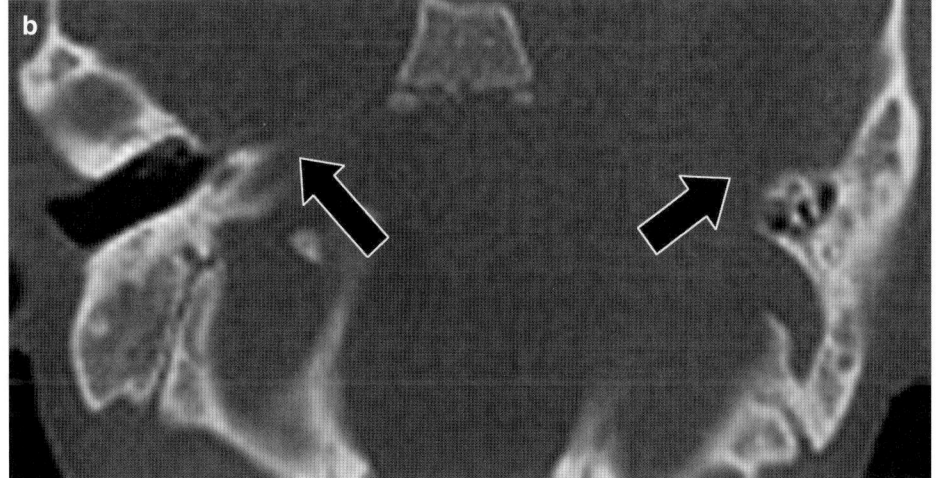

4.2.3.2 Cochlear Aplasia

The cochlea is absent. The vestibule and semicircular canals may be normal or malformed and are located posterolateral to the fundus of the internal auditory canal (Fig. 29). Cochlear implantation is not possible.

4.2.3.3 Common Cavity

The cochlea and the vestibule are seen as a round or ovoid single cavity. The semicircular canals may be normal or malformed. The internal auditory canal usually reaches the common cavity at its centre (Fig. 30). The cavity contains

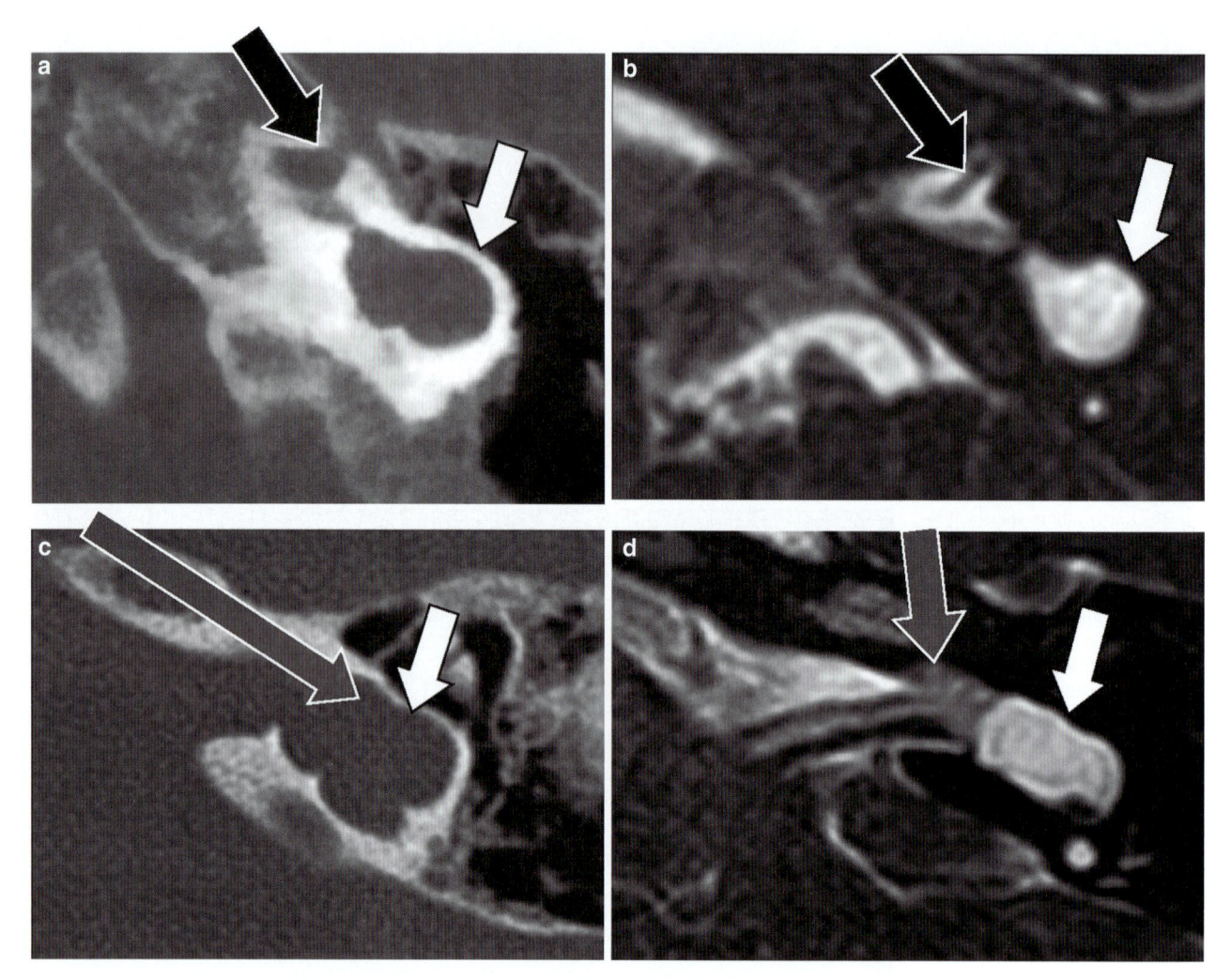

Fig. 29 Cochlear aplasia. **a–b** Axial CBCT (**a**) and 3D-TSE T2-weighted image (**b**) through the left labyrinth. The cochlea is absent and the fundus of the internal auditory canal (IAC) can be seen anterior to the abnormal cystic vestibular labyrinth, which consists of a cystic vestibule (*white arrows*) and a posterior semicircular canal. A separate facial nerve canal branches anteriorly from the fundus of the IAC (*black arrows*). **c–d** Axial CBCT (**c**) and 3D T2-weighted DRIVE image (**d**) showing a facial nerve and a not dividing cochleovestibular nerve in a not bifurcating fundus of the IAC (*grey arrows*). The IAC is again located completely anterior to the abnormal enlarged cystic vestibule (*white arrows*). Images 29 **c, d** Courtesy Dr. S. Vaid, Star Imaging and Research Center, Pune, India

both cochlear and vestibular neural structures, but of course the presence of the cochleovestibular nerve or the cochlear branch of the VIIIth nerve must be demonstrated before cochlear implantation is considered. But even in the presence of an VIIIth nerve, these patients often perform poor after cochlear implantation. A common cavity must be distinguished from cochlear aplasia with a vestibular dilatation. The latter is located posterolateral to the fundus of the internal auditory canal and stimulation with a cochlear implant is not possible at all in these patients.

4.2.3.4 Incomplete Partition Types I, II and III

In these patients, abnormalities inside the cochlea affecting the modiolus and the interscalar septa can be found.

Type I: In this type of cochlea, the complete modiolus and all interscalar septa are absent. The cochlea looks like an empty cystic structure and therefore this cochlear abnormality has also been called the "cystic cochleovestibular malformation" (Sennaroglu and Saatci 2002) (Fig. 31). The external dimensions of the cochlea are normal. The exact location of the ganglion cells is not known, but must be located at the periphery of the cystic cochlea and hence a non-hugging electrode with complete rings should be used. The vestibule is dilated and the vestibular aqueduct is most often normal but a defect exists between the cochlea and the fundus of the internal auditory canal due to the absence of the modiolus. Due to this defect, the CSF pressure is transmitted to the perilymph spaces and can cause a gusher

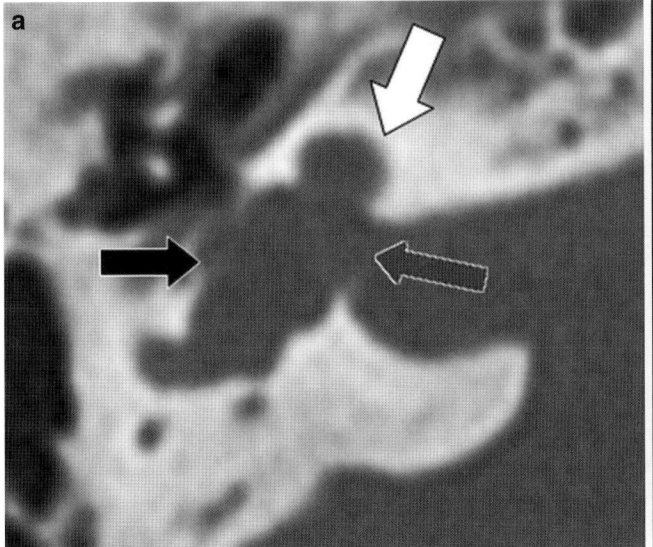

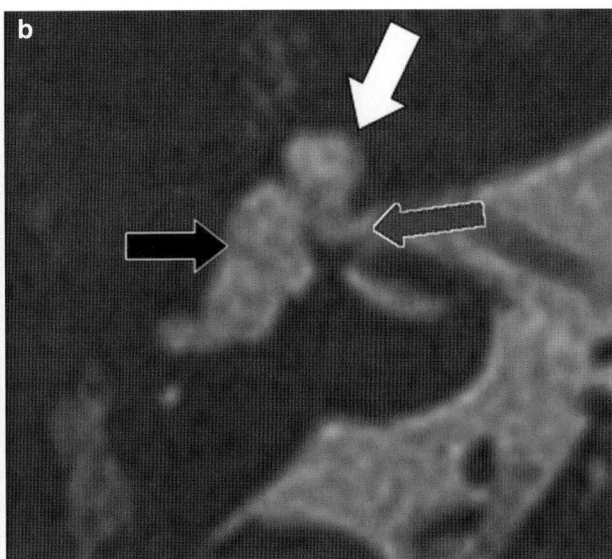

Fig. 30 Common cavity. **a–b** Axial CBCT (**a**) and 3D-TSE T2-weighted image (**b**) through the inner ear. A rudimentary cochlea and malformed vestibule are represented by a single chamber. The fundus of the internal auditory canal (IAC) (*grey arrows*) enters the common cavity at its centre, between the abnormal anterior cochlear (*white arrows*) and posterior vestibular part of the cavity (*black arrows*). In other cases, the IAC can also enter a single round or ovoid common cavity at their centre. The position of the fundus of the IAC is crucial to distinguish cochlear aplasia (completely anterior to the abnormal labyrinth) from a common cavity (entering the abnormal labyrinth at its centre)

ear during cochlear implant placement. Therefore, the surgeon can use a custom-made electrode with a 'cork' type silicon ring.

Type II: Only the basal part of the modiolus is present in a type II cochlea, the apical part of the modiolus and the interscalar septa of the apical part of the cochlea are absent. This results in a cystic appearance of the cochlear apex due to the confluence of the apical and middle turns (Fig. 32). The same cochlear changes were described by Mondini and were called the Mondini deformity when this cochlear abnormality was associated with a dilated vestibule and a large vestibular aqueduct. Spiral ganglion cells are present in the normal basal part of the modiolus and therefore good stimulation with all kind of electrodes placed in the normal basal turn is possible in IP-II patients.

Type III: This cochlear abnormality is seen in patients with X-linked deafness. The modiolus is completely absent, the interscalar septa are present at the lateral wall of the cochlea. The cochlea has normal external dimensions and is located at the lateral end of the fundus of the internal auditory canal and not in its normal position anterolateral to the fundus of the internal auditory canal (Fig. 33). Full-ring short electrodes, making one turn around the cochlea should be used, normal longer electrodes risk to enter the internal auditory canal.

4.2.3.5 Cochlear Hypoplasia

In cochlear hypoplasia, the external dimensions of the cochlea are smaller than normal. It is difficult to count the exact number of turns on CT and MR. Shorter electrodes should be used in these patients. Three types of cochlear hypoplasia can be distinguished in the Sennaroglu classification.

Type I or bud-like cochlea: The cochlea looks like a small bud placed at the lateral end of the internal auditory canal. The modiolus and interscalar septa are absent (Fig. 34a).

Type II or cystic hypoplastic cochlea: The dimensions of the cochlea are smaller than normal, but its external architecture is normal. The modiolus and interscalar septa are absent and a wide connection exists between the cochlea and the internal auditory canal, the vestibular aqueduct is enlarged and the vestibule is slightly dilated (Fig. 34b). In these patients, a gusher ear can be expected and there is also the risk that the electrode might enter the internal auditory canal.

Type III or cochlea with less than two turns: The modiolus is smaller and the length of the scalar septa is diminished, resulting in less than two turns (Fig. 34c). For

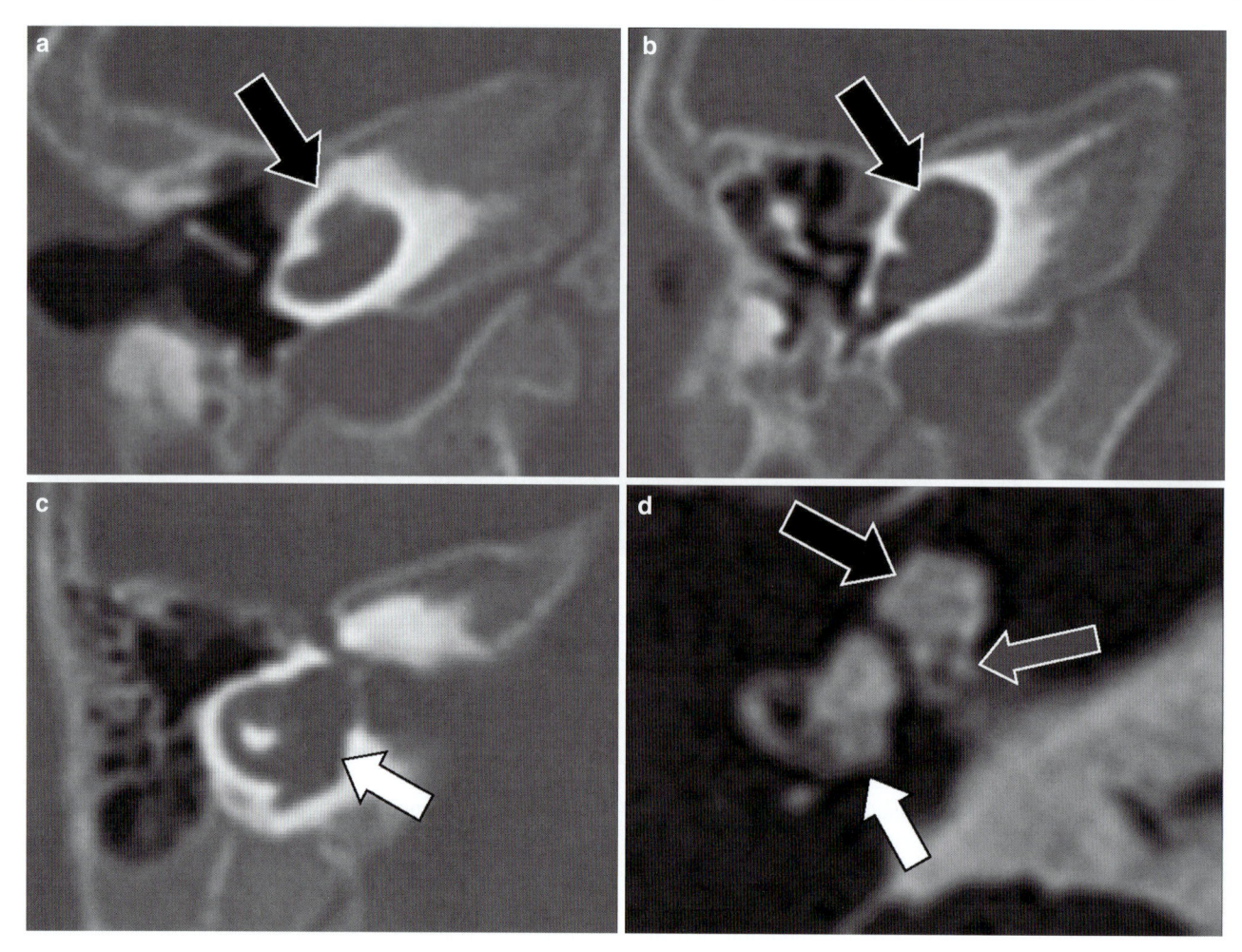

Fig. 31 Incomplete partition type I. **a–d** Axial MDCT through the right inner ear from the lower part (**a**) to the upper part (**c**) of the labyrinth and axial submillimetric T2-weighted 3D TSE image through the labyrinth (**d**). The interscalar septa and modiolus are absent and hence the cochlea has a cystic appearance (*black arrows*). This type of cochlear malformation is accompanied by a cystic dilatation of the vestibule (*white arrows*). The absence of the modiolus and abnormal development of the cochlear foramen causes a defect between the cochlea and the fundus of the internal auditory canal (*grey arrow*)

the rest, the cochlea has a normal internal and external architecture and is associated with vestibular and semicircular canal hypoplasia.

4.2.4 Large Vestibular Aqueduct

The vestibular aqueduct can be evaluated on CT and is considered enlarged when its diameter is larger than 1.5 mm (Valvassori and Clemis 1978). This diameter should be measured at the mid-point between the place where the aqueduct comes out of the vestibule and where it enters the posterior fossa. The diameter is best measured in the paracoronal plane perpendicular to the long axis of the petrous apex (Fig. 35). 1.5 mm corresponds to the diameter of the adjacent posterior semicircular canal which can be used as a quick reference to detect a large vestibular aqueduct (LVA). A LVA is one of the most frequent malformations of the inner ear and represents 13 % of all congenital malformations of the labyrinth and is occurring bilaterally in 46.7 % of the cases (Veillon et al. 2014). The diagnosis can also easily be made on heavily T2-weighted submillimetric images. On these images, the fluid-filled large endolymphatic duct and sac (LEDS) can be seen and even the extension of the sac in the posterior fossa, which remains most often invisible on CT, can be seen on MR. The reason for this is that heavily T2-weighted submillimetric MR images can show the hypointense wall of the sac between the CSF and the endolymph inside the sac and because the signal intensity of the endolymph is often higher than the signal intensity of the CSF as the endolymph is not dephased by fast flow. Sometimes low-signal intensity regions can be seen inside a LEDS (Fig. 36a, b). This low signal may represent fibrous tissue, loose vascular subepithelial connective tissue/cuboidal or columnar epithelial cells as found in the rugose part of a normal sac which can also be found in the normal

Congenital Malformations of the Temporal Bone

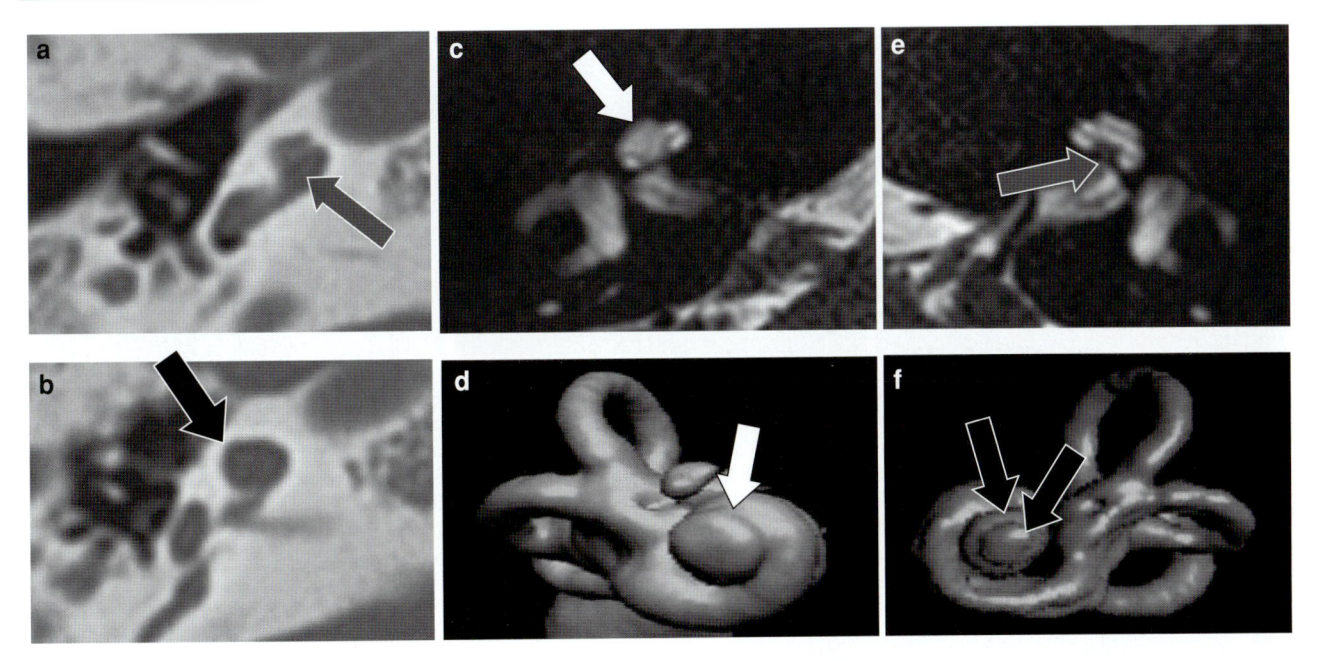

Fig. 32 Incomplete partition type II. **a–b** Axial MDCT through the right inner ear in a patient with incomplete partition type II. The basal turn has a normal appearance and the osseous spiral lamina between the scala tympani and scala media/vestibuli can be recognised (*grey arrow*). The apical part of the modiolus and corresponding interscalar septa are absent and therefore the apical and second turn can be seen as a cystic empty cavity (*black arrow*). **c–f** Axial heavily T2-weighted submillimetric 3D TSE DRIVE images through the abnormal right (**c**) and normal left inner ear (**e**) and corresponding 3D surface renderings (**d, f**). The absence of the upper part of the modiolus and interscalar septa results in a single fluid-filled cavity (**c**). This can be seen as single cavity on top of the basal turn on the 3D surface reconstruction (**d**) (*white arrows*). Compare with the normal left ear where the apical and second turn can be distinguished from each other (*black arrows*) and where a normal modiolus can be seen at the base of the cochlea (*grey arrow*)

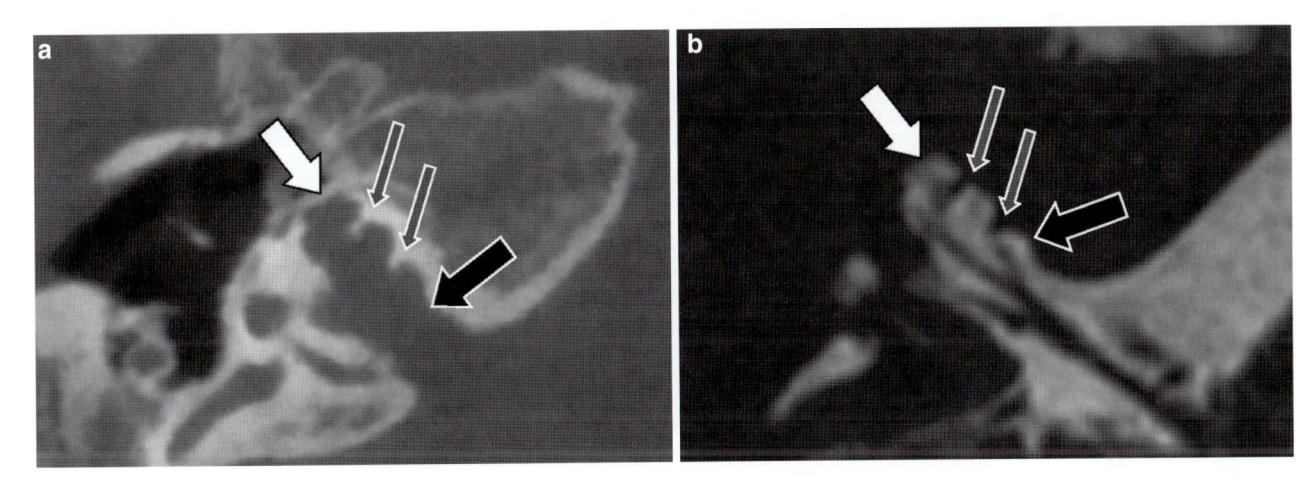

Fig. 33 Incomplete partition type III. **a–b** Axial CBCT (**a**) and axial heavily T2-weighted submillimetric 3D TSE DRIVE image (**b**) through the right internal auditory canal (IAC) and cochlea. The modiolus is absent (*white arrows*) but the interscalar septa are present (*grey arrows*). The cochlea is centred on the lateral end of the IAC and there is no barrier between the cochlea and the IAC (*black arrows*) due to the absence of the modiolus

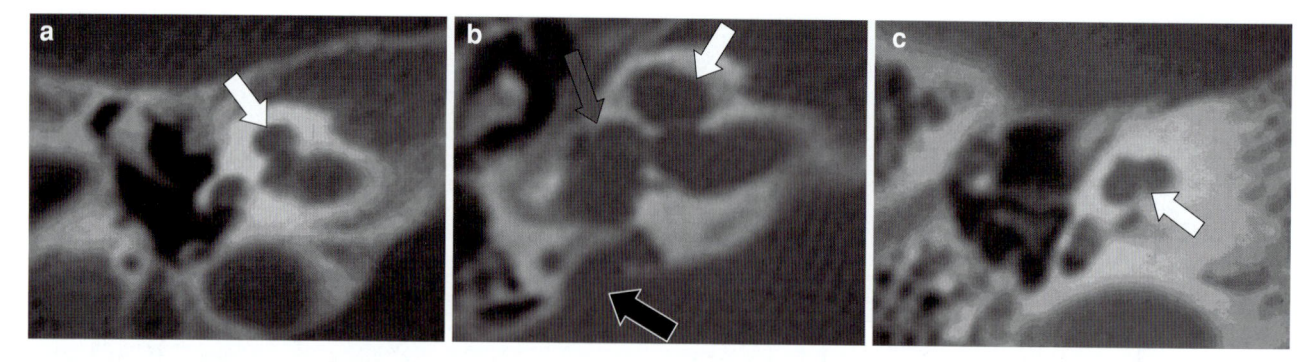

Fig. 34 Cochlear hypoplasia type I-II-III. **a–c** Axial MDCT image through the right cochlea in patients with a type I (**a**), type II (**b**) and type III (**c**) cochlear hypoplasia. **a** In type I cochlear hypoplasia, the cochlea appears as a small bud (*white arrow*), situated on the lateral end of the internal auditory canal (IAC). The modiolus and interscalar septa are absent. **b** In type II cochlear hypoplasia the cochlea is still smaller than normal (*white arrow*) and again the modiolus and interscalar septa are absent. The vestibule is slightly dilated (*grey arrow*) and the vestibular aqueduct is enlarged (*black arrow*). In these patients, cochlear implantation surgery can result in a gusher ear or unintentional electrode entry in the IAC. **c** In type III cochlear hypoplasia, the modiolus is smaller (*white arrow*) and the interscalar septa are shorter resulting in a cochlea with less windings but with a normal internal and external architecture

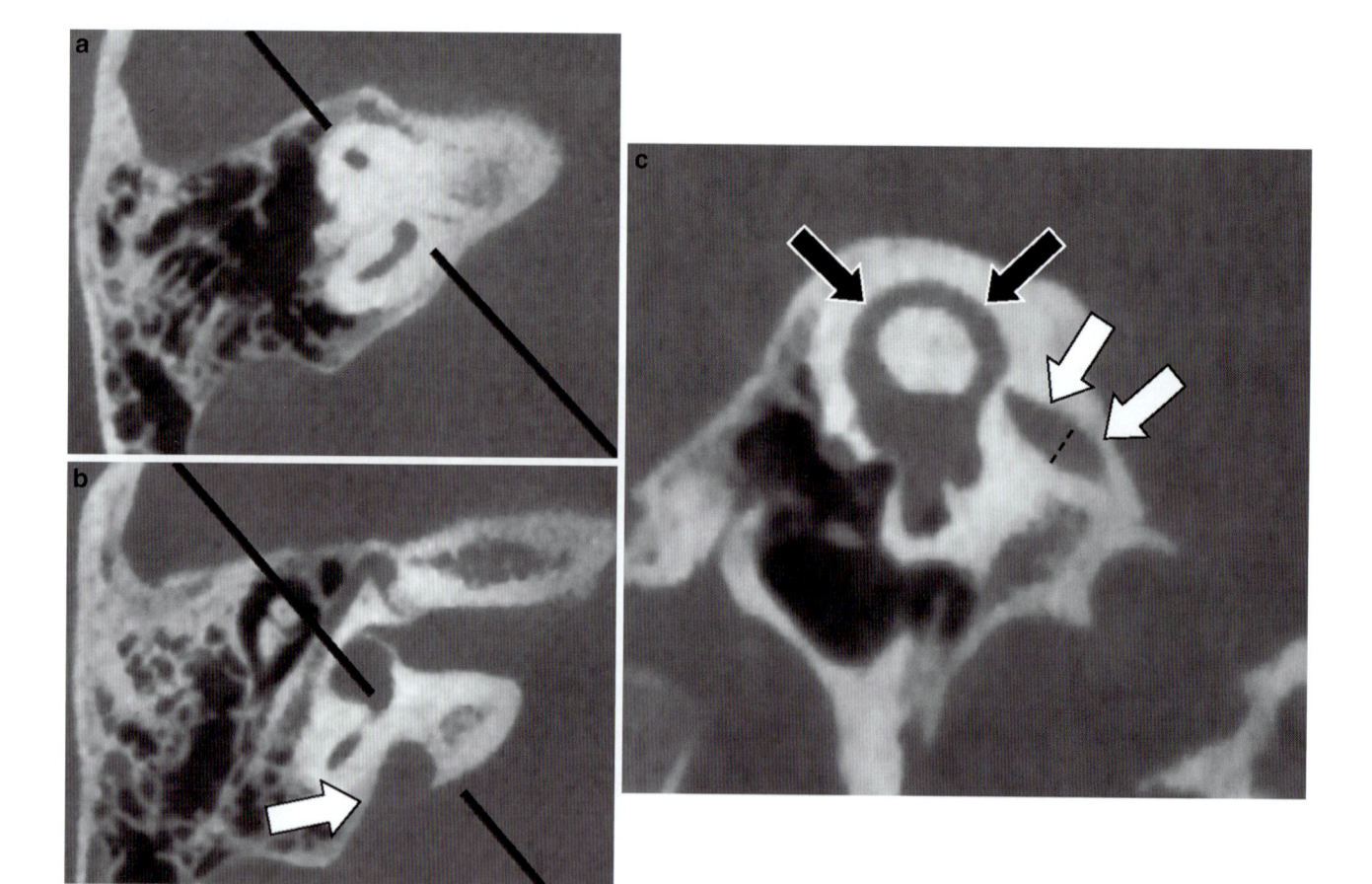

Fig. 35 Large vestibular aqueduct—measurement. **a–c** Axial CBCT image through the right superior semicircular canal (**a**) and large vestibular aqueduct (LVA) (**b**) and paracoronal reconstruction along the *black line* in **a** and **b** (**c**) passing through the mid-point of the LVA between the place where the aqueduct comes out of the vestibule and where it enters the posterior fossa. The diameter is best measured in the paracoronal plane (**c**) perpendicular to the long axis of the petrous bone along the *black line* in (**a-b**). Paracoronal reformatted images along this axis will show the entire superior semicircular canal (*black arrows*) and are located at the mid-point of the LVA, where measurements are reliable. At this point, the vestibular aqueduct must be wider than 1.5 mm (*dotted black line*) or wider than the adjacent posterior semicircular canal in order to be an LVA (*white arrows*)

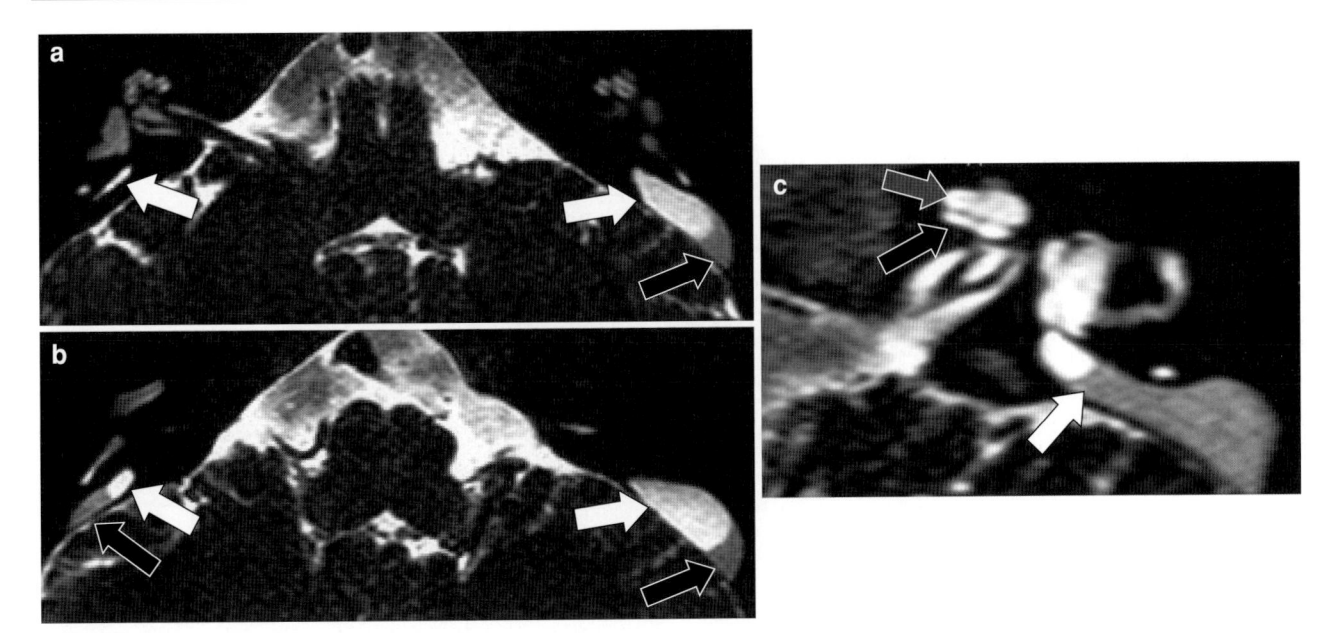

Fig. 36 Large vestibular aqueduct. **a–b** Axial T2-weighted TSE DRIVE images through the upper part (**a**) and lower part (**b**) of bilateral large endolymphatic ducts and sacs (LEDS's). On both sides, a fluid-filled LEDS can be seen (*white arrows*), which are much wider than the diameter of the fluid-filled adjacent posterior semicircular canals. The extension of the posterior part of the LEDS in the posterior fossa can be seen and in this patient they have a lower signal intensity (*black arrows*) representing fibrous tissue, loose vascular subepithelial connective tissue and cuboidal or columnar epithelial cells. **c** Axial T2-weighted TSE DRIVE image in another patient with a LEDS and a coexisting cochlear anomaly on the left side. LEDS with a dominant low signal intensity region and small fluid-filled part (*white arrow*). Asymmetry of the scala tympani (*black arrow*) and scala vestibuli (*grey arrow*), the latter is twice as large while normally they have the same size

endolymphatic duct and sac. High-resolution CT and MR studies have shown that a LVA or LEDS coexists with cochlear anomalies in up to 76 % of the cases (Davidson et al. 1999). In these patients, modiolar deficiencies, scalar asymmetries, gross cochlear dysmorphism, etc. were found (Fig. 36c). The majority of these patients presents with SNHL, although some of them present with conductive or mixed hearing loss. The conductive component of this hearing loss is probably a pure cochlear conductive loss (Govaerts et al. 1999) and there seems to be no correlation between the size of the LVA/LEDS and the hearing loss (Naganawa et al. 2000). It is very important to recognize these congenital malformations, especially in children. The presence of a LVA/LEDS indicates that these children have "fragile" labyrinths which can be damaged by trauma, causing progressive SNHL and eventually deafness in bilateral cases (Harnsberger 2004). Hence early diagnosis is necessary to protect these children against head trauma.

4.2.5 Internal Auditory Canal and Cochlear Foramen

The internal auditory canal (IAC) can be atretic (Fig. 28) and in these cases, there is no cochleovestibular nerve present. The normal IAC is 2–8 mm wide and is stenotic when the diameter is less than 2 mm at the IAC mid-point (Fig. 37). The relationship between stenotic IACs and SNHL is unpredictable (Shelton et al. 1989) and relies on the presence of a normal nerve and deformities of the membranous labyrinth, the latter are often invisible on CT and MR. The cochlear foramen through which the cochlear branch of the cochleovestibular nerve passes from the cochlea into the IAC normally measures 2.13 ± 0.44 mm and is considered stenotic below 1.5 mm (Veillon et al. 2014) (Fig. 38). Stenosis of this canal is rare and atresia is extremely rare. Studies showed that smaller cochlear foramina are associated with SNHL (Fatterpekar et al. 2000). It is obvious that the presence of a cochleovestibular nerve and cochlear branch of the cochleovestibular nerve must be checked on MR in patients with a stenotic IAC and/or stenotic cochlear foramen.

4.2.6 Cochleovestibular Nerve Aplasia and Dysplasia (CNAD)

The integrity of the cochleovestibular nerve (CVN) must be checked in patients with congenital deafness and especially in cochlear implant candidates (Casselman et al. 1997). Neuroblasts of the cochlear ganglion separate from the developing otic epithelium and fibers from these ganglion cell bodies grow peripherally back into the otic epithelium and centrally into the brainstem and will form the CVN.

Fig. 37 Stenotic internal auditory canal. **a** Axial MDCT image through the right internal auditory canal (IAC)—patient with a unilateral IAC stenosis. The right IAC is less than 2 mm wide at the mid-point of the IAC (*black arrows*) and hence is stenotic. **b–c** Coronal MDCT (**b**) and heavily T2-weighted TSE DRIVE image (**c**) in a patient with bilateral IAC stenosis, bilateral normal labyrinth and bilateral VIIIth nerve aplasia. The left and right IAC are less than 2 mm wide at the mid-point of the IAC (*white arrows*), only the fundus is wider on both sides. Images 37 **b, c** *Courtesy* Dr. S. Vaid, Star Imaging and Research Center, Pune, India

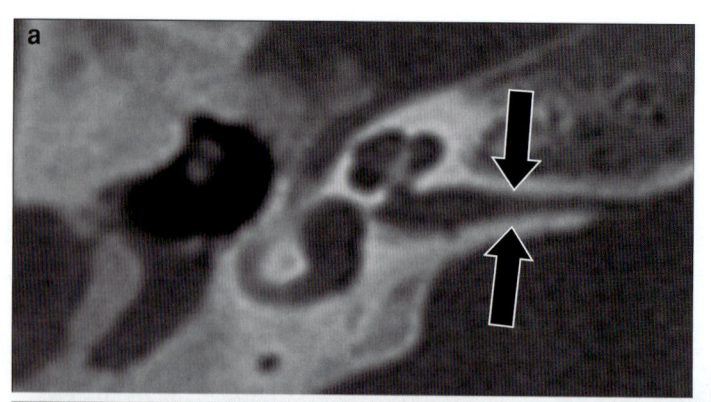

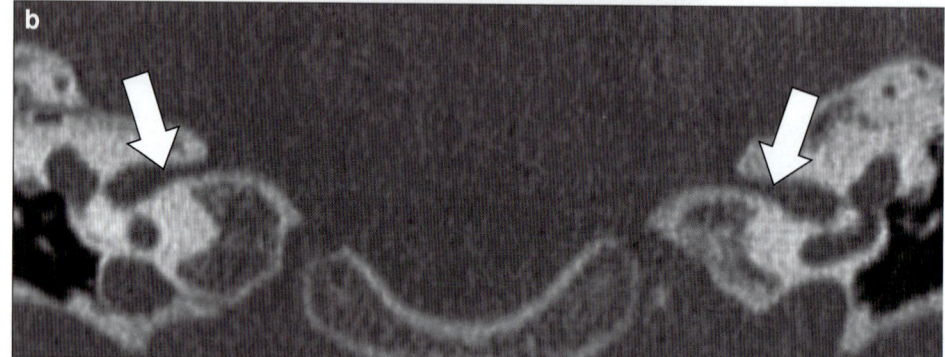

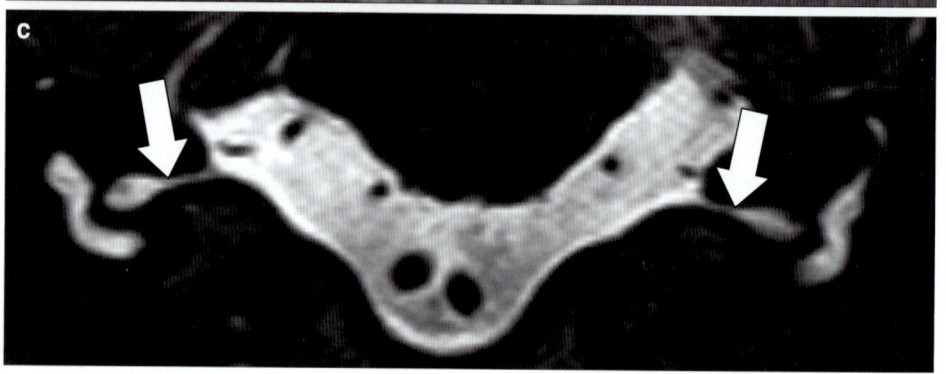

Therefore, there will be no nerve development when there is labyrinthine aplasia. On the other hand, it has been proven that the development of the cochlea does not depend on the presence of a CVN. Hence, one can find a normal cochlea in association with an absent CVN. An absent CVN is often associated with a stenosis of the IAC and a possible hypothesis is that the IAC is formed only in the presence of a normal nerve. Differentiation between aplasia, hypoplasia and a normal size of the cochlear branch can be very difficult and requires the highest possible resolution. The presence of a small internal auditory canal can make the diagnosis even more difficult and it increases the chance that a nerve lies against the wall of the IAC and becomes difficult to depict or becomes invisible. Therefore, imaging with the highest possible quality is required and therefore imaging at 3.0 Tesla using a heavily T2-weighted sequence with the highest possible resolution is preferred. For this indication, the voxel size is even reduced to 0.25 × 0.25 × 0.25 which results in an acquisition time of 7–9 min and in young children, this is of course only possible under general anesthesia (Fig. 39). When an abnormality is seen or suspected on these axial images, then direct parasagittal images with the same heavily T2-weighted sequence are made perpendicular on the nerves in the internal auditory canal and cerebellopontine angle (Casselman et al. 2001). This is done on both sides, so that bilateral pathology can be recognised or comparison with a normal side is possible. These direct images have a better resolution and are sharper than reconstructed images, which are acquired using the original axial images. The angulation perpendicular on the nerves is set out on the original axial series and on coronal low-resolution localizer images (Fig. 39). The presence of a normal, stenotic or

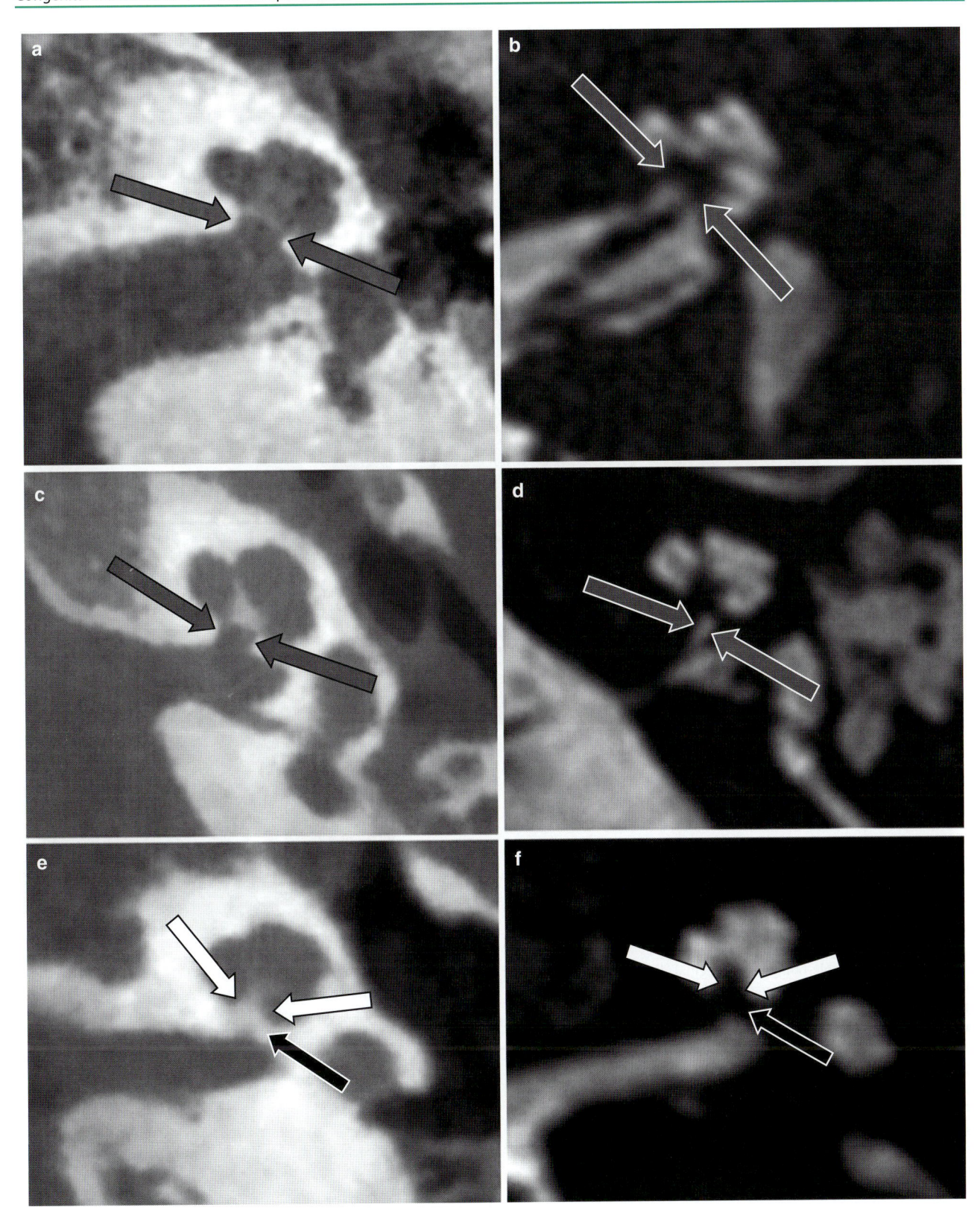

Congenital Malformations of the Temporal Bone

Fig. 38 Normal, stenotic and atretic cochlear foramen. **a–b** Axial CBCT (**a**) and axial heavily T2-weighted TSE DRIVE image (**b**) through a normal cochlear foramen at the base of the cochlea. The normal cochlear foramen (*grey arrows*), where the cochleovestibular nerve passes from the cochlea in the IAC, can be seen at the base of the calcified modiolus and normally measures 1.7–2.6 mm. It measures 2.0 mm in this patient. The cochlear foramen is stenotic when it is smaller than 1.7 mm. **c–d** Axial CBCT (**c**) and axial heavily T2-weighted TSE DRIVE image (**d**) through a stenotic cochlear foramen at the base of the cochlea. In this patient, the cochlear foramen (*grey arrows*) at the base of the modiolus measured 1.2 mm, below the minimum normal value of 1.7 mm. Therefore, this cochlear foramen is stenotic and this can be associated with a hypoplastic or absent cochlear branch of the VIIIth nerve. **e–f** Axial CBCT (**e**) and axial heavily T2-weighted TSE DRIVE image (**f**) through an atretic cochlear foramen at the base of the cochlea. The modiolus is too small and has an abnormal shape. There is no fluid at the base of the cochlea (*white arrows*) and there is even bone between the base of the cochlea and the fundus of the IAC (*black arrow*). Hence, the cochlear foramen is atretic and in these patients the cochlear branch of the VIIIth nerve is absent

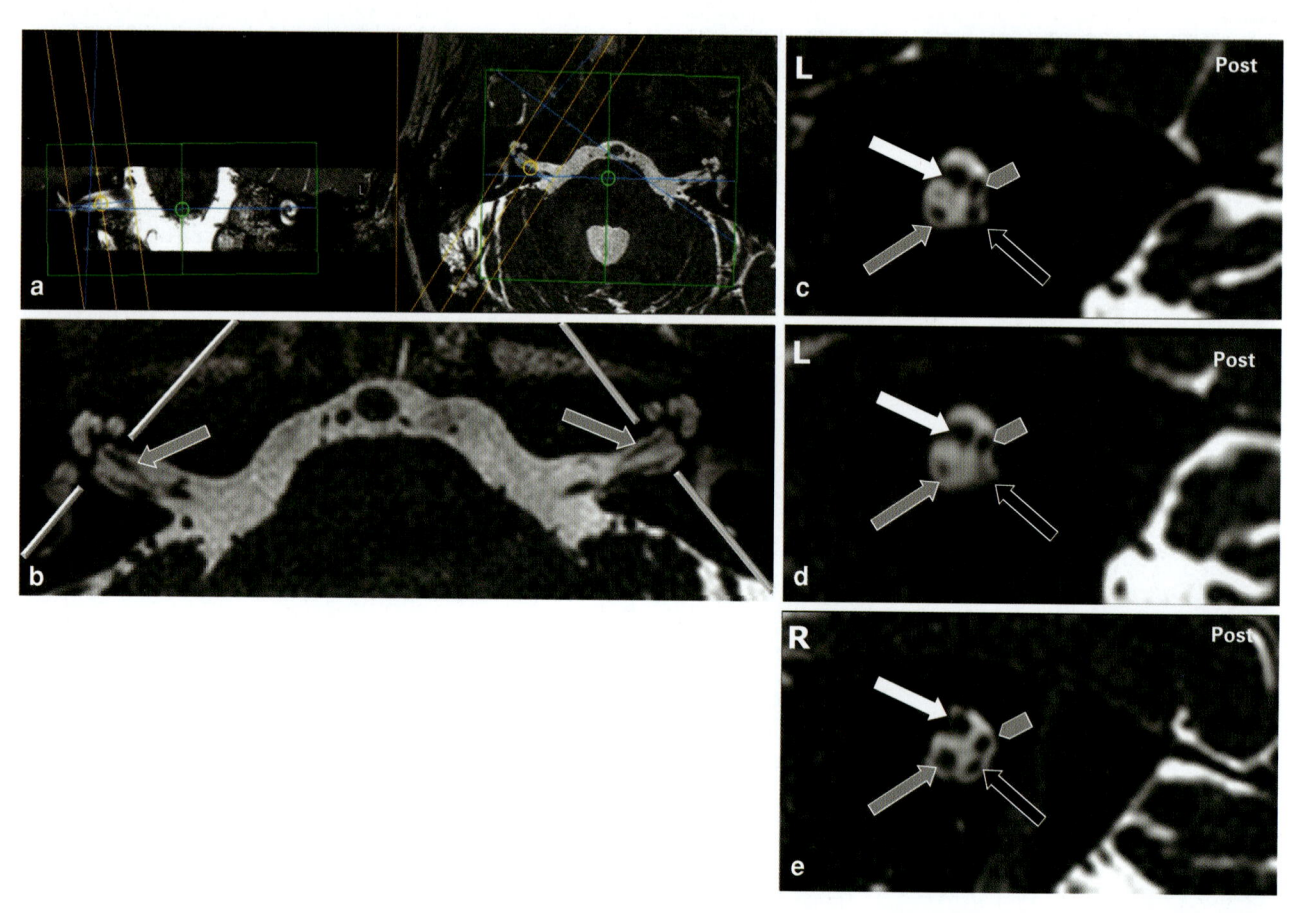

Fig. 39 Direct double-oblique parasagittal high-resolution images through the internal auditory canal. **a–b** Coronal and axial T2-weighted localizer images (**a**) and axial 0.25 × 0.25 × 0.25 mm heavily T2-weighted TSE DRIVE image through the IAC's. The double-oblique images are angled perpendicular to the axis of the IAC in both the axial and coronal plane (*yellow lines*) in order to acquire a perpendicular cross-section through the cochleovestibular nerve and its cochlear branch (**a**). The cochlear branches (*grey arrows*) can be evaluated in detail on these high-resolution images and the left cochlear branch is smaller or hypoplastic (**b**). **c–e** Double-oblique direct (**c**) and reformatted (**d**) high-resolution heavily T2-weighted TSE DRIVE image through the fundus of the left IAC and similar double-oblique direct image through the fundus of the right IAC (**e**). The mages at the fundus of the IAC were made along the white lines in (**b**) The facial nerve (*white arrow*) and superior vestibular nerve (*grey arrowhead*) have a normal appearance. The cochlear branch (*grey arrow*) is hypoplastic on the left side and clearly smaller than on the right side. The cochlear branch normally has the same size as the facial nerve as can be seen on the right side. The hypoplastic cochlear branch is much smaller than facial nerve on the left side. Notice that all nerves are unsharper on the reformatted image (**d**) than on the direct double-oblique image (**c**) and that the cochlear and especially the inferior vestibular nerve (*black arrows*) are almost disappearing on the reformatted image, illustrating the value of "direct double oblique" images

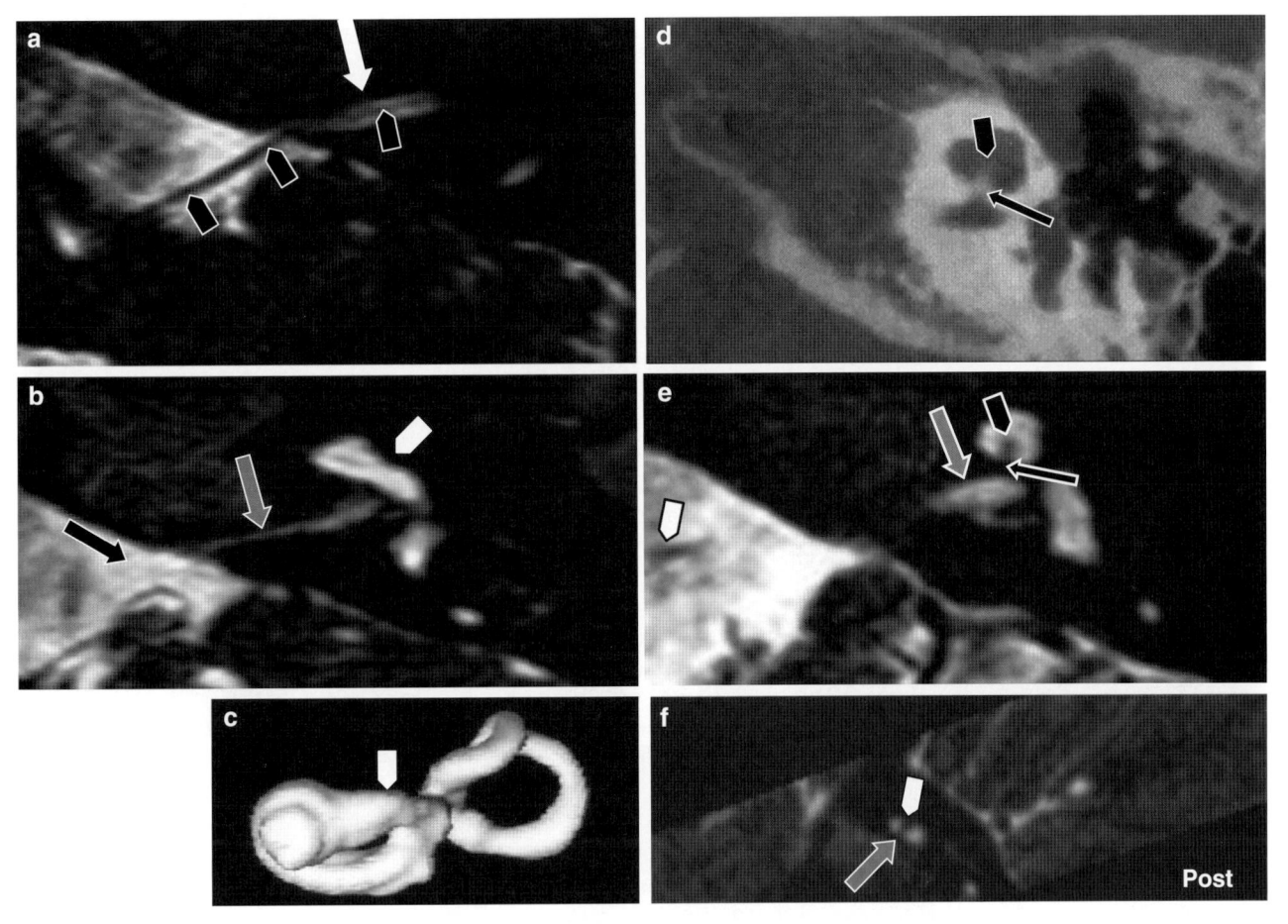

Congenital Malformations of the Temporal Bone

Fig. 40 Cochleovestibular nerve aplasia—Type 1A & 1B CNAD. **a–c** Axial heavily T2-weighted TSE DRIVE images through the upper (**a**) and middle (**b**) part of the left labyrinth and 3D surface rendering of the abnormal left labyrinth (**c**). The facial nerve (*black arrowheads*) can be seen in a separate facial nerve canal (*white arrow*) parallel to and above the extremely narrow internal auditory canal (IAC) (*grey arrow*). The latter is empty as there is cochleovestibular nerve aplasia (*black arrow*) and connects with a malformed labyrinth (*white arrowheads*). An abnormal connection between the cochlea and the vestibule can be seen (*white arrowhead*) and only 2 semicircular canals are present. Therefore, this is a CNAD type 1A. Similar findings were seen on the right side (note shown). **d–f** Axial CBCT (**d**) and heavily T2-weighted TSE DRIVE image (**e**) through the IAC and parasagittal reformatted image through the fundus of the IAC (**f**) in a different patient. A small modiolus can be seen at the base of the cochlea (*black arrowhead*) and bone is separating the base of the cochlea from the fundus of the IAC (*black arrow*): atretic cochlear foramen. The IAC is very thin (*grey arrow*) and the only nerve inside the IAC is the facial nerve (*white arrowhead*) which can be seen in the IAC on the parasagittal reformatted image and in the cerebellopontine angle on the axial T2-weighted image. The cochleovestibular nerve cannot be found, VIIIth nerve aplasia. This is a CNAD type 1B as the labyrinth was normal

absent cochlear foramen for the cochlear nerve between the fundus of the IAC and the modiolus at the base of the cochlea can also be helpful to find out if a cochlear branch is present or not (Fig. 38). This is better seen at high resolution and can best be done with the lowest possible radiation burden as the patients are often very young. For both reasons, Cone-Beam CT is preferred over MultiDetector conventional CT and is boosting the resolution from 0.625/0.5 mm for MDCT to 0.15 mm for CBCT. Again, in young children, this is best performed under anesthesia and CT and MR should be performed during the same anesthesia. However, when a high-end CBCT is not available, then it is better to use MDCT as most of the regular dental CBCT systems are not even able to provide the quality of MDCT.

4.2.6.1 Cochleovestibular Nerve Aplasia: Type 1 CNAD

Complete cochleovestibular nerve aplasia or a "Type 1 CNAD" is rare and represents in our series 15 % of all CNAD cases. Bilateral cases are more frequent (Fig. 37) and these children of course present as cochlear implant candidates. When the labyrinth on the side of the Type 1 CNAD is abnormal, then it is a Type 1A CNAD (Fig. 40). It is a Type 1B CNAD when the labyrinth is normal (Fig. 37). In these patients, only the facial nerve will be found in the normal or narrowed IAC, although one can often find a separate facial nerve canal parallel to and above the IAC in these patients. It is clear that cochlear implantation is not possible in these patients and that an auditory brainstem implant (ABI) should be considered in bilateral cases.

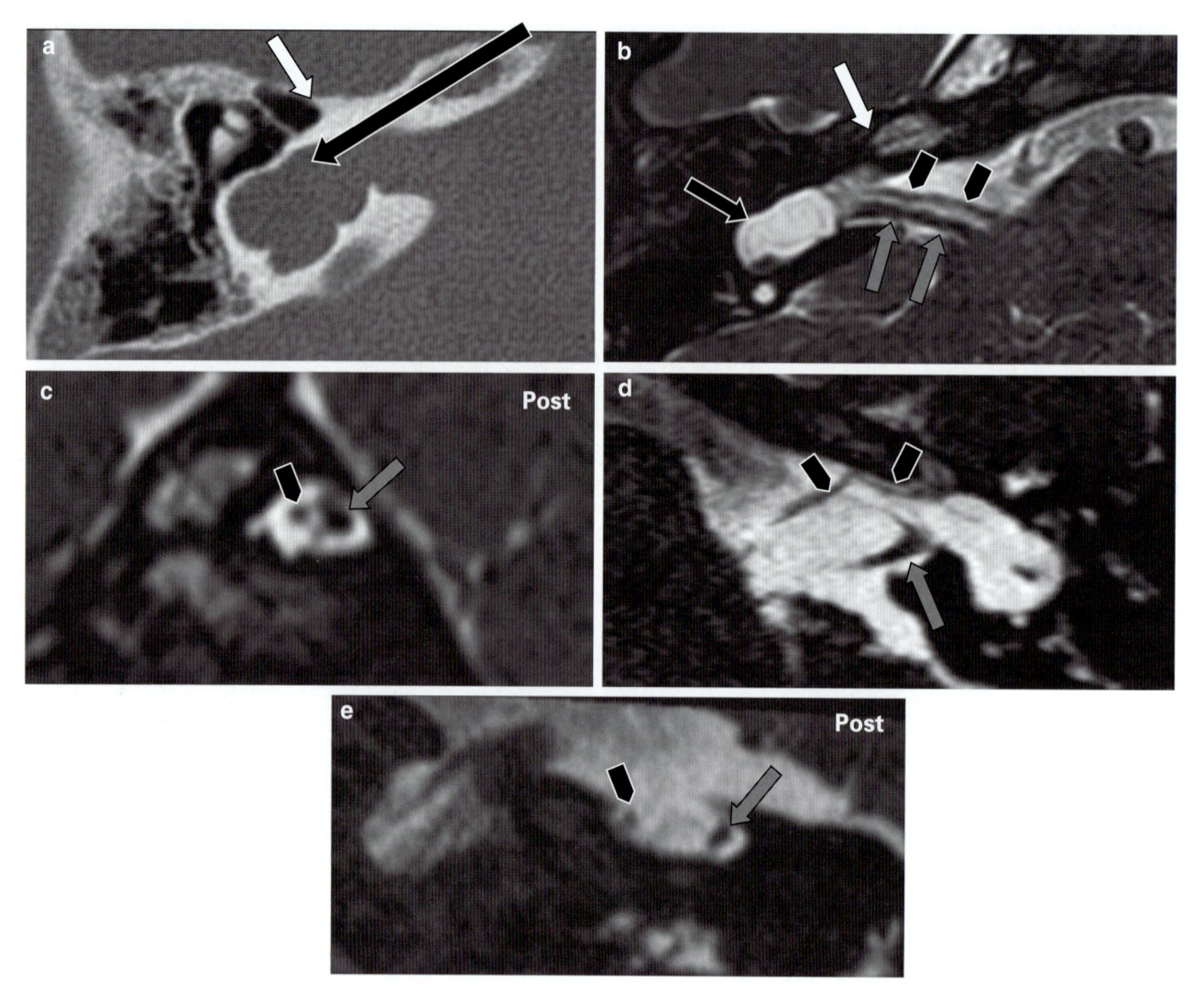

Fig. 41 Cochleovestibular nerve dysplasia—Type 2 CNAD, undivided cochleovestibular nerve or UCN. **a–c** Axial MDCT (**a**) and heavily T2-weighted TSE DRIVE image (**b**) through the internal auditory canal (IAC) and parasagittal reformatted image through the middle part of the IAC (**c**) in a patient with cochlear aplasia. The IAC reaches the labyrinth at the anterior border of an abnormal vestibule (*long black arrow*). The cochlea is not present in its usual location (*white arrow*). The facial nerve (*black arrowheads*) and the not dividing cochleovestibular nerve (*grey arrows*) are the only 2 nerves that can be depicted in the IAC. Therefore, this patient has a Type 2A UCN CNAD (abnormal labyrinth, undivided VIIIth nerve). **d–e** Axial (**d**) and parasagittal reformatted (**e**) heavily T2-weighted TSE DRIVE images through the left IAC and abnormal labyrinth. The facial nerve (*black arrowheads*) is fixed against the anterior wall of the IAC and makes an angle. The undivided VIIIth nerve (*grey arrows*) can be followed to the fundus of the IAC. This explains why only the facial nerve and undivided VIIIth nerve can be seen on the parasagittal image. Classification: Type 2A UCN CNAD. Images 41 **a–c** *Courtesy* Dr. S. Vaid, Star Imaging and Research Center, Pune, India

4.2.6.2 Cochleovestibular Nerve Dysplasia: Type 2 CNAD

Again, a Type 2A and 2B can be distinguished based on the presence of an abnormal or normal labyrinth. In these patients, a CVN is present but the nerve is not normal. Three subgroups can be distinguished (Casselman et al. 1997, 2014a).

Undivided Cochleovestibular Nerve "UCN":

The nerve is present but is not dividing in its three-end branches (superior vestibular, inferior vestibular and cochlear branch). This is most frequently associated with more severe labyrinth malformations like a common cavity or cochlear aplasia and therefore most of the UCN cases are Type 2A CNAD patients (Fig. 41). Cochlear implantation is technically possible in these patients but the clinical result is often disappointing and also depends on the kind of associated labyrinth malformation.

Absent Cochlear Branch or "ACB":

The VCN splits in a superior and inferior vestibular nerve at the fundus of the IAC but there is aplasia of the

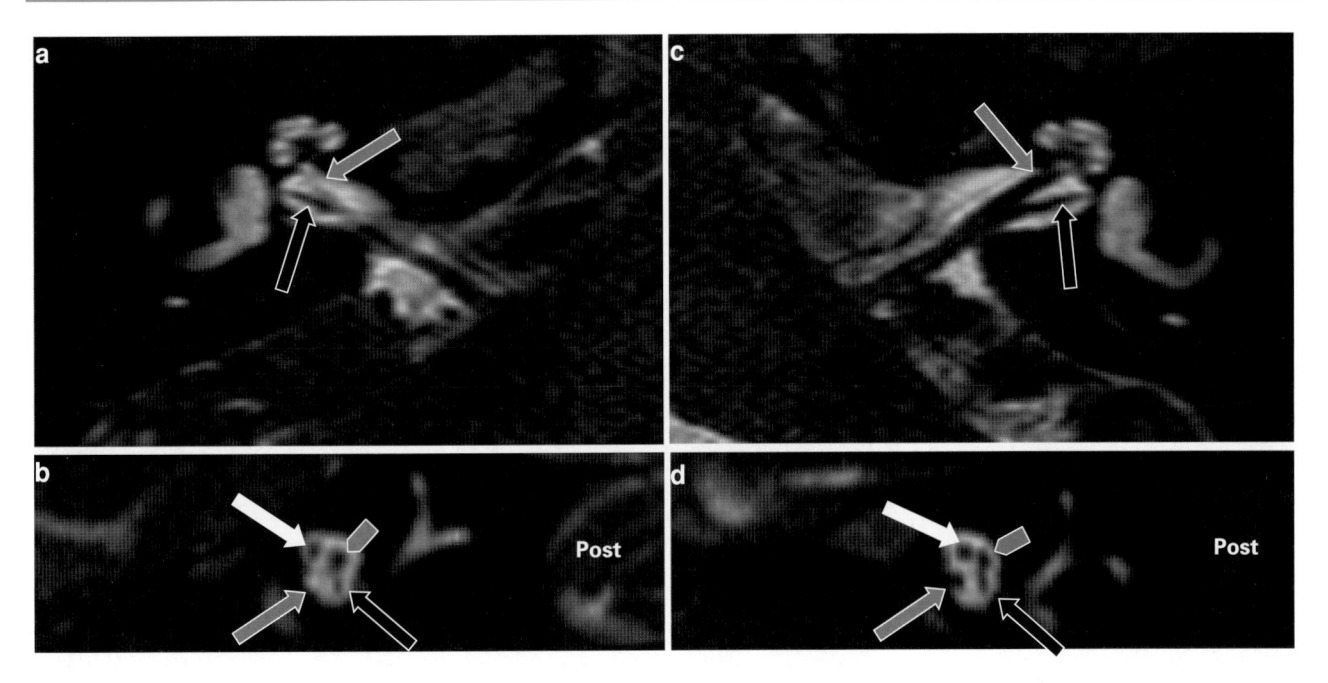

Fig. 42 Cochleovestibular nerve dysplasia—Type 2 CNAD, absent cochlear branch or ACB. **a–d** Axial (**a, c**) and parasagittal (**b, d**) heavily T2-weighted TSE DRIVE images through the right (**a, b**) and left (**c, d**) internal auditory canal (IAC) and inner ear. The labyrinth is normal. The cochlear branch of the VIIIth nerve (*grey arrow*) is absent on the right side but has a normal appearance on the left side. The other nerve branches are normal on both sides and there is no stenosis of the IAC. Classification: Type 2B ACB CNAD on the right side. Inferior vestibular nerve (*black arrow*), superior vestibular nerve (*grey arrowhead*), facial nerve (*white arrow*)

cochlear branch (Fig. 42). In these patients, the cochlea can still be normal but then the cochlear foramen is absent or stenotic. Hence, it is important to realise that a perfectly normal cochlea does not warrant the presence of a cochlear branch. Cochlear implantation is not possible in these patients.

Hypoplastic Cochlear Branch or "HCB":

In HCB cases, the VCN splits normally in its three-end branches but the cochlear branch is too small or hypoplastic (Fig. 39). Cochlear implantation is possible but the results depend on the number of available fibers in the hypoplastic cochlear branch(es) and on the kind of associated labyrinth malformation in Type 2A cases.

4.2.7 Syndromes with Congenital Ear Malformations

Mesenchyma is involved in the development of the outer ear, middle ear and inner ear. This explains why in some of the otocraniofacial dysplasias and toxic embryopathies (e.g. thalidomide), all three ear compartments can be involved simultaneously. Malformations in the three compartments have been described in the Alagille, Branchio-Oto-Renal (Fig. 43), DiGeorge's, Goldenhar's, Klippel-Feil, Moebius, Pierre Robin, Stickler, Treacher Collins and Wildervanck syndromes and in the CHARGE association, cleidocranial dyostosis, craniometaphyseal dysplasia and trisomy 13–15, 18 and 21. Only one or two compartments of the ear are involved in the Apert's, Chromosome 18 deletion, Pendred's, Refsum's and Waardenburg's syndromes and in patients with Achondroplasia, Crouzon's disease, Frontometaphyseal dysplasia, Hemifacial microsomia, X-linked deafness and Osteogenesis imperfecta (Phelps et al. 1981, 1998; Ceruti et al. 2002; Swinnen et al. 2013; Veillon et al. 2014; Curtin et al. 2011). Other organs and skeletal structures can be involved as is the case with the kidneys (Branchio-Oto-Renal syndrome), eye-retina (Usher's and Refsum's syndrome), maxillofacial structures (Hemifacial microsomia, Goldenhar's syndrome…), vertebra (Cleidocranial dyostosis, Hemifacial microsomia, Goldenhar's syndrome…), etc. Some syndromes, like Pendred's (otothyroid), Usher's (oto-ocular) and Jervell and Lange-Nielsen (oto-cardiac) syndrome initially present with only hearing loss and routine screening is needed to detect these syndromes at an early stage. Finally, in some of the syndromes, imaging remains normal and the diagnosis is made clinically and by genetic screening. This is for instance the case in patients with Usher's and Jervell and Lange-Nielsen syndrome and in patients with connexin 26 disorder/mutations.

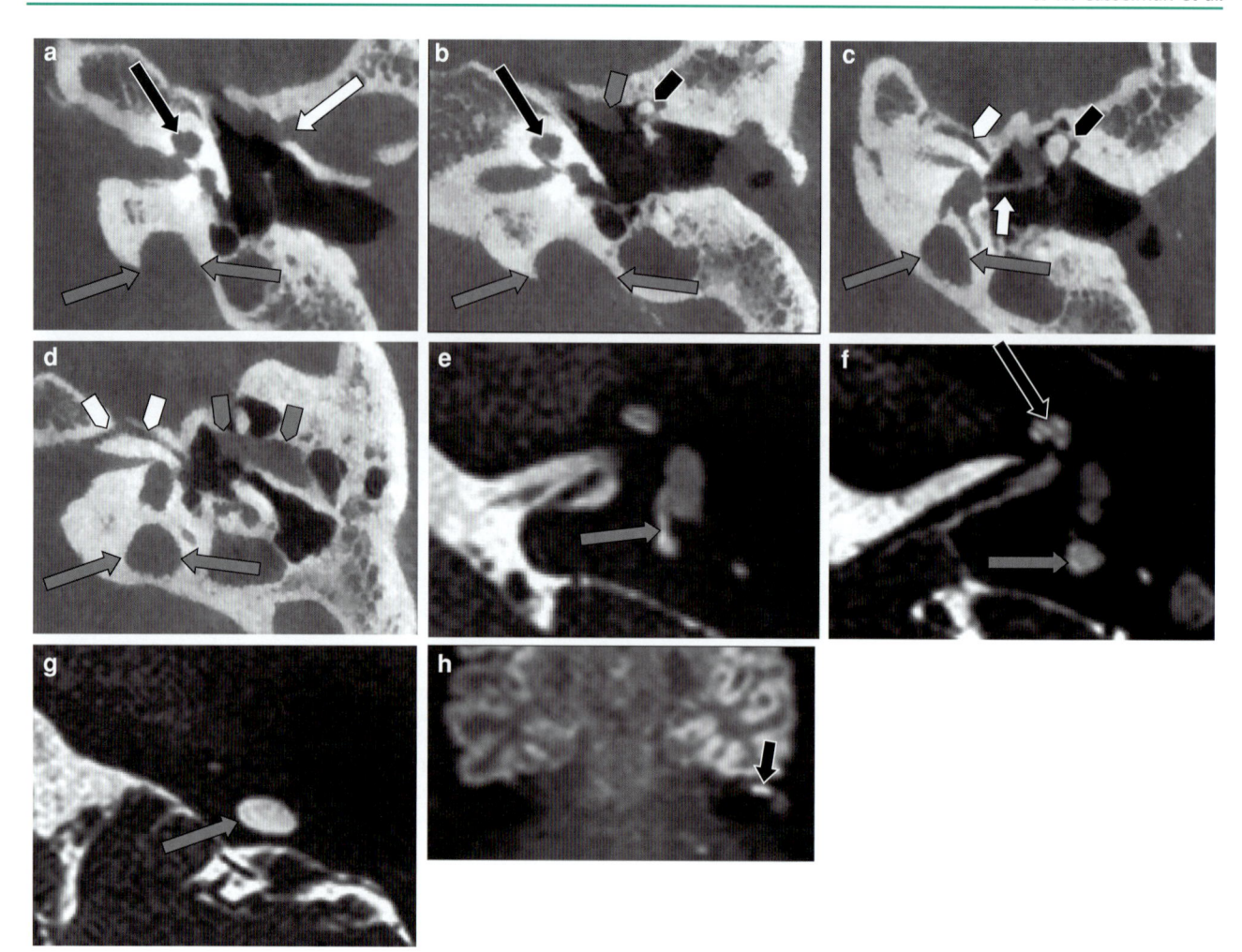

Fig. 43 Branchio-Oto-Renal syndrome—involvement of outer-middle-inner ear. **a–d** Axial CBCT images through the floor (**a**), lower part (**b**), upper part (**c**) and roof (**d**) of the left external auditory canal and middle ear. Outer ear: Foramen of Huschke or persistent foramen tympanicum (*white arrow*). This dehiscence in the anteroinferior portion of the tympanic bone can be considered as a normal variant. The anterior process of the malleus, which differentiates unlike the rest of the ossicles from the primitive tympanic ring, is fixed to the tympanic ring (*black arrowheads*). Middle ear: The malleus head and incus body are fused (*black arrowheads*) and a monopodal stapes is seen (*small white arrow*). The tensor tympani muscle is wide and has an abnormal course in the lateral part of the tympanic cavity (*grey arrowheads*). The cochleariform process is absent and the muscle never comes in contact with the promontory. Inner ear: Incomplete Partition type II malformation with confluence of the apical and second turn of the cochlea and absence of the upper part of the modiolus (*black arrows*). Large endolymphatic duct and sac (*grey arrows*). Obtuse angle between the labyrinthine and tympanic segment of the facial nerve canal (*white arrowheads*). The latter two findings should warn the surgeon for a gushing or oozing ear, known to be more frequent in patients with Incomplete Partition type II (and even more frequent in patients with IP type I). **e–g** Axial heavily T2-weighted TSE DRIVE images at the level of upper (**e**), middle (**f**) and lower (**g**) part of the labyrinth. The apical part of the modiolus and corresponding interscalar septa are absent, compatible with IP-II cochlear malformation (*black arrows*). Fluid-filled Large endolymphatic sac and duct (*grey arrows*). **h** Coronal non-EPI DWI b-1,000 image through both middle ears showing a high-signal intensity cholesteatoma (*small black arrow*) in the region of the widened tensor tympani muscle, indistinguishable from the muscle on CBCT

References

Anson B, Donaldson J (1981) Auditory ossicles of aberrant form encountered in malformation of the middle ear. In: Anson B, Donaldson J (eds) Surgical anatomy of the temoral bone. Saunders, Philadelphia, pp 398–399

Anson BJ, Davies J, Duckert LG (1991) Developmental anatomy of the ear. In: Paparella MM (ed) Otolaryngology. WB Saunders, Philadelphia, pp 3–21

Arey LB, Real RL (1974) Developmental anatomy: a textbook and laboratory manual of embryology. Saunders, Philadelphia, pp 236–238, 546–548

Bast T, Anson B (1949) The temporal bone and ear. Charles C Thomas, Springfield Illinois

Bellucci RJ (1981) Congenital aural malformations: diagnosis and treatment. Otolaryngol Clin North Am 14:95–124

Benton C, Bellet PS (2000) Imaging of congenital anomalies of the temporal bone. Neuroimaging Clin North Am 10:35–53

Brogan M, Chakeres DW, Schmalbrock P (1991) High resolution 3DFT MR imaging of the endolymphatic duct and soft tissues of the otic capsule. AJNR 12:1–11

Carey JP, Minor LB, Nager GT (2000) Dehiscence or thinning of bone overlying the superior semicircular canal in a temporal bone survey. Archives of Otolaryngology—Head and Neck 126:137–147

Casselman JW, Kuhweide R, Deimling M et al (1993a) Constructive interference in steady state-3DFT MR imaging of the inner ear and cerebellopontine angle. AJNR 14:47–57

Casselman JW, Kuhweide R, Ampe W et al (1993b) Pathology of the membranous labyrinth: comparison of T1- and T2-weighted and gadolinium-enhanced spin-echo and 3DFT-CISS imaging. AJNR 14:59–69

Casselman JW, Kuhweide R, Ampe W et al (1996) Inner ear malformations in patients with sensorineural hearing loss: MRI diagnosis. Neuroradiology 38:278–286

Casselman JW, Offeciers FE, Govaerts PJ et al (1997) Aplasia and hypoplasia of the vestibulocochlear nerve: diagnosis with MR imaging. Radiology 202:773–781

Casselman JW, Offeciers EF, de Foer B et al (2001) CT and MR imaging of congenital abnormalities of the inner ear and internal auditory Canal Eur J Radiol 40:94–104

Casselman JW, Vaid S, Zarowski A et al (2014a) Imagerie des implants cochléaires. In: Veillon F, Casselman JW, Meriot P, Cahen-Riehm S, Sick H (eds) Imagerie de l'oreille et de l'os temporal—Pediatrie. Lavoisier, Paris, pp 1377–1424

Casselman JW, Gieraerts K, Volders D et al (2014b) Cone Beam CT: non-dental applications. JBR/BTR 96:333–353

Ceruti S, Stinckens C, Cremers CWRJ et al. (2002) Temporal bone anomalies in the Branchio-Oto-Renal (BOR) syndrome: detailed CT and MRI findings Otol Neurotol 23:200-207

Clack JA (2002) Patterns and processes in the early evolution of the tetrapod ear. J Neurobiol 53:251–264

Cole RR, Jahrsdoerfer RA (1990) The risk of cholesteatoma in congenital aural atresia. Laryngoscope 100:576–578

Curtin HD, Gupta R, Bergeron RT (2011) Embryology, anatomy, and imaging of the temporal bone. In: Som P, Curtin H (eds) Head and neck imaging, 5th edn. Mosby-Year Book Inc, St. Louis, pp 1053–1096

Dahmani-Causse M, Marx M, Deguine O et al (2011) Morphologic examination of the temporal bone by cone beam computed tomography: comparison with multislice helical computed tomography. Eur Ann Otorhinolaryng Head and Neck diseases 128: 230–235

Davidson HC, Harnsberger HR, Lemmerling MM et al (1999) MR evaluation of vestibulocochlear anomalies associated with large endolymphatic duct and sac. AJNR Am J Neuroradiol 20:1435–1441

Dayal VS (1973) Embryology of the ear. Can J Otolaryngol 2:136

De Foer B et al (2010) Value of non echo-planar diffusion-weighted MR imaging versus delayed post gadolinium T1-weighted MR imaging for the detection of middle ear cholesteatoma. Radiology 255:866–872

Dubrulle F, Kohler B, Vincent C et al (2009) Two particular cases of superior semicircular canal dehiscence related to a procidence of the superior petrous sinus. J Neuroradiol 36:240–243

Evans AK, Kazahaya K (2007) Canal atresia: "surgery or implantable hearing devices? The expert's queston is revised". Int J Pediatr Otorhinolaryngol 71:367–374

Fatterpekar GM, Mukherji SK, Alley J et al (2000) Hypoplasia of the bony canal for the cochlear nerve in patients with congenital sensorineural hearing loss: initial observations. Radiology 215:243–246

Govaerts PJ, Casselman J, Daemers K et al (1999) Audiological findings in large vestibular aqueduct syndrome. Int J Pediatr Otorhinolaryngol 51:157–164

Gulya AJ (2003) Developmental anatomy of the temporal bone and skull base. In: Glasscock ME, Gulya AJ (eds) Glasscock-Shambaugh surgery of the ear, 5th edn. BC Decker, Hamilton Ont, pp 3–33

Gulya AJ (2007) Guly and Schuknecht's anatomy of the temporal bone with surgical implications. Informa Healthcare, New York

Harnsberger R (2004) Large endolymphatic sac anomaly. In: Harnsberger R (ed) Diagnostic imaging, head and neck. Amirsys, Salt Lake City, p 109

Hemond SG, Delanty FJ (1991) Formation of the cochlea in the chicken embryo: sequence of innervation and localization of basal lamina-associated molecules. Brain Res Dev Brain Res 61:87–90

Jackler R, Luxford W, House W (1987) Congenital ear malformations of the inner ear: a clarification based on embryogenesis. Laryngoscope 97:2–14

Jafek BW, Nager GT, Strife J et al (1975) Congenital aural atresia: an analysis of 311 cases. Trans Am Acad Ophthalmol Otolaryngol 98:807–812

Jahrsdoerfer RA (1981) The facial nerve in congenital middle ear malformations. Laryngoscope 91:1217–1225

Jahrsdoerfer RA (1988) Embryology of the facial nerve. Am J Otol 9:423–426

Kollias SS, Ball WS, Prenger EC, Myers CM III (1995) Dermoids of the Eustachian tube: CT and MR findings with histologic correlation. Am J Neuroradiol 16:663–668

Lagundoye SB, Martinson FD, Fajemisin AA (1975) The syndrome of enlarged vestibule and dysplasia of the lateral semicircular canal in congenital deafness. Radiology 115:377–378

Lambert PR, Dodson E (1996) Congenital malformations of the external auditory canal. Otolaryngol Clin North Am 29:741–760

Levenson MJ, Michaels L, Parisier SC (1989) Congenital cholesteatomas of the middle ear in children: origin and management. Otolaryngol Clin North Am 22:941–954

McGill TJ, Merchant S, Healy GB et al (1999) Congenital cholesteatoma of the middle ear in children: a clinical and histopathological report. Laryngoscope 1001:606–613

Minor LB, Solomon D, Zinreich J et al (1998) Sound- and/or pressure-induced vertigo due to bone dehiscence of the superior semicircular canal. Archives of Otolaryngology—Head & Neck Surgery 124:249–258

Miura M, Sando I, Thompson S (2003) Congenital anomalies of the external and middle ears. In: Bluestone CD (ed) Pediatric otolaryngology, 4th edn. Saunders, Philadelphia, pp 389–419

Mukherji SK, Tart RP, Slattery WH et al (1993) Evaluation of first branchial anomalies by CT and MR. J Comput Assist Tomogr 17:576–581

Naganawa S, Koshikawa T, Fukatsu H et al (2000) MR imaging of the enlarged endolymphatic duct and sac syndrome by use of a 3D fast asymmetric spin-echo sequence: volume and signal-intensity measurement of the endolymphatic duct and sac and area measurement of the cochlear modiolus. AJNR Am J Neuroradiol 21:1664–1669

Nager G (1993) Dysplasia of the external and middle ear. In: Nager G (ed) Pathology of the ear and temporal bone. Williams & Wilkins, Baltimore, pp 83–118

Penninger RT, Tavassolie TS, Carey JP (2011) Cone-beam volumetric tomography for applications in the temporal bone. Otol Neurotol 32:453–460

Phelps P, Coffey R, Trembath R et al (1998) Radiological malformations of the ear in Pendred syndrome. Clin Radiol 53:268–273

Phelps P, Poswillo I, Lloyd G (1981) The ear deformities in mandibulofacial dysostosis (Treacher-Collins syndrome). Clin Otolaryngol 6:15–28

Romo L, Casselman JW, Robson CD (2011) Temporal Bone: congenital anomalies. In: Som P, Curtin H (eds) Head and neck imaging. Mosby-Year Book, St. Louis, pp 1097–1165

Sando I, Shibahara Y, Takagi A et al (1988) Frequency and localization of congenital anomalies of the middle and inner ears: a human temporal bone histopathological study. Int J Pediatr Otorhinolaryngol 16:1–22

Schmalbrock P, Brogan MA, Chakeres D et al (1993) Optimization of submillimeter resolution MR imaging methods for the inner ear. J Magn Reson Imaging 3:451–459

Schmalbrock P, Pruski J, Sun L et al (1995) Phased array RF coils for high resolution MRI of the inner ear and brainstem. J Comput Assist Tomogr 19:8–14

Schuknecht HF (1989) Congenital aural atresia. Laryngoscope 99:908–917

Schuknecht HF (1993) Pathology of the ear. Lea and Febiger, Philadelphia

Sennaroglu L, Saatci I (2002) A new classification for cochleovestibular malformations. Laryngoscope 112:2230–2241

Shelton C, Luxford WM, Tonokawa LL et al (1989) The narrow internal auditory canal in children: a contraindication to cochlear implants. Otolaryngol Head Neck Surg 100:227–231

Swartz JD, Faerber EN (1985) Congenital malformations of the external and middle ear: high resolution CT findings of surgical importance. AJR 144:501–506

Swinnen F, Casselman JW, De Leenheer EMR et al (2013) Temporal bone imaging in osteogenesis imperfecta patients with hearing loss. Laryngoscope 123:1988–1995

Thompson H, Ohazama A, Sharpe PT et al (2012) The origin of the stapes and the relationship to the otic capsule and footplate. Dev Dynam 241:1396–1404

Tien RD, Felsberg GJ, Macfall J (1993) Three-dimensional MR gradient recalled echo imaging of the inner ear: comparison of FID and echo imaging techniques. Magn Reson Imaging 11:429–435

Triglia JM, Nicollas R, Ducroz V et al (1998) First branchial cleft anomalies: a study of 39 cases and a review of the literature. Arch Otolaryngol Head Neck Surgery 124:291–295

van de Water TR (1976) Effects of removal of the statoacoustic ganglion complex upon the growing otocyst. Ann Otol Rhinol Laryngol 85:2–31

Valvassori GE, Glemis JD (1978) The large vestibular aqueduct syndrome. Laryngoscope 88:723–728

Veillon F, Rock B, Cahen-Riehm S et al (2014) Malformations de l'oreille. In: Veillon F, Casselman JW, Meriot P, Cahen-Riehm S, Sick H (eds) Imagerie de l'oreille et de l'os temporal – Pediatrie. Lavoisier, Paris, pp 1175–1254

Verbist BM, Mancuso AA, Antonelli (2011) Developmental abnormalities of the external and middle ear (aural atresias) and cranial nerve VII. In: Mancuso AA, Hanafee WN (eds) Head and neck radiology. Lippincott Williams & Wilkins, Philadelphia, pp 669–689

Vercruysse JP, Casselman J, De Foer B et al (2006) Congenital bilateral oval and round window aplasia with a hypoplastic stapes. Otol Neurotol 27:441–442

Vissers LELM, van Ravenswaaij CMA, Admiraal R et al (2004) Mutations in a new member of the chromodomain gene family cause CHARGE syndrome. Nat Genet 36:955–957

Williams GH (1992) Developmental anatomy of the ear. In: English GM (ed) Otolaryngology. Lippincott, Philadelphia, pp 1–67

Work WP, Proctor CA (1963) The otologist and first branchial cleft anomalies. Ann Otol Rhinol Laryngol 72:584

Yeakly JW, Jahrsdoerfer RA (1996) CT evaluation of congenital aural atresia: what the radiologist and surgeon need to know. J Comput Assist Tomogr 20:724–731

Zeifer B, Sabini P, Sonne J (2000) Congenital absence of the oval window: radiologic diagnosis and associated anomalies. AJNR Am J Neuroradiol 9:423–426

Imaging of Cerebellopontine Angle and Internal Auditory Canal Lesions

Bert de Foer, Ken Carpentier, Anja Bernaerts, Christoph Kenis, Jan W. Casselman, and Erwin Offeciers

Contents

1 Introduction	155
2 Imaging Protocol and Imaging Anatomy	158
3 Congenital Lesions	164
3.1 Epidermoid Cysts	164
3.2 Arachnoid Cysts	170
3.3 Lipomas	170
3.4 Dermoid Cysts	171
3.5 Neurenteric Cysts	171
4 Tumoral Lesions	173
4.1 Vestibulocochlear Schwannomas	173
4.2 Meningiomas	177
4.3 Other Cranial Nerve Schwannomas	182
4.4 Metastasis	184
4.5 Brain Stem and Cerebellar Tumoral Lesions	185
5 Petrous Bone and Skull Base Lesions	186
5.1 Chordomas	186
5.2 Chondrosarcomas	189
5.3 Cholesterol Granulomata	190
5.4 Endolymphatic Sac Tumors	194
5.5 Paragangliomas	194
6 Vascular Lesions	203
6.1 Megadolichobasilaris: Basilar Artery Aneurysms	203
6.2 Vascular Loops and Neurovascular Conflicts	203
References	217

Abstract

Imaging of the cerebellopontine angle and internal auditory canal has become one of the cornerstones of modern head and neck imaging. Due to advances in imaging techniques with newer magnetic resonance (MR) sequences using thinner slice thickness and a higher resolution, the scala of detectable pathologies has increased tremendously. In this chapter, the lesions in and around the cerebellopontine angle cistern (CPA) are discussed, trying to emphasize some characteristic imaging features of most lesions. After illustrating the imaging protocol and imaging anatomy, pathological entities in this chapter will be discussed upon origin and/or location.

1 Introduction

The cerebellopontine angle cistern is a cerebrospinal fluid (CSF) filled space containing mainly nerves and vessels and some embryological remnants. It is bordered medially by the pons and brainstem, posteromedially by the anterior delineation of the cerebellar hemisphere and anterolaterally by the petrous bone apex which is covered by dura. The upper limit is formed by the 5th cranial nerve and the lower border is formed by the 9th, 10th, and 11th cranial nerve complex, also called the mixed nerves (Bonneville 2007a; Mohan et al. 2012).

Any structure in and around the CPA can give rise to lesions.

Signs and symptoms are highly aspecific and are not related to a single type of lesion itself but are mainly related to the compression of surrounding structures.

B. de Foer (✉) · K. Carpentier · A. Bernaerts · J. W. Casselman
Department of Radiology, GZA Hospitals Sint-Augustinus,
Oosterveldlaan 24, 2610 Wilrijk, Belgium
e-mail: bert.defoer@GZA.be

C. Kenis
Department of Radiology, Sint-Franciskus Hospital,
Pastoor Paquaylaan 129, 3550 Heusden-Zolder, Belgium

J. W. Casselman
Department of Radiology, AZ Sint-Jan AV Hospital,
Ruddershove 10, 8000 Brugge, Belgium

J. W. Casselman
University of Ghent, Ghent, Belgium

E. Offeciers
European Institute for ORL, GZA Hospitals Sint-Augustinus,
Oosterveldlaan 24, 2610 Wilrijk, Belgium

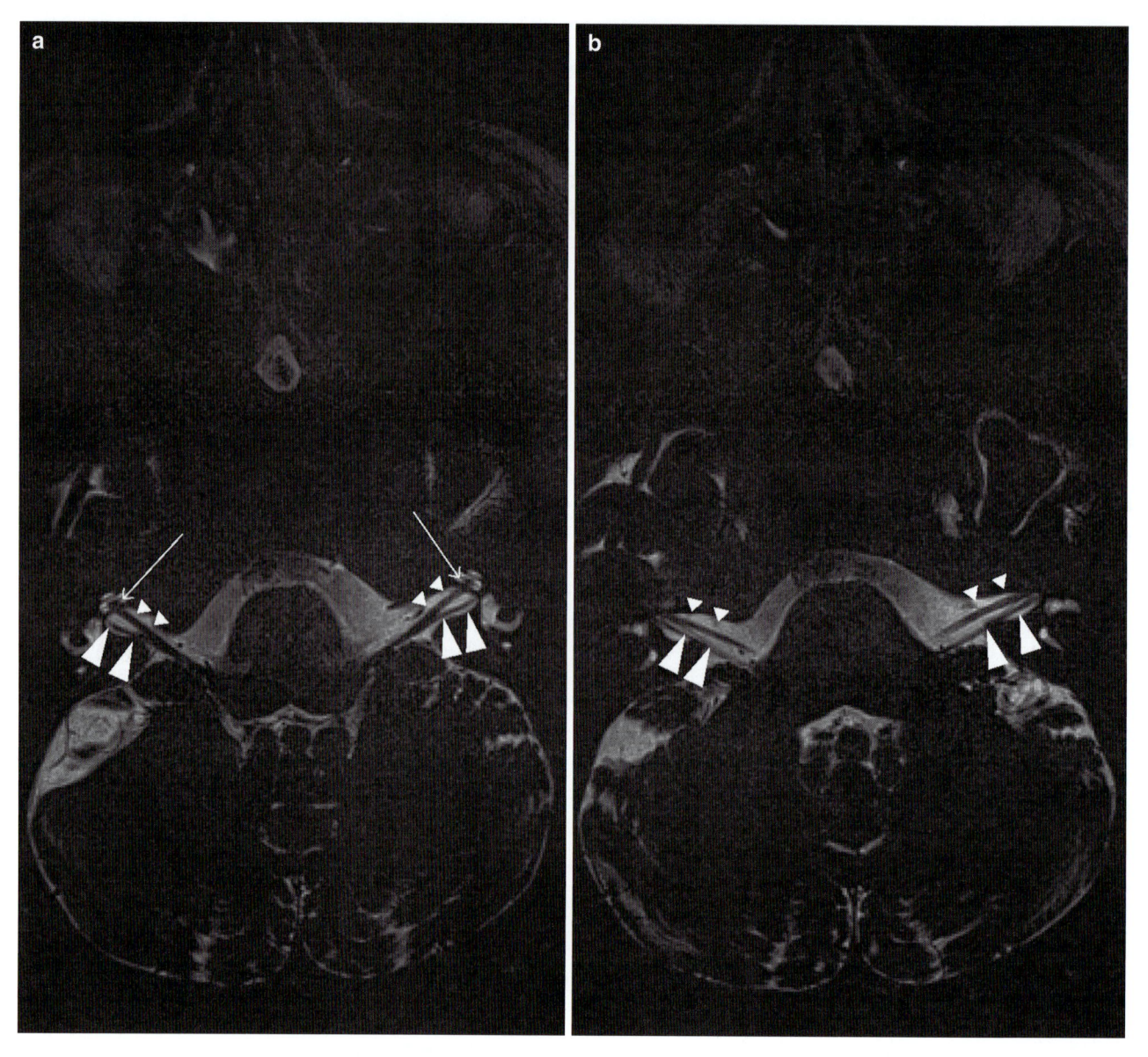

Fig. 1 16-year-old girl investigated for mixed hearing loss on both sides by CBCT and MRI. **a** Axial 0.4 mm thick 3D TSE T2-weighted image through the lower level of the IAC. On both sides a Y-shaped configuration of the nerves in the IAC can be found. The anterior division of the Y consists of the cochlear branch of the vestibulocochlear nerve (*small arrowheads*), running toward the modiolus of the cochlea (*thin arrow*). The posterior division of the Y consists of the inferior vestibular branch of the vestibulocochlear nerve (*large arrowheads*), running toward the fundus of the IAC. **b** Axial 0.4 mm thick 3D TSE T2-weighted image through the upper level of the IAC. On both sides a parallel configuration (compare to the Y-shaped configuration in figure a) of the nerves in the internal auditory can be found. The anterior nerve consists of the facial nerve (*small arrowheads*) running toward its separate canal. The posterior nerve consists of the superior vestibular branch of the vestibulocochlear nerve (*large arrowheads*) running toward the fundus of the IAC. Conclusion: Normal findings on both sides

Depending on its location, the compression of the various cranial nerves will give signs and symptoms. If located high in the CPA and around the petrous apex as such, trigeminal neuropathy may be the presenting symptom. If located and centered in or over the internal auditory canal (IAC), symptoms are mainly due to compression of the vestibulocochlear nerve causing sensorineural hearing loss (SNHL). This SNHL is in most cases gradual but in about

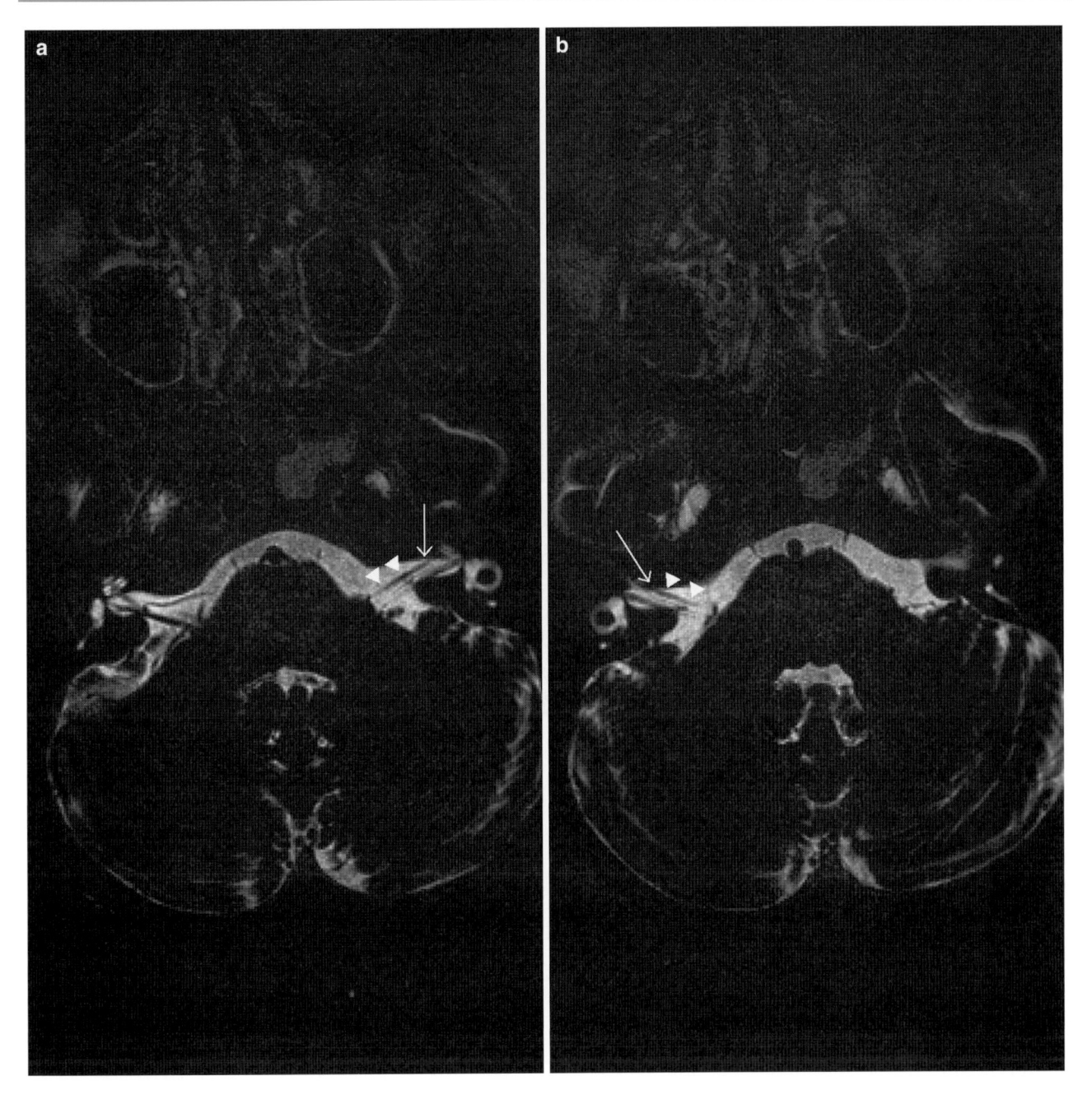

Fig. 2 54-year-old woman investigated for SNHL on the right side. Patient is in a slightly asymmetrical position. **a** Axial 0.4 mm thick 3D TSE T2-weighted image through the upper level of the IAC on the left side. Note the almost parallel configuration of the nerves in the IAC on the left side and the Y-shaped configuration of the nerves on the right side. On the left side the facial nerve (*small arrowheads*) is leaving the IAC at a more medial level (*small arrow*). This can be regarded as a normal variant. Compare to Fig. 1b. **b** Axial 0.4 mm thick 3D TSE T2-weighted image through the upper level of the IAC on the right side. Note the parallel configuration of the nerves in the IAC. The facial nerve (*small arrowheads*) is leaving the IAC at a more medial level (*small arrow*). This can be regarded as a normal variant. Compare to Fig. 1b. Conclusion: Normal variant on both sides

20 % a sudden onset of deafness is noted. Vertigo is a less frequent complaint and facial nerve palsy is rarely seen in cases of CPA lesions due to the higher resistance of the facial nerve to compression (Bonneville 2007a).

If CPA lesions become big, symptoms may be caused due to brainstem and cerebellar compression such as gait disturbance and headache due to supratentorial hydrocephalus.

The three most frequent CPA lesions are vestibulocochlear schwannomas (70–80 %), meningiomas (10–15 %), and epidermoid cysts (5 %). The remaining lesions account for less than 1 % each and are derived from a wide scale of unusual lesions (Bonneville 2007a; Mohan et al. 2012; Verbist 2012; Juliano 2013).

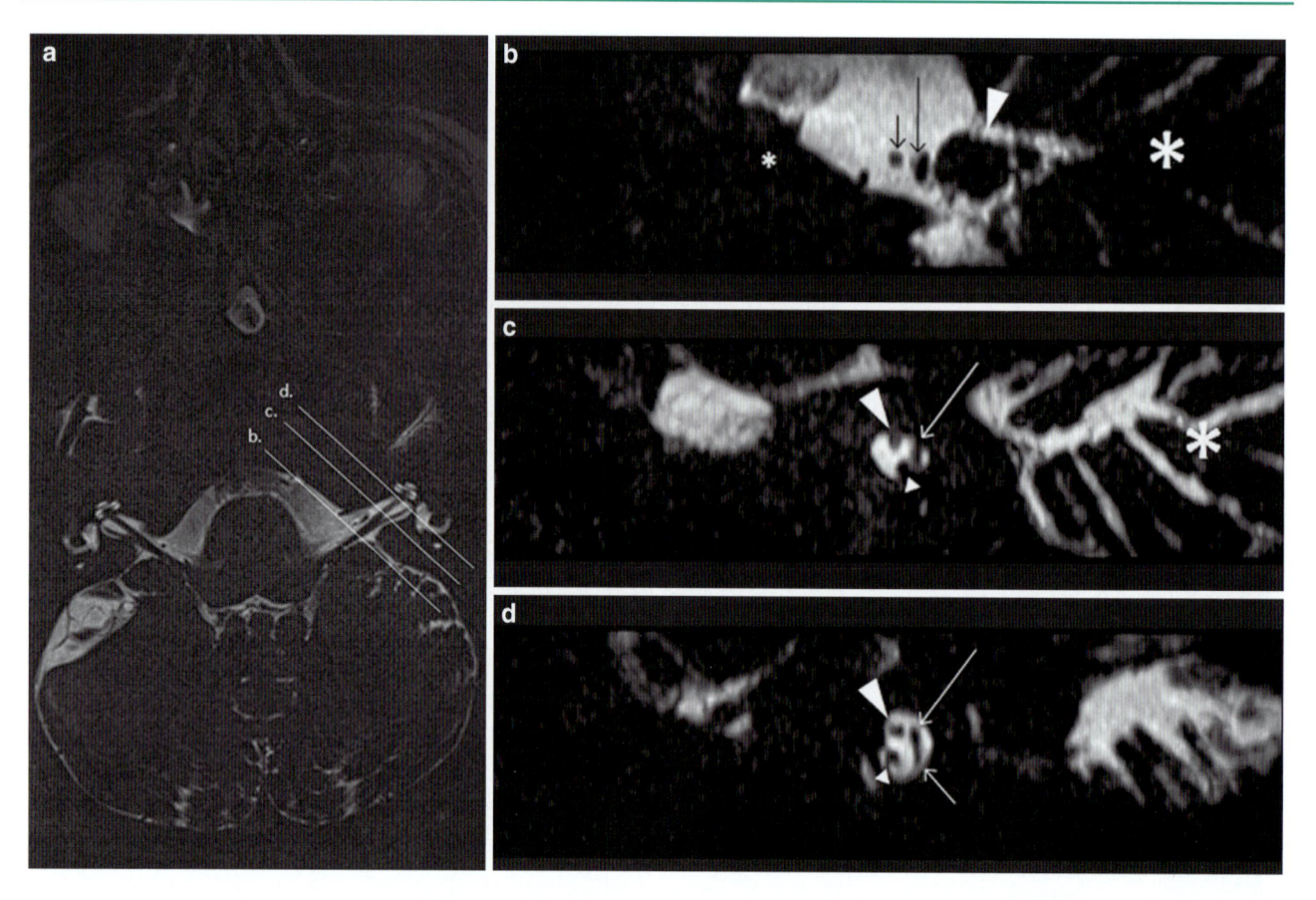

Fig. 3 24-year-old male investigated for SNHL on the left side. **a** Axial 0.4 mm thick 3D TSE T2-weighted image at the lower level of the IAC displaying the three levels of parasagittal reformation: (b) at the level of the CPA, (c) at the level of the mid IAC and (d) at level the fundus of the IAC, displaying a normal situation at the three different levels demonstrating a normal vestibulocochlear nerve and its branches. **b** Sagittal reformation at the level of the CPA. The cerebellum (*large asterisk*) is noted posterior and the brain stem is noted anterior (*small asterisk*). Three consecutive nodular structures are noted from anterior to posterior in the CPA cistern. The facial nerve is the smallest structure and is located most anterior (*small arrow*), the vestibulocochlear nerve is—in size—the intermediate structure (*large arrow*) and the largest structure located posterior is the flocculus cerebelli (*large arrowhead*). Note that the size relation between the normal vestibulocochlear nerve and the facial nerve is 2 to 1 in a normal situation. **c** Sagittal reformation at the level of the mid IAC. The cerebellum (*large asterisk*) is noted posterior. In the anterior-superior aspect of the IAC, the facial nerve is noted (*large arrowhead*). In the anterior-inferior aspect of the IAC, the cochlear branch of the vestibulocochlear nerve can be seen (*small arrowhead*). In the posterior aspect of the IAC, the vestibular nerve (*arrow*) dividing in its inferior and superior vestibular branch can be seen. **d** Sagittal reformation at the level of the fundus of the IAC. In the anterior-superior aspect of the IAC, the facial nerve can be seen (*large arrowhead*). In the anterior-inferior aspect of the IAC, the cochlear branch of the vestibulocochlear branch is running toward the modiolus (*small arrowhead*). In the posterior aspect of the IAC, the vestibular nerve is seen dividing in the inferior (*small arrow*) and the superior vestibular branch (*large arrow*). Conclusion: Normal findings on both sides

2 Imaging Protocol and Imaging Anatomy

As most patients present with SNHL, Magnetic Resonance Imaging (MRI) is the first imaging tool. Contrast-enhanced computed tomography (CT) of the posterior fossa in case of SNHL is considered no longer state-of-the-art. The only indication to perform contrast-enhanced CT of the posterior fossa is in patients with contraindication for MRI in order to exclude posterior fossa mass lesions. In all other cases, CT is reserved in a preoperative setting as an anatomical mapping and to highlight potential anatomical variants.

A standard MRI protocol for SNHL consists of three major parts (Mohan et al. 2012; Verbist 2012; Lakshmi 2009; Silk 2009).

A T2-weighted sequence or FLAIR sequence covering the entire brain is required to exclude centrally located lesions causing SNHL. A diffusion-weighted (DW) sequence is added in case an ischemic insult is suspected as cause of the hearing loss.

A small field of view (10–14 cm) submillimeter (0.4–1 mm) heavily T2-weighted sequence is performed covering the CPA, IAC, and the membranous labyrinth.

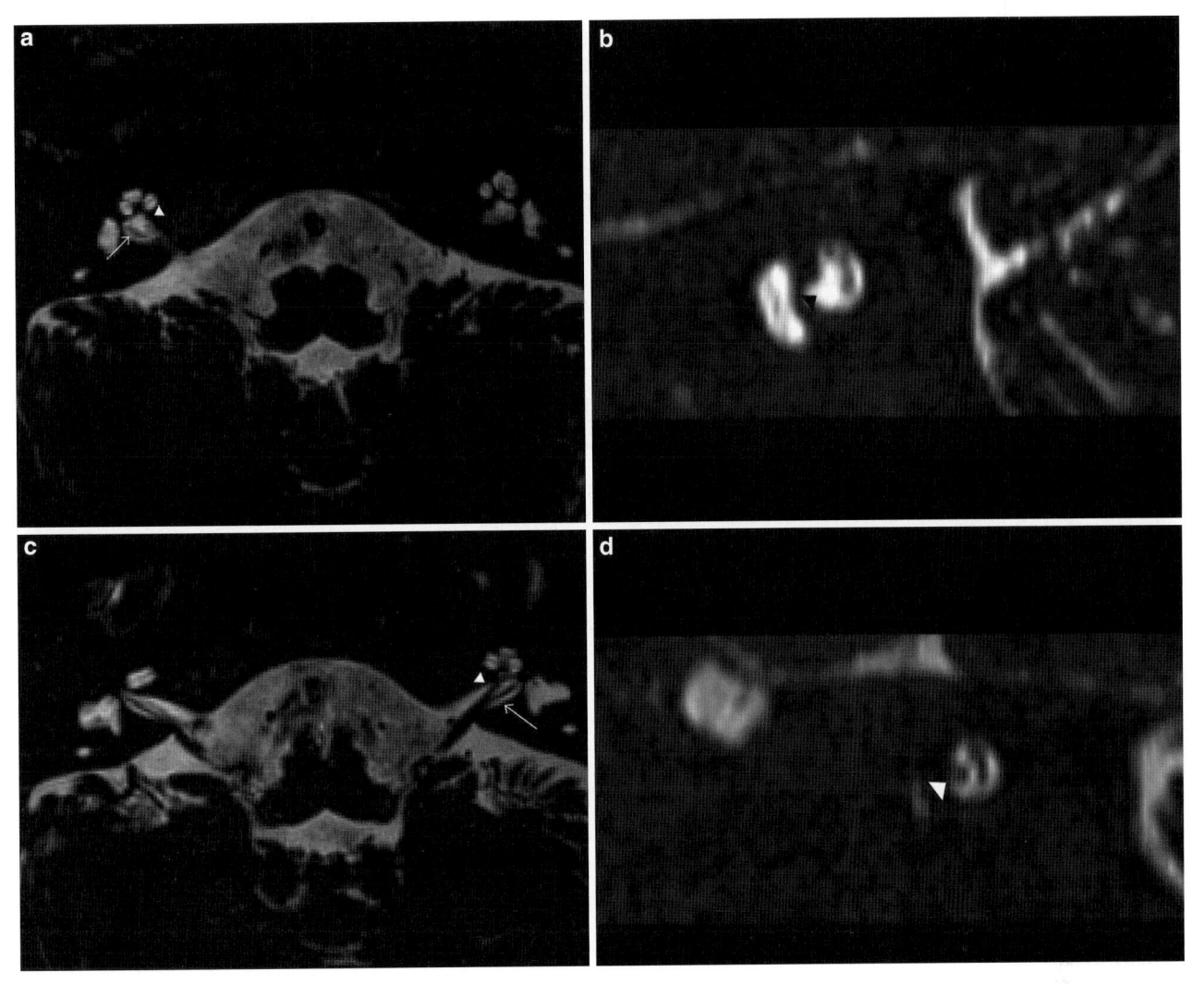

Fig. 4 6-year-old girl investigated for sensorineural deafness on the right side. Patient in a slightly asymmetrical position. **a** Axial 0.4 mm thick 3D TSE T2-weighted image at the lower level of the IAC on the right side. The inferior vestibular branch is clearly visible located posteriorly in the IAC (*arrow*). In the anterior aspect of the IAC, there is no visible cochlear branch running toward the modiolus (*arrowhead*). Compare to figure 4c. **b** Sagittal reformation at the level of the fundus of the IAC on the right side. In the fundus of the IAC, no visible cochlear branch can be seen running toward the modiolus (*arrowhead*). Compare to Fig. 4d. **c** Axial image at the lower level of the IAC on the left side. The inferior vestibular branch is clearly visible located posteriorly in the IAC (*arrow*). In the anterior aspect of the IAC, there is a clearly visible cochlear branch running toward the modiolus (*arrowhead*). Compare to Fig. 4a. **d** Sagittal reformation at the level of the fundus of the IAC on the left side. In the anterior-inferior aspect of the IAC, a cochlear branch is clearly visible running toward the modiolus (*arrowhead*). Compare to Fig. 4b. Conclusion: Agenesis of the cochlear branch on the right side

On this sequence, the delineation and volume of the nerves and different branches in the CPA and IAC needs to be evaluated.

In the upper part of the IAC, 2 parallel lines can be found in the IAC, caused by the facial nerve and the superior vestibular nerve (Fig. 1). The facial nerve is running in the anterior superior part of the IAC running toward its separate canal. As a variant, the facial nerve may leave the IAC at an earlier level (Fig. 2). The superior vestibular nerve is running in the posterior superior part of the IAC.

In the lower part of the IAC, a Y-shaped configuration can be found, caused by the divisions of the vestibulocochlear nerve. The anterior branch of the Y-shaped configuration is the cochlear nerve running toward the cochlear aperture. The posterior branch of the Y-shaped configuration is the inferior vestibular nerve (Fig. 1). Often, the ganglion of Scarpa can be seen as a small nonenhancing nodular thickening on the course of the inferior vestibular nerve in the internal auditory canal.

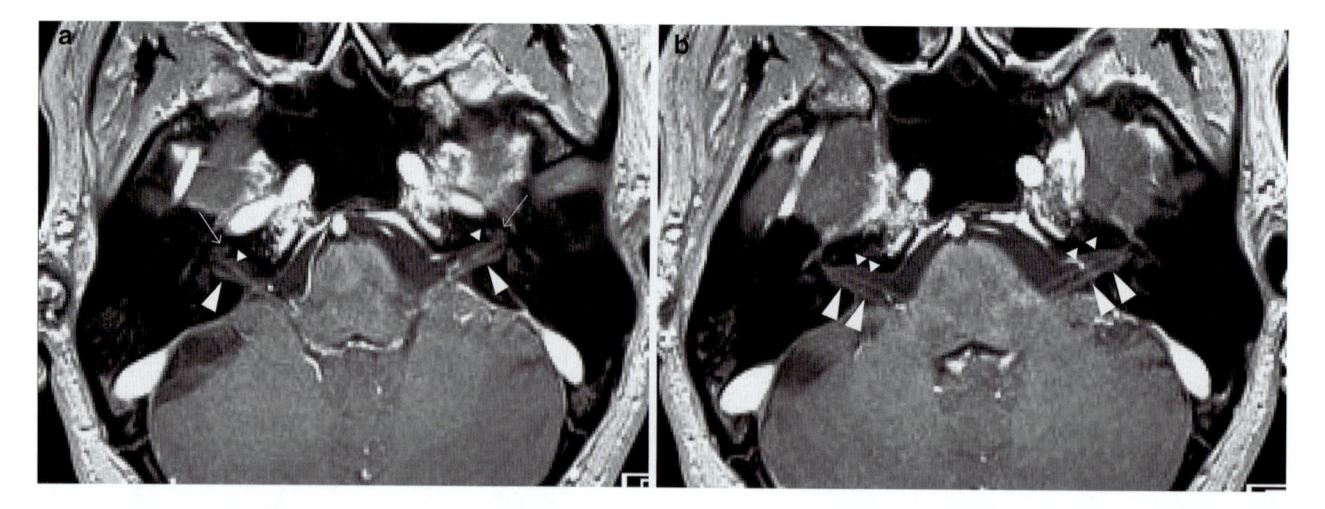

Fig. 5 45-year-old male investigated for SNHL on the left side. **a** Axial gadolinium-enhanced 0.7 mm thick 3D GRE T1-weighted image through the lower level of the IAC on both sides displays a Y-shaped configuration of the nerves in the IAC. The anterior division of the Y consists of the cochlear branch of the vestibulocochlear nerve (*small arrowheads*), running toward the modiolus of the cochlea (*thin arrow*). The posterior division of the Y consists of the inferior vestibular branch of the vestibulocochlear nerve (*large arrowheads*), running towards the fundus of the IAC. Compare to Fig. 1a. **b** Axial gadolinium-enhanced 0.7 mm thick 3D GRE T1-weighted image through the upper level of the IAC on both sides. Note the clear parallel configuration (compare to the Y-shaped configuration in figure a) of the nerves in the internal auditory on both sides. The anterior nerve consists of the facial nerve (*small arrowheads*) running toward its separate canal. The posterior nerve consists of the superior vestibular branch of the vestibulocochlear nerve (*large arrowheads*) running toward the fundus of the IAC. Compare to Fig. 1b. Conclusion: Normal findings on both sides

In case of enhancement of this small nodular structure, a small schwannoma must be considered and follow-up MRI investigations are mandatory.

It is of utmost importance to evaluate the facial nerve and the vestibulocochlear nerve and its branches in the CPA as well as in the IAC in a sagittal plane, perpendicular to the axis of the IAC (Casselman et al. 1996). In the sagittal plane, the normal volume relation of the vestibulocochlear nerve to the facial nerve is 2 to 1 meaning that the vestibulocochlear nerve is twice as thick as the facial nerve (Fig. 3). In case the vestibulocochlear nerve has the same volume as the facial nerve in the sagittal plane in the CPA, one has to evaluate all different branches of the vestibulocochlear nerve as agenesis of one of these branches will be highly likely.

In the fundus of the IAC, the facial nerve should be found in its anterosuperior position running toward its separate canal (Fig. 3). The cochlear branch will be found in its anteroinferior position (Fig. 3). The vestibular superior and inferior branches will be found posterior in the fundus with the superior vestibular nerve in the upper part of the IAC and the inferior vestibular nerve in the lower part of the IAC (Fig. 3). By evaluating the parasagittal reconstructions, one will easily detect abnormalities of one of the branches (Fig. 4) (Casselman et al. 1997; Aschenbach et al. 2005).

The different structures of the membranous labyrinth should also be evaluated in order to exclude congenital abnormalities or fibrosis as a sequel of labyrinthitis. This is however beyond the scope of this chapter and will be discussed elsewhere in this book.

Signal intensities in the membranous labyrinth should also be compared on both sides as some pathologies may cause a drop in signal intensity (see below).

Depending on the manufacturer, these heavily T2-weighted sequences are called DRIVE (Philips), FIESTA (General Electric), and 3D TSE T2 (Siemens). For the evaluation of the membranous labyrinth 3D-CISS sequences are less frequently used because of the artifacts in this sequence running through the membranous labyrinth. Due to its homogeneous peri-pontine signal intensity, the 3D-CISS sequence is much better suited to evaluate the pre- and peri-pontine cisterns.

In most cases, parallel imaging techniques are used: SENSE (Philips), ASSET (General Electric), and GRAPPA (Siemens).

For T1-weighted imaging either a submillimeter (0.7–1 mm) 3D gradient-echo (GRE) T1-weighted sequence can be performed or separate coronal and axial thin slice (2 mm at maximum) spin echo (SE) T1-weighted sequences can be scanned. Images should be acquired without and with gadolinium.

On these images the same configuration—Y-shaped and parallel lines—can be found in the IAC (Fig. 5).

Discussion still exists whether or not gadolinium should be administered. Some groups advocate evaluation of the heavily T2-weighted sequences alone in order to evaluate

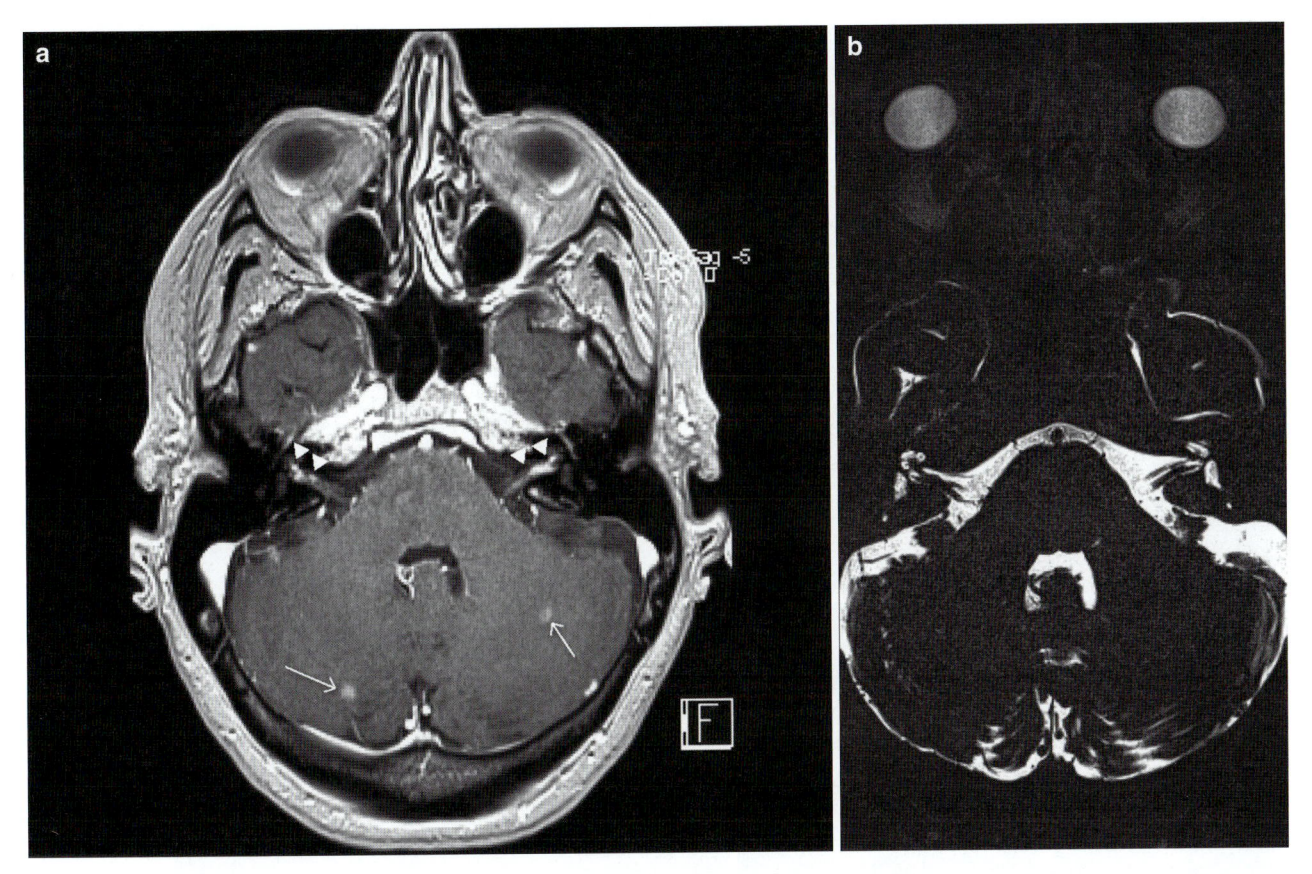

Fig. 6 42-year-old female with sudden onset of sensorineural hearing loss on both sides. Prior history of breast carcinoma. **a** Axial gadolinium-enhanced 0.7 mm thick 3D GRE T1-weighted image through the posterior fossa at the level of the IAC. There is diffuse enhancement of the IAC on both sides, more pronounced on the left side than on the right side (*arrowheads*). Discrimination of the different nerve structures in the IAC is no longer possible (compare to Fig. 5a and b). Note that there are two nodular enhancing lesions in both cerebellar hemispheres (*arrows*). **b** Axial 0.4 mm thick 3D TSE T2-weighted image through the posterior fossa at the level of the IAC. Note that the nerve structures are still discernable in the IAC on both sides (compare to Fig. 6a). No clear abnormalities can be found. Conclusion: Metastatic disease from prior breast carcinoma with parenchymal metastatic deposits in both cerebellar hemispheres and meningeal metastatic involvement in both IACs. If this patient would have been evaluated by heavily T2-weighted sequences alone, pathology would have been missed

the nerve and membranous labyrinth either looking for nodular thickening of the nerves or a zone of signal drop in the membranous labyrinth to demonstrate tumors of the vestibulocochlear nerve or intralabyrinthine schwannomas. It is, however, generally accepted that several entities can be missed using heavily T2-weighted sequences alone (Goebell et al. 2005). The enhancement in the acute phase of labyrinthitis for example can be missed. Enhancing foci of otospongiosis around the membranous labyrinth will also be missed. Metastatic lesion in the IAC may present without any changes on heavily T2-weighted images and can be missed as well, if gadolinium is not administered (Fig. 6). Very small intracanalicular schwannomas can also be missed (Jackler 1996). Also, volume measurements of vestibulocochlear schwannomas are measured more accurately on gadolinium-enhanced 3D GRE T1-weighted sequences than on heavily 3D T2-weighted sequences (Van de Langenberg et al. 2009).

In the future, there may be a growing role for 3D-FLAIR sequences. 3D-FLAIR sequences carry a higher sensitivity for subtle compositional changes in lymph fluid of the inner ear, demonstrating a possible spontaneous higher intensity on unenhanced images in the IAC and membranous labyrinth. These subtle changes may be encountered in cases of labyrinthitis or intralabyrinthine hemorrhage.

Also, increased signal intensity of the diseased inner ear can be observed on these sequences after gadolinium administration. These findings have been reported in many different pathologies, such as sudden SNHL, cholesteatoma with fistulisation, cochlear otospongiosis and vestibular schwannoma (Yamazaki et al. 2009, 2010).

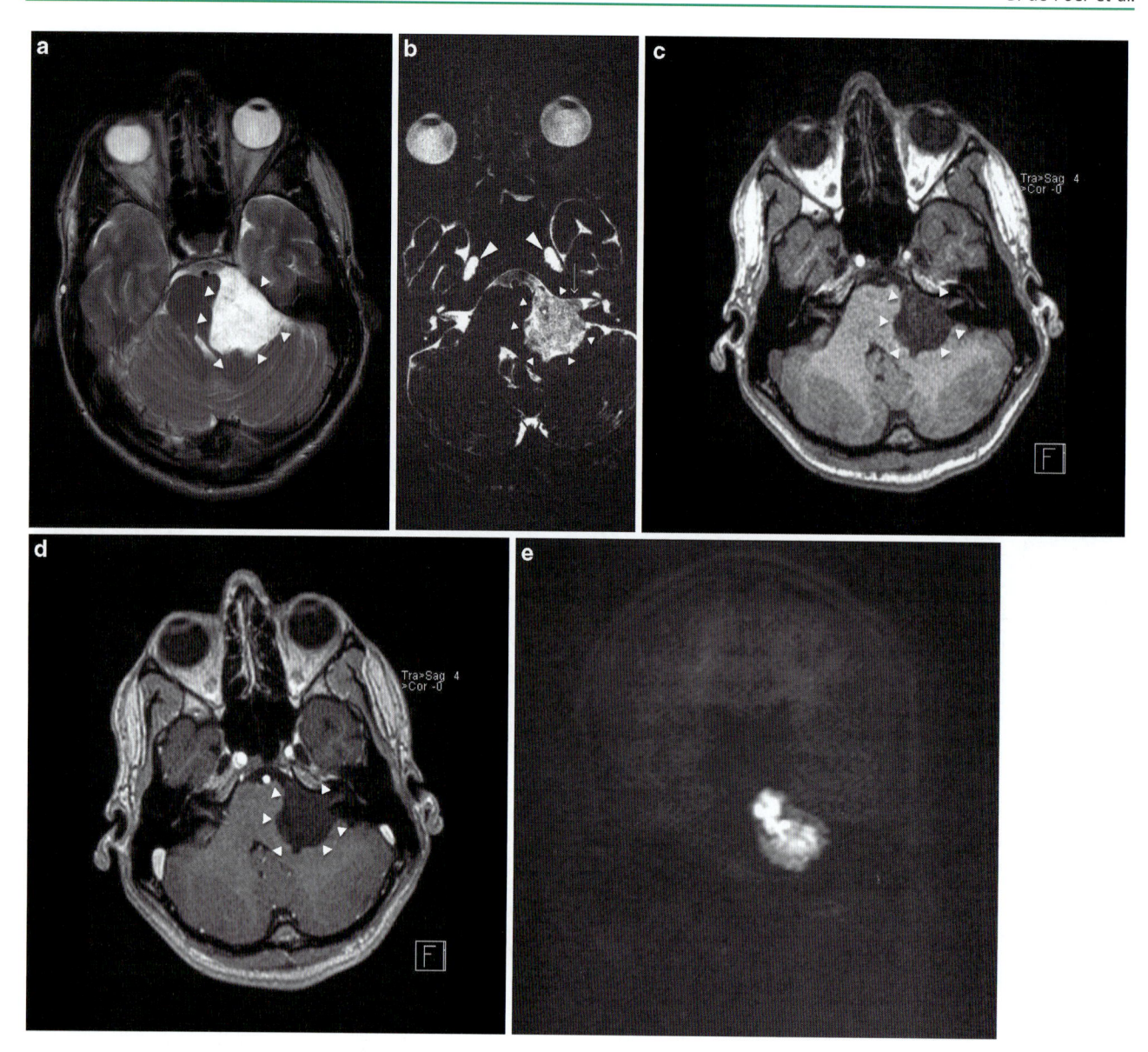

Fig. 7 20-year-old male investigated for headache. A CT scan (not shown) of the brain demonstrated a cystic lesion in the left CPA. MRI was performed for further differentiation. **a** Axial 4 mm thick TSE T2-weighted image of the brain. There is a large hyperintense lesion (*arrowheads*) in the left CPA compressing the brain stem and middle cerebellar peduncle. Note that the lesion has a slightly inhomogeneous aspect compared to the fluid signal of the globe. **b** Axial 0.7 mm thick 3D TSE T2-weighted image at the level of the IAC demonstrating a mixed hyperintense/hypointense lesion (*small arrowheads*) in the left CPA with clear extension in the left IAC (*arrow*). Note that the lesion shows a clearly inhomogeneous signal intensity compared to the fluid signal in both Meckel's cave (*large arrowheads*). **c** Axial unenhanced 2 mm thick SE T1-weighted image through the posterior fossa at the level of the IAC. There is a slightly inhomogeneous hypointense mass lesion (*arrowheads*) in the left CPA, extending in the left IAC. Note again that the lesion has a slightly inhomogeneous aspect compared to the fluid signal of the globe. **d** Axial gadolinium-enhanced 2 mm thick SE T1-weighted image through the posterior fossa at the level of the IAC (same level as Fig. 7c). The lesion shows no clear enhancement (*arrowheads*). **e** Coronal 2 mm non-EP DW *b*1000 image (HASTE diffusion) clearly demonstrating the homogeneous hyperintense aspect of the lesion. Conclusion: The pseudo-cystic aspect of the lesion on standard sequences with the characteristic hyperintense aspect on *b*1000 non-EP DW sequence is highly typical for an epidermoid

3D-FLAIR imaging 24 h after intratympanic gadolinium injection has been reported to be able to visualize perilymphatic and endolymphatic fluid separately. Recently, 3D-FLAIR sequences performed 4 h after IV gadolinium injection also has been reported to visualize perilymphatic and endolymphatic fluid separately, enabling the visualization of endolymphatic hydrops in Menière patients (Yamazaki et al. 2012; Barath et al. 2014), but this is also beyond the scope of this chapter and will be discussed elsewhere in this book.

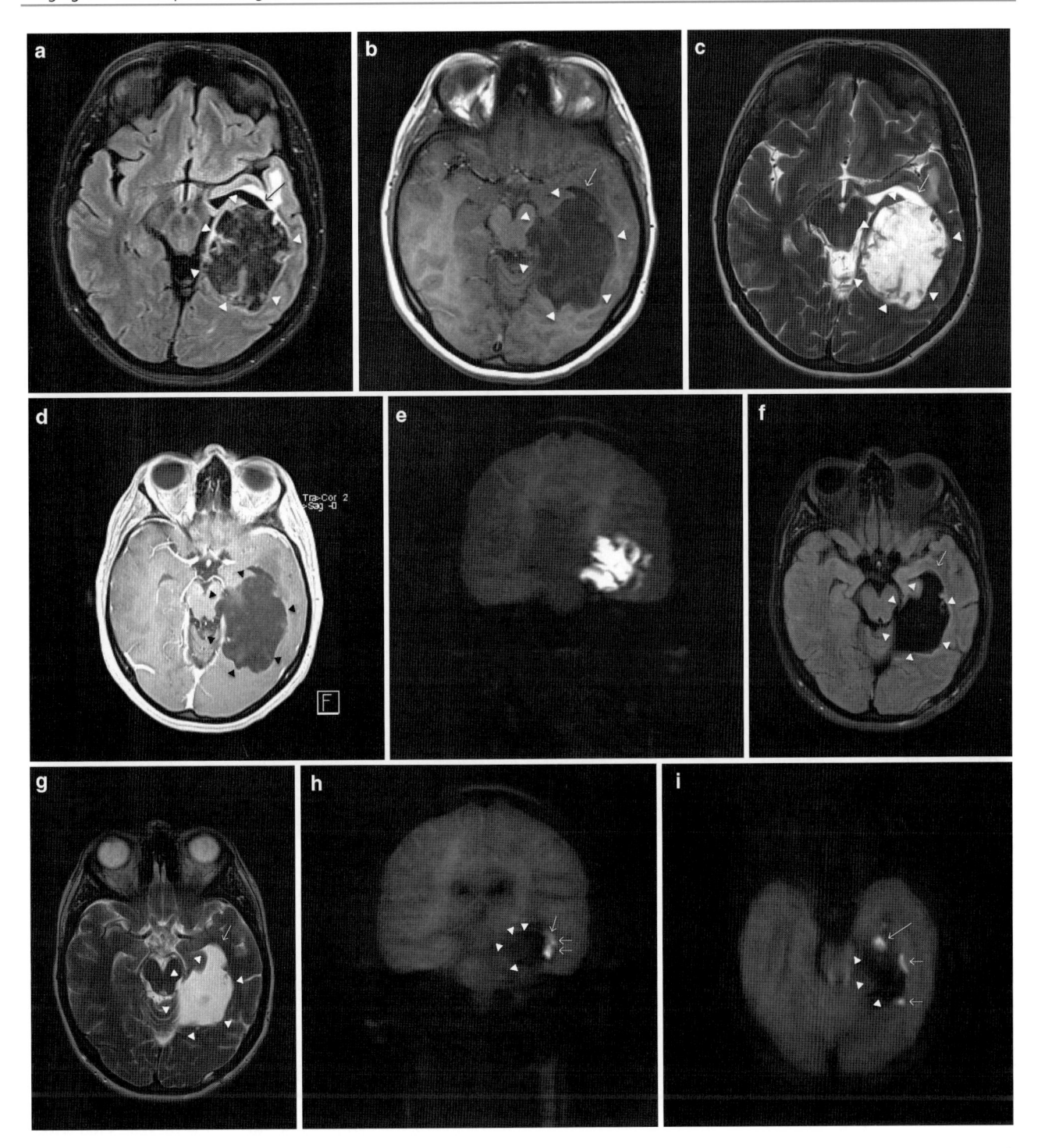

Fig. 8 34-year-old female admitted to hospital with grand mal epilepsy at the emergency department. CT scan (not shown) demonstrated a left-sided deep temporal located hypodensity. MRI was performed for further differentiation. **a** Axial 4 mm thick FLAIR image of the brain demonstrates an inhomogeneous moderately hypointense lesion deep in the left temporal lobe (*arrowheads*), located posterior to the left temporal horn (*small arrow*). Note the slightly higher intensity of the lesion compared to the low intensity of the CSF in the temporal horn. **b** Axial unenhanced 4 mm thick SE T1-weighted image (same level as figure a) demonstrates the moderately hypointense lesion deep in the left temporal lobe (*arrowheads*), located posterior to the left temporal horn (*small arrow*). Note again the slightly higher intensity of the lesion compared to the CSF in the temporal horn. **c** Axial 4 mm thick TSE T2-weighted image (same level as a and b) demonstrates the lesion as a slightly inhomogeneous hyperintense lesion deep in the left temporal lobe (*arrowheads*), located posterior to the left temporal horn (*small arrow*). Compare to the homogeneous signal of the CSF in the left temporal horn. **d** Axial 4 mm thick gadolinium-enhanced SE T1-weighted image (same level as a, b, and c). The lesion demonstrates no contrast enhancement (*arrowheads*). **e** Coronal 2 mm thick *b*1000 HASTE DW image. The lesion has a very high signal intensity. The high signal intensity of the

lesion is nearly pathognomonic for an epidermoid, located in a supratentorial position. **f** Postoperative axial 4 mm thick FLAIR image (same level as a, b, c, and d). The resection cavity (*arrowheads*) displays a homogeneous low signal intensity, comparable to the signal intensity of the left temporal horn (*small arrow*). Compare to the inhomogeneous signal intensity of the lesion prior to surgery in figure a. **g** Postoperative axial 4 mm thick TSE T2-weighted image (same level as a, b, c, d and f) also displaying a homogeneous high signal intensity (*arrowheads*) comparable to the signal intensity of the left temporal horn (*small arrow*). Compare to the inhomogeneous signal intensity of the lesion prior to surgery in figure c. **h** Postoperative coronal 2 mm thick *b*1000 HASTE DW image (same level as e). The resection cavity (*arrowheads*) has a homogeneous low signal intensity. On this sequence, the residual epidermoid is nicely visible as small high signal intensity nodular lesions lateral in the resection cavity (*small arrows*). **i** Postoperative axial 2 mm thick *b*1000 HASTE DW image (same level as a to d). The resection cavity (*arrowheads*) has a homogeneous low signal intensity. Again, the residual epidermoid is nicely visible as small high signal intensity nodular lesions lateral in the resection cavity (*small arrows*) Conclusion: Large epidermoid in a rather unusual supratentorial location. Note the value of the *b* 1000 HASTE sequence in diagnosing the lesion and its strength in detecting residual lesions after surgery

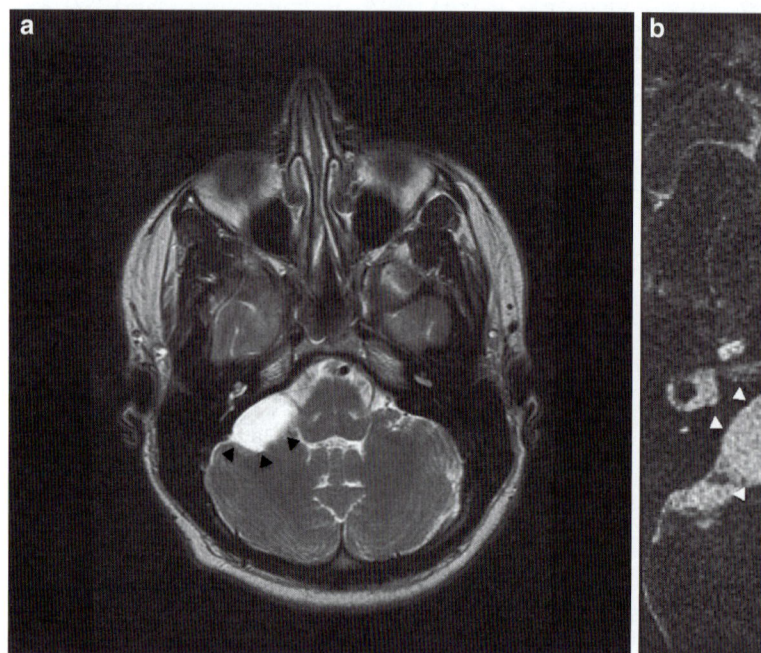

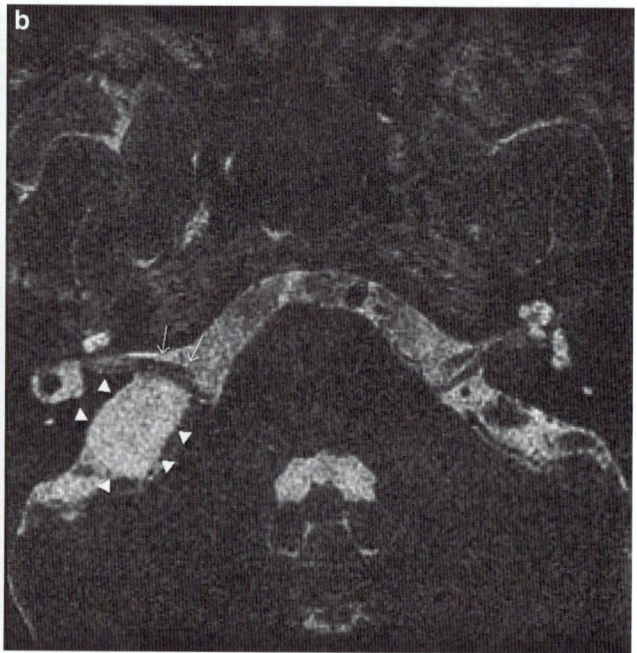

Fig. 9 22-year-old male investigated for SNHL on the left side. **a** Axial 4 mm thick FSE T2-weighted image of the brain through the posterior fossa. Note the presence of a large oval hyperintense lesion in the right CPA. Note the slight impression on the right cerebellar hemisphere (*arrowheads*). **b** Axial 0.7 mm thick FSE T2-weighted image through the posterior fossa demonstrating the homogeneous hyperintense lesion in the right CPA (*arrowheads*), located posterior to the right vestibulocochlear nerve with slight anterior displacement of the nerve (*arrows*). Conclusion: Arachnoid cyst in the right CPA with slight anterior displacement of the nerve. Note that the clinical symptoms of the patient are located on the left side

3 Congenital Lesions

3.1 Epidermoid Cysts

Epidermoid cysts or epidermoid tumors are part of the scala of pathologies such as epidermoid lesions and congenital cholesteatoma. This lesion is not a tumor as such but it should rather be regarded as a congenital lesion caused by inclusion of ectoderm—the later skin—into the skull. If the ectoderm gets entrapped intradurally in the skull, the lesion is called an epidermoid tumor. If the ectoderm gets entrapped extradurally, in the temporal bone, the lesion is called a congenital cholesteatoma. Histologically the lesions are exactly the same, consisting of included skin. Symptoms arise when the skin starts to exfoliate and the lesion enlarges with compression of the surrounding structures. The epidermoid contains keratin and it is that keratin as such which is responsible for the high signal intensity of the lesion on diffusion-weighted MRI.

Epidermoid cysts are the third most frequent lesions in the CPA, after vestibulocochlear schwannoma and meningioma (Bonneville et al. 2007a; Verbist 2012; Holman et al. 2013).

Epidermoid cysts are most frequently found in the CPA (Fig. 7) but can extend in the IAC or toward Meckel's cave. The lesion can be quite large and compress surrounding

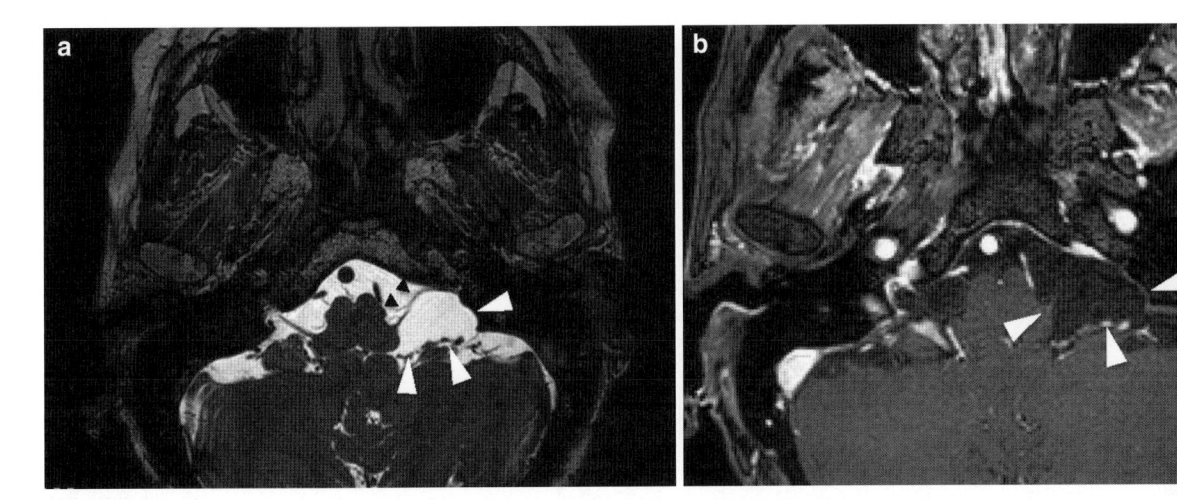

Fig. 10 54-year-old male with swallowing difficulties. **a** Axial 0.8 mm thick FSE T2-weighted image through the posterior fossa demonstrating the homogeneous hyperintense lesion in the lower left CPA (*large arrowheads*). The lesion is stretching the 9th, 10th, and 11th nerve complex anteriorly (*small arrowheads*). **b** Axial gadolinium-enhanced 1.2 mm thick GRE T1-weighted image through the posterior fossa (same level as Fig. 10a). The lesion (*large arrowheads*) is demonstrating a homogeneous CSF-like intensity and displays no contrast enhancement. Conclusion: Arachnoid cyst in the lower left CPA with anterior displacement of the nerves. Decompressive surgery resolved the patient's symptoms

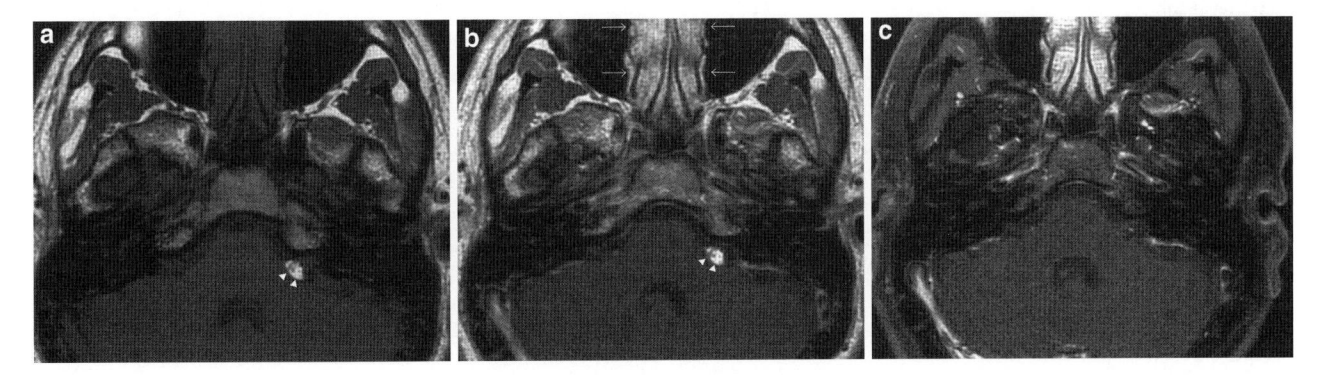

Fig. 11 17-year-old male investigated for headache. **a** Axial unenhanced 2 mm thick SE T1-weighted image through the posterior fossa at the level of the base of the IAC. Note the small nodular spontaneous hyperintense lesion in the left CPA (*small arrowheads*). **b** Axial gadolinium-enhanced 2 mm thick SE T1-weighted image through the posterior fossa (same level as a). The lesion demonstrates a persistent high signal intensity (*small arrowheads*). Note the clear enhancement of the nasal mucosa (*arrows*). **c** Axial gadolinium-enhanced 2 mm thick SE fat saturated T1-weighted image through the posterior fossa (same level as a and b). The lesion has apparently disappeared. Conclusion: Small spontaneous hyperintense lesion in the left CPA compatible with a small CPA lipoma. Note the linear hypointense structures running through the lesion, compatible with nerves, veins and arteries. The fact that the lesion apparently disappears on fat saturated T1-weighted lesions confirms the fact that the lesion is a lipoma. These lesions should be considered as leave-me-alone lesions as performing surgery on these patients will cause more harm due to the fact that nerves, veins, and arteries are running through these lesions

structures before even causing symptoms. Supratentorial extension may exist and epidermoid cysts can even occur in a completely supratentorial position (Fig. 8).

On MR imaging, the lesion demonstrates as a CSF-like signal intensity on standard T1- and T2-weighted images making differential diagnosis with an arachnoidal cyst sometimes difficult. Both the arachnoid cyst and epidermoid tumor display high signal intensity on standard T2-weighted sequences and a low signal intensity on T1-weighted images without any enhancement on gadolinium-enhanced T1-weighted images. However, signal intensities differ significantly on various other sequences making differential diagnosis with an arachnoidal cyst possible. On FLAIR sequences, signal intensities of an epidermoid cyst are mixed, compared to the homogeneous low signal intensity of CSF. Also on heavily T2-weighted sequences, signal intensities of an epidermoid cyst are mixed with a predominant component of low signal intensities compared to the homogeneous high signal intensity of CSF on heavily T2-weighted sequences (Bonneville et al. 2007a; Mohan et al. 2012; Verbist 2012). Apart from this, the major advantage of submillimeter heavily T2-weighted sequences is that the exact extension of the epidermoid cyst can be done on these sequences (Figs. 7 and 8).

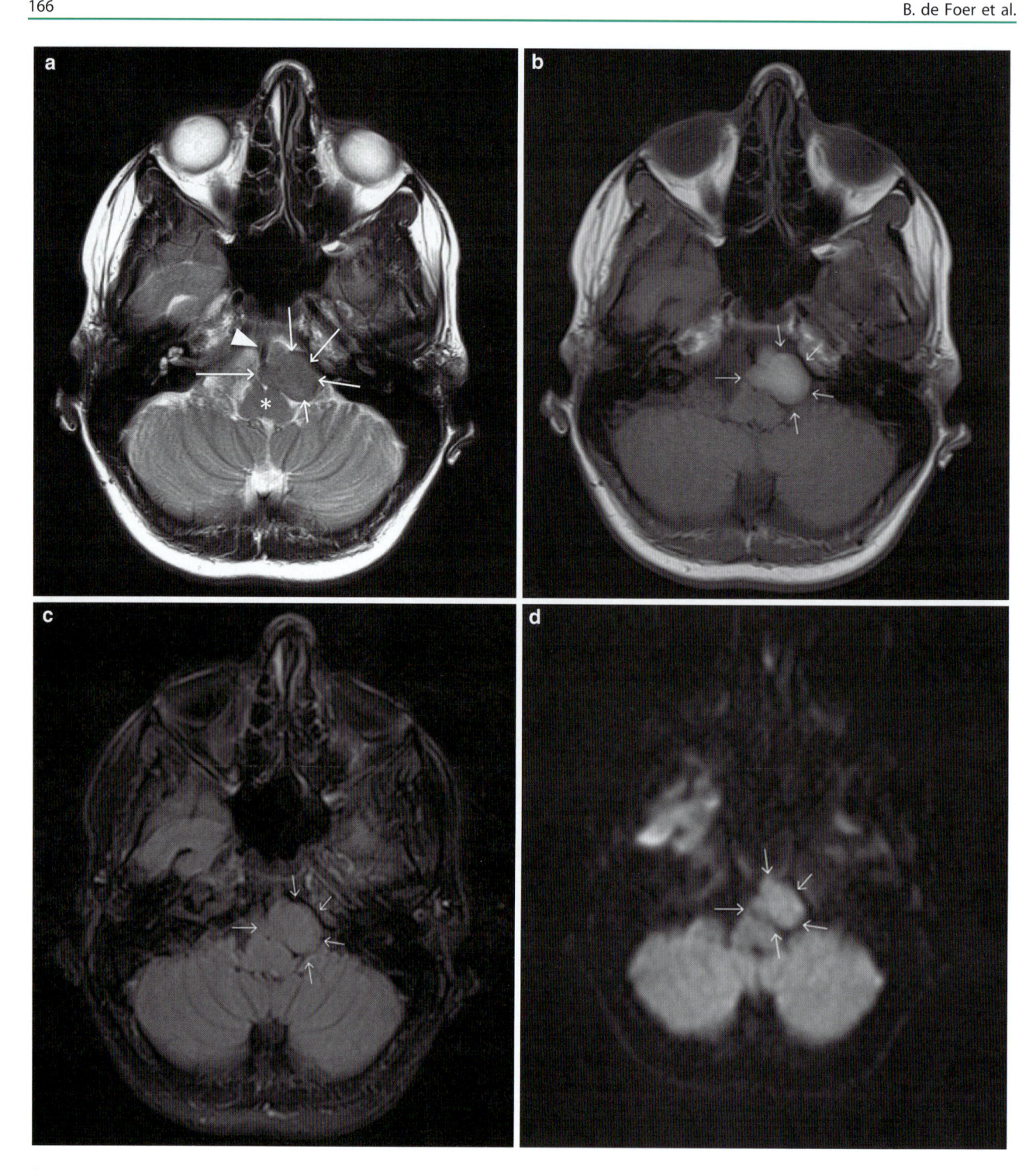

Fig. 12 23-year-old female investigated for quadrant anopsia at the left eye. **a** Axial 4 mm thick TSE T2-weighted image through the lower CPA demonstrating homogeneous rather low intense sharply delineated mass lesion in the lower left-sided CPA (*arrows*). The lesion is abutting the medulla oblongata (*asterisk*) and is slightly displacing the basilar artery (*arrowhead*). Note that the lesion is almost isointense to the medulla oblongata. **b** Axial unenhanced 4 mm thick SE T1-weighted image (same level as Fig. 12a). The lesion displays a homogeneous high signal intensity (*arrows*). There was no visible enhancement (not shown). **c** Axial 4 mm thick FLAIR image (same level as Fig. 12a and b). The lesion displays no fluid signal intensity (*arrows*). Signal intensity is comparable to the signal intensity of the brainstem. **d** Axial 4 mm thick *b*1000 EP DW image (same level as Fig. 12a, b and c). The lesion displays no frank hyperintensity (*arrows*). Conclusion: Location and signal intensity is compatible with a neurenteric cyst. Surgery and pathology confirmed the diagnosis of a neurenteric cyst (*Courtesy* Prof. P. M. Parizel, Prof. J. Van Goethem, Antwerp, Belgium)

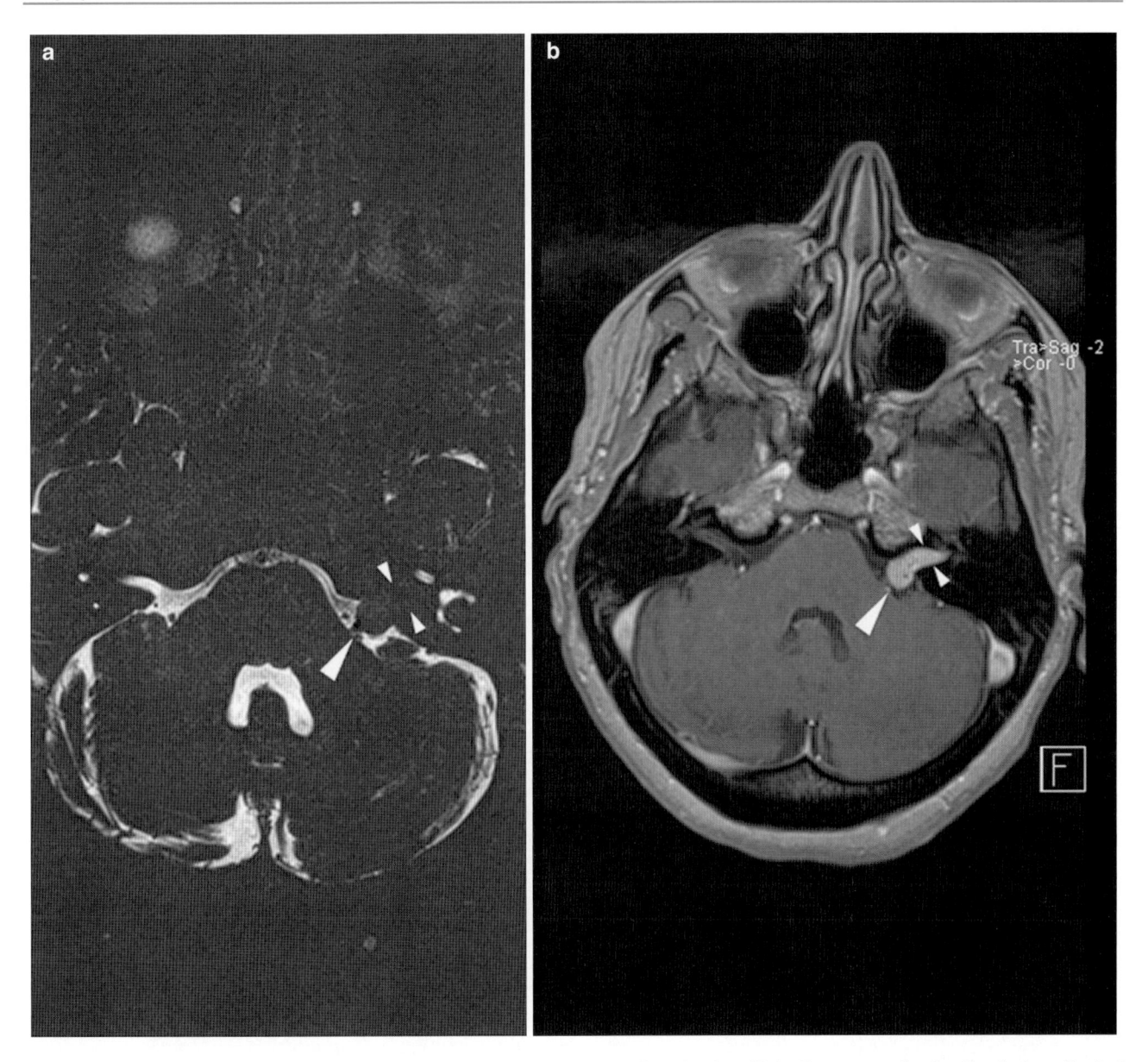

Fig. 13 46-year-old female investigated for SNHL on the left side. **a** Axial 0.4 mm thick 3D TSE T2-weighted image through the posterior fossa. Mass lesion displacing the normal hyperintense fluid signal in the IAC (*small arrowheads*) with a small component protruding in the left CPA (*large arrowhead*). **b** Axial gadolinium-enhanced 0.7 mm thick GRE T1-weighted image (same level as Fig. 13a). The mass lesion displays a homogeneous enhancement and has a component in the IAC (*small arrowheads*) and a component protruding in the CPA (*large arrowhead*). Conclusion: Typical appearance of a vestibulocochlear schwannoma with a component in the IAC and a component in the CPA (*ice cream cone appearance*). There is no residual fluid in the IAC, which can be regarded as a negative predictive sign for hearing preservation surgery. The signal intensity in the membranous labyrinth is normal: this can, however, be regarded as a positive predictive sign for hearing preservation surgery

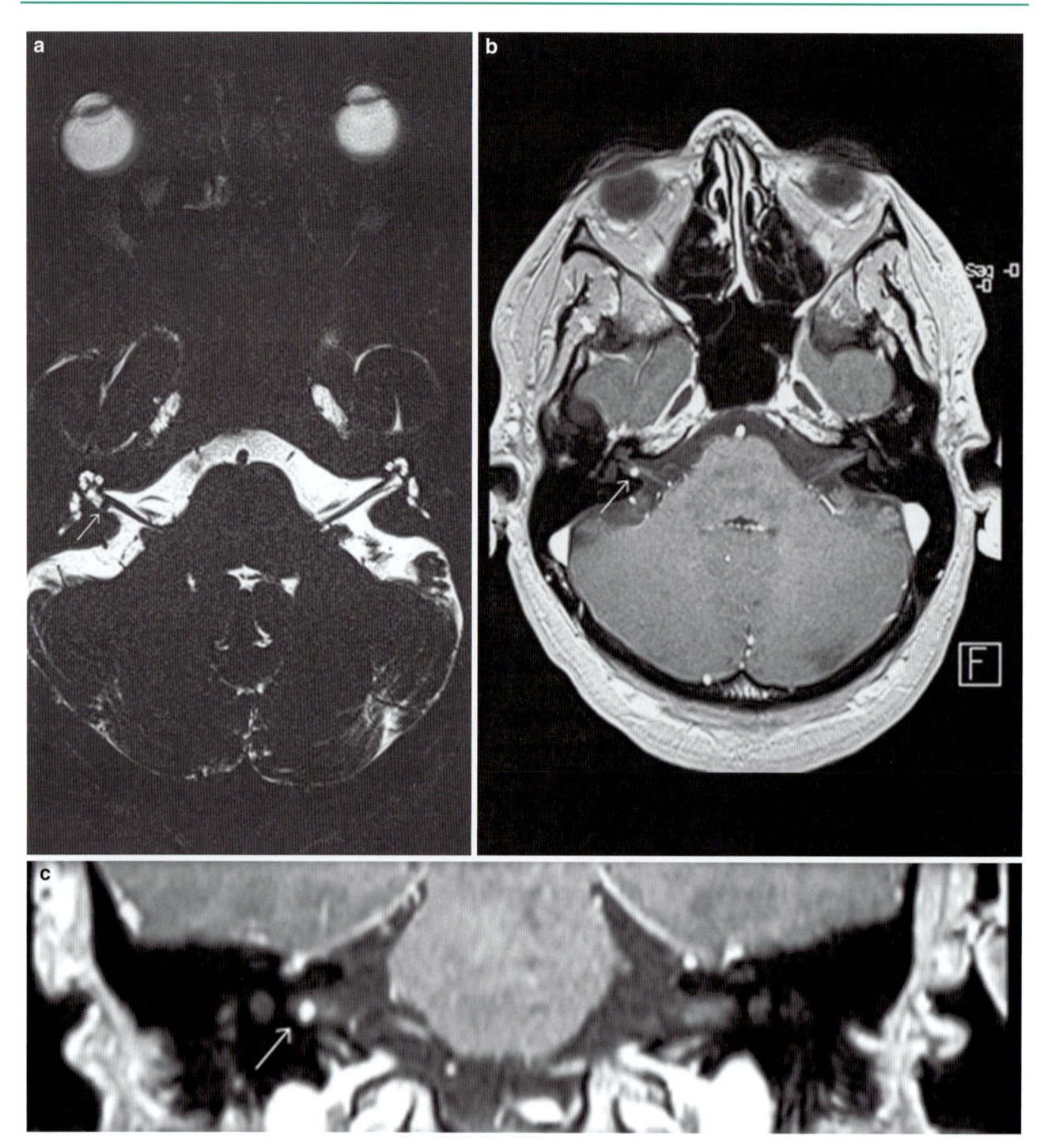

Fig. 14 44-year-old female investigated for SNHL on the right side. Patient also complained of tinnitus. **a** Axial 0.4 mm thick 3D TSE T2-weighted image through the posterior fossa. On the left side, the normal Y-shaped appearance of the dividing vestibulocochlear nerve in its cochlear branch and in its vestibular inferior branch is clearly seen. On the right side, a very small hypointense nodule can be noted posteriorly in the IAC (*arrow*) behind the cochlear nerve. **b** Axial gadolinium-enhanced 0.7 mm thick 3D GRE T1-weighted image (same level as Fig. 14a) displaying the lesion as a small strongly enhancing nodule posterior in the right IAC (*arrow*). **c** Coronal gadolinium-enhanced 1 mm thick multiplanar reformation (MPR) of a 3D GRE T1-weighted data set showing the lesion as a small nodule low in the right IAC (*arrow*). Conclusion: Small intra-canalicular vestibulocochlear schwannoma in the right IAC located on the inferior vestibular nerve. A wait-and-scan approach in this patient was advocated

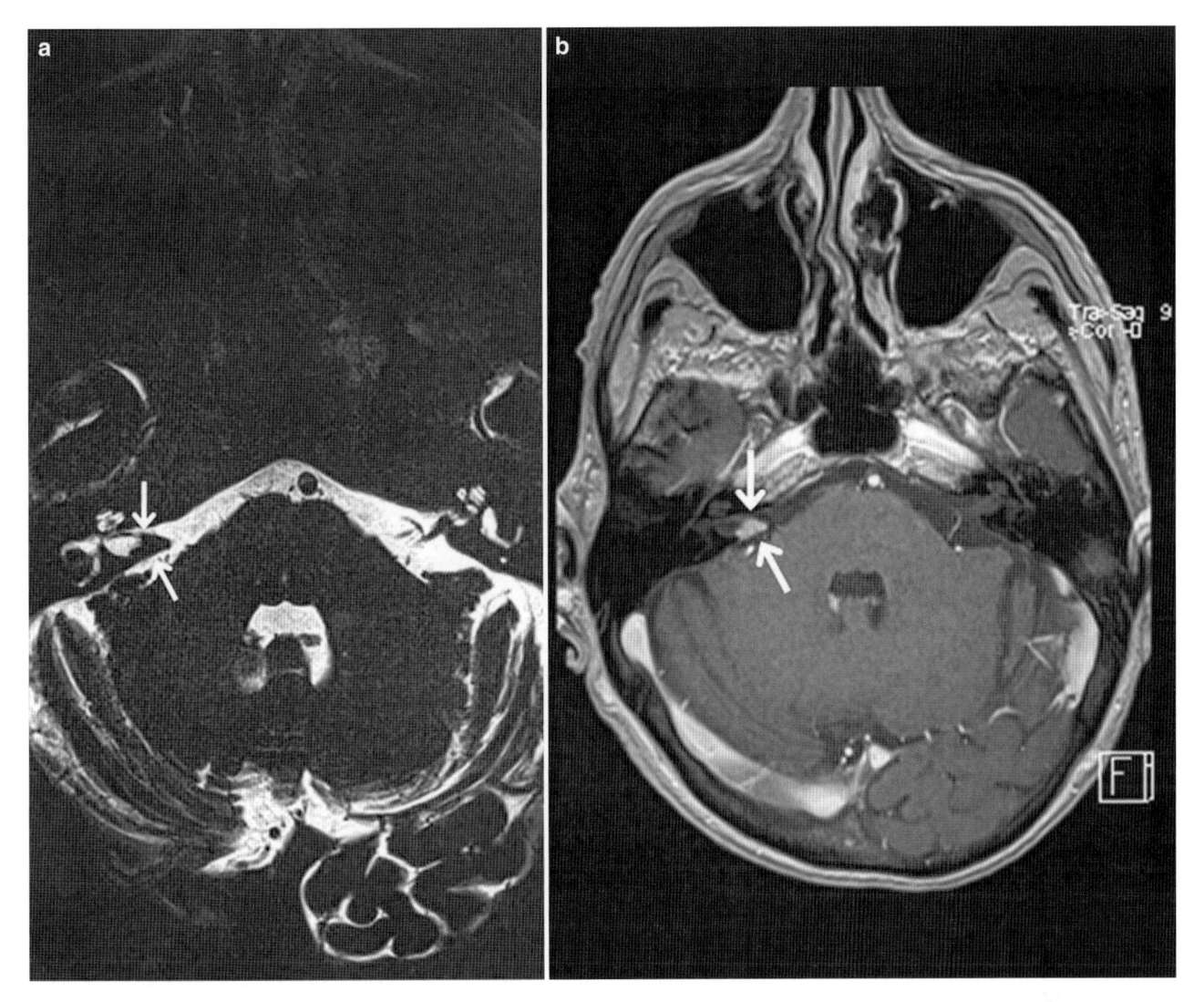

Fig. 15 68-year-old female investigated for vertigo. Audiogram also demonstrated SNHL on the right side. **a** Axial 0.4 mm thick 3D TSE T2-weighted image through the posterior fossa. On the right side a triangular hypointense mass lesion is found located on the porus acusticus internus without clear extension into the right IAC (*arrows*). **b** Axial gadolinium-enhanced 0.7 mm thick 3GRE T1-weighted image (same level as Fig. 15a) shows the lesion as a homogeneous enhancing mass lesion located over the porus acusticus internus without extension into the IAC (*arrows*). Conclusion: Presumed vestibulocochlear schwannoma over the porus acusticus internus on the right side. Patient was not treated. Wait-and-scan policy was adapted and the lesion remained unchanged for the past 10 years. Whereas most vestibulocochlear schwannomas display the classical ice cream cone appearance (see Fig. 13), some lesions only display an exofytic growth over the porus acusticus internus

DW sequences are able to make the differential diagnosis as epidermoid tumors display a homogeneous high signal intensity on high *b*-value DW images as opposed to the low signal intensity of the arachnoid cyst on high *b*-value DW images. This high signal intensity is caused by the keratin in the epidermoid tumor causing a restriction in diffusion with a subsequent low signal on Apparent Diffusion Coefficient (ADC) maps (Mohan et al. 2012; Juliano 2013; Bonneville 2007b).

Using DW sequences, preference should be given to non-echo planar (EP) DW sequences over standard EP DW sequences as the non-EP sequences display a higher signal-to-noise ratio, a higher resolution, a thinner slice thickness, and a complete lack of susceptibility artifacts at the air-bone interface of the temporal bone (de Foer et al. 2010).

Non-EP sequences are very valuable in particular in the postoperative situation as it accurately displays residual epidermoid lesions as hyperintense nodular lesions (Fig. 8).

Malignant transformation of an epidermoid is extremely rare and is characterized by areas of contrast enhancement within the lesion (Kano et al. 2010). Unusual appearances of epidermoids have been reported and included the

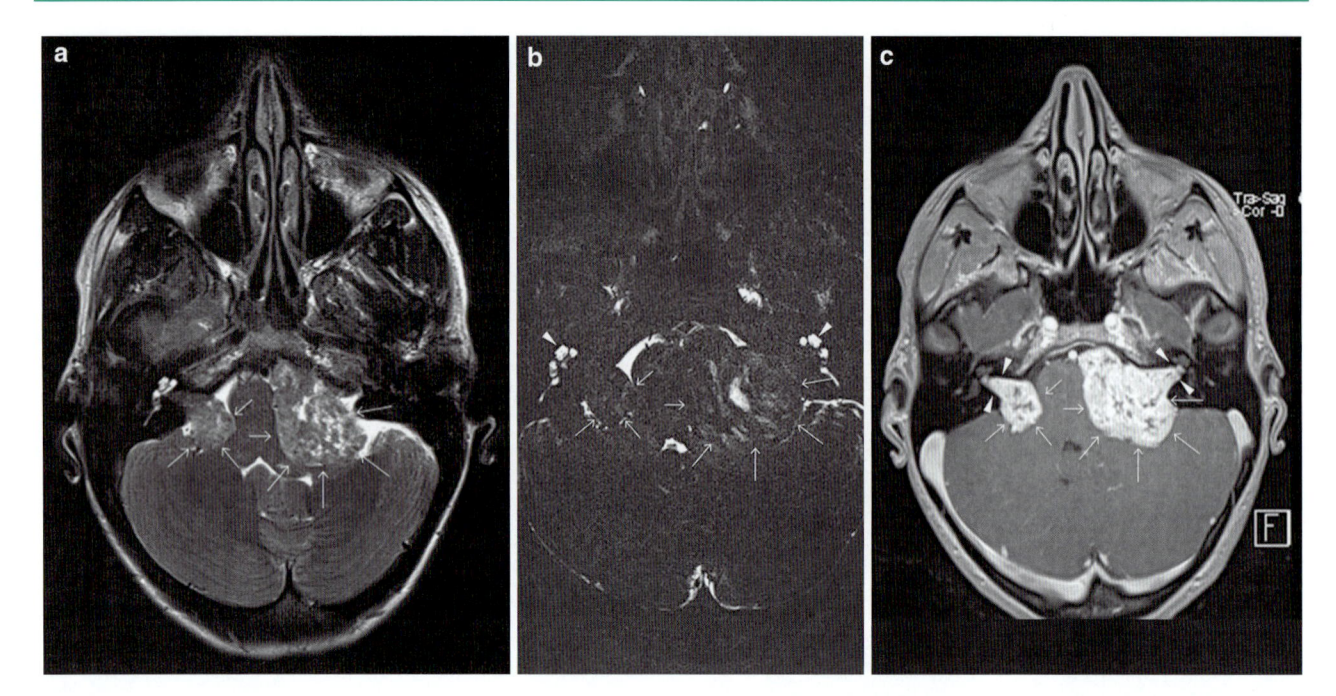

Fig. 16 20-year-old female with progressive SNHL on both sides, most pronounced on the left side. There is a familial history of NF2 with a niece diagnosed with bilateral vestibulocochlear schwannoma upon occurrence of a sudden deafness, a few years before. **a** Axial 4 mm thick TSE T2-weighted image of the brain. Large nodular inhomogeneous mass lesions in both CPAs (*arrows*). **b** Axial 0.4 mm thick 3D TSE T2-weighted image through the posterior fossa demonstrating bilateral hypointense mass lesions in both CPAs, completely filling up both IACs (*arrows*). Note the normal signal of both cochlea (*arrowheads*). **c** Axial gadolinium-enhanced 0.7 mm thick 3D GRE T1-weighted image through the posterior fossa demonstrating the inhomogeneous enhancing mass lesions in both CPAs (*arrows*) extending in the IAC on both sides (*arrowheads*). Conclusion: Bilateral large vestibulocochlear schwannomas in a patient diagnosed with NF2. Patient was treated with resection of the left-sided schwannoma via retrosigmoidal approach and is planned for a brain stem implant

so-called white epidermoids. These epidermoid show inversed signal intensities meaning they have high signal intensity on T1-weighted sequences and low signal intensity on T2-weighted images caused by their high proteinaceous content (Bonneville 2007b).

3.2 Arachnoid Cysts

Arachnoid cysts comprise the most frequent differential diagnosis of epidermoid tumor. These cysts are uniloculated CSF collections, resulting from a congenital focal defect or duplication of the arachnoid membrane. They are frequently found in the CPA but can also be found in the middle cranial fossa, against the hemispheric convexities, in the suprasellar cistern and the cisterna magna. Arachnoid cysts are thin-walled lesions containing only CSF, showing no enhancement with facilitated diffusion. In the CPA, they can compress the brainstem but most frequently they can give displacement of cranial nerves. Most frequently, cranial nerves 7 and 8 are displaced (Fig. 9). If located low in the CPA, displacement of cranial nerves 9, 10, and 11 is more likely to be the case (Fig. 10). There is still an ongoing debate why this displacement is giving rise to symptoms in few cases and why it is mostly an incidental finding without any symptoms. Imaging features have been described above with emphasis on the use of DW sequences being able to make the differential diagnosis between an arachnoid cyst and an epidermoid (Mohan et al. 2012; Juliano 2013; Bonneville 2007b).

3.3 Lipomas

Lipomas are benign lesions believed to result from a maldifferentiation of the primitive meninx. The majority of intracranial lipoma is located around the corpus callosum but some of them also occur in the CPA and even in the IAC. These lesions have a characteristic high signal intensity on unenhanced T1-weighted images with subsequent signal loss on fat-suppressed images while no enhancement is observed after contrast administration (Fig. 11). In the CPA, lipomas encase very often the neurovascular structures, as nicely demonstrated by the linear low signal intensities running through the lesion. They are usually asymptomatic and are often an incidental finding on MR

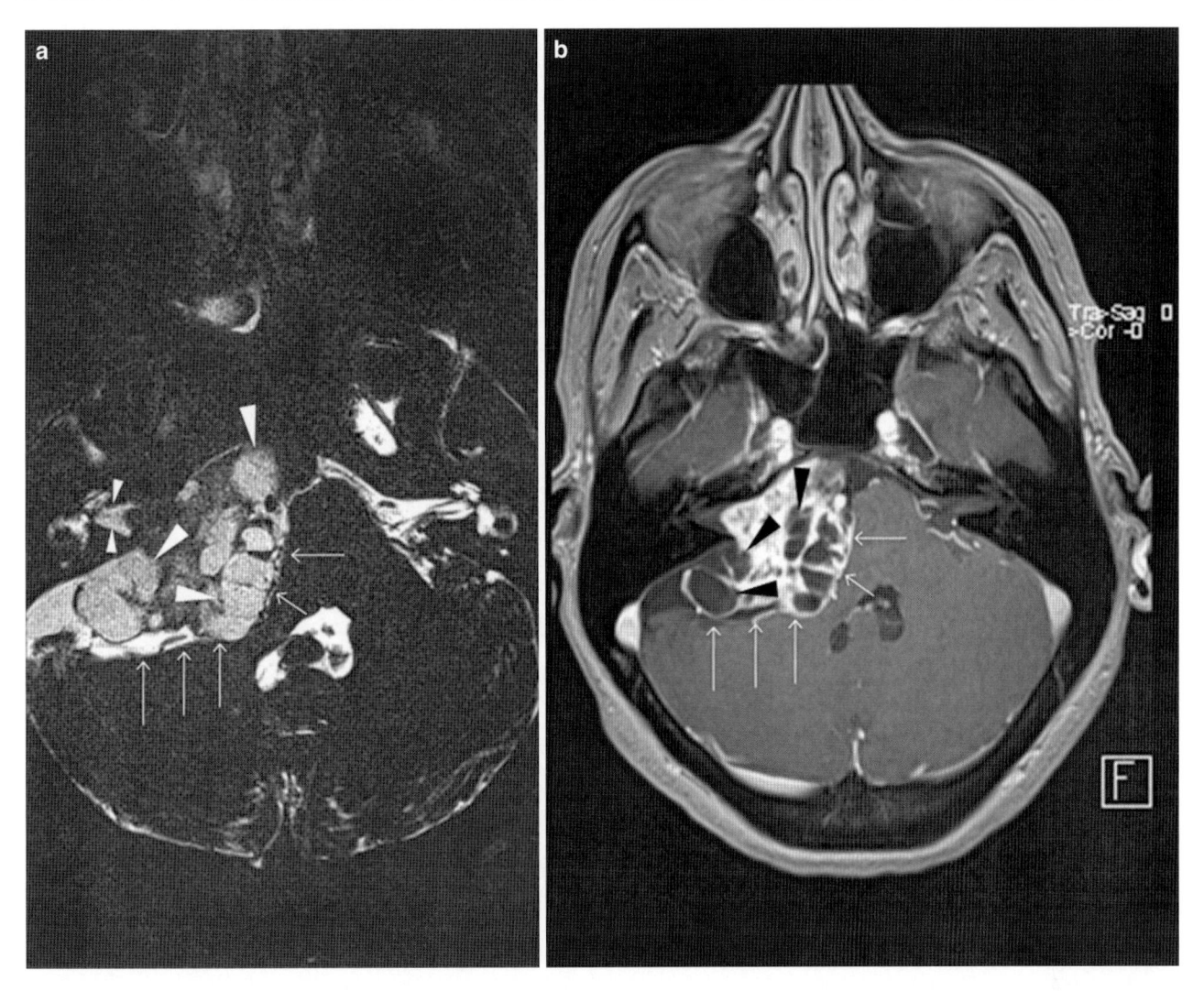

Fig. 17 52-year-old female investigated for severe SNHL on the right side. **a** Axial 0.4 mm thick 3D TSE T2-weighted image through the posterior fossa. Note the presence of a large mass lesion (*arrows*) with multiple cystic components (*large arrowheads*) in the right CPA with extension into the IAC (*small arrowhead*). **b** Axial gadolinium-enhanced 0.7 mm thick 3D GRE T1-weighted image (same level as Fig. 17a) through the posterior fossa showing the enhancing mass lesion (*arrows*) with the multiple nonenhancing cystic components in the lesion (*large arrowheads*). Note the severe compression of the brainstem and cerebellum. Conclusion: Large mainly cystic vestibulocochlear schwannoma in the right CPA with compression of the brainstem and cerebellum. Patient was treated by surgery via a translabyrinthine approach because of the fact that the patient was almost completely deaf and the large volume of the lesion

imaging of the brain or posterior fossa. One of the most important messages is that intracranial lipomas are regarded as leave-me-alone lesions which definitely should not be operated upon (Mukherjee 2011).

3.4 Dermoid Cysts

Dermoid cysts are similar to epidermoid cysts in that it is the result of a congenital inclusion of cutaneous ectoderm. Dermoid cysts may contain fat, hair, teeth, and calcification. On imaging, a dermoid cysts appears as a well-circumscribed fatty round mass with a thick peripheral capsule. It is mostly located supratentorial near the midline. In case of rupture, the characteristic appearance of scattered fat droplets—presenting as small T1 hyperintense nodules—in the CSF space with the clinical image of a chemical meningitis can be found (Bonneville 2007b).

3.5 Neurenteric Cysts

Neurenteric cysts are congenital cystic masses lined by a mucin-producing epithelium of endodermal origin, closely resembling gastrointestinal tract mucosa. Most of the

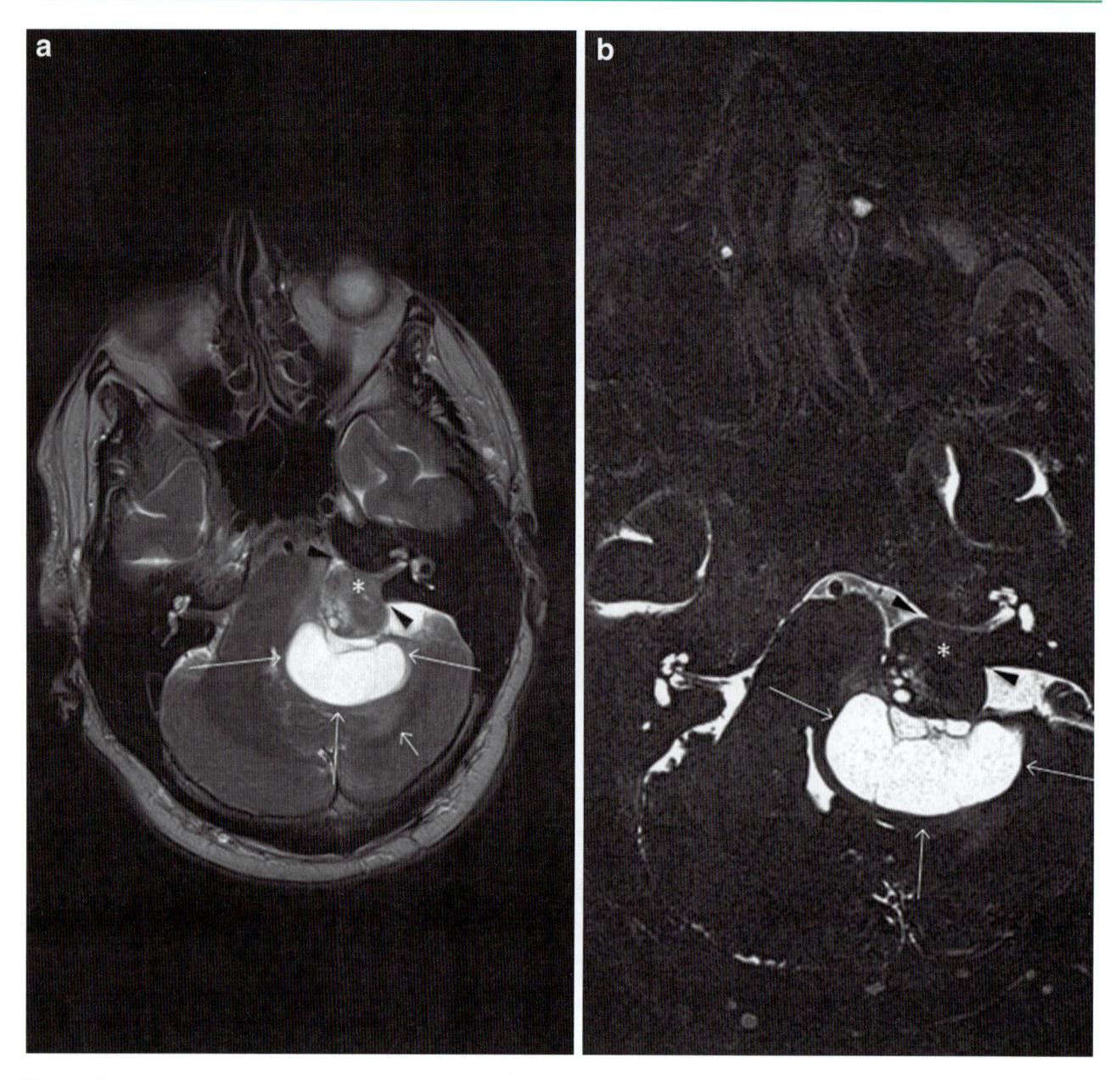

Fig. 18 48-year-old male with a sudden onset of profound SNHL on the left side. **a** Axial 4 mm thick TSE T2-weighted image of the brain. Large nodular isointense lesion (*asterisk*) in the left CPA, centered over the IAC with sharp angles with the posterior side of the temporal bone pyramid (*arrowheads*). Note that the mass displays very small cystic components inside. There is a large cystic component—apparently completely different from the VC schwannoma—in the left middle cerebellar peduncle (*large arrows*). There is also some edema in the brain stem (*small arrow*). **b** Axial 0.7 mm thick 3D TSE T2-weighted image of the posterior fossa at the level of the IAC. This image essentially displays the same findings as Fig. 18a: the large vestibulocochlear schwannoma (*asterisk*), centered over the left IAC with sharp angles (*arrowheads*) with the posterior wall of the left temporal bone pyramid. The large cystic lesion in the left middle cerebellar peduncle (*large arrows*) and the small cystic components in the vestibulocochlear schwannoma are easily discriminated on this heavily T2-weighted image. **c** Axial unenhanced 2 mm thick SE T1-weighted image displays the large isointense vestibulocochlear schwannoma (*asterisk*) and the large cystic lesion in the left middle cerebellar peduncle (*large arrows*). **d** Axial gadolinium-enhanced 2 mm thick SE T1-weighted image (same level as Fig. 18c) showing the enhancement of the VC schwannoma (*asterisk*). Note the small nonenhancing cystic components in the schwannoma and the large nonenhancing cystic lesion in the middle cerebellar peduncle (*large arrows*). Conclusion: Large left-sided partially cystic vestibulocochlear schwannoma compressing the brain stem and the left cerebellar peduncle. The large cystic lesion in the left cerebellar peduncle was found to be entrapped CSF at surgery. The sharp angles of the lesion with the posterior side of the temporal bone pyramid as well as it center over and in the IAC are highly typical for a vestibulocochlear schwannoma

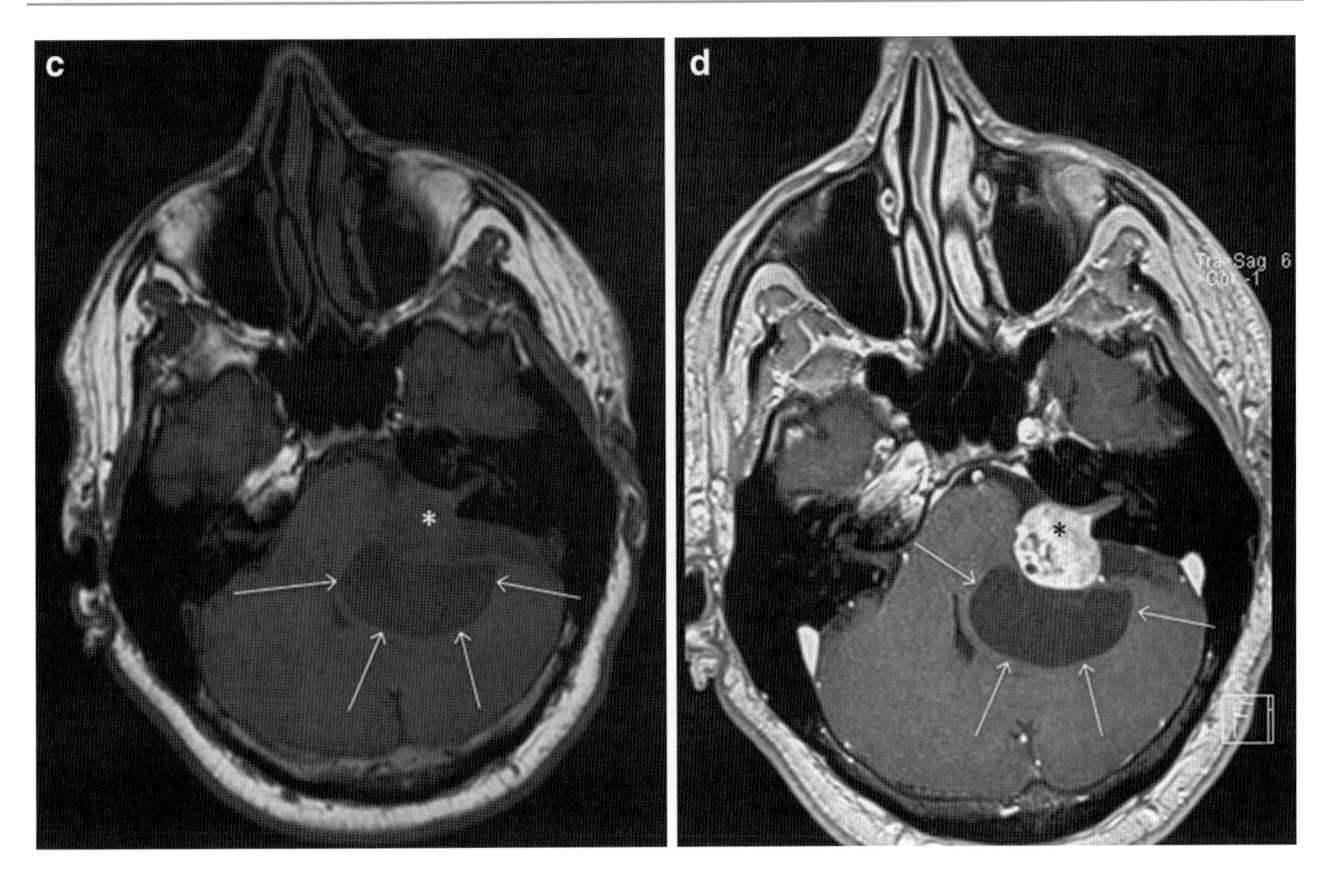

Fig. 18 continued

neurenteric cysts in the central nervous system are located within the spinal canal, ventral to the spinal cord. Intracranial neurenteric cysts are very rare, mainly located near the midline in the posterior fossa or in the CPA. Signal intensities on MRI depend on its protein content and concentration. In case of low protein content, it can mimic CSF signal intensities. It is often isointense to hyperintense relative to brain parenchyma on T1-weighted images and hyperintense on T2-weighted images when the protein concentration is high. They very rarely show peripheral rim enhancement (Fig. 12). On DW MR sequences, neurenteric cysts have a predominantly low signal intensity as opposed to the characteristic high signal intensity of epidermoid cysts (Bonneville 2007b).

4 Tumoral Lesions

4.1 Vestibulocochlear Schwannomas

Vestibulocochlear schwannomas (formerly called acoustic neuromas) are benign slowly growing neoplasms accounting for at least three quarters of all CPA lesions and for about one-tenth of all intracranial tumors. Vestibular schwannomas develop from the Schwann sheath of the inferior vestibular nerve. Most frequently they originate at the opening or mouth of the IAC growing secondary into the IAC and into the CPA giving rise to the typical ice cream cone appearance (Fig. 13).

They also can originate in the fundus of the IAC and give rise to a completely intracanalicular lesion (Fig. 14). A third less common variant is a purely intracisternal component growing from the external opening in the porus, completely into the cistern (Fig. 15).

Most patients with vestibulocochlear schwannoma present with progressive SNHL. About 20 % of patients, however, present with sudden deafness.

Other—less frequent—symptoms are vertigo and tinnitus. Facial nerve palsy as a symptom is virtually nonexisting as the facial nerve is much more resistant to chronic pressure (Bonneville 2007a; Mohan et al. 2012; Verbist 2012; Juliano 2013).

When the lesion becomes large, symptoms of cerebellar and brainstem compression may complicate the clinical findings. Bilateral vestibulocochlear schwannomas can be considered the handmark of neurofibromatosis type 2 and can be the first manifestation of the disease (Fig. 16).

On MRI, they show T1 isointensity and T2 high signal intensity with strong enhancement after gadolinium injection.

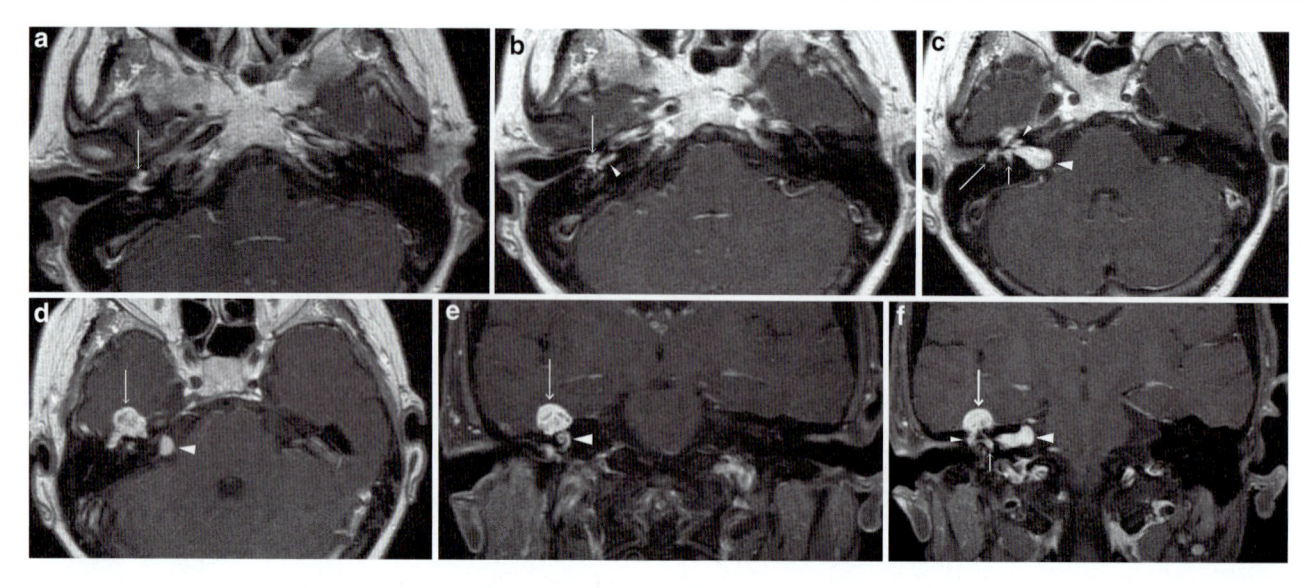

Fig. 19 44-year-old male with known NF-1 presenting with facial nerve palsy on the right side. **a** Axial gadolinium-enhanced 2 mm thick SE T1-weighted MR image at the level of the hypotympanon. There is a small enhancing lesion (*arrow*) visible, apparently located in the lower part of the middle ear. **b** Axial gadolinium-enhanced 2 mm thick SE T1-weighted MR image at the level of the basal turn of the cochlea. Scan level is slightly higher than Fig. 19a. Note that part of the lesion is located in the lower part of the middle ear (*arrow*). There is extension in the basal turn of the cochlea (*arrowhead*). **c** Axial gadolinium-enhanced 2 mm thick SE T1-weighted MR image at the level of the IAC. Note the enhancement of nearly the entire membranous labyrinth with an enhancing component in the IAC (*large arrowhead*), in the mid and apical turn of the cochlea (*small arrowhead*), the vestibule and lateral semicircular canal (*small arrow*). The component in the middle ear is also visible (*large arrow*). **d** Axial gadolinium-enhanced 2 mm thick SE T1-weighted MR image at the level of the geniculate ganglion. Note the large lesion centered on the geniculate ganglion (*arrow*) and the small component in the CPA (*arrowhead*). **e** Coronal gadolinium-enhanced 2 mm thick SE T1-weighted MR image with fat sat at the level of the cochlea. Large lesion centered on the geniculate ganglion (*arrow*). Note the extension in the cochlea (*arrowhead*). **f** Coronal gadolinium-enhanced 2 mm thick SE T1-weighted MR image with fat sat at the level of the IAC. Mass lesion centerd on the geniculate ganglion (*large arrows*). Note the component in the IAC (*large arrowhead*), the component along the tympanic segment of the facial nerve (*small arrowhead*) and the component in the membranous labyrinth (*small arrow*). Conclusion: Large plexiform neurofibroma of the facial nerve centered on the geniculate ganglion with extension along all the segments of the facial nerve and invasion into the membranous labyrinth

On heavily T2-weighted images, they replace the fluid signal of CSF. The enhancement pattern is either homogeneous (50–60 %), heterogeneous (30–40 %), and cystic (5–15 %).

Vestibulocochlear schwannomas are by definition centered on the IAC and have sharp angles with the posterior side of the temporal bone. A dural tail may occur but is rather unfrequent (Bonneville 2007a; Mohan et al. 2012; Verbist 2012; Juliano 2013).

Small vestibular schwannomas are usually homogeneous and histologically composed of Antony type A pattern, while heterogeneous and cystic vestibular schwannomas are larger and harbor Antoni B pattern or a mix of type A and B.

Vestibulocochlear schwannomas always become heterogeneous in lesions larger than 25 mm because of the occurrence of those additional cystic or necrotic components (Figs. 17 and 18). Larger lesions may entrap fluid between the tumor and the brainstem giving rise to rapidly progressive symptoms (Fig. 18).

Some other lesions might resemble vestibulocochlear schwannomas. Facial nerve schwannomas as such usually originates in the region of the geniculate ganglion and can extend along the different nerve segments. Extension into the IAC is not uncommon but a facial nerve schwannoma located only in the IAC as such is virtually nonexisting (Fig. 19) (Wiggins et al. 2006).

In children, in case of a lesion filling up the IAC without a history of neurofibromatosis, diagnose of a more aggressive lesion such as rhabdomyosarcoma should be considered (Fig. 20) (Holman et al. 2013).

The treatment of vestibulocochlear schwannomas depends on various factors: the degree of SNHL, the age of the patient, the size, and aspect of the lesion and its degree of extension in the IAC.

At first, the 'wait and scan' option can be preferred in case of a small lesion. In order to do so, volume calculation of the lesion can be done on most computer work stations. Volume calculation can be regarded as much more accurate than diameter measurement in the axial plane. A first control examination after 6 months can be followed by an annual MRI control examination. If the lesion remains stable, later on a bi-annual MRI control examination can be advocated.

About half of all vestibulocochlear schwannomas grow (Fig. 21), about half of them remain stable (Fig. 22) and less than 1 % diminishes in size spontaneously (Fig. 23).

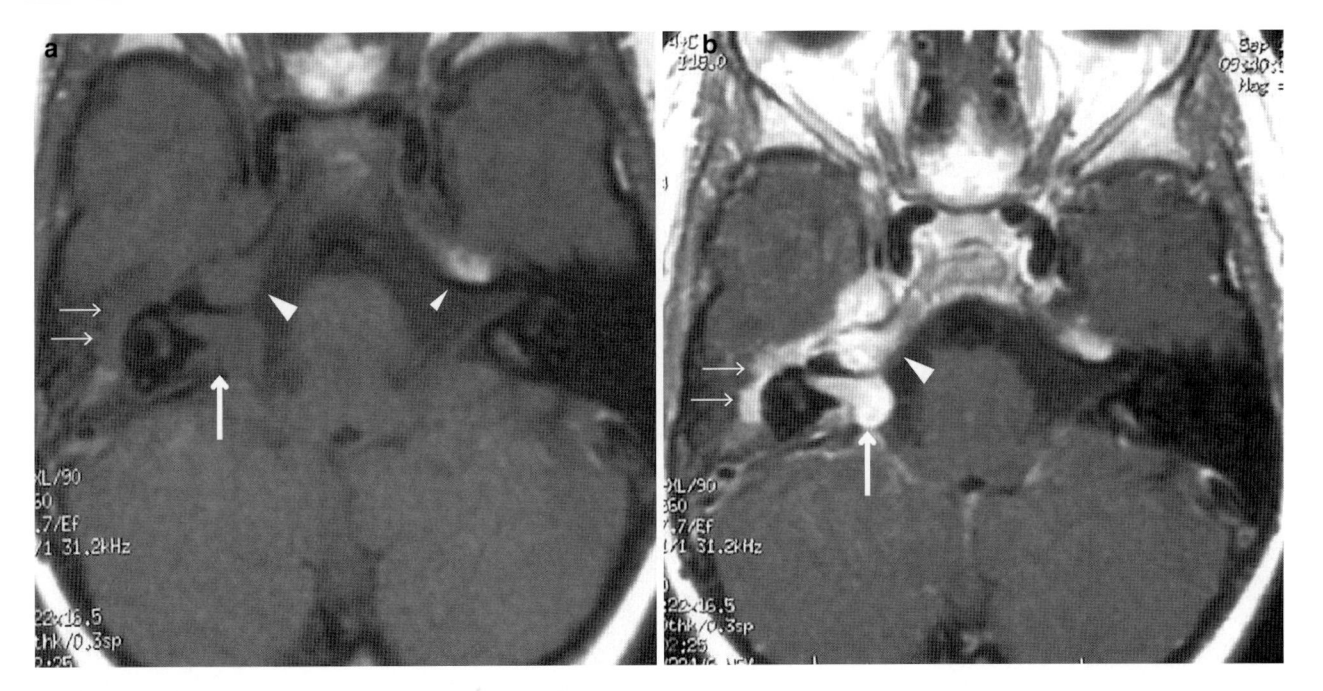

Fig. 20 6-year-old girl with deafness on the right side and a sudden onset of facial nerve palsy on the right side. **a** Axial 3 mm thick SE T1-weighted MR image through the posterior fossa at the level of the IAC. Note the isointense mass lesion in the right IAC (*large arrow*) with a component in the CPA. Asymmetrical aspect of the petrous bone apex with loss of high fat signal on the right side (*large arrowhead*). Compare to the fat signal in the left petrous apex (*small arrowhead*). There is component of the mass extending along the tympanic segment of the facial nerve (*small arrows*). **b** Axial gadolinium-enhanced 3 mm thick SE T1-weighted MR image through the posterior fossa at the level of the IAC (same level as Fig. 20a). The lesion is filling the IAC (*large arrow*), invading in the petrous bone apex (*large arrowhead*) and extending along the tympanic segment of the facial nerve (*small arrows*). Conclusion: Aggressive looking lesion with alarm symptoms (deafness and facial nerve palsy) with imaging characteristics of a facial nerve schwannoma. In the absence of neurofibromatosis, a facial nerve schwannoma at this age is highly unlikely. Biopsy revealed a rhabdomyosarcoma

Further treatment options consist of surgical removal either by a retrosigmoidal approach or a translabyrinthine approach. The retrosigmoidal approach is performed in case hearing preservation is preferred. Drawback of this technique is that no direct visualization of the IAC can be obtained (Silk 2009).

There are two features that may predict the postoperative outcome after retrosigmoidal approach and that is the presence of residual fluid in the fundus of the IAC and the signal intensities of the fluid in the membranous labyrinth.

The presence of residual fluid in the fundus of the IAC and a normal signal of the membranous labyrinth on heavily T2-weighted sequences can be regarded as positive predictive signs for hearing preservation surgery. A loss of residual fluid in the fundus of the IAC associated to a decreased signal in the membranous labyrinth on heavily T2-weighted sequences can be regarded as a negative predictive sign for hearing preservation surgery.

It should be stressed that these signal alterations are dependent on the type of sequences used (Somers et al. 2001). If the signal loss is doubtful, MIP reconstructions can be helpful (Fig. 24).

In case of serious SNHL or complete deafness or in case of a very large tumor, translabyrinthine approach is preferred as this technique allows direct visualization of the CPA and the nerves. In those cases, the created defect of the petrosectomy is usually filled up with abdominal fat and—if needed—a facial nerve anastomosis is constructed (Fig. 25) (Silk 2009). On postoperative imaging follow-up, linear enhancement can very often be noted and can be regarded as normal (Fig. 26). It should be noted that this linear enhancement can persist for months and even years after surgery. Nodular enhancing components should always be regarded as a possible residual and/or recurrent tumor and should always be followed carefully (Fig. 27). Follow-up imaging will be able to demonstrate growth of a possible lesion (Silk 2009).

Focalized radiotherapy or so-called gamma knife surgery can also be used as treatment (Pollock et al. 2006). It should be kept in mind that the lesion at first might display a volume augmentation due to swelling of the lesion and that loss of volume of the lesion can take up to 2 years before taking place. Also, long-term effects such as sarcomatous degeneration of the lesion—although extremely rare—should be considered.

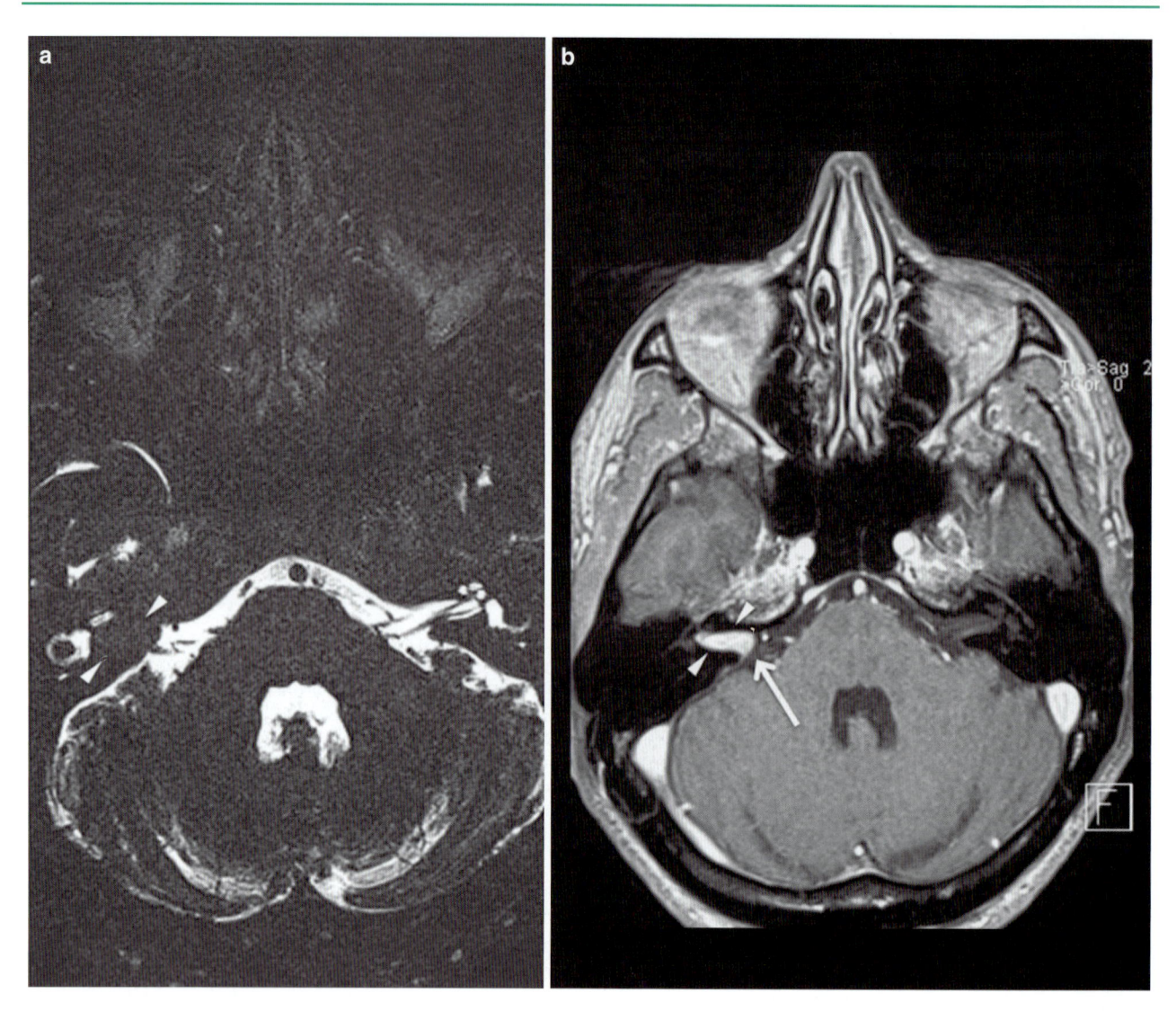

Fig. 21 62-year-old male investigated for SNHL on the right side. **a** Axial 0.4 mm thick 3D TSE T2-weighted image at the level of the IAC. There is a lesion filling up nearly the entire IAC on the right side (*arrowheads*). **b** Axial gadolinium-enhanced 0.7 mm thick 3D GRE T1-weighted image at the level of the IAC (same level as Fig. 21a) demonstrating the enhancing lesion in the right IAC. Note that at that time there was virtually no component protruding into the CPA (*arrow*). **c** axial 0.4 mm thick 3D TSE T2-weighted image at the level of the IAC (same level as Fig. 21a and b). This examination was performed 2 years after the first diagnosis. The lesion is filling up the entire IAC on the right side (*arrowheads*) with a clear component protruding into the CPA (*arrow*). **d** Axial gadolinium-enhanced 0.7 mm thick 3D GRE T1-weighted image at the level of the IAC (same level as Fig. 21a, b, and c). The lesion is filling up the entire IAC on the right side (*arrowheads*) with a clear component protruding into the CPA (*arrow*). Conclusion: Right-sided vestibulocochlear schwannoma with volume gain over a period of 2 years. Patient was treated with surgery via a retrosigmoidal approach with preservation of hearing

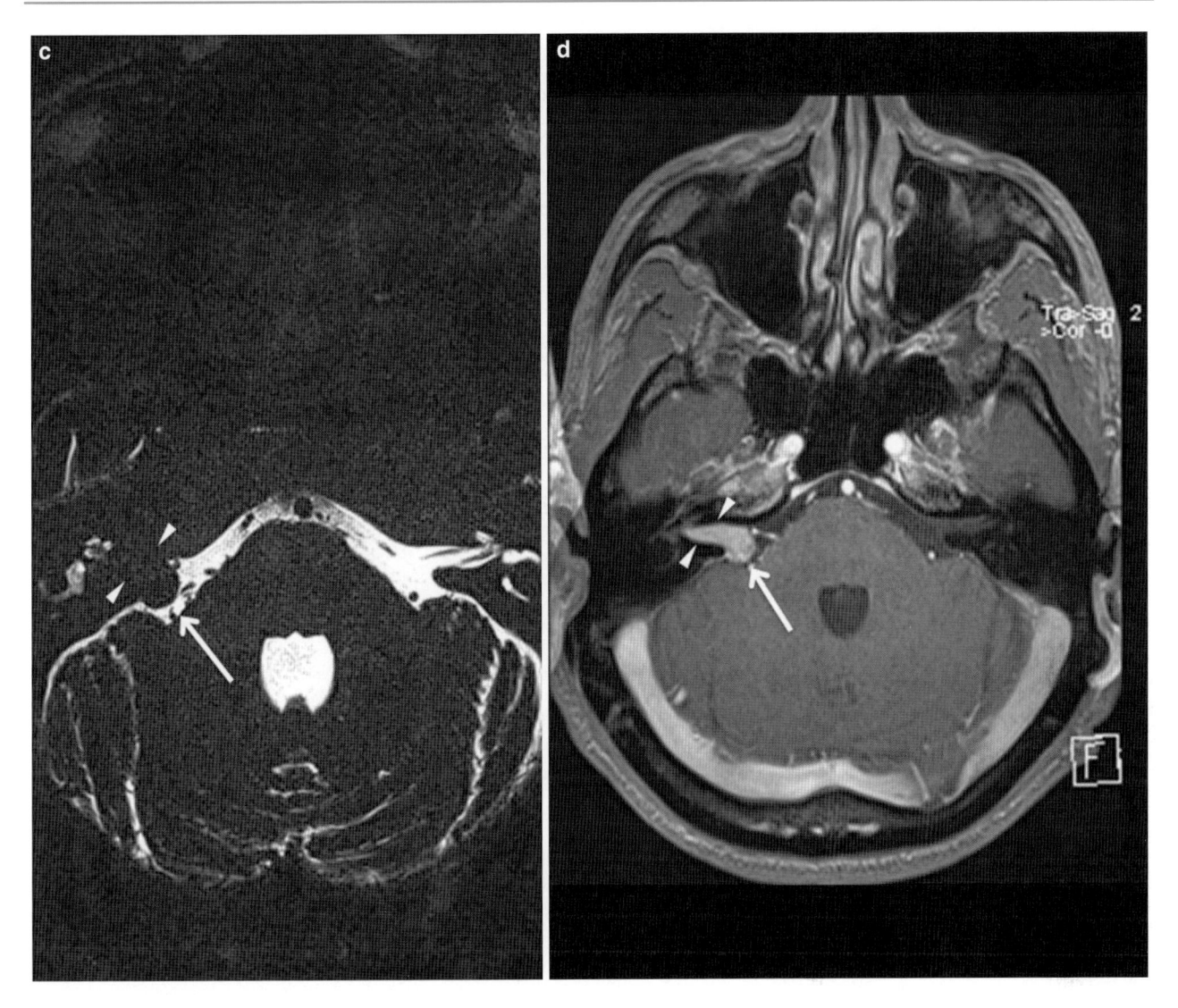

Fig. 21 continued

The choice of therapy depends on multiple factors such as the age of the patient, the general condition of the patient, the degree of hearing loss, the size and location of the lesion, the presence of residual fluid in the fundus of the IAC and the signal intensity of the membranous labyrinth, and most important the presence of the required surgical and/or radiotherapeutic skills in the proximity of the patient.

4.2 Meningiomas

Meningioma is the second most frequent lesion in the CPA after vestibular schwannoma, representing 10–15 % of all tumors in this location. Meningioma is the most common intracranial extra-axial tumor in adults, arising from arachnoid meningoepithelial cells, growing slowly in the CPA.

In and around the middle ear, various forms and presentations of meningioma have been described. Most frequently, they arise from the dura of the dorsal aspect of the petrous temporal bone. In these cases, they may be eccentric over the IAC but they can be centered over the IAC with extension into the IAC, but without enlargement of the porus. They usually form obtuse angles with the posterior side of the temporal bone and a dural tail may be present (Fig. 28). Dural tails can, however, be encountered in numerous other pathologies (Bonneville 2007a; Mohan et al. 2012; Verbist 2012; Juliano 2013; Hamilton et al. 2006).

Very frequently, meningioma can also be found as a coincident finding in various types of other pathologies (Fig. 29). Other frequent locations around the temporal bone are the petrous bone apex and the tentorium.

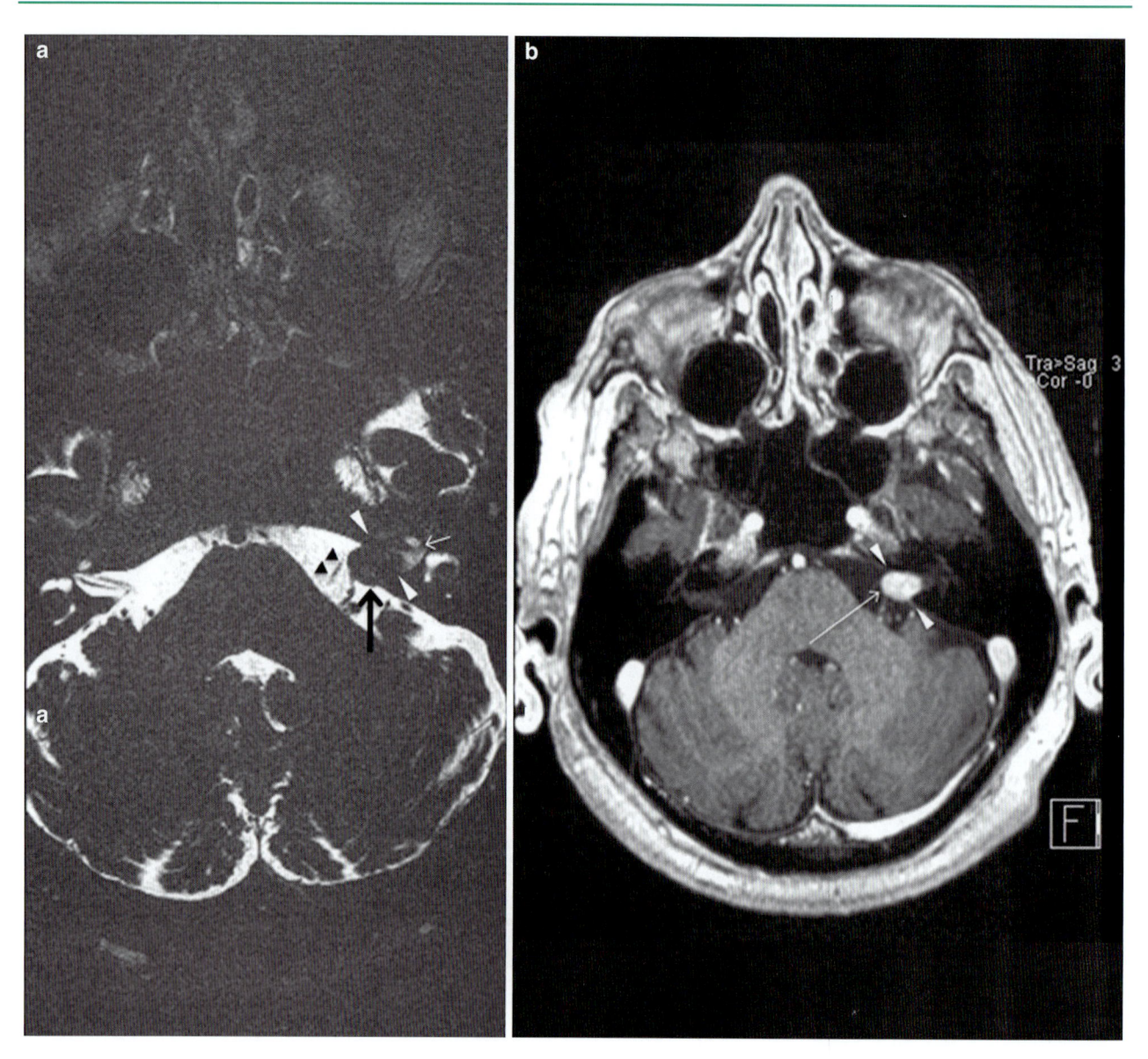

Fig. 22 52-year-old male investigated for SNHL on the left side. Figures a and b are from an MRI examination performed in December 2005, figures c and d are from an MRI examination performed in December 2006 and figures e and f are from an MRI examination performed in May 2008. **a** Axial 0.4 mm thick 3D TSE T2-weighted image at the level of the IAC demonstrating a lesion in the left IAC (*large arrowheads*) with a component protruding into the CPA (*large arrow*). Note that the facial nerve and the vestibulocochlear nerve seem to be running towards the anterior delineation of the tumor (*small arrowhead*). There is some residual fluid in the IAC on the left side but this signal has dropped (*small arrow*). **b** Axial gadolinium-enhanced 0.7 mm thick 3D GRE T1-weighted image at the level of the IAC (same level as Fig. 22a) shows the lesion as an enhancing mass lesion in the left IAC (*large arrowheads*) and a small component protruding into the CPA (*large arrow*). **c** Axial 0.4 mm thick 3D TSE T2-weighted image at the level of the IAC 1 year after the first examination, demonstrating again the lesion in the left IAC (*large arrowheads*) with a component protruding into the CPA (*large arrow*) (same level as Fig. 22a and b). The lesion has remained unchanged. **d** Axial gadolinium-enhanced 0.7 mm thick 3D GRE T1-weighted image at the level of the IAC (same level as Fig. 22a, b, and c) 1 year after the first examination, shows again the lesion as an enhancing mass lesion in the left IAC (*large arrowheads*) and a small component protruding into the CPA (*large arrow*). The lesion has remained unchanged, which was confirmed by volume measurement (not shown). **e** Axial 0.4 mm thick 3D TSE T2-weighted image at the level of the IAC two and a half years after the first examination demonstrating again the lesion in the left IAC (*large arrowheads*) with a component protruding into the CPA (*large arrow*) (same level as Fig. 22a, b, c, and d). The lesion has remained unchanged. **f** Axial gadolinium-enhanced 0.7 mm thick 3D GRE T1-weighted image at the level of the IAC (same level as Fig. 22a, b, c, d and e) two and a half years after the first examination shows again the lesion as an enhancing mass lesion in the left IAC (*large arrowheads*) and a small component protruding into the CPA (*large arrow*). The lesion has remained unchanged which was confirmed by volume measurement (not shown). Conclusion: Vestibulocochlear schwannoma remaining unchanged for 2.5 years. As hearing loss was not worsening, patient was left untreated and follow-up scans demonstrated a lack of growth

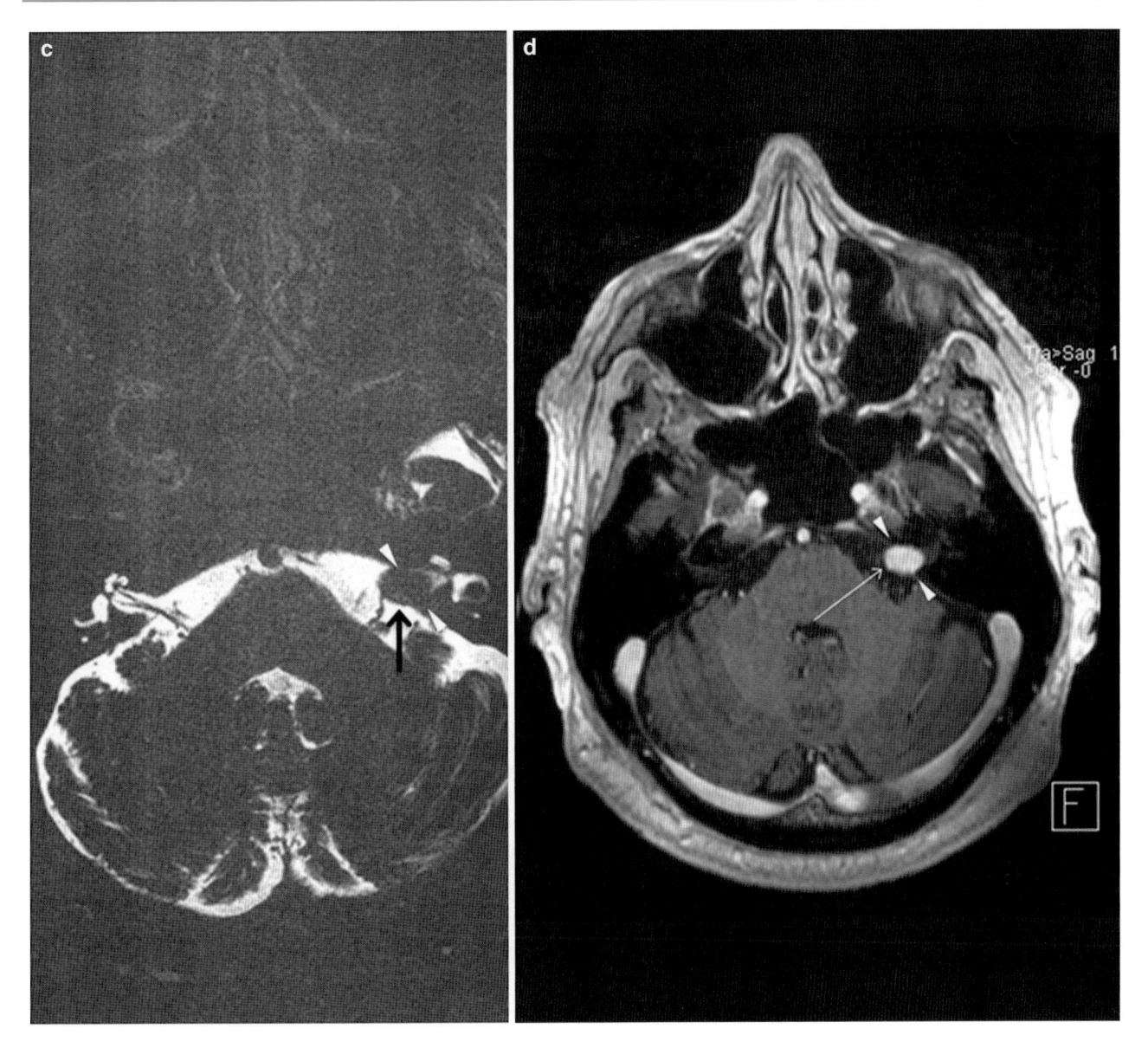

Fig. 22 continued

Petrous bone apex meningiomas may remain undetected for some time and can have a large volume before symptoms are presented (Fig. 30). It should be kept in mind that a meningioma originating from the tentorium may hang down in the CPA. By doing so, the meningioma may present as a nodular lesion resembling vestibulocochlear schwannoma at imaging (Fig. 31).

In rare cases, they can present as a completely intracanalicular lesion, making differentiation with a vestibulocochlear schwannoma impossible. These meningiomas can also invade the membranous labyrinth and grow secondarily in the CPA (Fig. 32) (Hamilton et al. 2006).

Other specific but less frequent temporal bone locations have also been reported.

Meningiomas may occur in the tegmen tympani, usually presenting as meningioma-en-plaque growing in the bone of the tegmen tympani and invading both the middle fossa and the middle ear. The bone of the tegmen tympani is very often thickened and sclerotic but internal trabecular architecture of the involved bone is preserved. On MRI, a typical enhancement of the bone as well as the thickened dura can be noted. It is usually the middle ear component causing symptoms of conductive hearing loss due to impingement on the ossicles (Fig. 33) (Hamilton et al. 2006; Ayache et al. 2006).

A possible other temporal bone location is the jugular foramen. These meningiomas can invade the bone of the skull base, giving rise to sclerosis but with preservation of

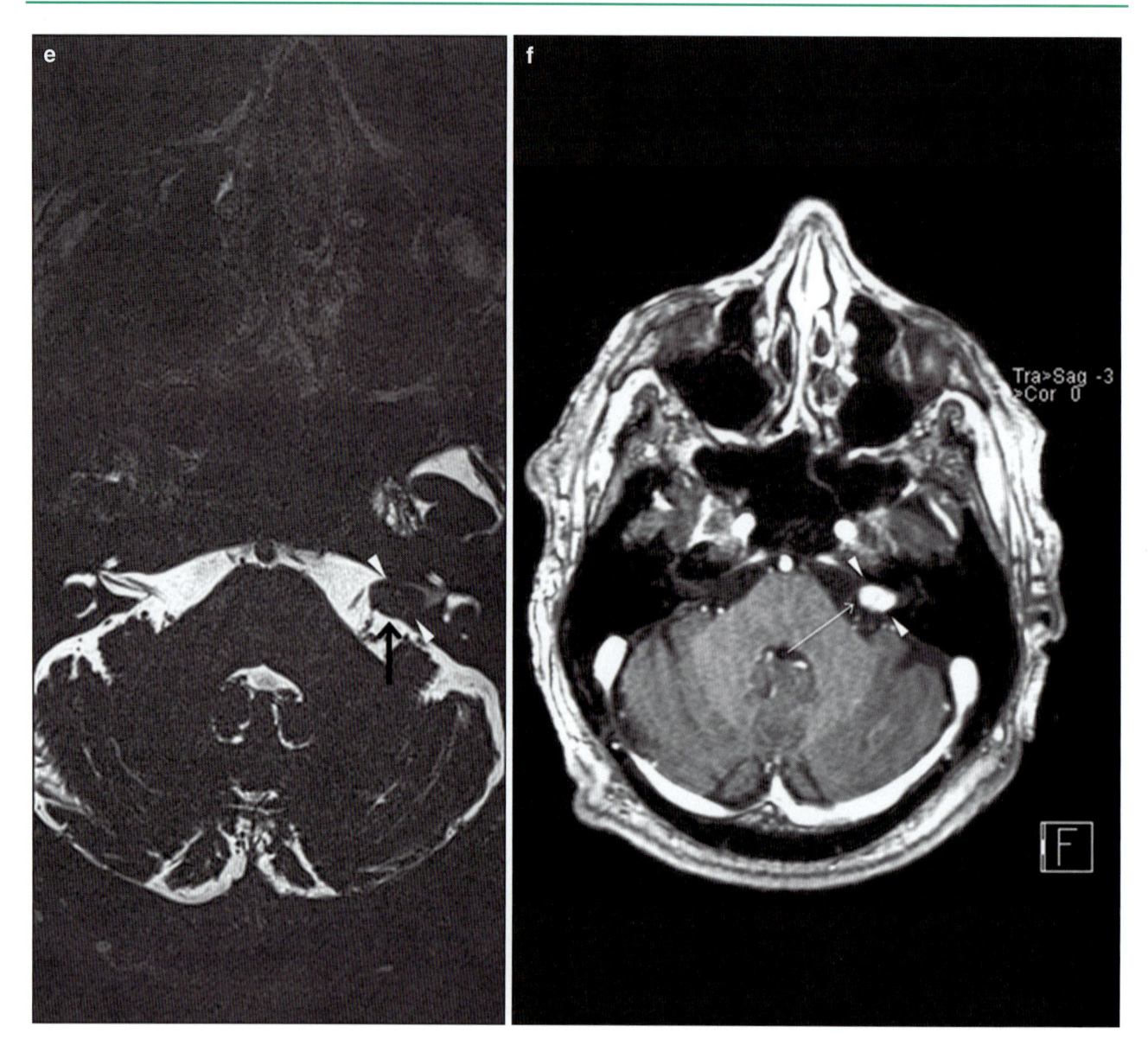

Fig. 22 continued

the internal trabecular architecture. From there on, invasion into the middle ear can be noted (Hamilton et al. 2006).

However, meningiomas of the jugular foramen may also grow up in the CPA without bony invasion in the skull base. Clinical signs in these cases can be swallowing difficulties due to compression of the 9th, 10th, and 11th nerve complex but also hearing loss due to pressure of the growing lesion on the vestibulocochlear nerve (Fig. 34). Differential diagnosis with a schwannoma of these mixed nerves can be sometimes difficult if not impossible (see below).

Other clinical signs can be tinnitus due to the high degree of vascularization and possible headache. In case of a large lesion, signs of cerebellar compression might predominate as well as signs of trigeminal neuropathy.

On CT, CPA meningioma present as slightly hyperdense lesions on unenhanced images. The lesion can be calcified (Fig. 35) and frequently shows adjacent bone reaction such as hyperostosis and an enostotic spur (Hamilton et al. 2006).

MRI clearly depicts the lesion as a broad-based, dural, hemispheric mass attached to the posterior side of the temporal bone, or pendulating from the inferior aspect of the tentorium. Meningiomas are usually isointense to brain cortex on all sequences with strong enhancement after intravenous administration of gadolinium (Hamilton et al. 2006).

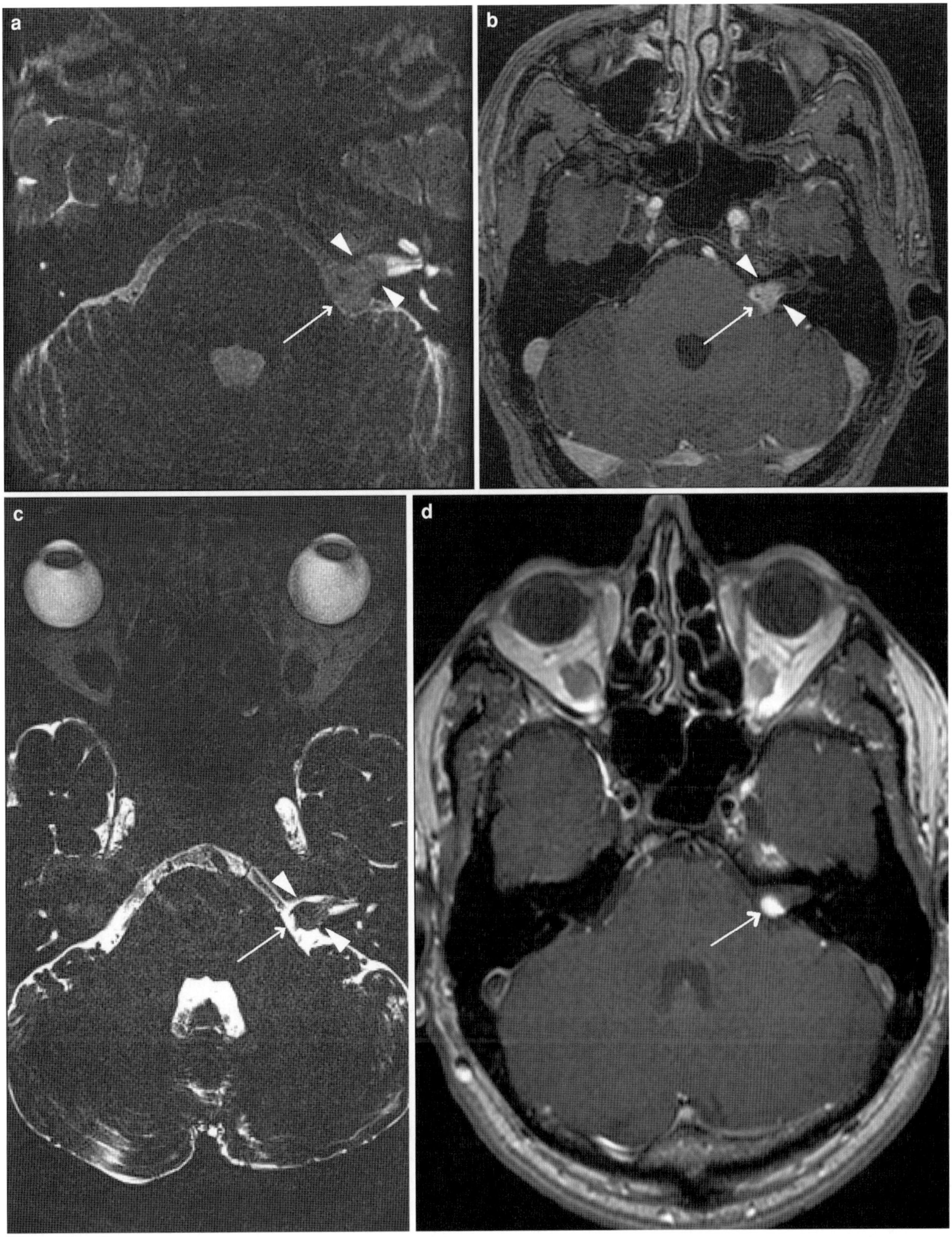
a
b
c
d

◀ **Fig. 23** 63-year-old male investigated for SNHL on the left side. Images a and b are from an MRI examination performed in December 2003. Images c and d are from an MRI examination performed in July 2007. **a** Axial 1 mm thick 3D TSE T2-weighted image at the level of the left IAC (patient is asymmetrically positioned). There is a hypointense mass lesion with a component in the left IAC (*large arrowheads*) and a component protruding into the left CPA (*large arrow*). **b** Axial gadolinium-enhanced 2 mm thick SE T1-weighted image with fatsat at the level of the left IAC (same level as Fig. 23a) demonstrating the mass as an enhancing nodular mass lesion with a component in the left IAC (*large arrowheads*) and a component protruding into the left CPA (*large arrow*). **c** Axial 0.4 mm thick 3D TSE T2-weighted image at the level of the IAC 3.5 years after the first examination demonstrating again the lesion in the left IAC (*large arrowheads*) with a component protruding into the CPA (*large arrow*) (same level as Fig. 23a and b). The lesion has clearly diminished in size. **d** Axial gadolinium-enhanced 1 mm thick SE T1-weighted image at the level of the IAC (same level as Fig. 23a, b and c) three and a half years after the first examination shows again the lesion as an enhancing mass lesion in the left porus acusticus internus (*large arrow*). The lesion has clearly diminished in size. Conclusion: Vestibulocochlear schwannoma left untreated with a clear spontaneous reduction of size. About half of the vestibulocochlear schwannomas grow and about half of vestibulocochlear schwannomas remain unchanged. Less than 1 % of lesions diminish spontaneously in size

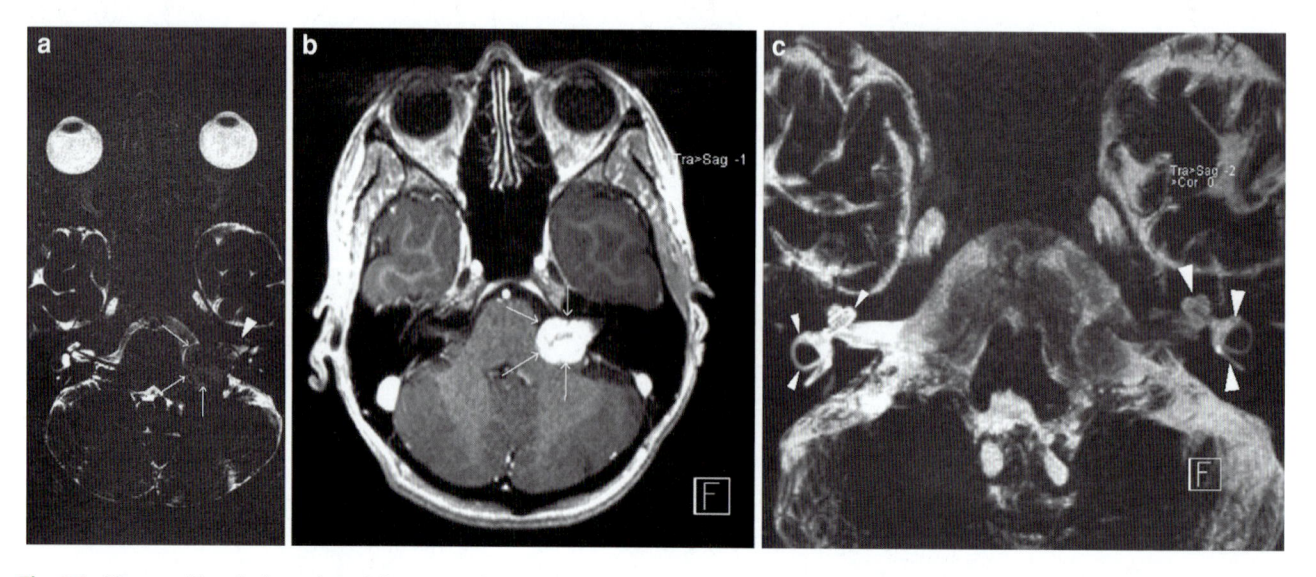

Fig. 24 22-year-old male investigated for severe SNHL on the left side. **a** Axial 0.4 mm thick 3D TSE T2-weighted image at the level of the IAC. Large mass lesion in the left IAC and CPA (*arrows*) on the left side. There is some fluid left in the fundus of the IAC (*arrowhead*). The signal of this residual fluid seems however to be low. **b** Axial gadolinium-enhanced 0.7 mm thick 3D GRE T1-weighted image (same level as Fig. 24a) demonstrating the lesion as a large homogeneously enhancing mass lesion in the left CPA and IAC (*arrows*). **c** Axial MIP reconstruction of the 3D TSE T2-weighted data set clearly displaying the signal loss of the left membranous labyrinth (*large arrowheads*). Compare to the normal signal of the right membranous labyrinth (*small arrowheads*). Conclusion: Large vestibulocochlear schwannoma on the left side with clear signal loss on the MIP reconstructions in the membranous labyrinth. Because of the signal loss and the severe SNHL, a surgical approach via a translabyrinthine approach was performed

4.3 Other Cranial Nerve Schwannomas

Although signal intensities and post-contrast behavior of nonvestibular schwannomas in the CPA look similar to those of vestibular schwannomas, they are easily distinguished by the fact that they present with different symptoms, location, shape, and relationship to the skull base neuroforamina and canals (Borges 2007).

The most frequent nonvestibular schwannoma is the trigeminal schwannoma located cephalad to the vestibular schwannoma with an anteroposterior axis in relation to the CPA and very often with extension into Meckel's cave. The clinical features are predominantly trigeminal neuropathy (Fig. 36) (Borges 2007).

Facial nerve schwannoma may be difficult to distinguish from vestibulocochlear schwannoma because of the similar anatomical location and clinical presentation. However, differentiation can very often be made due to the particular extension pattern of the facial nerve schwannoma along the different segments of the nerve (Fig. 19).

A facial nerve schwannoma that only exists and originates in the IAC is virtually nonexisting. The most frequent site of origin is the region of the geniculate ganglion. From there on, it can extend and grow along the labyrinthine segment and the tympanic segment of the facial nerve and even into the middle fossa (Fig. 19) (Wiggins et al. 2006; Borges 2007).

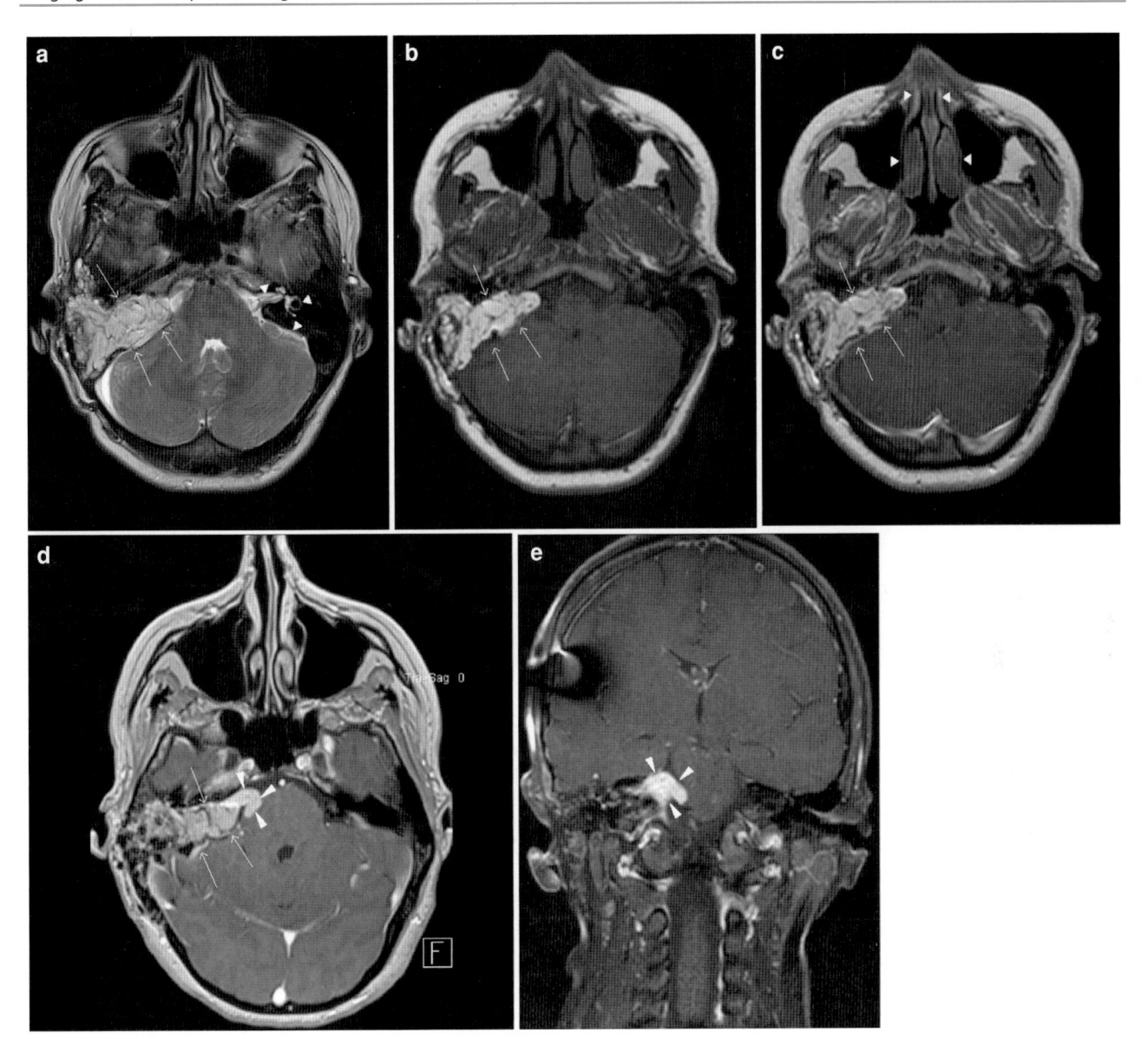

Fig. 25 30-year-old female with a prior history of a large right-sided vestibulocochlear schwannoma treated with translabyrinthine surgery. **a** Axial 4 mm thick TSE T2-weighted image through the posterior fossa. Note the normal aspect of the IAC and membranous labyrinth on the left side (*arrowheads*). On the right side, the entire temporal bone has been removed and the surgical defect has been filled up with (abdominal) fat (*arrows*). **b** Axial 2 mm thick SE T1-weighted image through the lower posterior fossa (slightly lower than Fig. 25a). The low signal of the right-sided temporal bone is replaced by the high signal of the abdominal fat (*arrows*). **c** Axial gadolinium-enhanced 2 mm thick SE T1-weighted image through the lower posterior fossa (same level as Fig. 25b). The signal intensity of the fat plug at the petrosectomy site remains unchanged (*arrows*) (compare to Fig. 25b). Note the clear enhancement of the turbinates (*arrowheads*) (compare to Fig. 25b). **d** Axial gadolinium-enhanced 2 mm thick SE T1-weighted image at the level of Meckel's cave. The level of this image is scanned at a higher level than Fig. 25b and c. The fat plug in the petrosectomy site is clearly seen (*arrows*). Medial to the fat plug an inversed C shaped enhancing nodule can be seen (*arrowheads*). This lesion is suspect of a residual vestibulocochlear schwannoma. **e** Coronal gadolinium-enhanced 2 mm thick SE T1-weighted image with fat sat. The signal intensity of the fat plug is homogeneously suppressed. Note the nodular enhancing remnant of the vestibulocochlear schwannoma (*arrowheads*) medial to the fat plug. Conclusion: Status post translabyrinthine surgery with filling up of the defect by abdominal fat and with a residual tumor focus in the depth of the defect

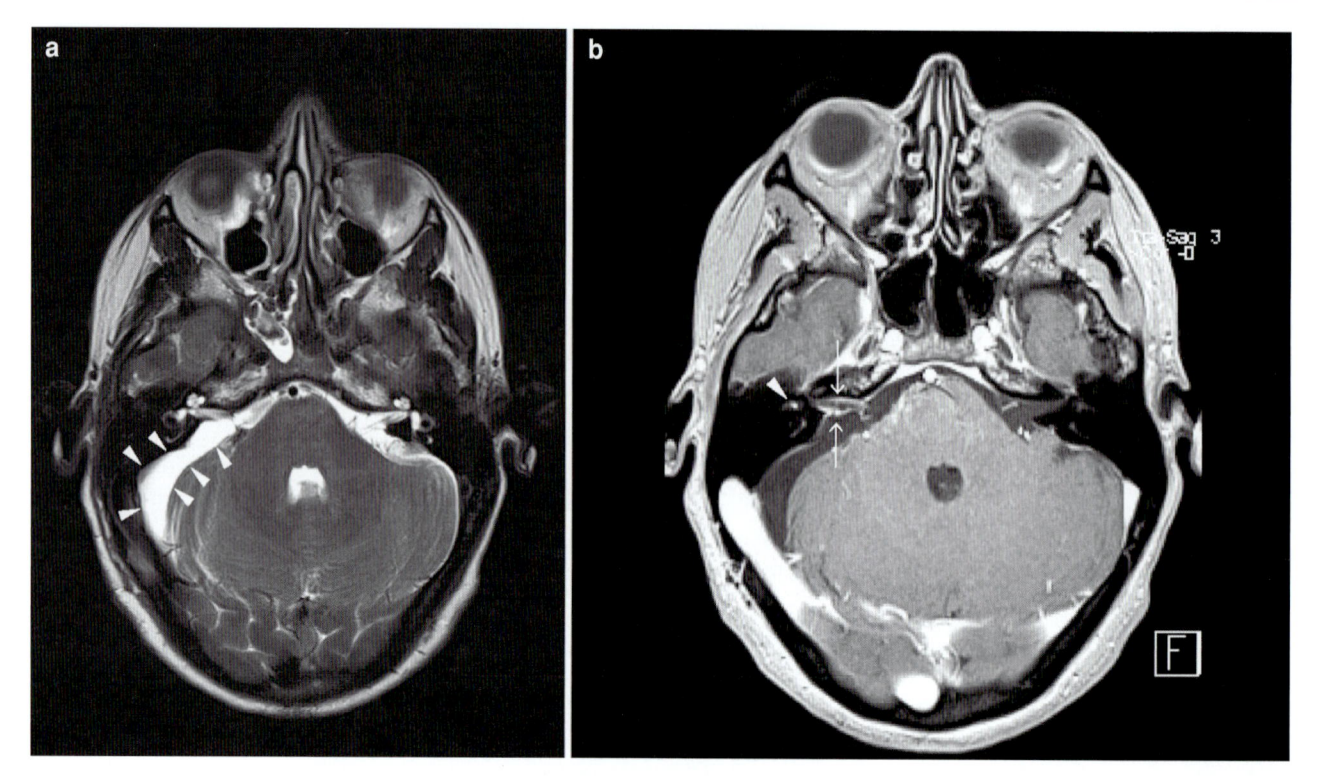

Fig. 26 56-year-old male with a prior history of right-sided surgery for vestibulocochlear schwannoma via retrosigmoidal approach. **a** Axial 4 mm thick TSE T2-weighted image through the posterior fossa. Note the subarachnoidal encapsulated fluid collection between the cerebellum and the posterior side of the temporal bone on the right side (*arrowheads*). **b** Axial gadolinium-enhanced 2 mm thick SE T1-weighted image through the posterior fossa at the level of the IAC. There is linear enhancement at the anterior en posterior delineation of the IAC on the right side (*arrows*). Note also the high intensity of the anterior limb of the superior semicircular canal on the right side, which (*arrowhead*) was already visible on unenhanced images (not shown): postoperative changes. Conclusion: Postoperative status via retrosigmoidal approach for a vestibulocochlear schwannoma. The linear enhancement in the IAC can be regarded as postoperative changes. This type of enhancement can last for years after surgery

Finally, glossopharyngeal, vagal, and spinal accessory nerve schwannomas may extend cranially into the CPA and may mimic an intracisternal vestibulocochlear schwannoma. However, a more caudad center and the extension towards and through an often enlarged jugular foramen can be clues to diagnosis. Differentiation with a jugular foramen meningioma can be difficult (Figs. 34 and 37). These lesions can be asymptomatic (Fig. 38) but can also present with swallowing difficulties (Fig. 37) or symptoms of pressure on the cerebellum and brain stem (Bonneville 2007a).

4.4 Metastasis

Meningeal enhancement can have various origins but causes are most frequently either metastatic (Figs. 6, 39, 40 and 41), infectious (Fig. 42), inflammatory (Figs. 43 and 44), reactive, or chemical.

Metastatic involvement of the CPA/IAC is not unfrequent. It is most frequently found in breast carcinoma (Figs. 6 and 39), bronchial carcinoma (Fig. 40) and melanoma (Fig. 41) (Bonneville 2007a; Warren et al. 2008).

Metastatic involvement can be hematogenic or by direct spread via CSF, the latter form being more frequent. In case of hematogenic spread, it often spreads into the skull base with moth-eaten lysis of the bones of the skull base (Fig. 45).

In case of CSF spread, differentiation should be made between leptomeningeal and pachymeningeal enhancement. In case of leptomeningeal enhancement (pia and arachnoid) the enhancement follows the convolutions of the gyri and involves the meninges around the basal cisterns. Pachymeningeal involvement is considered when the enhancement is thick, linear, and/or nodular along the inner surface of the calvarium, skull base and IAC, falx or tentorium without extension into the cortical gyri or basal cistern involvement (Kioumehr et al. 1995).

In case of metastatic disease, both types of enhancement can be seen but enhancement will most likely rather be pachymeningeal whereas leptomeningeal enhancement is more frequently seen in case of infectious origin (Bonneville 2007a; Warren et al. 2008).

Clinical symptoms are most frequently SNHL (Figs. 39, 40 and 41) and/or vertigo.

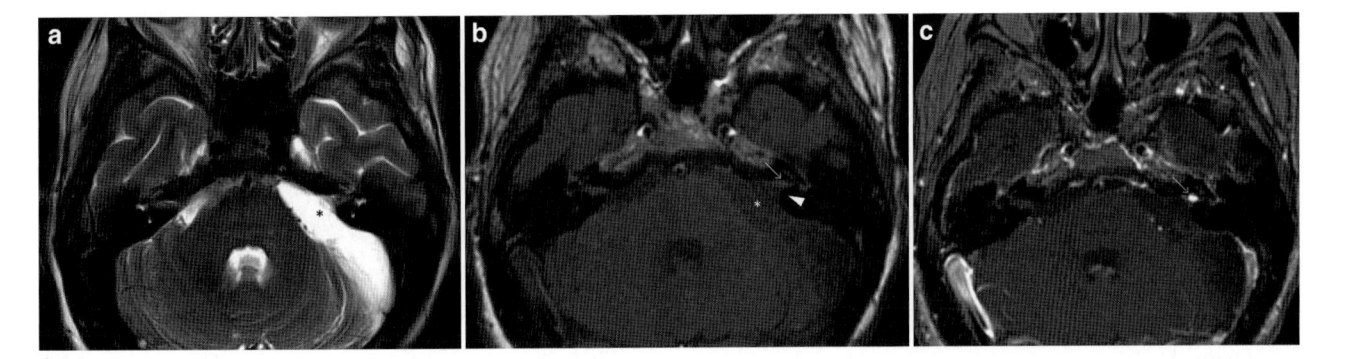

Fig. 27 58-year-old male with a prior history of vestibulocochlear schwannoma surgery via a retrosigmoidal approach on the left side. **a** Axial 4 mm TSE T2-weighted image through the posterior fossa demonstrating a large subarachnoidal encapsulated fluid collection (*asterisk*) as a sequel of the retrosigmoidal surgical approach. **b** Axial unenhanced 2 mm thick SE T1-weighted image through the posterior fossa. On the left side, the hypointense encapsulated subarachnoidal fluid collection is noted (*asterisk*) with amputation of the posterior side of the IAC (*arrowhead*). In the fundus of the IAC, a small isointense nodule can be found (*arrow*). **c** Axial gadolinium-enhanced 2 mm thick SE T1-weighted image with fat sat through the posterior fossa (same level as Fig. 27b): there is a small nodular enhancing lesion visible in the fundus of the IAC (*arrow*). The nodular aspect of the lesion makes it highly suspicious of a residual/recurrent vestibulocochlear schwannoma. Conclusion: Retrosigmoidal approach for a vestibulocochlear schwannoma with a small residual or recurrent schwannoma in the fundus of the IAC on the left side

Onset of symptoms is usually sudden (Figs. 39, 40 and 41) and can be unilateral or bilateral.

Sometimes, the clinical presentation of SNHL and/or vertigo can be the first manifestation of the disease (Fig. 40).

At imaging, the presence of multifocal cerebral/cerebellar lesions is highly suggestive of metastases, but CPA metastases may be solitary and mimic benign tumors of the CPA such as vestibulocochlear schwannomas (Figs. 39 and 41), or be bilateral, mimicking neurofibromatosis type 2 (Figs. 39 and 40) (Bonneville 2007a; Warren et al. 2008).

Imaging features are usually displacement of the fluid signal on heavily T2-weighted by hypointense tumoral tissue with enhancement after intravenous gadolinium administration on T1-weighted images. In case of pachymeningeal spread, enhancement can be more nodular and will follow posterior fossa bony surfaces. In case of leptomeningeal spread, enhancement will follow the cortical sulci.

Enhancement on T1-weighted images without any signal alteration on heavily T2-weighted sequences can also be found (Fig. 6).

In case of metastatic melanoma, a subtle intrinsic homogeneous T1 high signal intensity can be found due to the paramagnetic effect of the melanine contained in the tumor (Fig. 41) (Bonneville 2007a; Warren et al. 2008).

As mentioned above, differentiation of meningeal enhancement is difficult as many other infectious and inflammatory disease entities can cause meningeal thickening and enhancement. Differentiation should be made upon an extensive anamnesis, clinical and laboratory evaluation and can be extremely difficult (Kioumehr et al. 1995).

Various infectious entities can cause pachymeningitis such as tuberculosis and Cryptococcus infection (Fig. 42).

Other inflammatory disease entities that also can cause pachymeningitis are other granulomatous diseases such as rheumatoid disorders, sarcoidosis and Wegener granulomatosis (Fig. 43) (Kioumehr et al. 1995). Last but not least, if all other causes have been excluded, idiopathic pachymeningitis will be the final conclusion (Fig. 44).

4.5 Brain Stem and Cerebellar Tumoral Lesions

The vast majority of mass lesions in the CPA are extra-axial lesions of which the vestibulocochlear schwannomas and meningiomas are the most frequent lesions. In most cases, the extra-axial nature of a lesion is clear due to the fact that the lesions are separated from the brain parenchyma by a cleft of CSF. If large, they can also push the cranial nerves, the brain stem and even the cerebellum away as a sign of their extra-axial origin. However, if the CPA cistern is obliterated, the exact extra- or intra-axial origin of such a lesion sometimes cannot be determined.

Extensive peritumoral edema surrounding an enhancing lesion, centered on a significant mass effect obliterating the CPA cistern is highly likely to be an intra-axial lesion (Bonneville 2007b).

A large variety of tumoral lesions in the brain stem and cerebellum can be found such as medulloblastoma, ependymoma, papilloma, glioma, lymphoma, and medulloblastoma. The discussion of these different subtypes is beyond the scope of this chapter. Two examples presenting with an intra-axial tumoral lesion and SNHL will be illustrated.

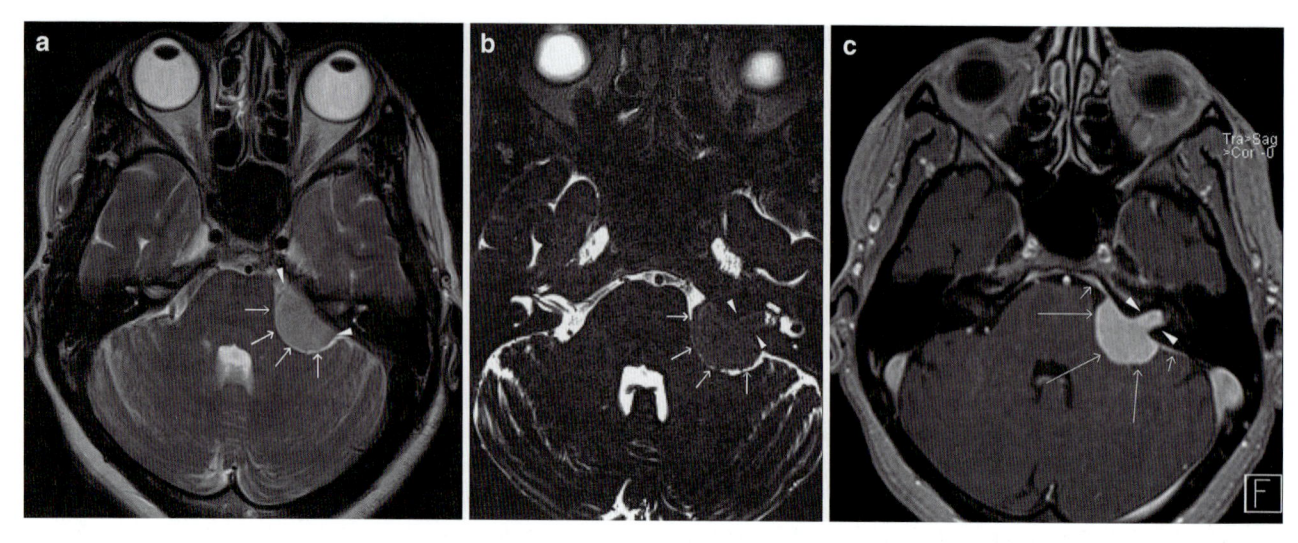

Fig. 28 26-year-old female investigated for left-sided facial numbness. **a** Axial 4 mm TSE T2-weighted image through the posterior fossa. A semi-lunar slightly hyperintense lesion is found in the left CPA (*arrows*). The lesion is broad-based against the posterior side of the temporal bone and has obtuse angles with the posterior side of the temporal bone (*arrowheads*). **b** Axial 0.4 mm thick 3D TSE T2-weighted image through the posterior fossa (same level as Fig. 28a) demonstrating the lesion against the posterior side of the temporal bone on the left side (*arrows*). Note the extension of the lesion in the IAC (*arrowheads*). **c** Axial gadolinium-enhanced 0.7 mm thick 3D GRE T1-weighted image through the posterior fossa (same level as Fig. 28a and b). The lesion (*large arrows*) is homogeneously enhancing with obtuse angles with the posterior side of the temporal bone. Note the extension into the IAC (*arrowheads*) as well as the dural tail on both sides of the lesion (*small arrows*). Conclusion: Surgically proven meningioma of the posterior fossa with extension into the IAC. The clinical findings in this patient could be explained by the fact that the meningioma was compressing the left trigeminal nerve at its anterior border

Glial tumors of the brain stem, and especially pilocytic astrocytomas in young adults can manifest as an asymmetrical expansion of the brain stem that even can be pedunculated in rare cases and be exophytic expanding in the CPA. Extension into and expansion of the IAC can also be found (Fig. 46). Usually the SNHL is not the major complaint, which is mainly caused by the mass effect of the lesion on the vestibulocochlear nerve. Imaging features are nonspecific: mass lesion with T2 hyperintensity, T1 hypointensity and variable enhancement depending on the glioma grade (Fig. 46) (Bonneville 2007b).

Primary central nervous system lymphomas may be either intra- or extra-axial in the CPA. However, except for the signs related to the location, imaging features are identical for both sides of origin. On MRI, they appear with an intermediate to low signal intensity on T1-weighted images with strong and homogeneous enhancement after gadolinium administration and a low signal intensity on T2-weighted images. The low signal intensity can be explained by the high cellularity of this type of tumor which also explains the diffusion restriction on ADC maps and the high signal on high *b*-value diffusion-weighted images. Intra-axial lesions may present as any other tumoral mass lesion in the brain stem, extra-axial lesions may mimic vestibulocochlear schwannomas (Fig. 47) (Bonneville 2007b).

5 Petrous Bone and Skull Base Lesions

The petrous apex forms the anterior and anterolateral border of the CPA. Several lesions originating in the petrous apex may extend into the CPA. These lesions can be incidental findings. Symptomatology is in most cases caused by compression of cranial nerves depending on its location. Most frequently the 5th, 7th, or 8th cranial nerve are compressed, giving rise to symptoms.

5.1 Chordomas

Chordomas are tumors of notochordal remnants. The two most common locations are the clivus and the sacrum. They usually are midline lesions, although lateral chordomas can occur. In most cases, extension to the CPA is limited. The relation to the clivus with its erosion is, however, crucial for the diagnosis (Fig. 48).

At CT, chordoma typically appears as a centrally located, well-circumscribed, expansile soft tissue mass associated to extensive lytic destruction of the clivus.

On MRI, chordomas display intermediate to low signal intensity on T1-weighted images with possible foci of T1 high signal intensity due to either residual ossified fragments, tumor calcification, or zones of high protein content or hemorrhage.

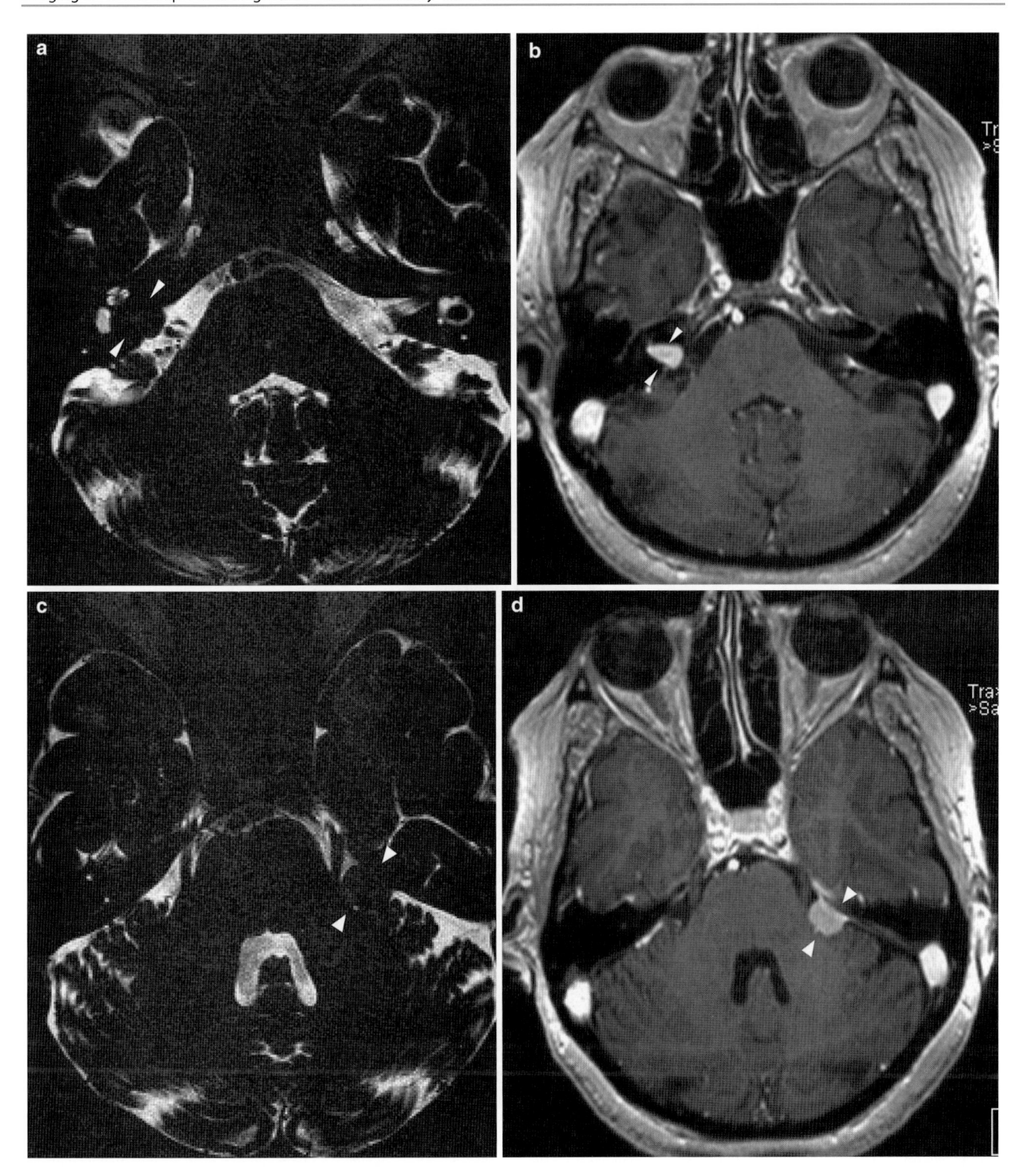

Fig. 29 70-year-old female investigated for SNHL on the right side and conductive hearing loss on the left side. **a** Axial 0.4 mm thick 3D TSE T2-weighted image through the posterior fossa demonstrating a lesion in the right IAC (*arrowheads*). **b** Axial gadolinium-enhanced 0.7 mm thick 3D GRE T1-weighted image through the posterior fossa shows the lesion as an enhancing lesion with a component in the IAC, slightly protruding in the CPA (*arrowheads*). **c** Axial 0.4 mm thick 3D TSE T2-weighted image through the posterior fossa at the level of the trigeminal nerve. There is a small nodular lesion against the posterior side of the temporal bone (*arrowheads*). **d** Axial gadolinium-enhanced 0.7 mm thick 3D GRE T1-weighted image through the posterior fossa shows the lesion as a small enhancing nodule (*arrowheads*). Note the obtuse angles of the lesion with the posterior side of the temporal bone. Conclusion: Right-sided vestibulocochlear schwannoma and left-sided meningioma. The meningioma was a coincident finding in this investigation for SNHL on the right side. The conductive hearing loss on the left side could be explained by otospongiosis, as diagnosed on CT scan (not shown). This patient also had a dehiscent superior semicircular canal (not shown)

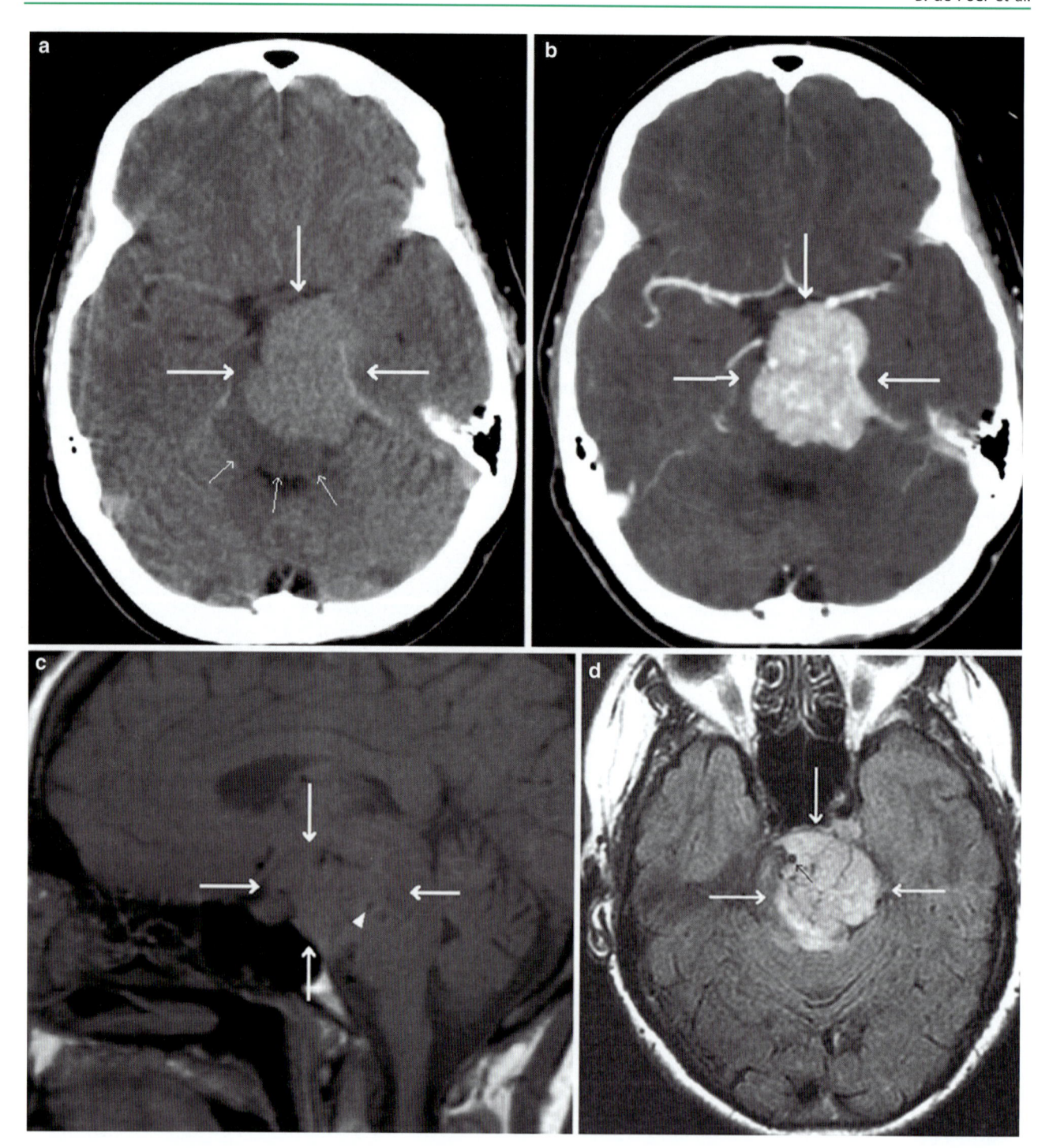

Fig. 30 59-year-old female presenting with swallowing difficulties. A barium swallow was considered normal. **a** Axial unenhanced CT scan of the brain showing a large nodular slightly hyperdense lesion (*large arrows*) with compression of the brain stem (*small arrows*). **b** Axial contrast-enhanced CT scan (same level as Fig. 30a) displays the strong enhancement of the lesion (*large arrows*). **c** Sagittal 5 mm thick unenhanced SE T1-weighted image displaying the isointense mass lesion (*large arrows*) with internal signal voids due to the supplying arteries (*small arrowhead*) compressing the brain stem. **d** Axial 5 mm thick FLAIR sequence showing the large hyperintense mass lesion (*large arrows*) partially encasing the basilar artery (*small arrow*). **e** Axial 5 mm thick FSE T2-weighted image. The lesion shows a moderate hyperintensity (*large arrows*). Note again the encasing of the basilar artery (*small arrow*). The linear hypointensities in the lesion represent arteries in the lesion. **f** Axial 5 mm thick gadolinium-enhanced SE T1-weighted image showing the strong enhancement of the lesion (*large arrows*). The brainstem is compressed and the basilar artery is encased. **g** Sagittal 5 mm thick gadolinium-enhanced SE T1-weighted image (same level as Fig. 30c). The lesion is strongly enhancing (*large arrows*). **h** Coronal 4 mm thick gadolinium-enhanced SE T1-weighted image. Strong enhancement of the lesion (*large arrows*) centered over the petrous bone apex and extending as a large nodular lesion in the posterior fossa. Conclusion: Large petrous bone apex meningioma extending into the CPA and compressing the brainstem. Patient was treated by focalized radiotherapy which stabilized the lesion and has lead to a reduction in size after 5 years (not shown)

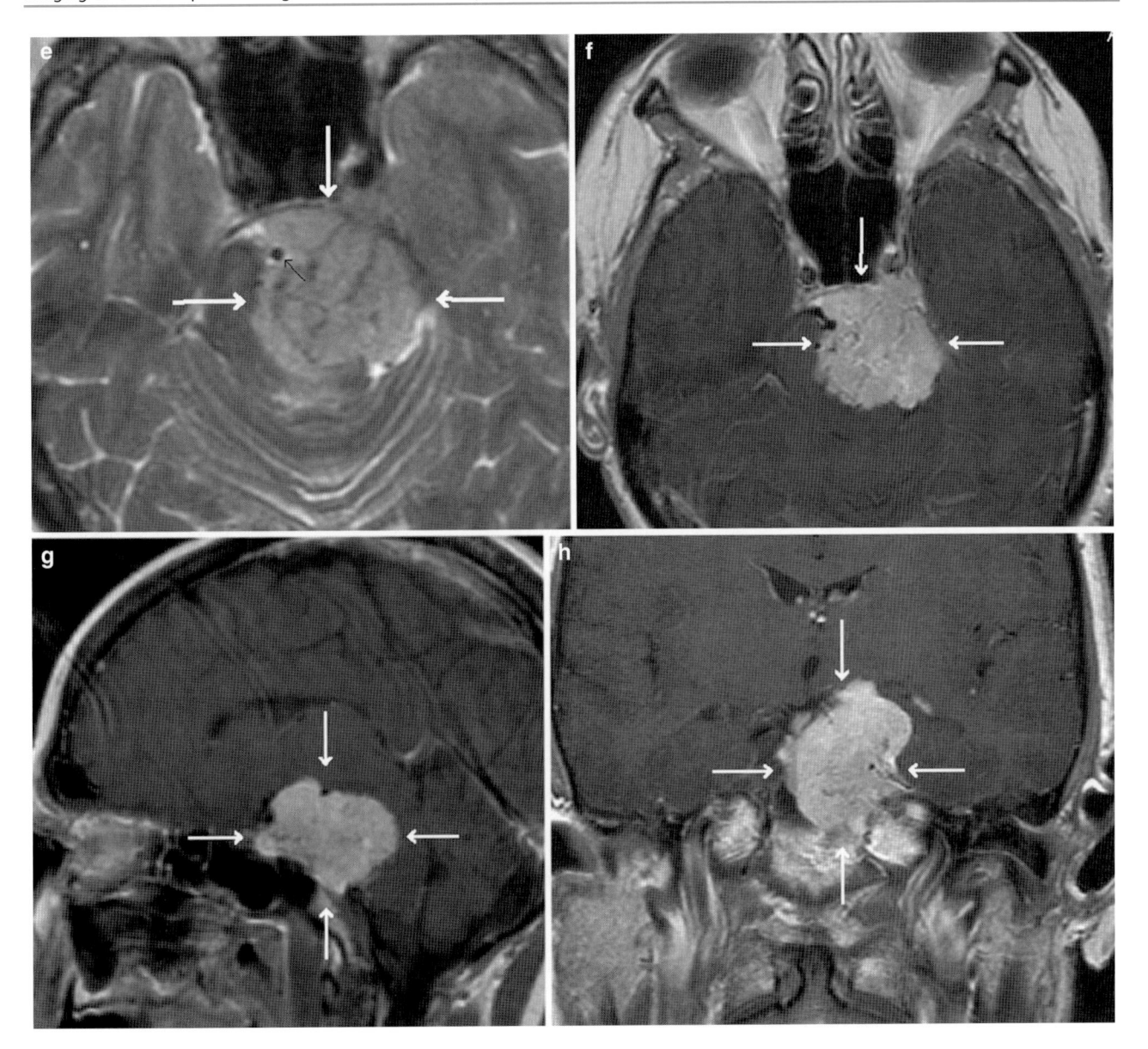

Fig. 30 continued

On T2-weighted MRI, they demonstrate very high signal intensity and septae of low signal intensity. Slight enhancement after contrast administration can be found (Bonneville 2007b; Mohan et al. 2012; Juliano 2013).

5.2 Chondrosarcomas

Chondrosarcomas are malignant tumors composed of cartilage producing cells arising from persistent islands of embryonal cartilage that occur near the skull base synchondroses. They are rare entities, representing 0.15 % of all intracranial tumors and 6 % of all skull base tumors. These tumors usually originate off midline at the petro-occipital fissure or near the jugular foramen with subsequent possible invasion into the CPA. They can be asymptomatic but when becoming large, they may cause symptoms of cranial nerve palsies such as diplopia, hoarseness, swallowing difficulties, facial dysesthesia, hearing loss, headache, and gait disturbances. The malignant potential of these lesions is associated not only with histological subtypes and grade of differentiation but also with the location of the tumor in the skull base and its proximity to vital neurovascular structures (Bonneville 2007b; Mohan et al. 2012; Juliano 2013).

On CT, cartilaginous tumors are hypo- to iso-attenuating with intratumoral calcifications. On MRI, intensities are low

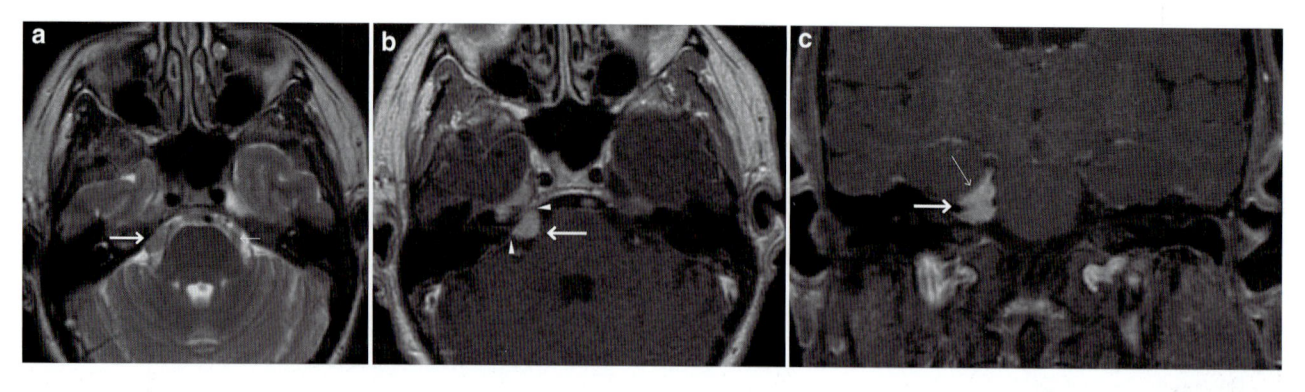

Fig. 31 74-year-old male with right-sided trigeminal neuropathy. **a** Axial 4 mm thick FSE T2-weighted image. Nodular slightly hyperintense lesion in the upper part of the right CPA (*large arrow*) with loss of delineation of the right trigeminal nerve. Note the normal trigeminal nerve on the left side (*small arrow*). **b** Axial 4 mm thick gadolinium-enhanced SE T1-weighted image. Nodular lesion (*arrow*) with sharp borders with the posterior side of the temporal bone (*arrows*). **c** Coronal 4 mm thick gadolinium-enhanced SE T1-weighted image with fatsat. The nodular lesion (*large arrow*) is hanging down from the tentorium where it is originating (*small arrow*). Conclusion: Small meningioma originating from the tentorium and hanging in the CPA where it has—in the axial plane—imaging features of a schwannoma. However, the coronal plane is clearly showing the origin of the lesion, enabling the diagnosis of a meningioma

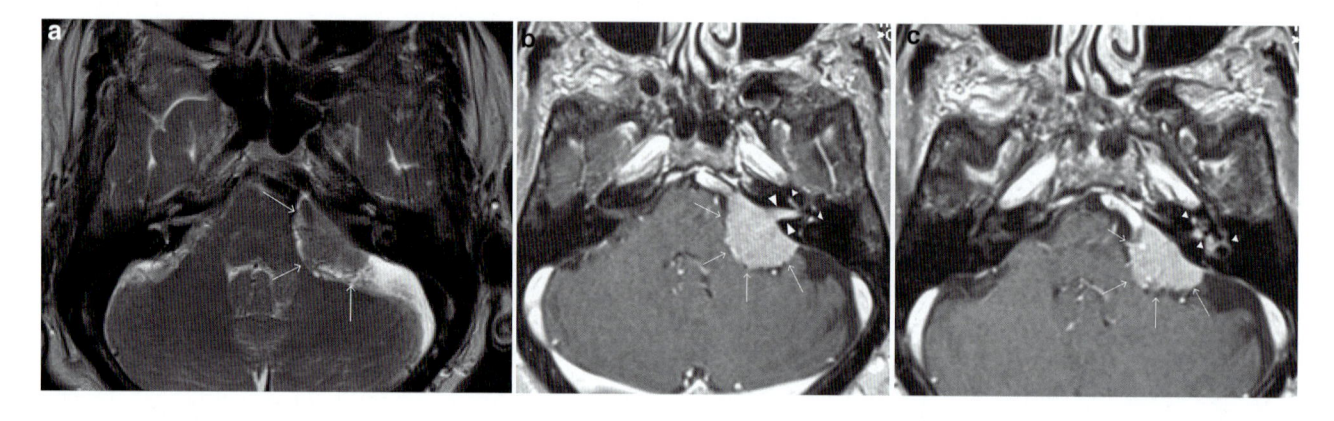

Fig. 32 80-year-old male investigated for a long standing progressive SNHL. **a** Axial 4 mm thick TSE T2-weighted image through the posterior fossa at the level of the IAC. Broad-based slightly hyperintense mass lesion in the left CPA (*arrows*) against the posterior side of the temporal bone pyramid. **b** Axial gadolinium-enhanced 1 mm thick GRE T1-weighted image at the level of the IAC. The lesion is homogeneously enhancing and broad-based over the posterior side of the temporal bone (*arrows*). Note the extension into the IAC (*large arrowheads*). Even the membranous labyrinth is filled up with enhancing tumor (*small arrowheads*). **c** Axial gadolinium-enhanced 1 mm thick GRE T1-weighted image at the upper level of the CPA (image position slightly higher than Fig. 32b). The mass lesion is broad-based against the posterior side of the temporal bone (*arrows*). Note the complete enhancement of the membranous labyrinth—cochlea, vestibule, and semicircular canals—due to tumor invasion (*arrowheads*). Conclusion: Large meningioma centered over the IAC and invading into the IAC with invasion into the entire membranous labyrinth

on unenhanced T1-weighted images with high signal intensity on T2-weighted images. Enhancement can be seen and the curvilinear aspect of the enhancement is called ring-and-arc pattern (Fig. 49).

5.3 Cholesterol Granulomata

The cholesterol granuloma is an expansile lesion of the petrous bone apex which can also be found in the middle ear. In the middle ear it is believed to be the consequence of chronic middle ear and otomastoid inflammation. In the petrous apex it is believed to be caused by inadequate ventilation of a pneumatized petrous apex, resulting in a negative pressure, reabsorption of air, mucosal edema, and hemorrhage with local tissue breakdown and cholesterol formation leading to a foreign body reaction.

A second—more recent—theory is based upon exposed bone marrow as a result of progressive and aggressive pneumatisation of the petrous bone apex that leads to coaptation of bone marrow and mucosa, eliciting hemorrhage that obstructs the apical outflow tract. This process leads to breakdown of the blood and foreign body reaction with subsequent cyst formation and bony expansion.

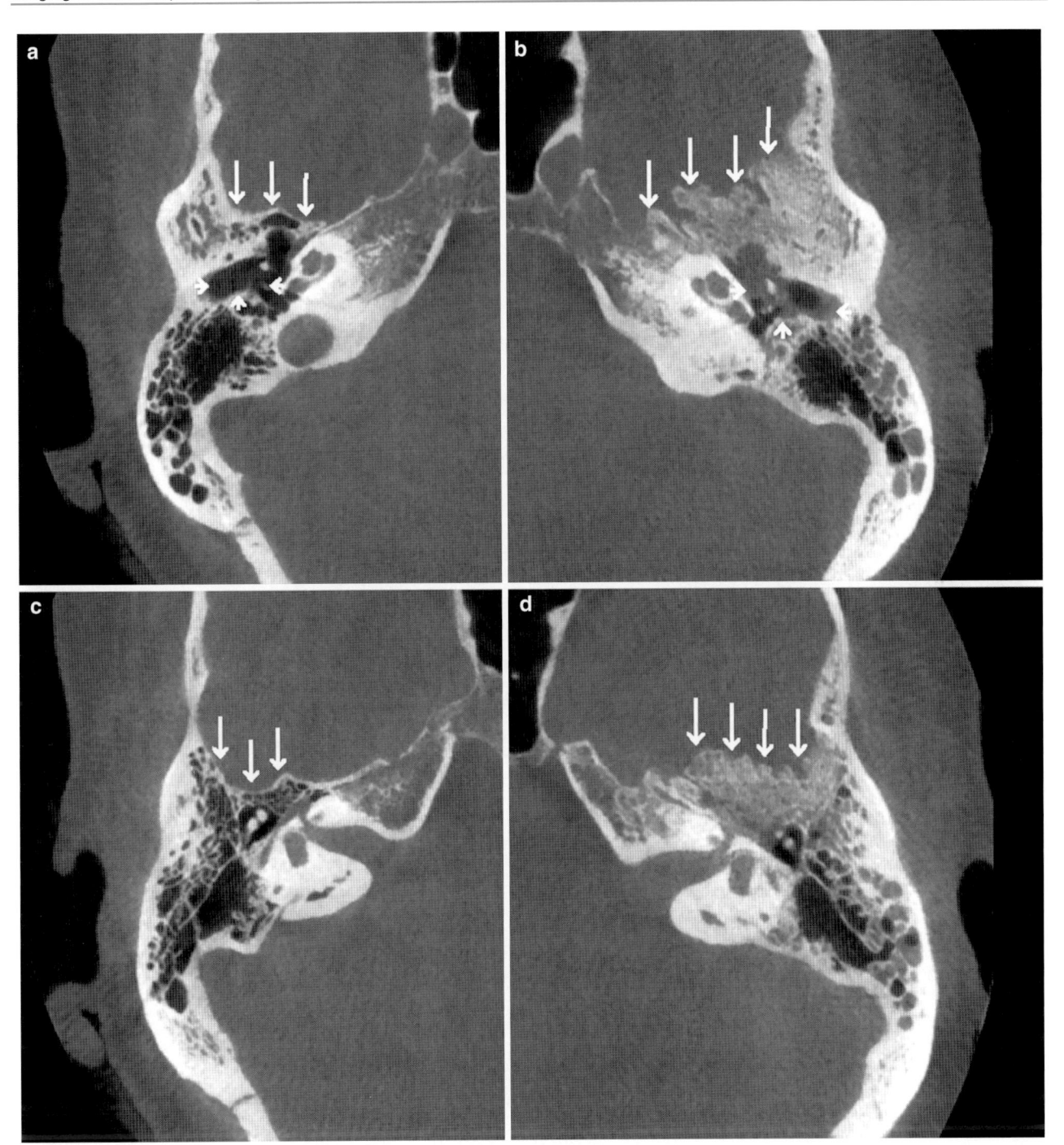

Fig. 33 44-year-old female investigated for signs of chronic otitis media on the left side and a clear conductive hearing loss. **a** Axial CBCT image at the level of the basal turn of the cochlea on the right side. The middle ear is well aerated without any signs of opacification (*small arrow*). Note the normal—very thin—delineation of the anterior wall of the middle ear (*large arrows*). **b** Axial CBCT image at the level of the basal turn of the cochlea on the left side (same level as Fig. 33a). Note the opacification of the middle ear (*small arrows*). Most striking, however, is the thickened and sclerotic aspect of the anterior wall of the middle ear (*large arrows*). Compare to the normal contralateral side in Fig. 33a. **c** Axial CBCT image at the level of the vestibule and labyrinthine segment of the facial nerve on the right side. Note the normal aspect of the anterior wall of the middle ear cavity (*large arrows*) and the nicely aerated aspect of the middle ear. **d** Axial CBCT image at the level of the vestibule and labyrinthine segment of the facial nerve (same level as Fig. 33c). Image acquisition is slightly higher than in Fig. 33a and b. Note again the striking sclerotic and thickened aspect of the anterior wall of the middle ear (*large arrows*). **e** Coronal CBCT image at the level of the anterior wall of the right middle ear. Normal aspect of the anterior wall of the middle ear. **f** Coronal CBCT at the level of the anterior wall of the left middle ear (same level as Fig. 33e). Note the thickened and sclerotic aspect of the anterior wall of the middle ear (*large arrows*). Compare to right side in Fig 33e. **g** Axial 4 mm thick TSE T2-weighted image through the posterior fossa. Note the hyperintense material in the left middle ear (*small arrows*) and the hypointense thickened aspect of the anterior wall of the middle ear

◀ (*large arrows*). **h** Axial 0.7 mm gadolinium-enhanced 3D GRE T1-weighted image (slightly higher than Fig. 33g). Note the global hypointense thickening of the anterior wall of the left-sided middle ear (*large arrows*) with clear enhancement (*small arrows*). Conclusion: Typical imaging features of an en-plaque-meningioma of the left middle ear in the anterior and cranial wall of the middle ear cavity. There is an associated inflammation in the middle ear causing the complaints and conductive hearing loss of the patient

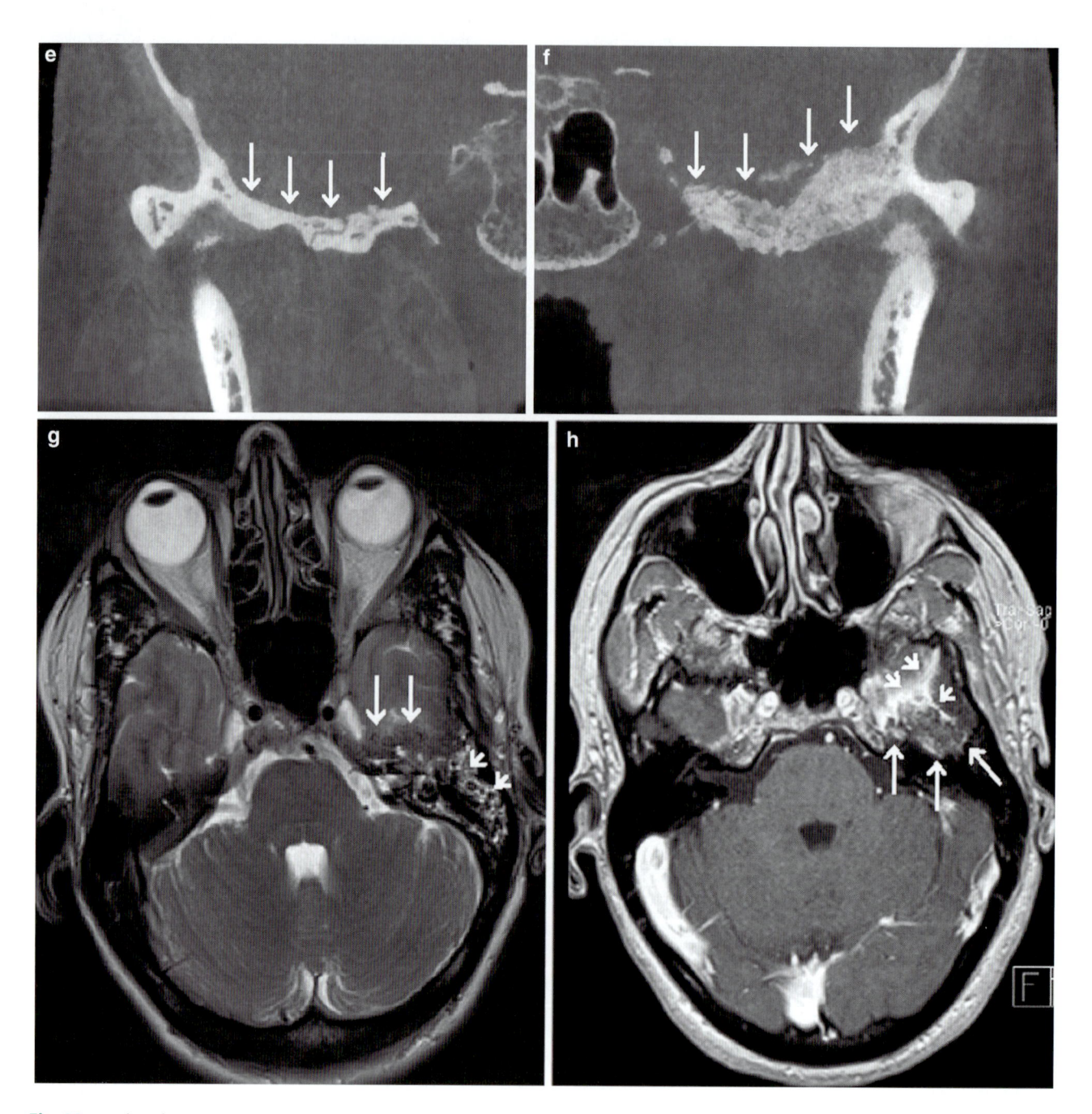

Fig. 33 continued

One of the most important features is that the lesion contains blood degradation products resulting in a characteristic high signal intensity on T1 and T2-weighted images. On CT, the lesion has a location in the petrous bone apex with an expansile aspect and a sharp delineation. A cholesterol granuloma develops almost always in a pneumatized petrous bone apex and as symmetry in pneumatization is usually the case, the presence of a contralateral highly

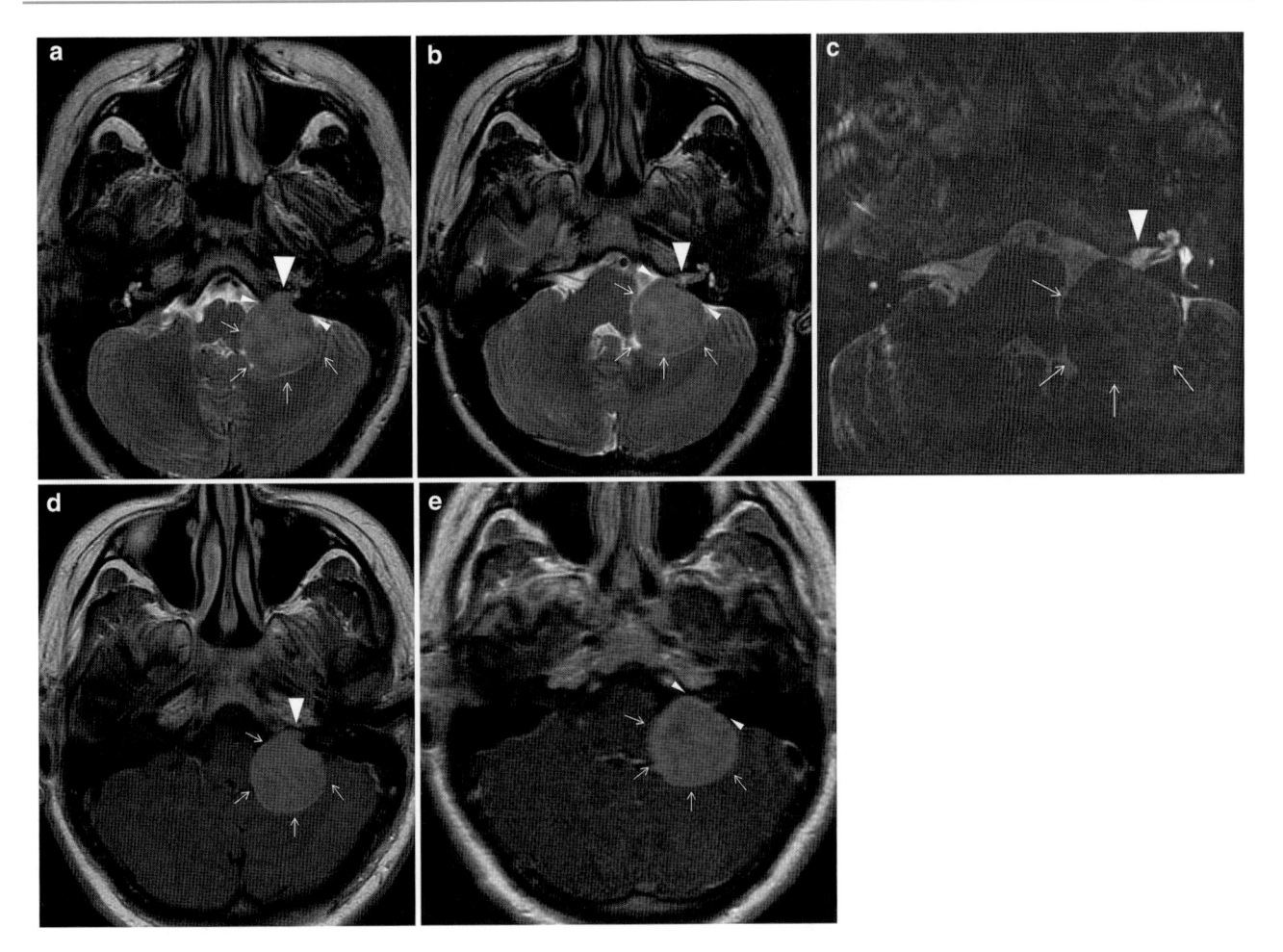

Fig. 34 42-year-old female investigated for sudden deafness on the left side. **a** Axial 3 mm TSE T2-weighted MR image through the posterior fossa. Moderately intense nodular lesion (*arrows*) in the lower left CPA with tail-like extension (*large arrowhead*) toward the jugular foramen. Note that the lesion has sharp borders with the posterior side of the lower petrous bone (*small arrowheads*). **b** Axial 3 mm TSE T2-weighted MR image trough the posterior fossa at the level of the IAC. The lesion (*arrows*) is located eccentric over the IAC (*large arrowhead*) and has sharp borders with the posterior side of the temporal bone (*small arrowheads*). **c** Axial 1 mm thick FSE T2-weighted image through the posterior fossa at the level of the IAC displaying the lesion (*arrows*) crossing the IAC (*large arrowhead*). Note that the cisternal course of the vestibulocochlear nerve and the facial nerve no longer can be seen. **d** Axial gadolinium-enhanced 2 mm thick SE T1-weighted image through the lower posterior fossa (same level as Fig. 34a). The lesion is homogeneously enhancing (*arrows*). Note the tail-like extension toward the jugular foramen (*large arrowhead*). **e** Axial gadolinium-enhanced 2 mm thick SE T1-weighted image through the posterior fossa at the level of the IAC (same level as Fig. 34b). Note the homogeneous enhancing lesion (*arrows*) with sharp margins against the posterior side of the temporal bone (*small arrowheads*) Conclusion: Mass lesion apparently originating in the lower CPA with extension toward the jugular foramen. Presumed diagnosis was a schwannoma of the mixed nerves due to its relationship with the jugular foramen and the sharp borders with the posterior side of the temporal bone pyramid. At surgery, a large meningioma—originating from the jugular foramen—was found. The presenting symptom of the patient—sudden left-sided deafness—could be explained by the pressure of the meningioma on the 7th and 8th cranial nerve

pneumatized petrous bone apex favors the diagnosis in a contralateral petrous bone apex. On CT the lesion is sharply delineated and expansile, with sometimes—in case of a large lesion—cortical tinning of the bone of the petrous apex (Fig. 50) (Bonneville 2007b; Mohan et al. 2012; Juliano 2013; de Foer et al. 2010).

Differential diagnosis lies in the asymmetrical petrous bone apex. An asymmetrical fat deposition is the most important differential diagnosis in which the petrous bone apex can display a high signal intensity on T1 as well as T2-weighted images. The solution is most likely presented by CT scan on which the lesion is completely filled with fatty bony marrow. Moreover, an asymmetrical fat deposition will never display an expansile aspect and its aspect on CT scan will display an homogeneous fat filled bony marrow instead of a lytic lesion (Mohan et al. 2012; de Foer et al. 2010).

One of the other most frequent differential diagnosis is the asymmetrical aerated petrous bone apex with fluid opacification and/or mucocele formation. In this entity

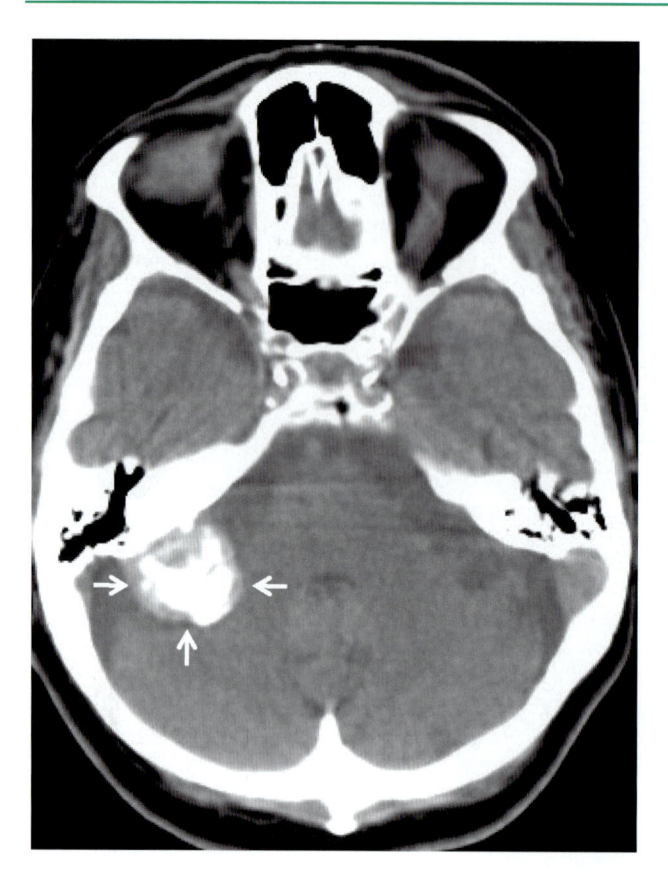

Fig. 35 98-year-old male admitted to hospital with suspicion of an acute cerebral infarction. Axial unenhanced CT image through the posterior fossa. Large calcificied broad-based lesion against the posterior side of the right temporal bone (*arrows*). Conclusion: Coincident finding of a large calcified meningioma of the posterior side of the right temporal bone

the petrous bone apex is aerated on one side and opacified presenting with a homogeneous signal intensity on T2-weighted images and a homogeneous low signal intensity on T1-weighted images with possible peripheral enhancement. In case of a mucocele, signal intensities on T1-weighted images may be higher depending on the protein composition of the fluid contents. However, intensity on T1-weighted images will not be as high as in case of a cholesterol granuloma.

A petrous bone cholesterol granuloma can be a coincident finding. If symptomatic—most likely in case of a cholesterol granuloma abutting the IAC or inner ear—SNHL and/or tinnitus can be found.

The clue of diagnosis is given by the fact that the lesion is expansile and that it displays a high signal intensity on both T1-weighted as well as T2-weighted MRI sequences (Fig. 50) (Mohan et al. 2012; de Foer et al. 2010).

Another differential diagnosis is the petrous bone apex cholesteatoma. Discussion still exists whether this is a primary or congenital cholesteatoma or an acquired cholesteatoma that has spread to an aerated petrous bone apex. Signal intensities are equal to the signal intensities of the much more common middle ear cholesteatoma that is low signal intensity on T1-weighted images, high signal intensity on T2-weighted images with some possible peripheral enhancement. Diffusion-weighted sequences will confirm diagnosis due to the high signal intensity on *b*1000 diffusion-weighted images. Preference should be given to non-EP diffusion-weighted sequences as they display no artifacts at the skull base.

5.4 Endolymphatic Sac Tumors

Endolymphatic sac tumor (ELST) also known as papillary adenomatous tumor of the temporal bone is a rare neoplasm that occurs as a locally invasive mass in a retrolabyrinthine location on the location of the endolymphatic sac. If large enough, they may extend into the middle ear and CPA and even compress the brain stem.

ELST occurs either isolated or in the context of von Hipple-Lindau disease.

SNHL is seen in nearly all patients. Other symptoms included facial nerve palsy, pulsatile tinnitus, and vertigo (Bonneville 2007b; Mohan et al. 2012; Juliano 2013).

ELST is an extradural tumor that erodes and destroys the retrolabyrinthine petrous bone. On CT, the lesion is aggressive looking with moth-eaten margins on CT and intratumoral calcifications. A thin rim of calcifications along the posterior margin of the tumor is common.

At MRI, the lesion is heterogeneous on both T1-weighted and T2-weighted images, with foci of high signal intensity due to intratumoral subacute hemorrhage. A T1- and T2-hyperintense cystic component, rich in blood and proteins, may be present and is suggestive of the diagnosis in this very specific location (Fig. 51). Flow voids can be seen when the tumor is larger than 2 cm. There is heterogeneous enhancement on contrast-enhanced MR imaging (Bonneville 2007b; Mohan et al. 2012; Juliano 2013).

5.5 Paragangliomas

Paragangliomas arise from the extra-adrenal neural crest-derived paraganglia, the glomus bodies. The glomus bodies can be found on various locations in the head and neck region. In the temporal bone these glomus bodies are located against the cochlear promontory in the middle ear giving rise to the glomus tympanicum. They can also be found in proximity of the jugular foramen giving rise to glomus jugulare tumors. When becoming large and extending into the middle ear, the term glomus jugulotympanicum is used. Most of these jugulotympanic tumors arise in association with the glomus formations of the inferior tympanic branch of the glossopharyngeaus nerve

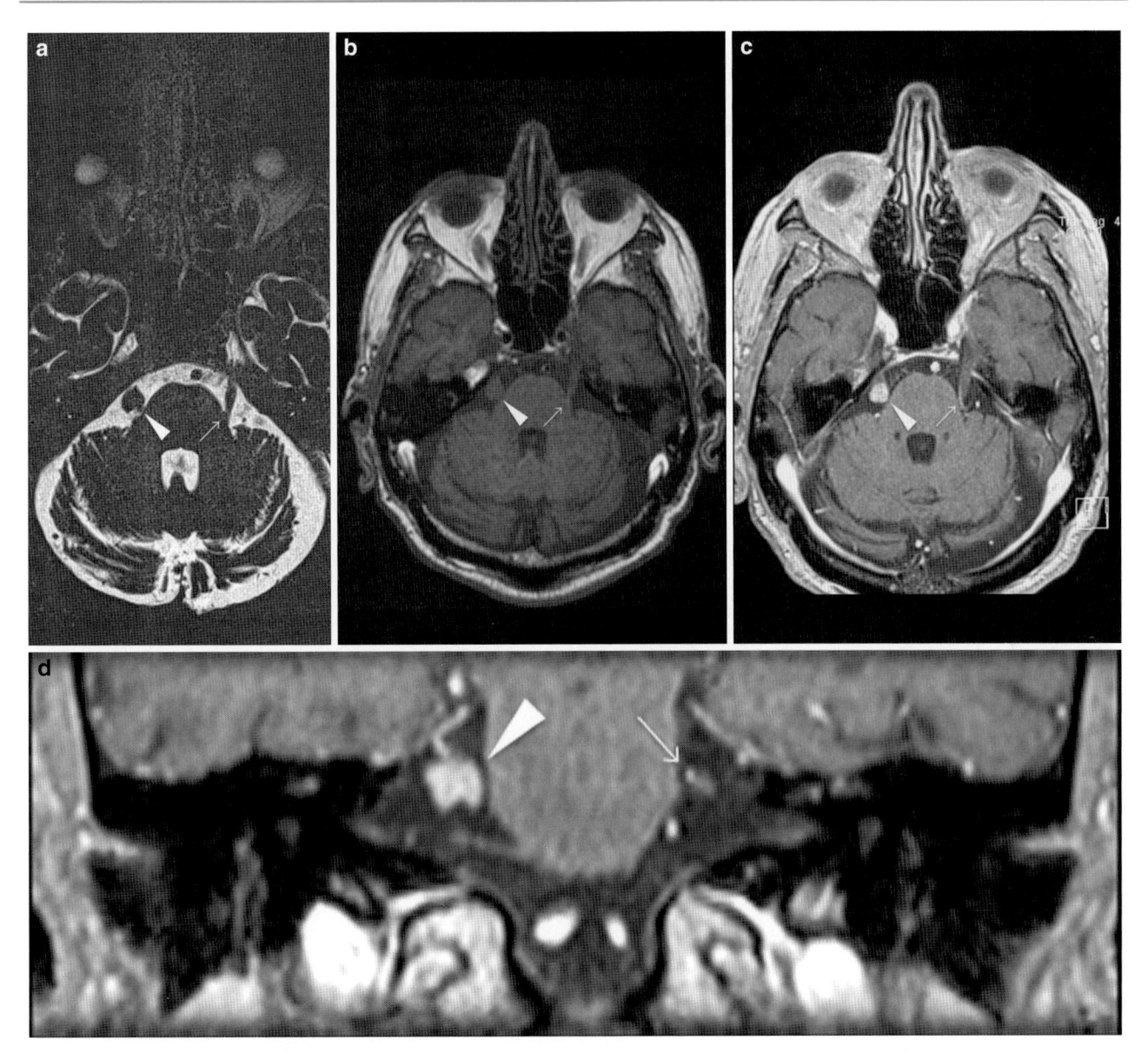

Fig. 36 75-year-old male with trigeminal neuropathy on the right side. **a** Axial 0.4 mm thick 3D TSE T2-weighted image through the posterior fossa at the level of the trigeminal nerve. There is a nodular lesion visible on the right trigeminal nerve (*arrowhead*). Compare to the normal trigeminal nerve on the left side (*arrow*). **b** Axial 2 mm thick SE T1-weighted image showing the nodular thickening of the right trigeminal nerve (*arrowhead*). Compare to the normal trigeminal nerve on the left side (*arrow*). **c** Axial gadolinium-enhanced 0.7 mm thick 3D GRE T1-weighted image. The lesion is homogeneously enhancing (*arrowhead*). Compare to the normal trigeminal nerve on the left side (*arrow*). **d** Coronal reformation of the 3D GRE T1-weighted dataset demonstrating the lesion on the right side (*arrowhead*). Compare to the normal trigeminal nerve on the left side (*arrow*). Conclusion: Schwannoma of the right sided trigeminal nerve

(Jacobson nerve) or the mastoid branch of the vagus nerve (Arnold's nerve).

Clinically, patients typically present with pulsatile tinnitus, conductive hearing loss, and possibly SNHL. In case of large tumors, multiple lower cranial neuropathies may occur (Bonneville 2007b; Mohan et al. 2012; Juliano 2013).

Glomus jugulotympanicum tumors present on CT as lesions centered on the jugular foramen with ill-defined moth-eaten. Soft tissue components may extend into the middle ear but also extracranially through the jugular foramen.

On MRI, the lesion is isointense on unenhanced T1-weighted images with multiple flow voids due to the vessels in the lesion causing the characteristic salt and pepper appearance where the pepper represents the hypointense dots caused by the flow voids of the feeding arteries

196   B. de Foer et al.

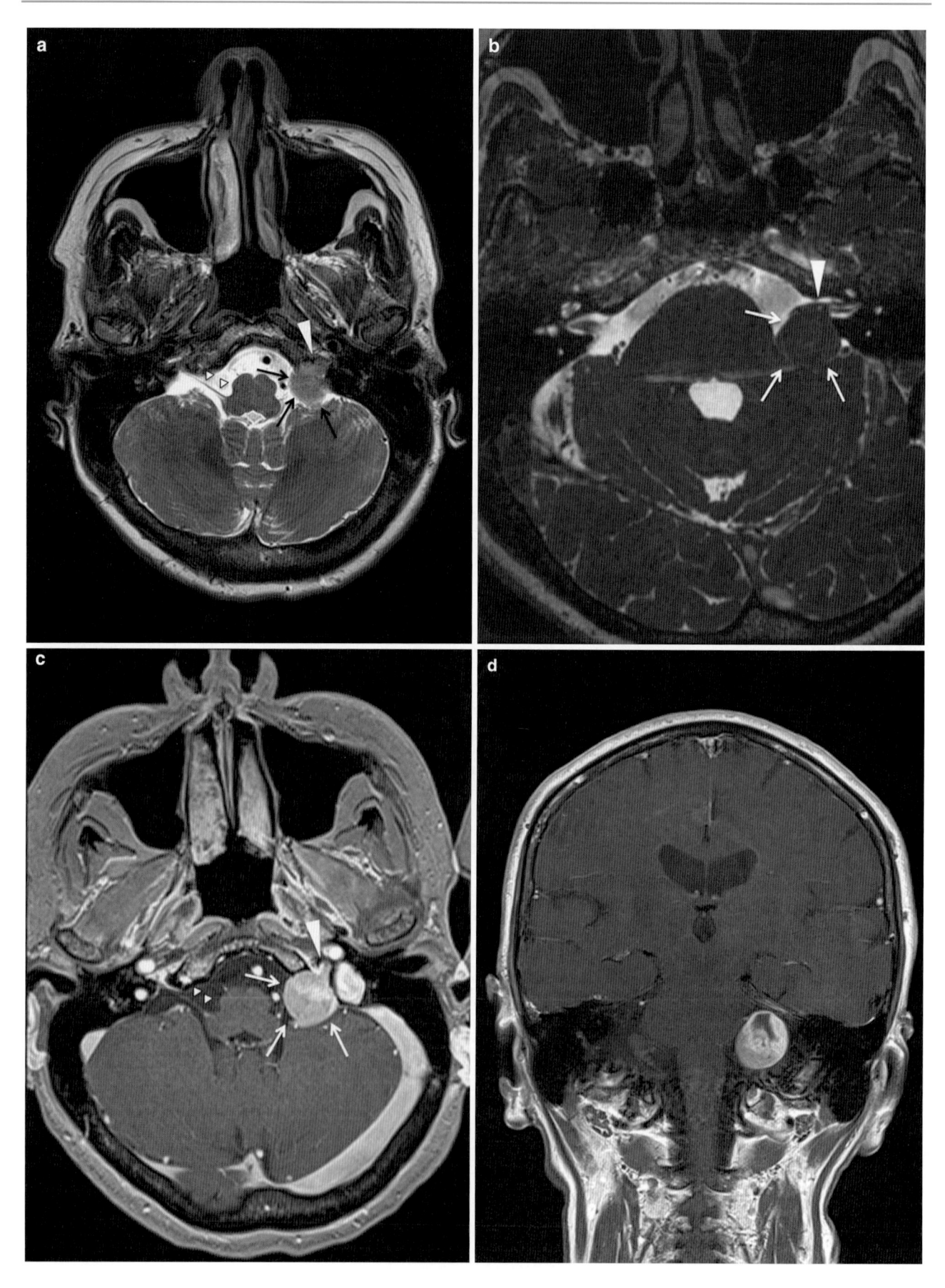

Fig. 37 62-year-old female investigated for swallowing difficulties. Clinical examination as well as a barium swallowing were considered negative. **a** Axial 2 mm thick TSE T2-weighted image through the lower posterior fossa at the level of the mixed nerves. Note a slightly more intense mass lesion in the left CPA (*arrows*) with a small extension towards the jugular foramen (*large arrowhead*). Note the normal 9th, 10th, and 11th nerves on the right side (*small arrowheads*). **b** Axial 1 mm thick CISS image at the level of the IAC. The upper pole of the mass lesion (*arrows*) is reaching the level of the IAC and is partially covering the porus acousticus internus (*arrowhead*). Patient had no SNHL. **c** Axial gadolinium-enhanced 2 mm thick SE T1-weighted image (same level as Fig. 37a) displaying the homogeneous enhancement of the lesion (arrows) with the small tail-like extension toward the jugular foramen (*large arrowhead*). Note again the normal mixed nerve on the right side (*small arrowheads*). **d** Coronal gadolinium-enhanced 2 mm thick SE T1-weighted image. The lesion is originating in the lower part of the left CPA with extension upwards into the left CPA. Conclusion: Schwannoma of the 9th, 10th, and 11th cranial nerves (mixed nerves) on the left side, confirmed at surgery

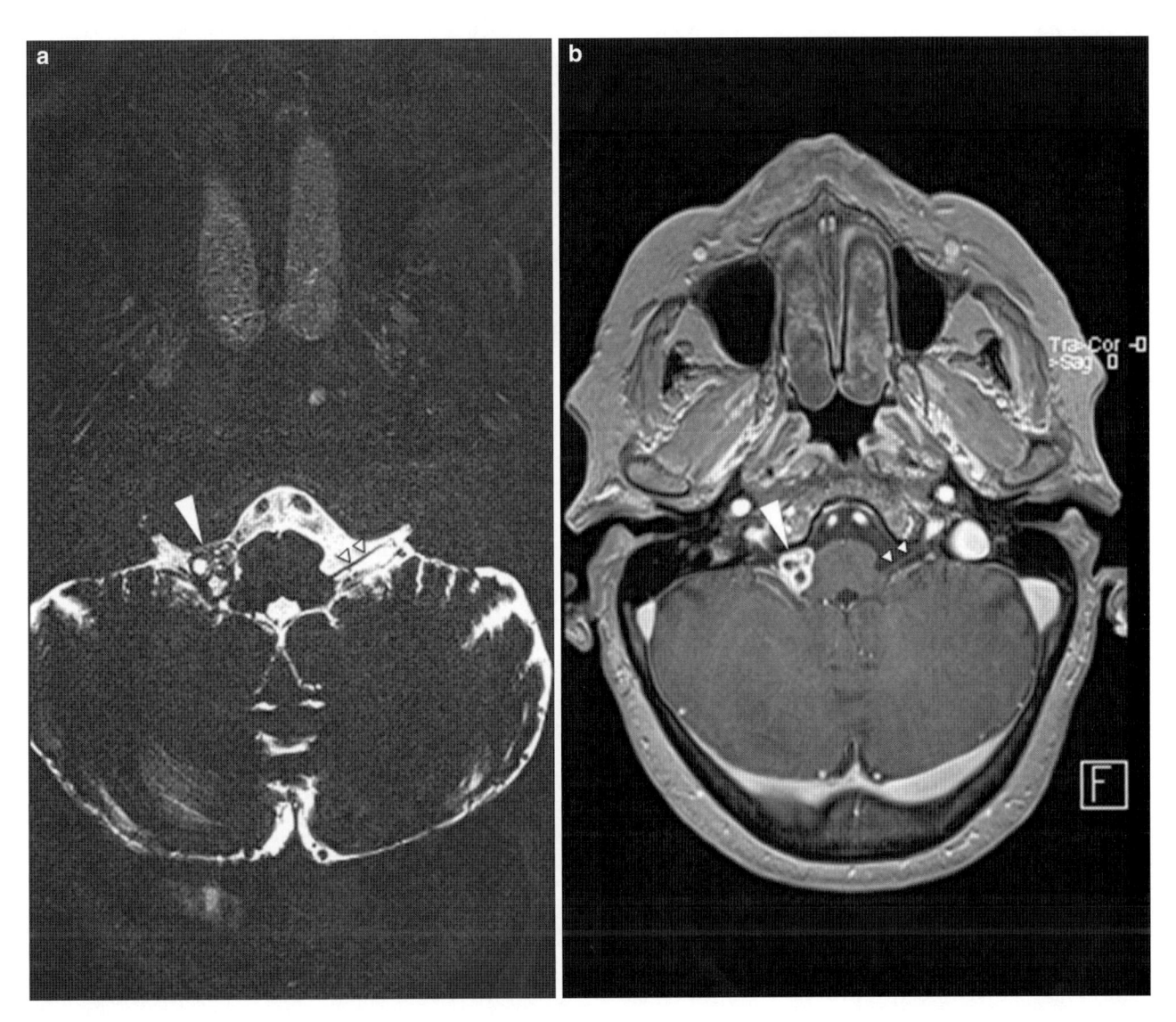

Fig. 38 36-year-old male investigated for SNHL on the right side. **a** Axial 0.4 mm thick TSE T2-weighted image through the lower CPA at the level of the mixed nerves. The nerves are clearly visible on the left side (*small arrowheads*). On the right side a small nodule (*large arrowhead*) containing small cysts is visible. **b** Axial gadolinium-enhanced 0.7 mm thick 3D GRE T1-weighted image. The lesion is clearly visible as a small enhancing nodule (*large arrowhead*) containing small cysts. Note again the normal mixed nerve on the left side (*small arrowheads*). Conclusion: Schwannoma of the mixed nerves on the right side. The lesion cannot explain the hearing loss of the patient. The lesion itself did not cause any complaints. Follow-up examinations revealed an unchanged aspect of the lesion

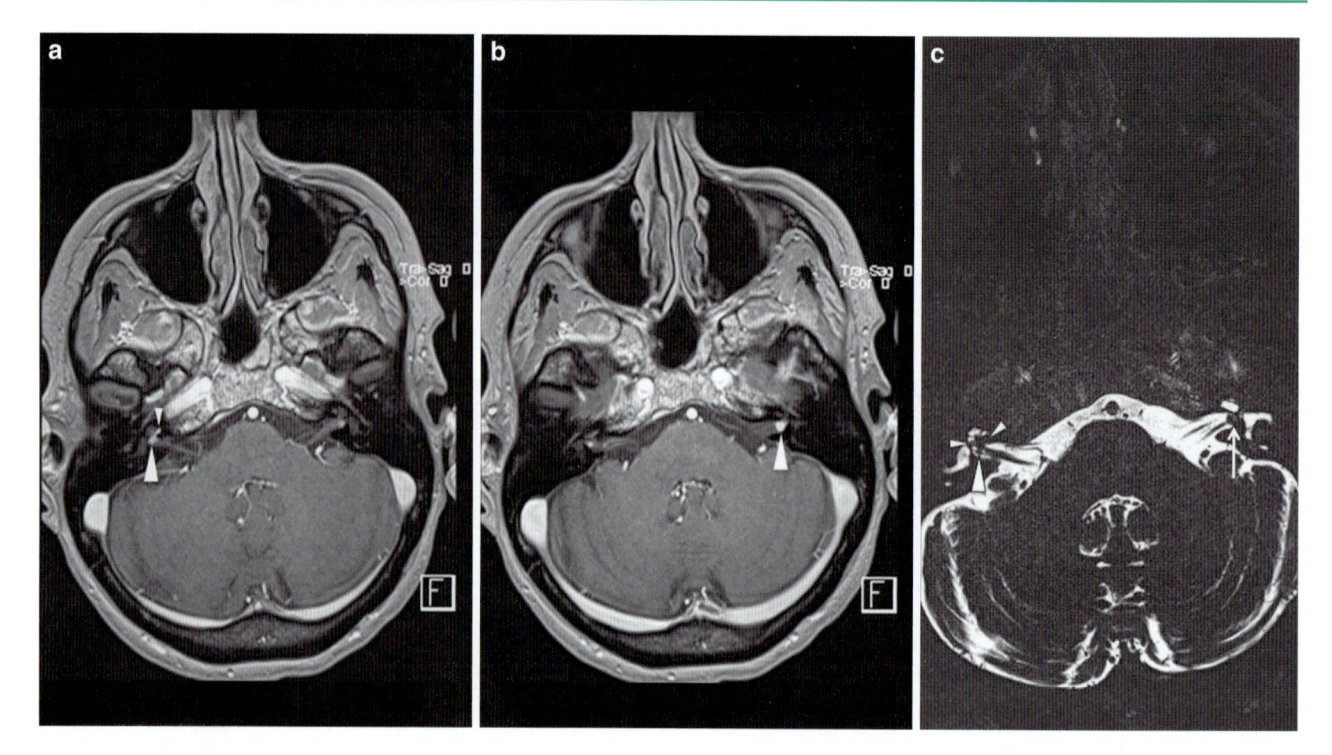

Fig. 39 57-year-old female with a prior history of invasive breast carcinoma, investigated for profound SNHL on both sides. **a** Axial gadolinium-enhanced 0.7 mm thick 3D GRE T1-weighted image through the right IAC demonstrating a small enhancing nodule in the fundus of the IAC (*large arrowhead*) with a small extension in the medial part of the midturn of the cochlea (*small arrowhead*). **b** Axial gadolinium-enhanced 0.7 mm thick 3D GRE T1-weighted image through the left IAC demonstrating a small enhancing nodule in the fundus of the IAC (*large arrowhead*). **c** Axial 0.4 mm thick 3D TSE T2-weighted image through the IAC. Note the small nodule in the fundus of the IAC on the left side (*large arrow*). On the right side there is a nodular thickening between the cochlear branch and the inferior vestibular branch (*large arrowhead*). There is also signal loss of the scala tympani of the midturn of the cochlea (*small arrowheads*). Conclusion: Evaluation of the CSF via lumbar puncture in this patient demonstrated malignant cells of the same type as the breast cancer in the CSF. The lesions in both IACs are compatible with metastatic leptomeningeal spread of disease. The extension pattern towards the scala tympani on the right side is an unusual pattern of spread of metastatic disease

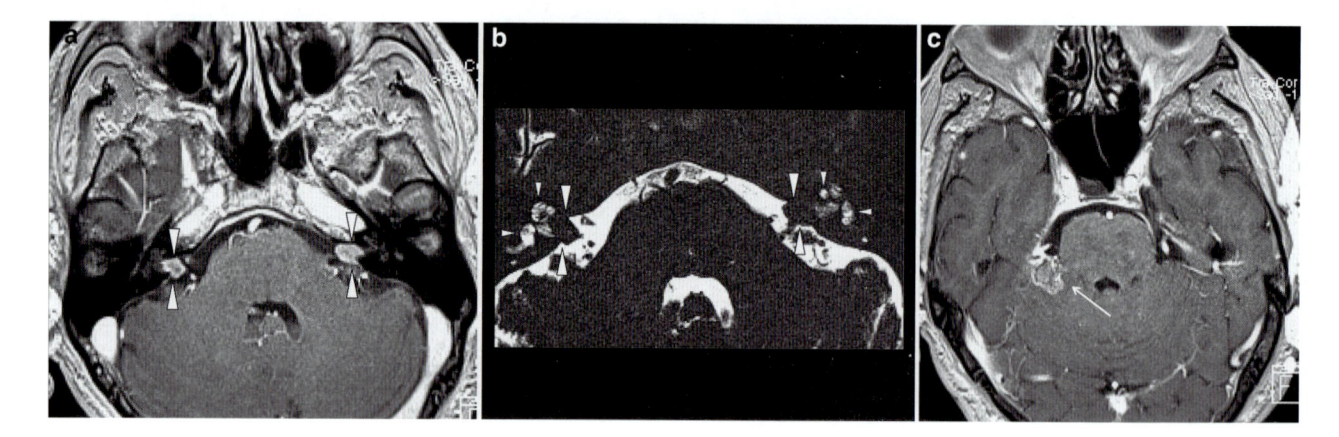

Fig. 40 61-year-old male investigated for profound SNHL with sudden onset on both sides. No prior medical history. **a** Axial gadolinium-enhanced 0.7 mm thick 3D GRE T1-weighted image through the posterior fossa demonstrates the enhancing lesions on both sides in the IAC (*arrowheads*). **b** Axial 0.4 mm thick 3D TSE T2-weighted image (same level as Fig. 40a). Bilateral hypointense lesions in the porus acousticus internus (*large arrowheads*). Note the signal loss in the fundus of the IAC and membranous labyrinth on both sides (*small arrowheads*). Compare to normal signal intensity of the CSF in the CPA on both sides. **c** Axial gadolinium-enhanced 0.7 mm thick 3D GRE T1-weighted image through the upper part of the posterior fossa. Inhomogeneous enhancing mass lesion in the upper part of the right cerebellar hemisphere (*arrow*). Conclusion: Metastatic lesions of a—until then undetected—lung carcinoma

Fig. 41 32-year-old male investigated for severe SNHL on the left side. Prior history of malignant melanoma. a Axial 3 mm thick SE T1-weighted image through the left IAC. Patient is in an asymmetrical position. Note the soft tissues in the left IAC with slightly higher signal intensity (*arrowheads*). b Axial 0.4 mm thick TSE T2-weighted image through the left IAC. On the left side, the IAC is entirely filled up with hypointense material (*large arrowheads*). Compare to the normal IAC on the right side with the visible nerves (*small arrowhead*). c Axial gadolinium-enhanced 0.7 mm thick 3D GRE T1-weighted image (same level as figure 41a). The IAC is entirely filled up with enhancing tumoral tissue (*arrowheads*). d Coronal gadolinium-enhanced GRE T1-weighted reformation showing an enhancing nodular lesion in the head of the caudate nucleus. Conclusion: Metastatic lesions of a malignant melanoma in the brain and in the left IAC. The slightly higher signal intensity of the lesion in the IAC on the left side is caused by the melanine in the metastatic lesion

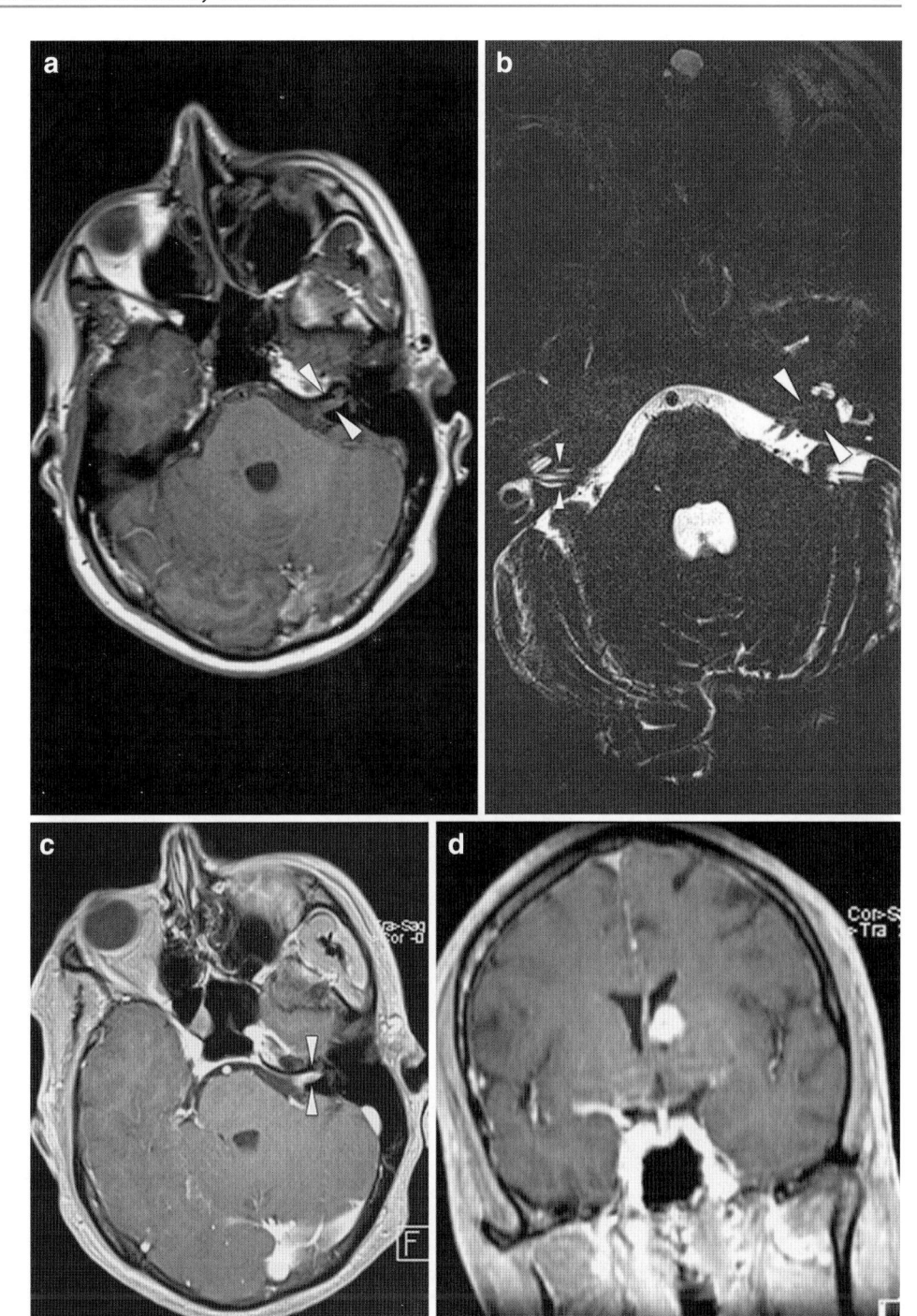

200   B. de Foer et al.

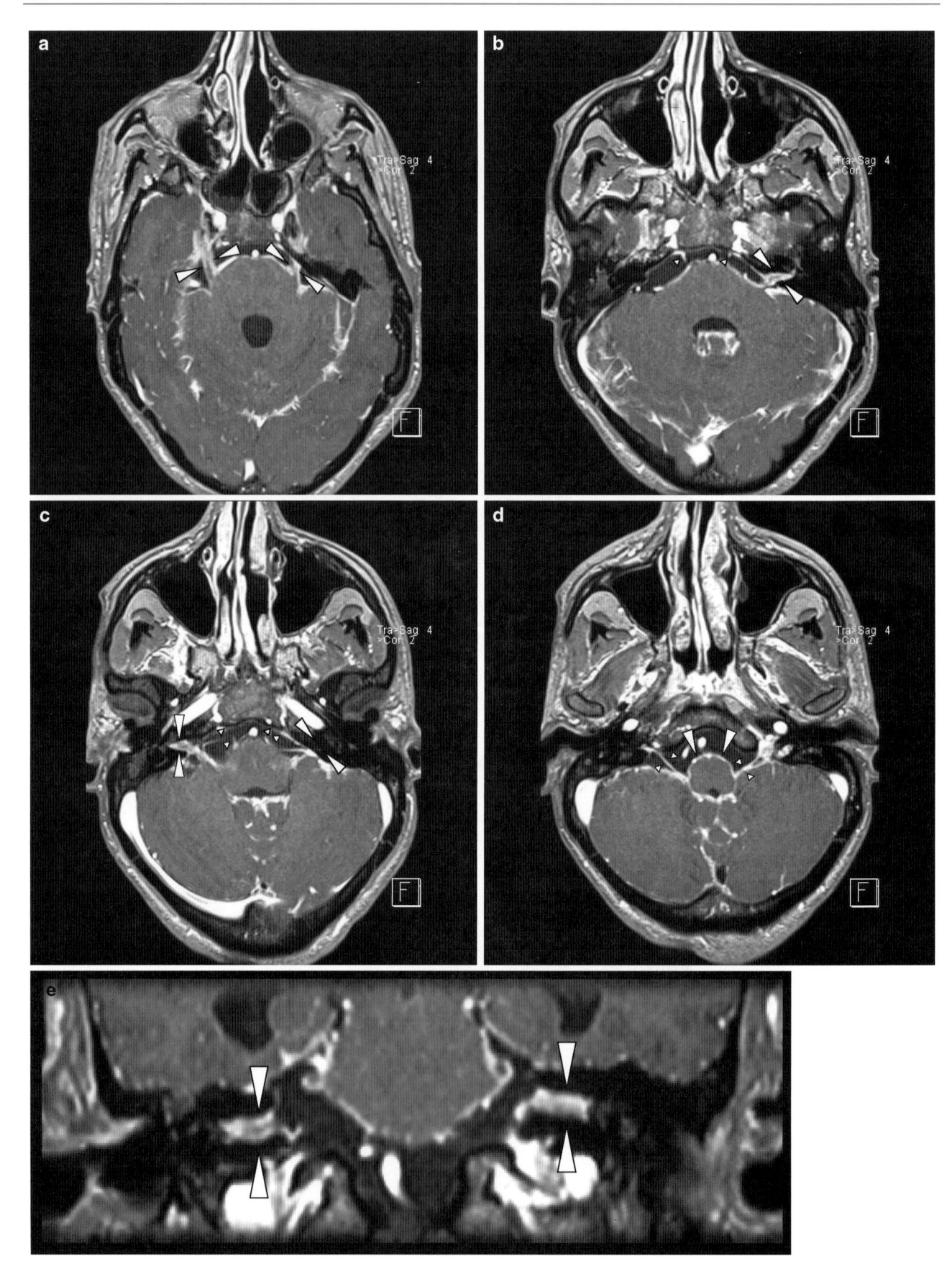

Fig. 42 28-year-old immuno-compromised patient with—after recuperation of a sudden coma onset—multiple cranial nerve deficits. **a** Axial gadolinium-enhanced 1 mm thick T1-weighted image through the posterior fossa at the level of the trigeminal nerve. There is a diffuse leptomeningeal and pachymeningeal enhancement. Note the extension of enhancement along the trigeminal nerve (*arrowheads*) on both sides. **b** Axial gadolinium-enhanced 1 mm thick T1-weighted image through the posterior fossa at the level of the IAC on the left side. There is a diffuse pachymeningeal enhancement extending into the left IAC (*large arrowheads*). Note also the enhancement along both 6th cranial nerves (*small arrowheads*). **c** Axial gadolinium-enhanced 1 mm thick T1-weighted image through the posterior fossa at the level of the IAC on the right side. Note the enhancement in the right IAC (*large arrowheads*) and along both 6th cranial nerves (*small arrowheads*). **d** Axial gadolinium-enhanced 1 mm thick T1-weighted image through the posterior fossa at the level of the 9th, 10th, and 11th cranial nerves on the right side. Note the diffuse enhancement around the brain stem (*large arrowheads*) and along the mixed nerves on both sides (*small arrowheads*). **e** Coronal gadolinium-enhanced 1 mm thick reformatted T1-weighted image through the posterior fossa at the level of the IAC showing the diffuse enhancement in the IAC (*large arrowhead*). Conclusion: CSF evaluation and hemoculture revealed a cryptococcal infection

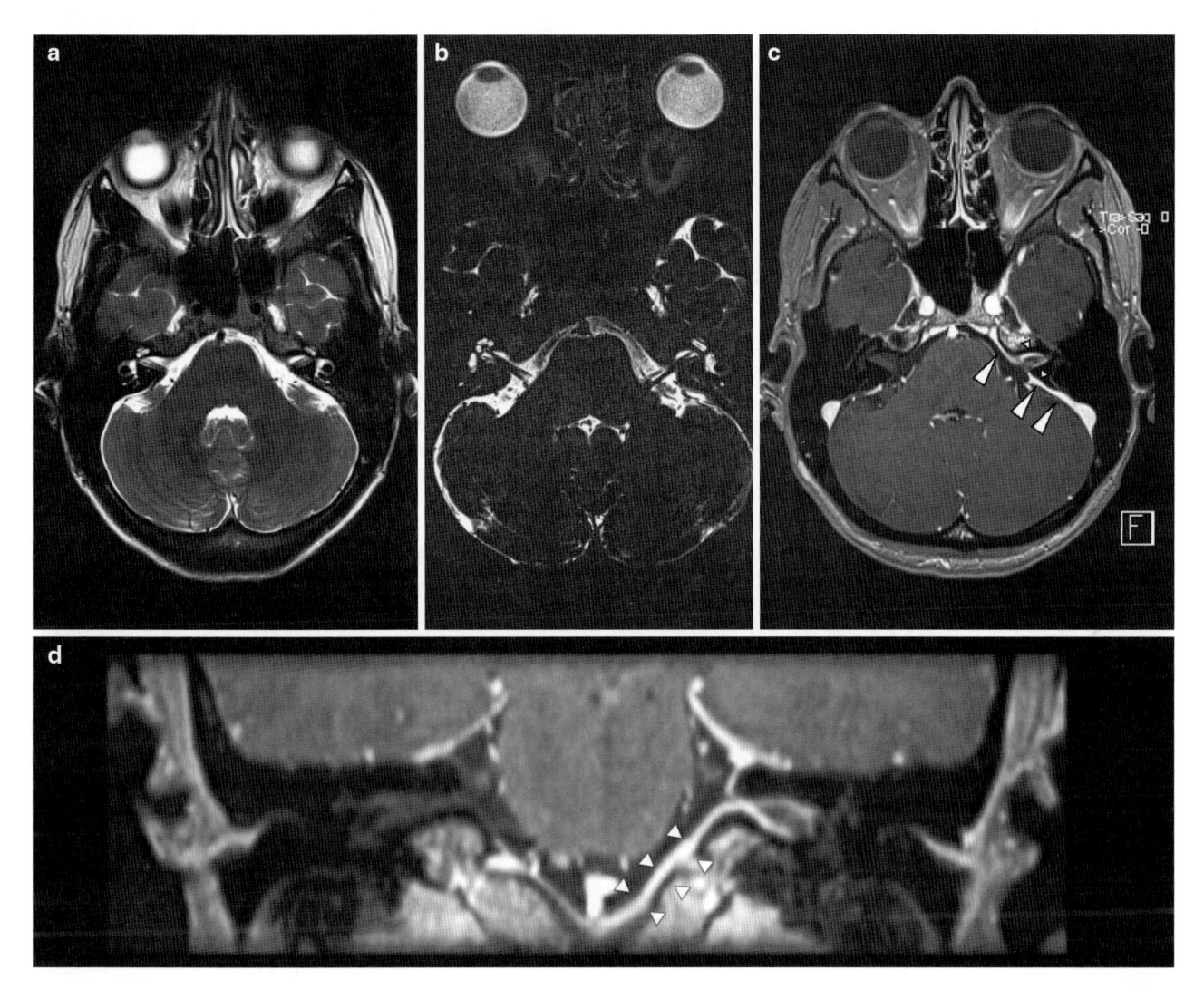

Fig. 43 33-year-old female investigated for Menière by a fossa posterior MRI. **a** Axial 3 mm thick TSE T2-weighted image through the posterior fossa revealing no clear abnormalities. **b** Axial 0.4 mm thick TSE T2-weighted image through the posterior fossa revealing no clear abnormalities. IAC, nerves, and membranous labyrinth look normal. **c** Axial gadolinium-enhanced 0.7 mm thick 3D GRE T1-weighted image through the posterior fossa revealing the clear meningeal thickening (*large arrowheads*) with extension into the IAC (*small arrowheads*) against the posterior side of the left-sided temporal bone. **d** Coronal gadolinium-enhanced reformatted GRE T1-weighted image through the posterior fossa. The thickened and enhancing meninges in the IAC and lower posterior fossa (*small arrowheads*) can clearly be seen. Conclusion: Pachymeningeal thickening and enhancement of the meninges in the left posterior fossa against the posterior side of the left-sided temporal bone, with extension in the IAC. Extensive investigation of this patient revealed Wegener's disease. After corticosteroid treatment this pachymeningeal thickening disappeared (not shown) as well as the Menièriform complaints

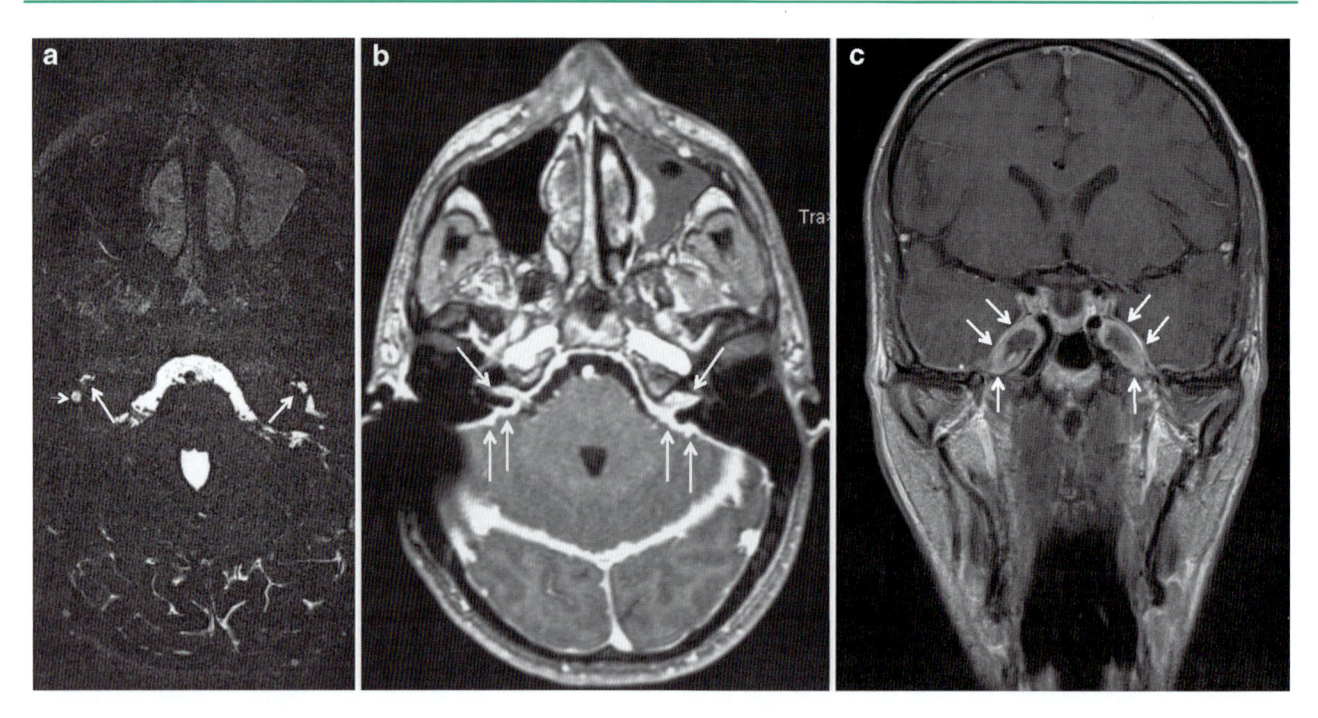

Fig. 44 32-year-old male with progressive SNHL and visual loss lasting for years, evolving into complete deafness and blindness. a Axial 0.4 mm thick 3D TSE T2-weighted image through the posterior fossa. There is complete loss of delineation of the IAC on both sides. There is partial loss of the vestibule on the right side (*small arrow*). There is also partial loss of delineation of the mid turn of the cochlea on both side (*large arrows*). b Axial 1 mm reformation of a 3D GRE T1 data set through the posterior fossa at the level of the IAC. There is diffuse pachymeningeal enhancement extending into the IAC on both side (*arrows*). c Coronal 2 mm thick gadolinium-enhanced SE T1-weighted image through Meckel's cave. There is diffuse pachymeningeal thickening along the periphery of Meckel's cave on both side (*arrows*). Conclusion: Idiopathic pachymeningitis extending along the course of nearly all cranial nerves

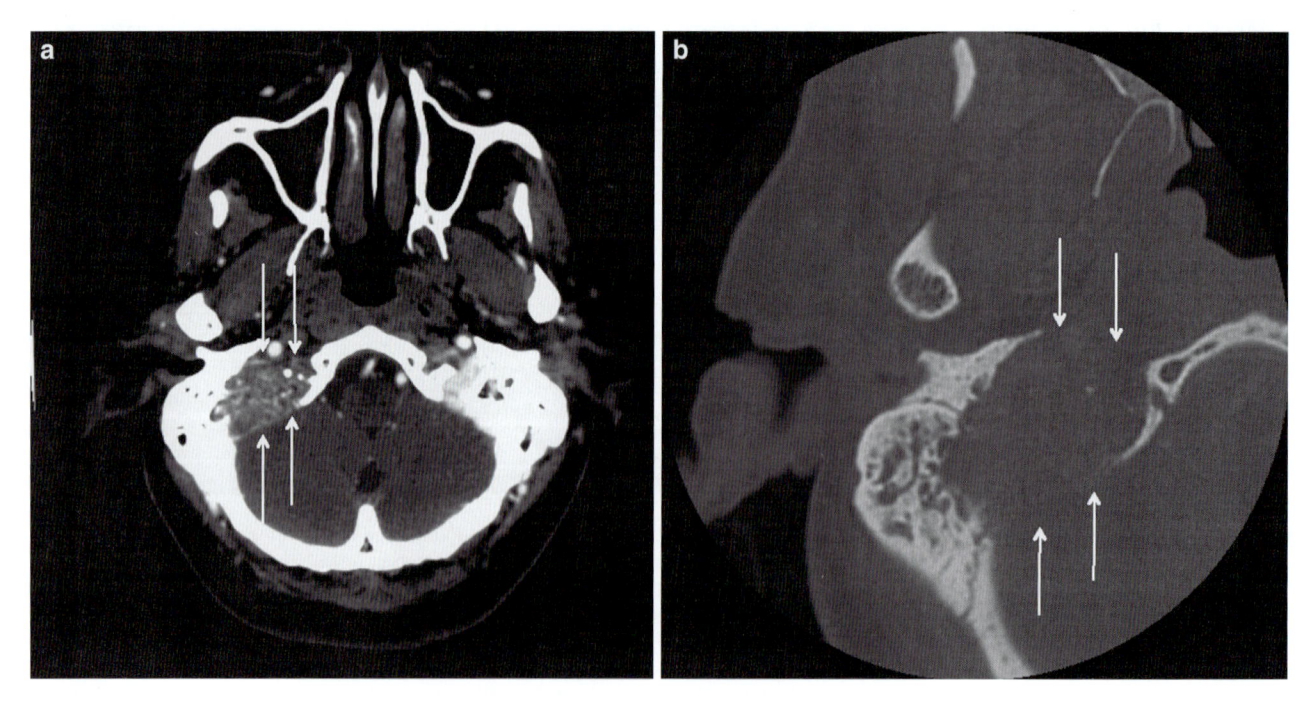

Fig. 45 62-year-old female investigated for tinnitus. a Axial post-contrast CT scan of the skull demonstrating an ill-defined enhancing lesion in the right side of the skull base (*arrows*), eroding the skull base. b Axial bone window setting (same level as Fig. 45a): large lytic lesion of the skull base (*arrows*). Conclusion: Metastatic lesion in the skull base from a—until then undetected—lung carcinoma. The symptom of tinnitus can be explained by the high degree of vascularisation of the lesion

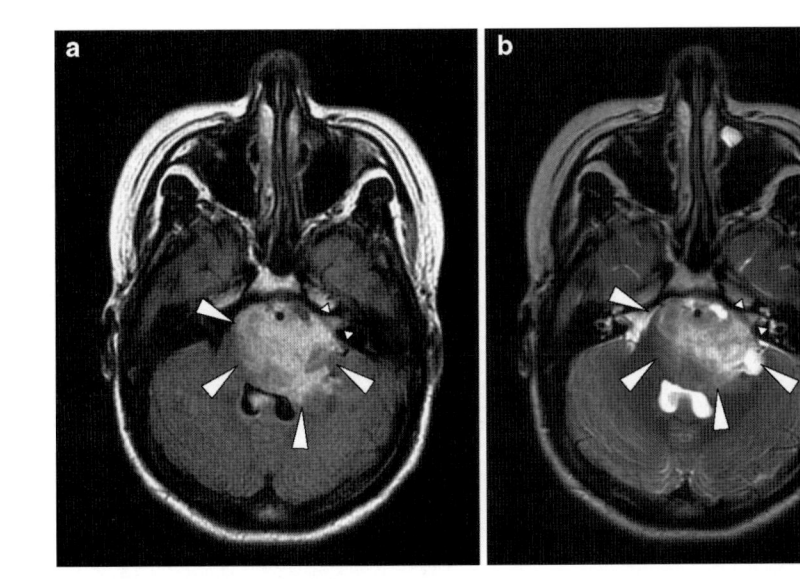

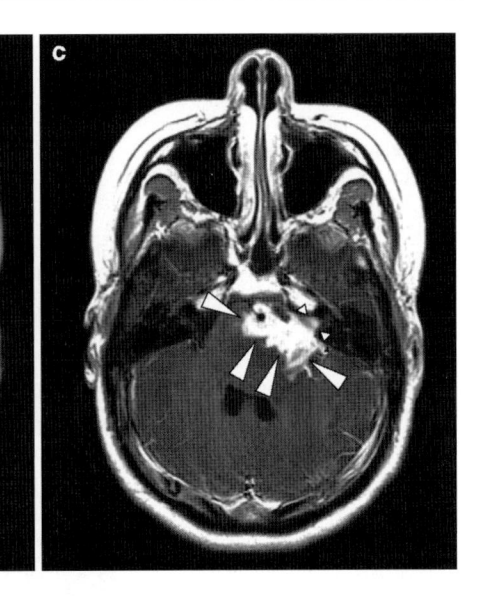

Fig. 46 12-year-old girl with sudden onset of gait disturbance, problems of equilibrium and left-sided deafness. **a** Axial 4 mm thick FLAIR image at the level of the posterior fossa. Large lesion in the brainstem with diffuse hyperintense signal in the brain stem (*large arrowheads*). Note the extension into the internal auditory canal (*small arrowhead*). **b** Axial 4 mm thick TSE T2-weighted image at the level of the posterior fossa demonstrating the enlargement of the brain stem with diffuse hyperintense signal (*large arrowheads*). Note again the extension into the IAC (*small arrowhead*). **c** Axial gadolinium-enhanced 4 mm thick gadolinium-enhanced SE T1-weighted image through the posterior fossa. Partial enhancement of the lesion (*large arrowheads*) with extension into the IAC (*small arrowhead*). Conclusion: High grade malignant brain stem glioma growing into the left CPA and IAC

and the salt is caused by subacute hemorrhage in the tumor. MR angiography sequences are very useful. On an unenhanced 3D time-of-flight MR angiography sequence, serpiginous high signal intensities can be found in the tumor representing the high-velocity flow of the large feeding arteries (Fig. 52). In the assessment of paragangliomas, the combination of conventional MR imaging and contrast-enhanced MR angiography is significantly superior to conventional MR imaging sequences alone (Bonneville 2007b; Mohan et al. 2012; Juliano 2013).

If the lesion becomes large, invasion into the CPA can be extensive (Fig. 52).

6 Vascular Lesions

6.1 Megadolichobasilaris: Basilar Artery Aneurysms

Dolichoectasia of the basilar artery can frequently be found in the elderly patient and can give rise to compression of the vestibulocochlear nerve at its root entry in the brain stem and is seldom associated to otological symptomatology or to tinnitus (Fig. 53).

Basilar artery aneurysms may resemble vestibulocochlear schwannoma on contrast-enhanced CT as they appear often as a strongly enhancing well-defined round or oval lesions. At MRI however, aneurysms without significant internal thrombus have obvious flow voids and pulsation artifacts on all spin echo sequences but demonstrate iso- to high signal intensities on unenhanced images and variable patterns of gadolinium uptake on post gadolinium T1-weighted images when intraluminal thrombus is present (Fig. 54). However, diagnosis should obviously be suspected when a round/oval lesion with low to no signal intensity is seen on T2-weighted sequences. MR angiography can confirm the diagnosis and depicts the parent artery which could be the posterior-inferior cerebellar artery (PICA), the anterior-inferior cerebellar artery (AICA), the vertebral artery or the basilar artery itself (Bonneville 2007a).

Thrombosed aneurysms may mimic tumoral lesions of the posterior fossa due to their very often mixed signal intensities (Fig. 54). MR angio sequences are in these cases helpful in diagnosis.

6.2 Vascular Loops and Neurovascular Conflicts

Neurovascular conflicts result from a conflict between a vessel and a nerve at vulnerable sites. Of particular vulnerability is the segment of central or glial myelination and the boundary or transitional zone between central and peripheral myelination, which is seen at a variable distance from the root entry/exit zone (REZ), for each individual nerve (Borges 2007).

Fig. 47 24-year-old male investigated for sudden hearing loss on the left side. **a** Axial 2 mm thick unenhanced SE T1-weighted image through the posterior fossa at the level of the IAC. There is a mass lesion visible in the left CPA (*arrowheads*) extending from the brain stem in the CPA cistern and filling up the entire IAC. The lesion is following the trajectory of the 7th and 8th cranial nerves. Both nerves can no longer be discriminated. **b** Axial gadolinium-enhanced 2 mm thick SE T1-weighted image through the posterior fossa at the level of the IAC (same level as Fig. 47a). The mass lesion (*arrowheads*) is displaying a homogeneous contrast enhancement. **c** Axial 1 mm thick TSE T2-weighted image through the posterior fossa at the level of the IAC (same level as Fig. 47a and b). Discrimination of the 7th and 8th cranial nerves is no longer possible due to the mass lesion (*large arrowheads*). Compare to the normal nerves on the right side (*small arrowheads*). *Courtesy*. Bert-Jan De Bondt, Zwolle, The Netherlands. Conclusion: Lymphoma involving the 7th and 8th cranial nerve on the left side. Although at first sight, the lesion mimicks a vestibulocochlear schwannoma, its elongated aspect along the entire course of the 7th and 8th cranial nerve is not typical for a vestibulocochlear schwannoma

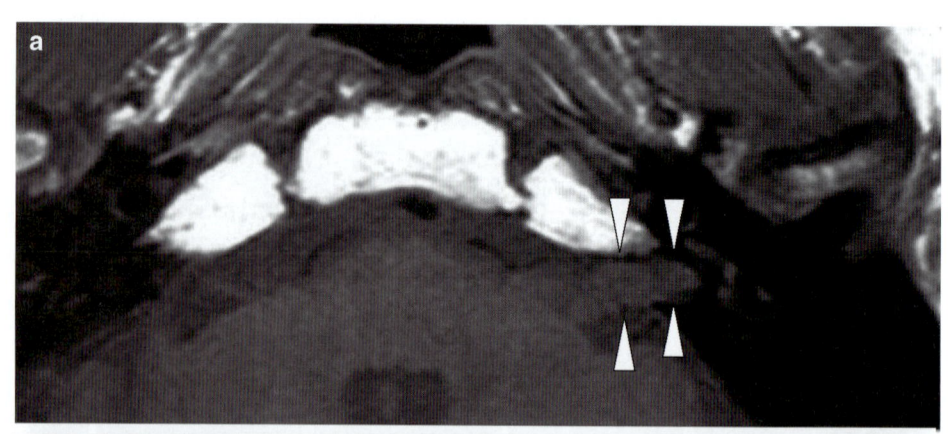

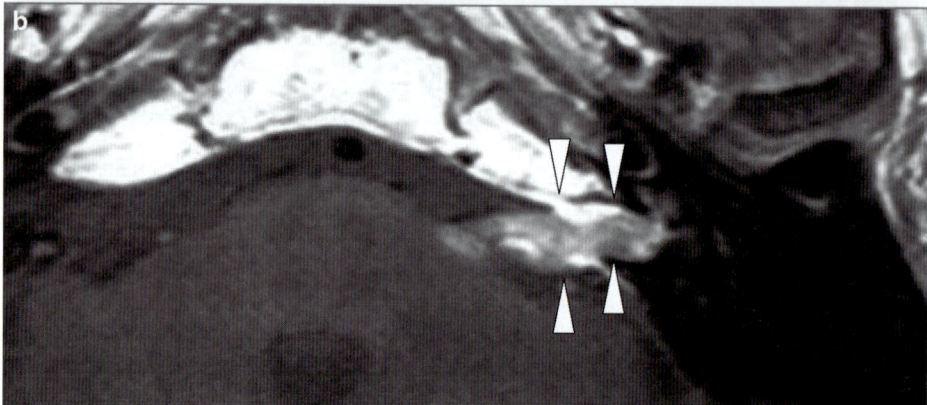

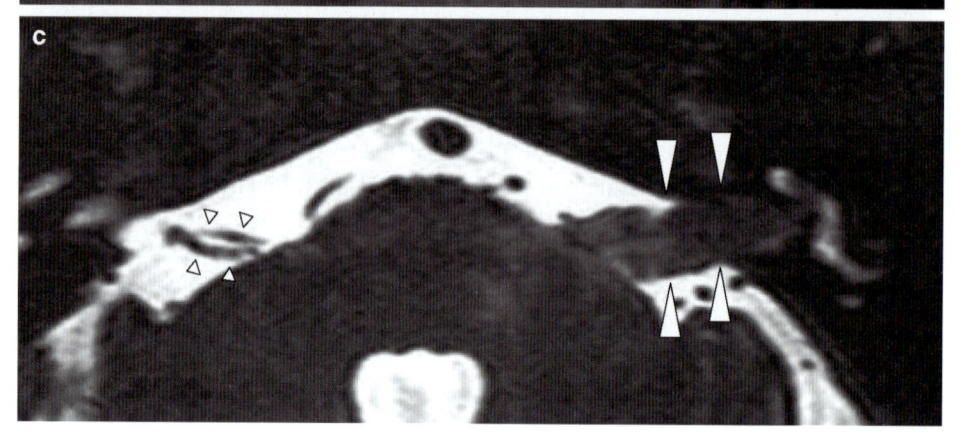

For the trigeminal nerve, this zone is at a mean distance of 3 mm from the root entry zone, for the facial nerve, it is a distance of 8 mm from the root entry zone.

Possible offending vessels are subject of controversy with some authors considering both arteries and veins as possible causes, while others deny the role of veins due to their plasticity, low pressure, and absent pulsatility. Strict criteria for neurovascular conflict state that the offending vessel must be an artery, the site of contact must be the root entry zone, the vessel must cross the nerve perpendicularly, and the nerve must be deviated or indented by the vessel or compressed or encased between two or more adjacent vessels in the appropriate clinical setting (Borges 2007). Usually the vessel at hand is the anterior- inferior cerebellar artery or the posterior inferior cerebellar artery. A megadolichobasilar artery may also cause compression (see above).

Discussion still exists as to whether vascular loops in contact with the vestibulocochlear nerve can cause otological symptoms through vascular compression. Some papers advocate a correlation between SNHL and compression of the vestibulocochlear nerve by a vascular loop or penetration of a vascular loop in the IAC (de Ridder et al. 2005). Vascular loops in contact with the vestibulocochlear nerve occur in up to a third of the normal population and may therefore

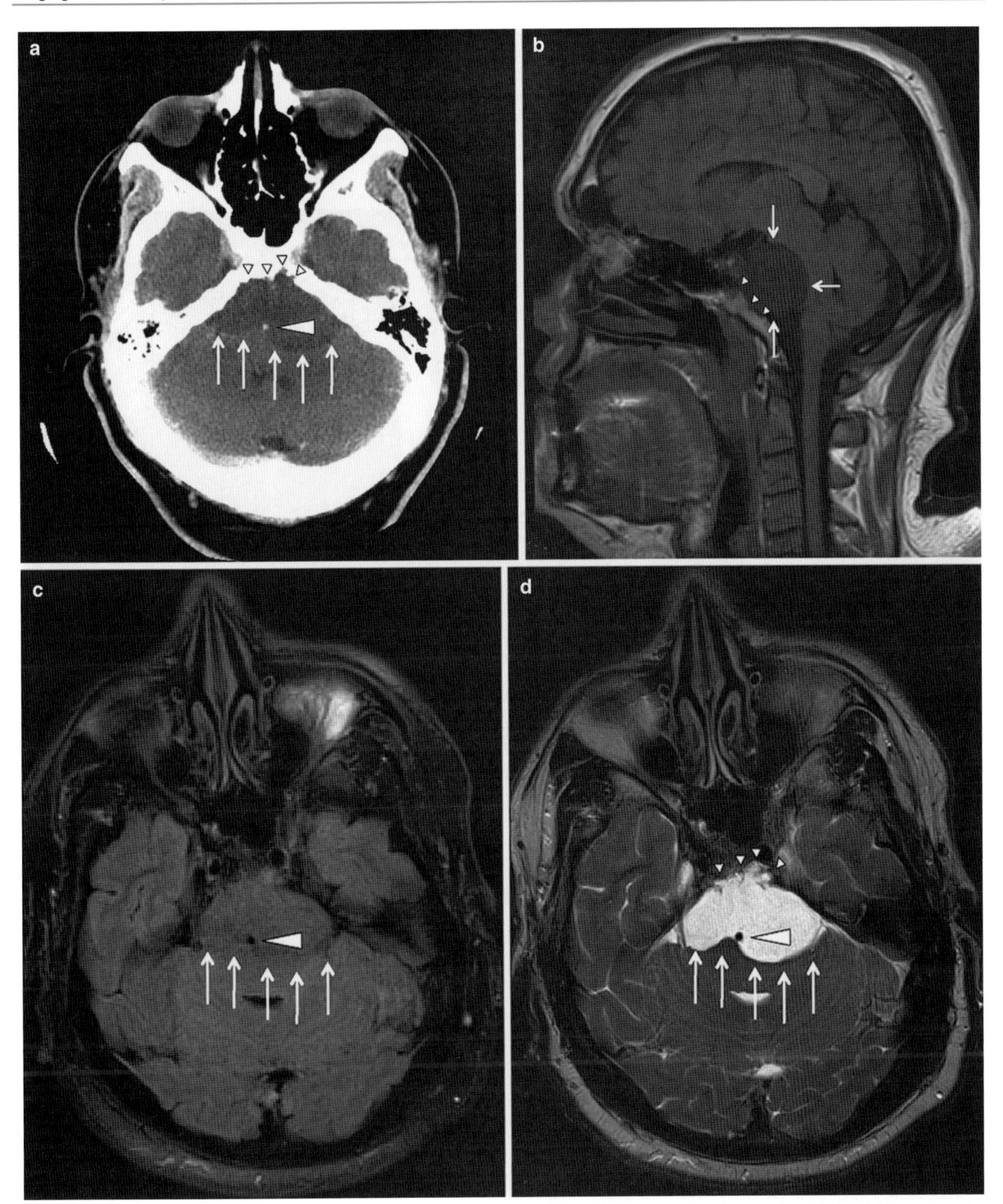

Fig. 48 48-year-old male investigated for headache. **a** Axial postcontrast CT scan through the posterior fossa demonstrating a large hypodense mass lesion nearly completely filling up the prepontine cistern and both CPA's (*arrows*). The lesion is encasing the basilar artery (*large arrowhead*). Note the relation to the skull base with signs of erosion of the skull base (*small arrowhead*). **b** Sagittal 3 mm thick unenhanced SE T1-weighted image shows the hypointense lesion in the prepontine cistern (*arrows*). Note the relationship of the lesion to the clivus, which seems to be eroded (*small arrowheads*). **c** Axial 3 mm thick FLAIR image through the posterior fossa. The mass lesion (*arrows*) has a homogeneous isointensity to gray tissue of the brain, encasing the basilar artery (*large arrowhead*). **d** Axial 3 mm thick TSE

◀ T2-weighted image. The lesion demonstrates a homogeneous high signal intensity (*arrows*), encasing the basilar artery (*large arrowhead*). Note again the relationship to the skull base (*small arrowhead*). **e** Axial 4 mm thick *b*1000 EP diffusion-weighted image demonstrating the isointensity of the lesion to brain tissue (*arrows*). There is no frank hyperintensity visible. **f** Axial gadolinium-enhanced 3 mm thick SE T1-weighted image through the posterior fossa shows that the lesion does not enhance (*arrows*). **g** Sagittal gadolinium-enhanced 3 mm thick SE T1-weighted image (same level as Fig. 48b): the lesion (*arrows*) does not demonstrate enhancement. Conclusion: Atypical appearance of a chordoma. Clue to diagnosis is given by its relationship to the clivus. The signal intensities of the lesion on standard MR sequences resemble an epidermoid cyst but the low signal intensity of the lesion on DW sequences excludes this diagnosis

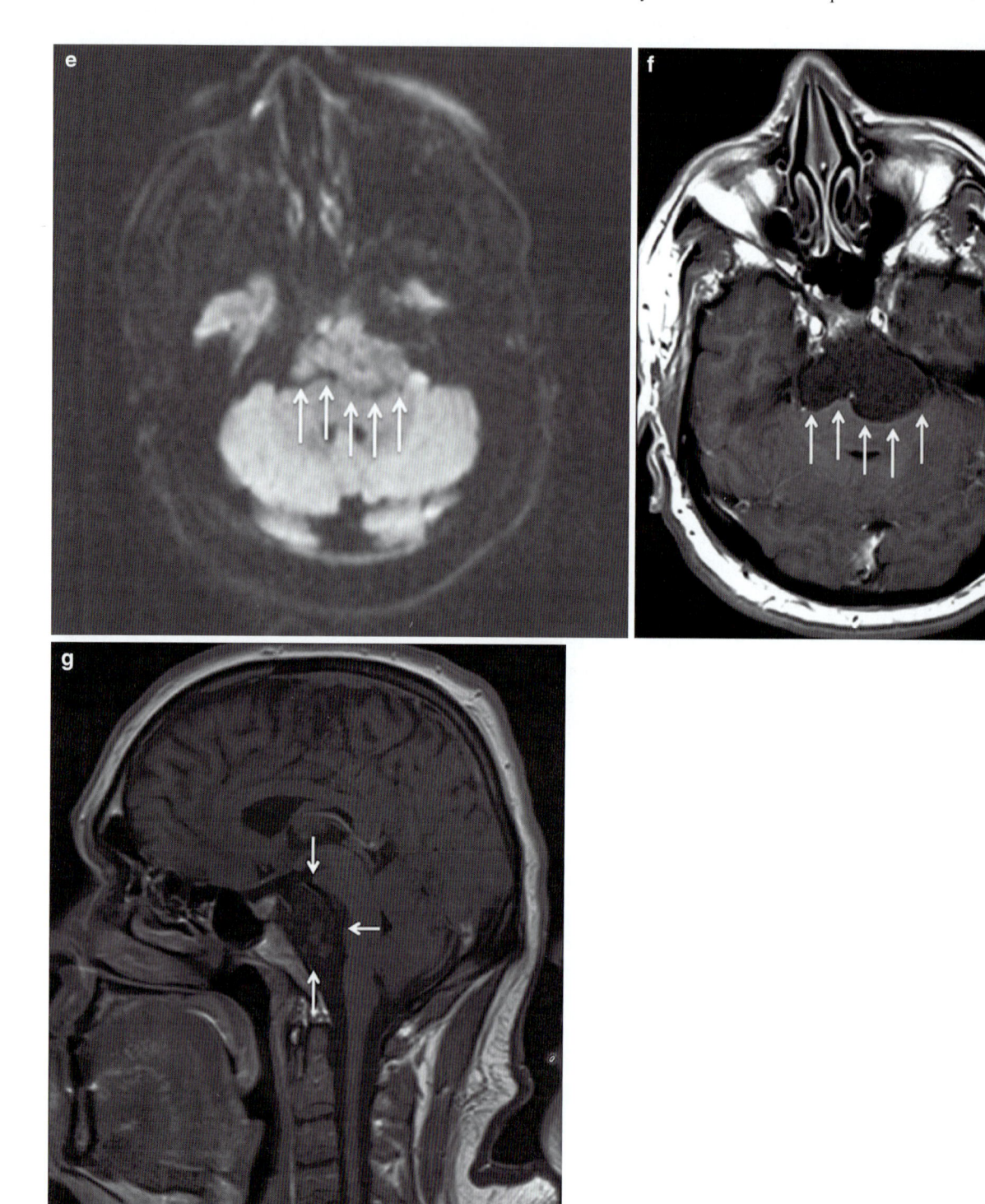

Fig. 48 continued

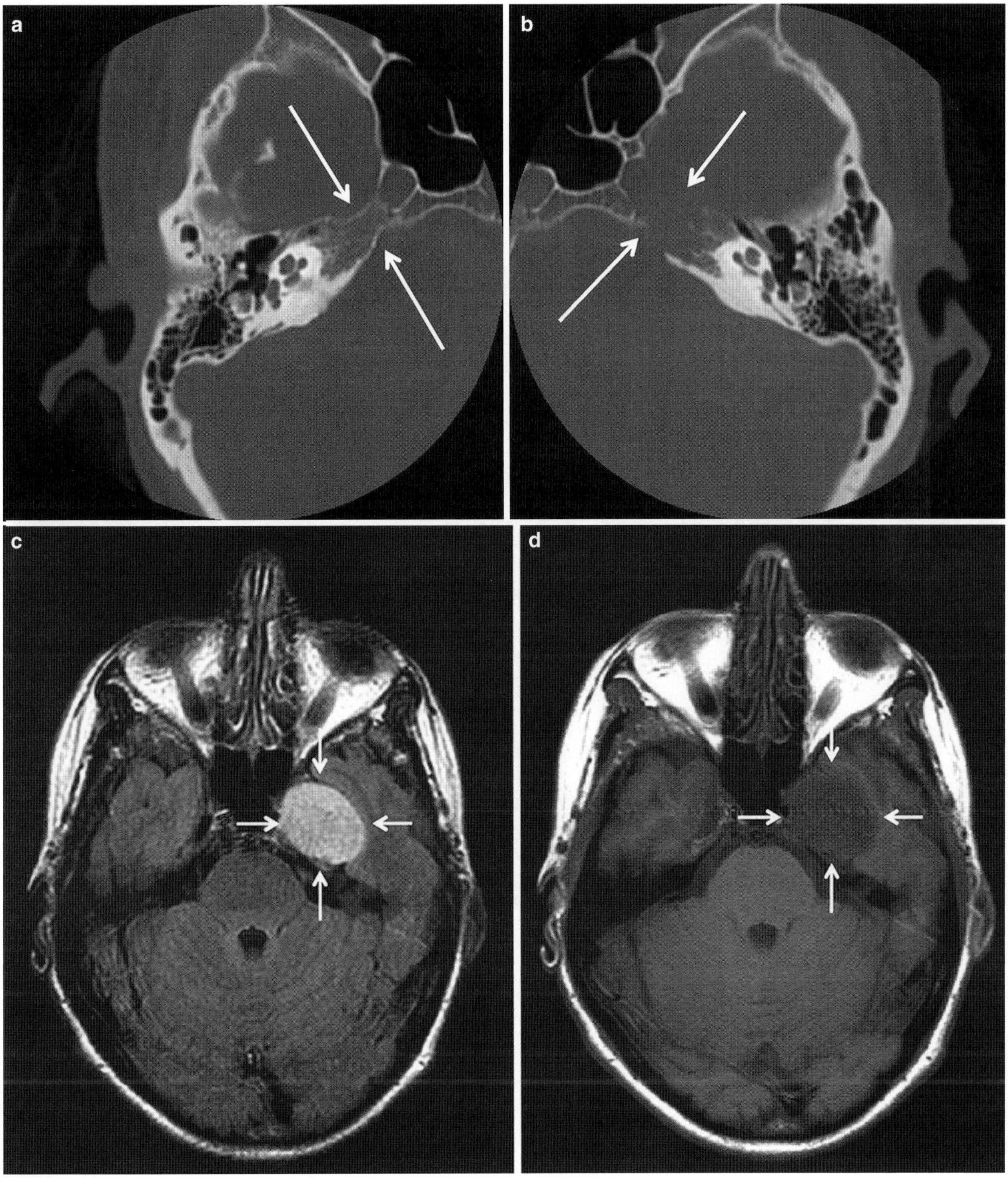
a
b
c
d

Fig. 49 50-year-old female investigated for headache. On a CT scan of the brain (not shown) a mass lesion against the petrous apex was found. **a** Axial CT scan of the right temporal bone at the level of the basal turn of the cochlea. Normal aspect of the petrous apex (*large arrows*). Compare to Fig. 49b. **b** Axial CT scan of the left temporal bone at the level of the basal turn of the cochlea. There is a lytic lesion of the petrous bone apex (*large arrows*). Compare to the normal findings in Fig. 49a. **c** Axial 4 mm thick FLAIR image through the skull base. Large hyperintense sharply delineated nodular lesion in the middle cranial fossa (*arrows*). **d** Axial 4 mm thick SE T1-weighted image (same level as Fig. 49c) demonstrating an isointense large nodular lesion in the middle cranial fossa against the petrous bone apex (*arrows*). **e** Axial gadolinium-enhanced 4 mm thick SE T1-weighted image (same level as Fig. 49c and d) shows the somewhat more pronounced peripheral curvilinear enhancement of the lesion (*arrows*). **f** Coronal gadolinium-enhanced 4 mm thick SE T1-weighted image at the level of Meckel's cave. Note the large enhancing lesion (*arrows*) with a tail-like extension towards the petrous bone apex (*arrowhead*). Conclusion: Chondrosarcoma of the left petrous bone apex

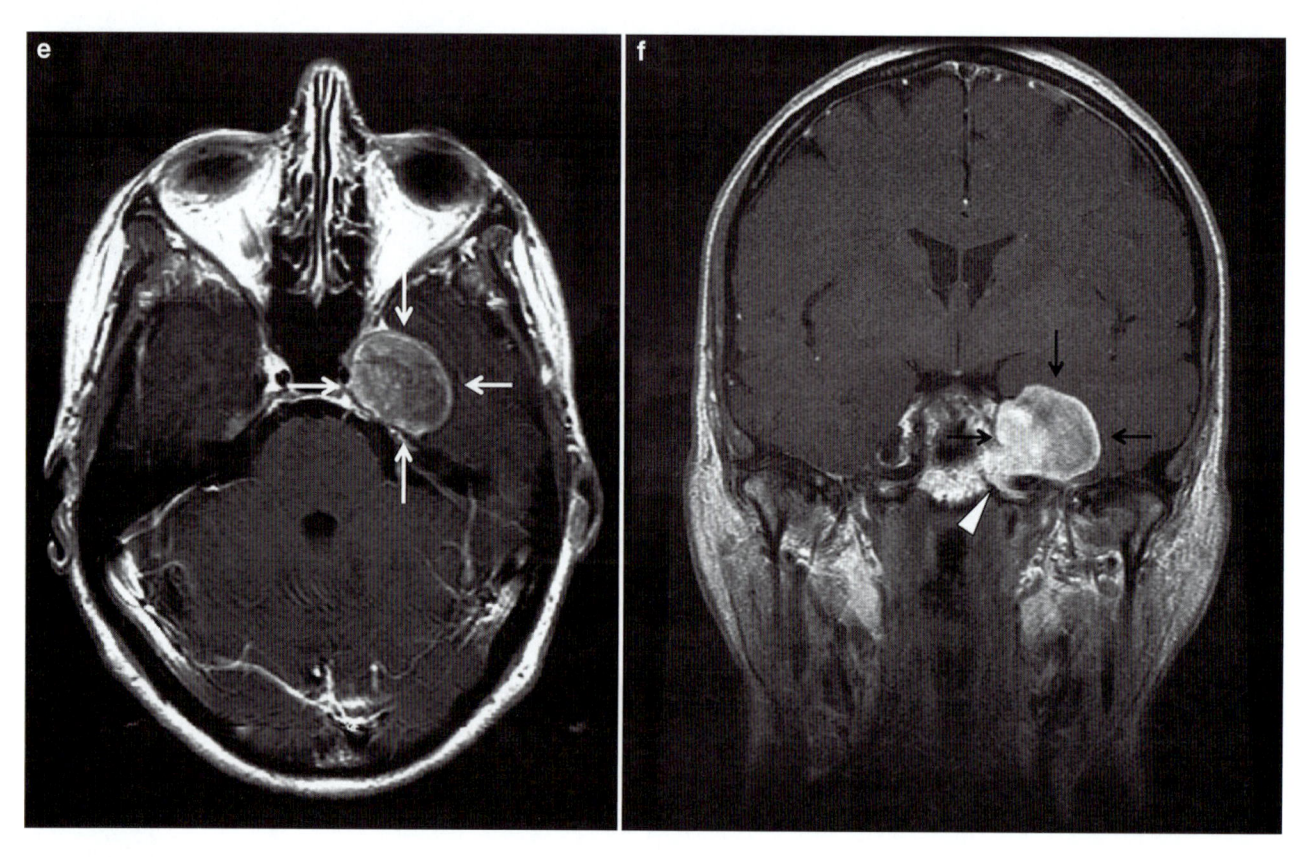

Fig. 49 continued

Fig. 50 25-year-old male investigated for bilateral severe SNHL. **a** Axial CT scan at the level of the horizontal carotid canal on both side. Note the presence of bilateral sharply delineated lytic lesions in the petrous bone apex on both sides (*arrows*). Note the thinning and/or disruption of the bone at the posterior side of the temporal bone on both sides. **b** Axial 3 mm thick TSE T2-weighted image at the level of the basal turn of the cochlea on both sides demonstrating sharply delineated hyperintense lesions in the petrous apex (*arrows*). **c** Axial 3 mm thick SE T1-weighted image at the level of the IAC showing both lesions with a high signal intensity (*arrows*). Note the invasion in both IACs. Conclusion: Pathognomonic aspect of cholesterol granuloma in the petrous apex on both sides with high signal intensity on T1 as well as T2-weighted images. Both lesions invade the IAC on both sides

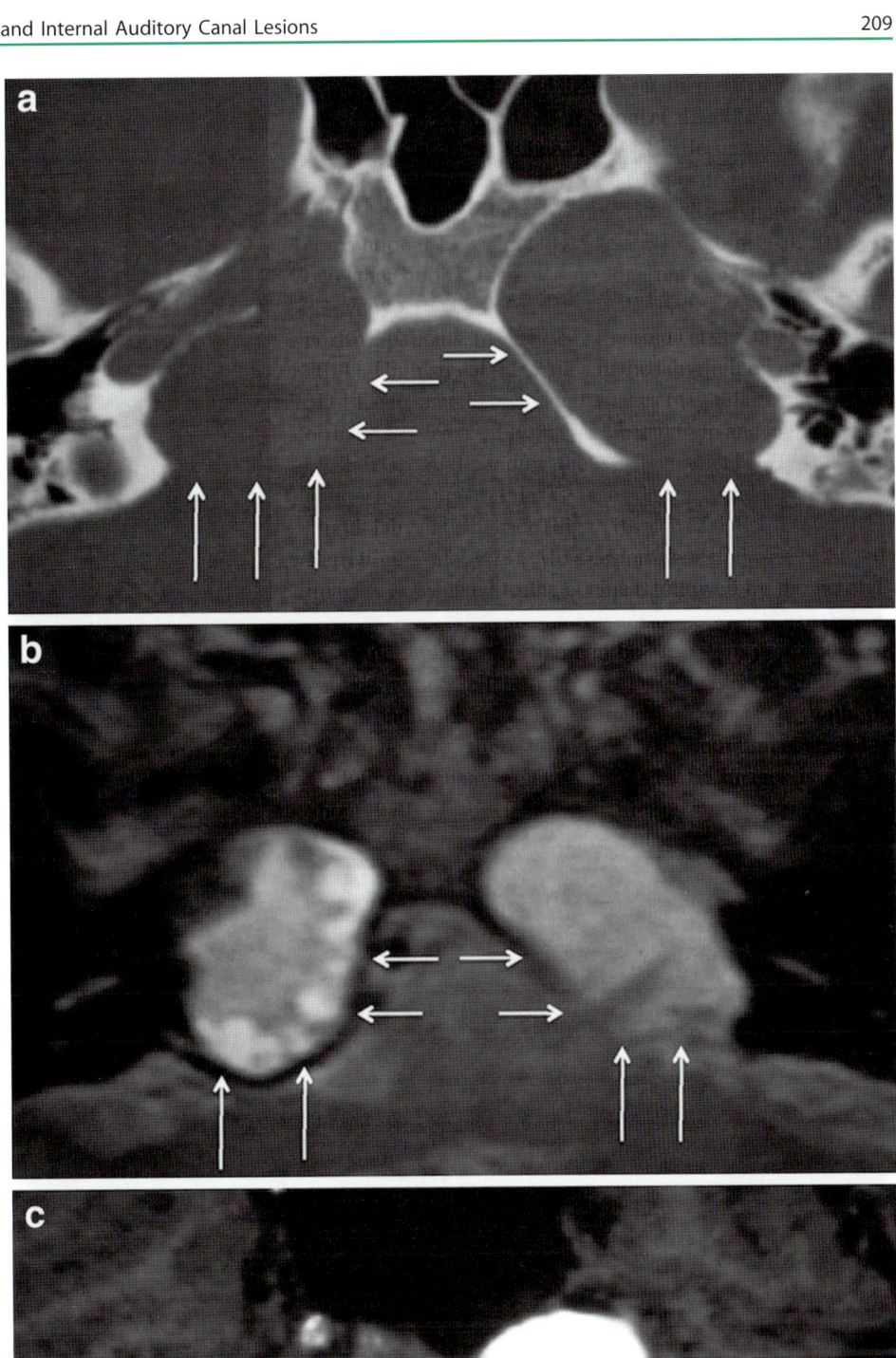

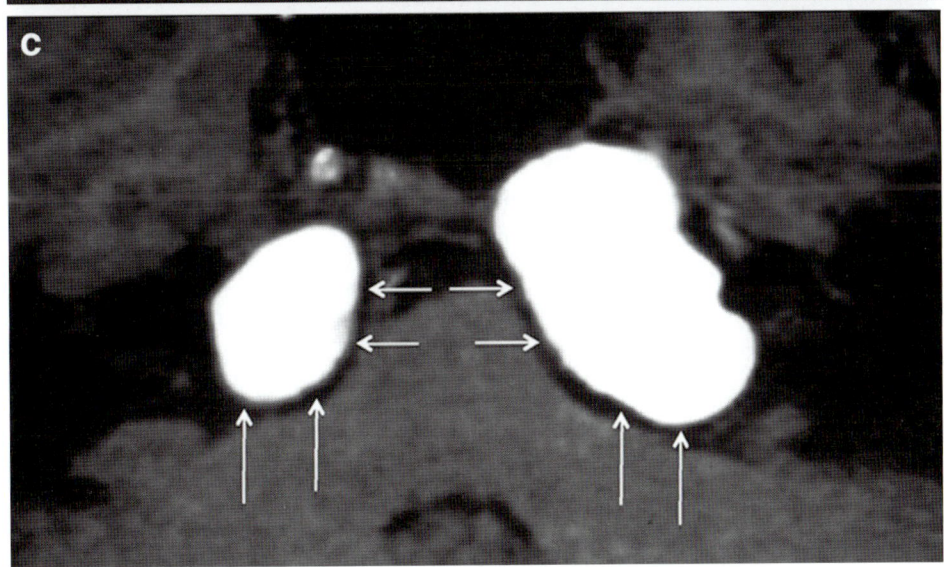

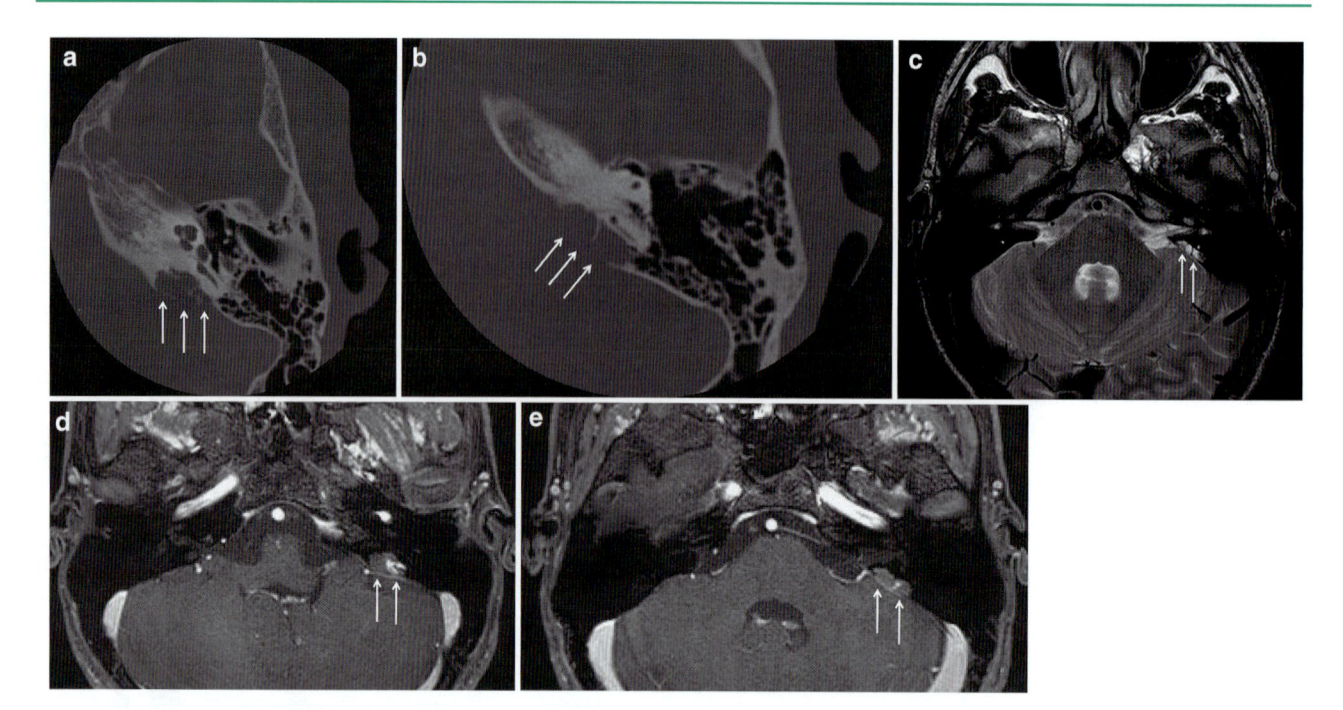

Fig. 51 18-year-old boy with von Hippel-Lindau disease investigated for SNHL **a** Axial CT scan of the temporal bone at the level of the oval window. Large rather sharply delineated lytic lesion in the posterior side of the temporal bone situated on the expected location of the endolymphatic sac and duct (*arrows*). **b** Axial CT scan of the temporal bone at the level of the superior semicircular canal. Sharply delineated lytic lesion located posteriorly in the temporal bone (*arrows*). **c** Axial 4 mm thick TSE T2-weighted image through the posterior fossa displaying a hyperintense lesion in a retrolabyrinthine position (*arrows*). **d** Axial gadolinium-enhanced 3 mm thick SE T1-weighted image with fatsat at the level of the lower posterior fossa demonstrating the mass lesion with a partial low intensity and a partial higher signal intensity (*arrows*). **e** Axial gadolinium-enhanced 3 mm thick SE T1-weighted image with fatsat at the level of the IAC demonstrating again the mass lesion (*arrows*) with a slightly higher intensity and a small enhancing component. Conclusion: Left-sided endolymphatic sac tumor in a boy with von Hippel-Lindau disease

be considered a normal variant (Fig. 55). It is also generally accepted that the presence of a vascular loop either in contact with the vestibulocochlear nerve and causing angulation of the cisternal component of the nerve or its penetration into the IAC does not correlate with tinnitus (Fig. 56) (Van der Steenstraten 2007; Chadha 2008; Gultekin 2008).

This is opposed to compression of the facial nerve in the CPA, in which it is generally accepted that vascular compression/displacement of the facial nerve may cause hemifacial spasm (Fig. 57). This condition, occurring most frequently in women, is characterized by unilateral, intermittent, and involuntary muscular twitches. The offending vessel is most often the AICA, PICA or the vertebrobasilar system (Borges 2007).

Compression of the glossopharyngeus nerve in its cisternal component can give rise to glossopharyngeus neuralgia (Fig. 58). This entity is characterized by unilateral, paroxysmal pain, which is sudden in onset and radiates from the oropharynx to the ear. Swallowing is the most common precipitating factor.

In most cases of neurovascular conflict, decompressive surgery with Teflon interposition may relieve symptoms (Figs. 57 and 58) (Borges 2007).

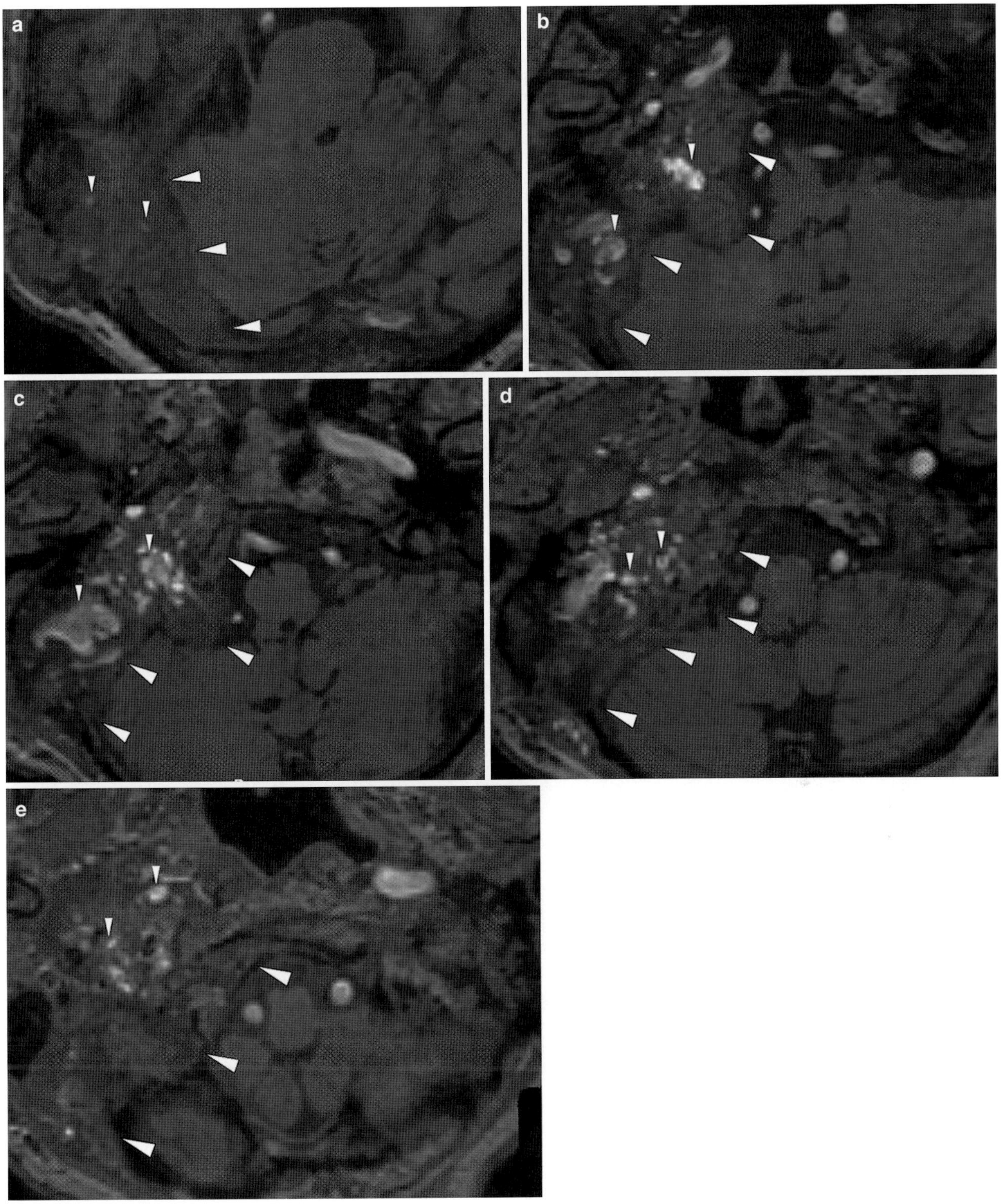
a
b
c
d
e

◄ **Fig. 52** 80-year-old female with a prior diagnosis of a large right-sided glomus jugulo-tympanicum, lost to follow-up for 10 years. Clinical history of pulsatile tinnitus and swallowing difficulties. Figures **a–e** Axial unenhanced 3D-TOF MR angio sequence demonstrating the large isointense mass lesion nearly invading the entire right petrous bone, with a large component invading the right CPA (*large arrowheads*). The lesion displays multiple high signal intensities (*small arrowheads*) inside compatible with high flow status arterial vessels in the glomus tumor. As this patient was lost to follow-up and was left untreated the glomus tumor has had time to develop and invade the entire temporal bone. *Courtesy* Hervé Tanghe, Erasmus MC, Rotterdam, The Netherlands. Conclusion: Huge glomus jugulo-tympanicum invading the entire petrous bone pyramid and invading the CPA

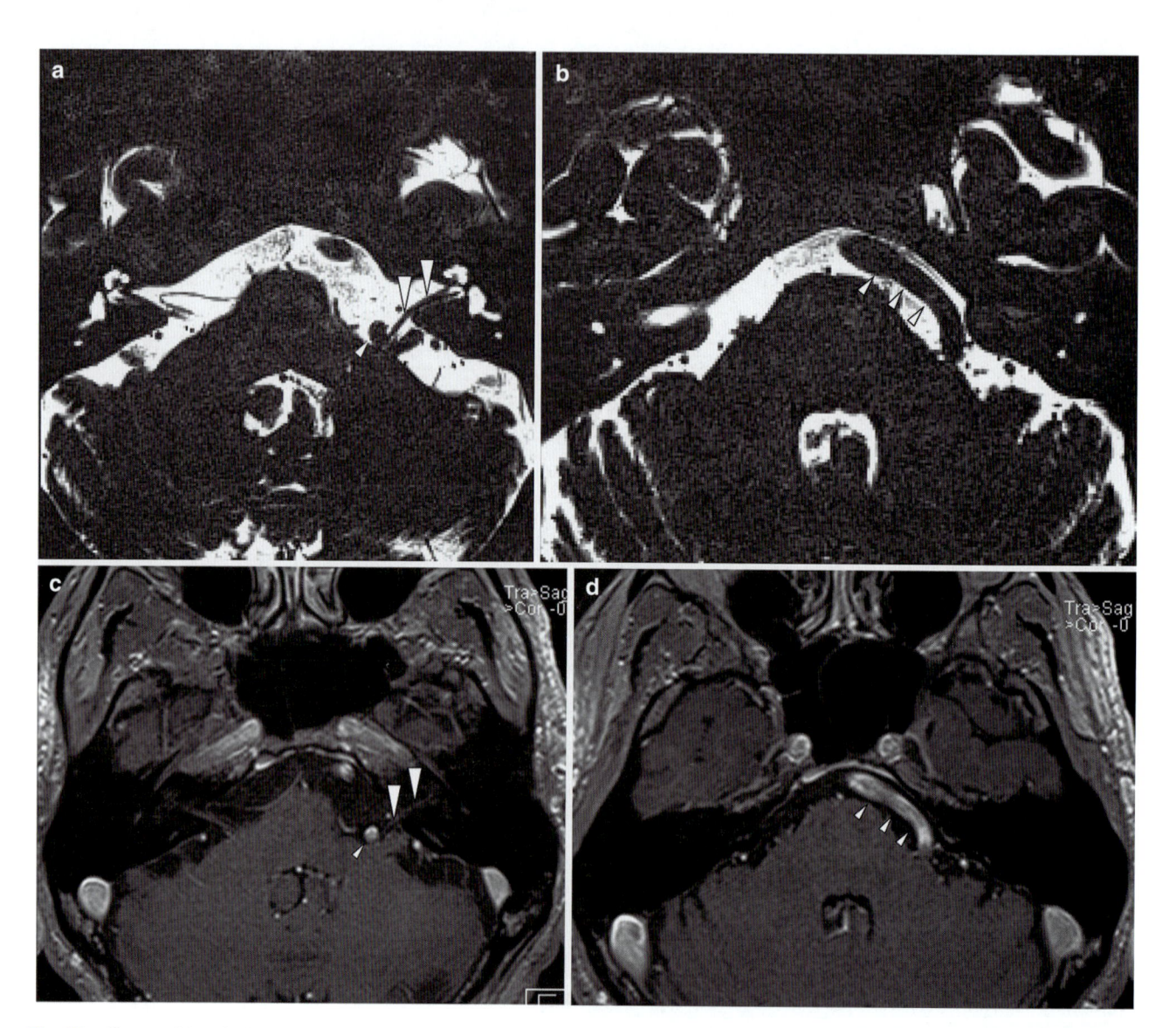

Fig. 53 63-year-old male investigate for SNHL on the right side. Patient had no complaints of tinnitus. **a** Axial 0.4 mm thick 3D TSE T2-weighted image through the posterior fossa at the level of the IAC. The left-sided vestibulocochlear nerve (*large arrowheads*) is compressed at its origin in the brainstem by the vertebrobasilar artery (*small arrowhead*). **b** Axial 0.4 mm thick 3D TSE T2-weighted image through the posterior fossa at a level a bit higher than Fig. 53a. Note the deviation of the basilar artery to the left side (*small arrowheads*). **c** Axial gadolinium-enhanced 0.7 mm thick GRE T1-weighted image (same level as Fig. 53a) demonstrating the enhancing basilar artery (*small arrowhead*) compressing the left vestibulocochlear nerve (*large arrowheads*). **d** Axial gadolinium-enhanced 0.7 mm thick GRE T1-weighted image (same level as Fig. 53b) demonstrating the elongated tortuous aspect of the enhancing basilar artery to the left (*small arrowheads*). Conclusion: Elongated tortuous basilar artery deviated to the left, compressing the vestibulocochlear nerve. Although this has been reported as a possible cause of tinnitus, this patient had no complaints of tinnitus

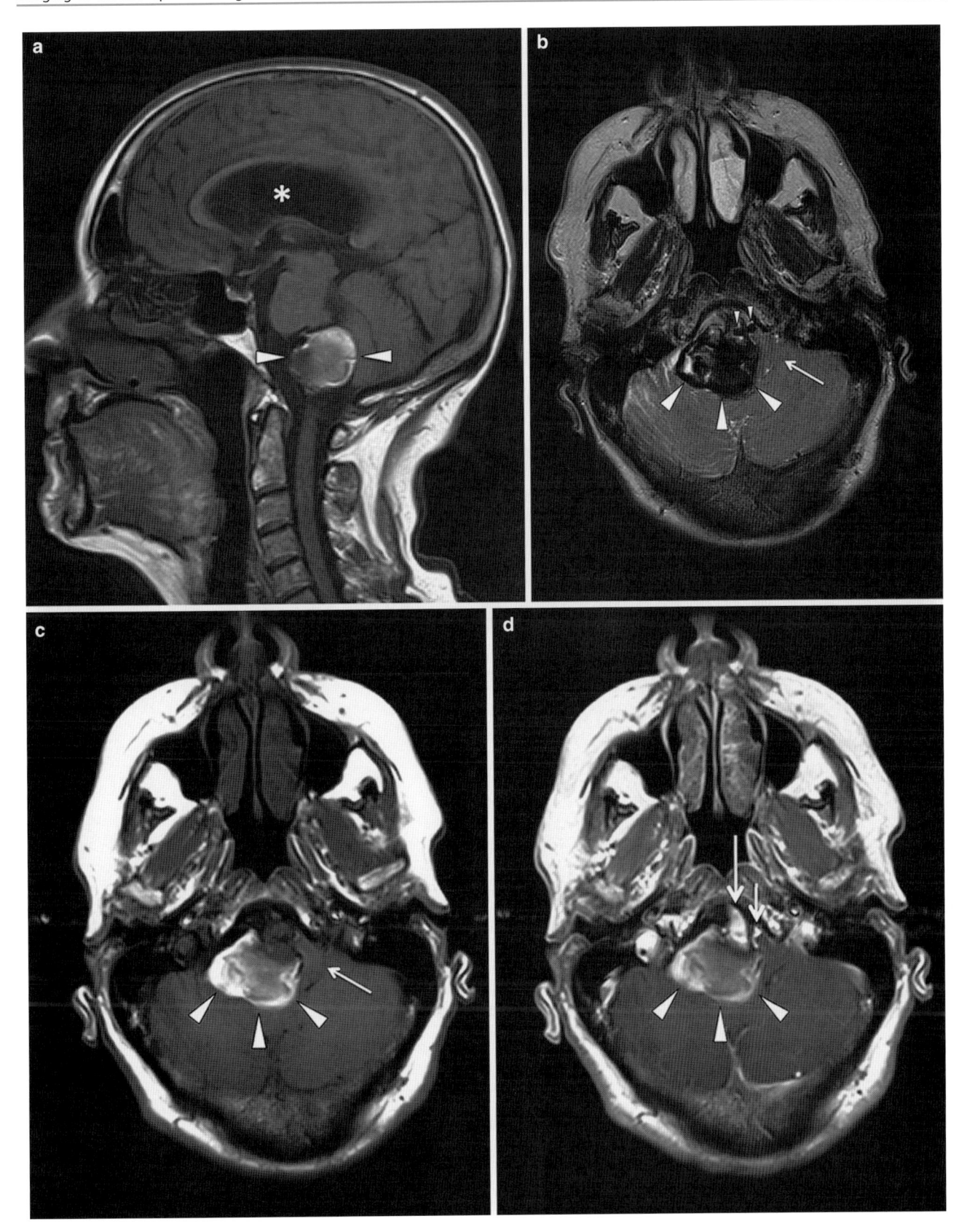

Imaging of Cerebellopontine Angle and Internal Auditory Canal Lesions

◀ **Fig. 54** 72-year-old female investigated for gait disturbance, with a rather sudden onset. **a** Sagittal 2 mm thick SE T1-weighted image. Large apparently somewhat layered mass (*arrowheads*) with a hyperintense aspect located nearly on the midline with impression on the brainstem and cerebellum. There is a clear enlargement of the third ventricle (*asterisk*). **b** Axial 3 mm thick TSE T2-weighted image through the posterior fossa. Large apparently extra-axially located mass lesion (*large arrowheads*) with compression of the cerebellum but mainly of the brainstem (*arrow*). Note the left-sided deviation of both vertebral arteries (*small arrowheads*). **c** Axial 2 mm thick SE T1-weighted image through the posterior fossa (same level as Fig. 54b). The lesion has a mainly high signal intensity (*large arrowheads*) and compresses the brainstem (*arrow*). **d** Axial gadolinium-enhanced 2 mm thick SE T1-weighted image through the posterior fossa (same level as Fig. 54b and c). The lesion does not demonstrate enhancement (*large arrowheads*). Note the fusiform enlargement of the right vertebral artery (*large arrow*). Compare to the normal sized left vertebral artery (*small arrow*). **e** Axial 1 mm unenhanced 3D TOF MR angio sequence (same level as Fig. 54b, c and d). The mass lesion displays an inhomogeneous high signal intensity (*large arrowheads*). The fusiform enlargement of the right vertebral artery is clearly demonstrated (*large arrow*). Compare to the normal sized left vertebral artery (*small arrow*). **f** 3D TOF MR angio reconstruction displays the lesion as a large nodular high signal intensity (*large arrowheads*) with vertebrobasilar artery deviation to the left side (*small arrowheads*). Conclusion: Thrombosed fusiform aneurysm of the right-sided vertebral artery, with mass effect on the cerebellum but mainly on the brainstem causing supratentorial hydrocephalus. The combination of cerebellar and brainstem compression is responsible for the supratentorial hydrocephalus causing the gait disturbance

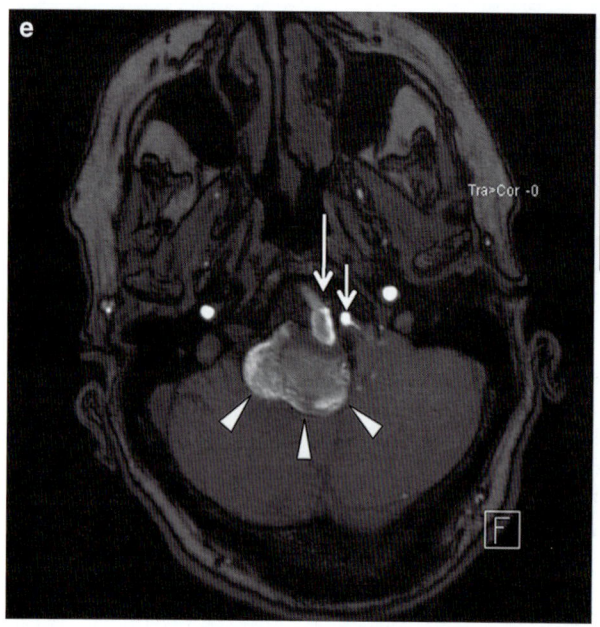

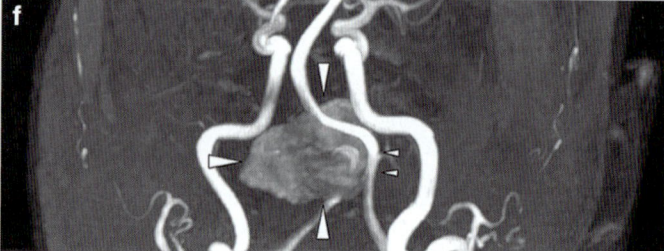

Fig. 54 continued

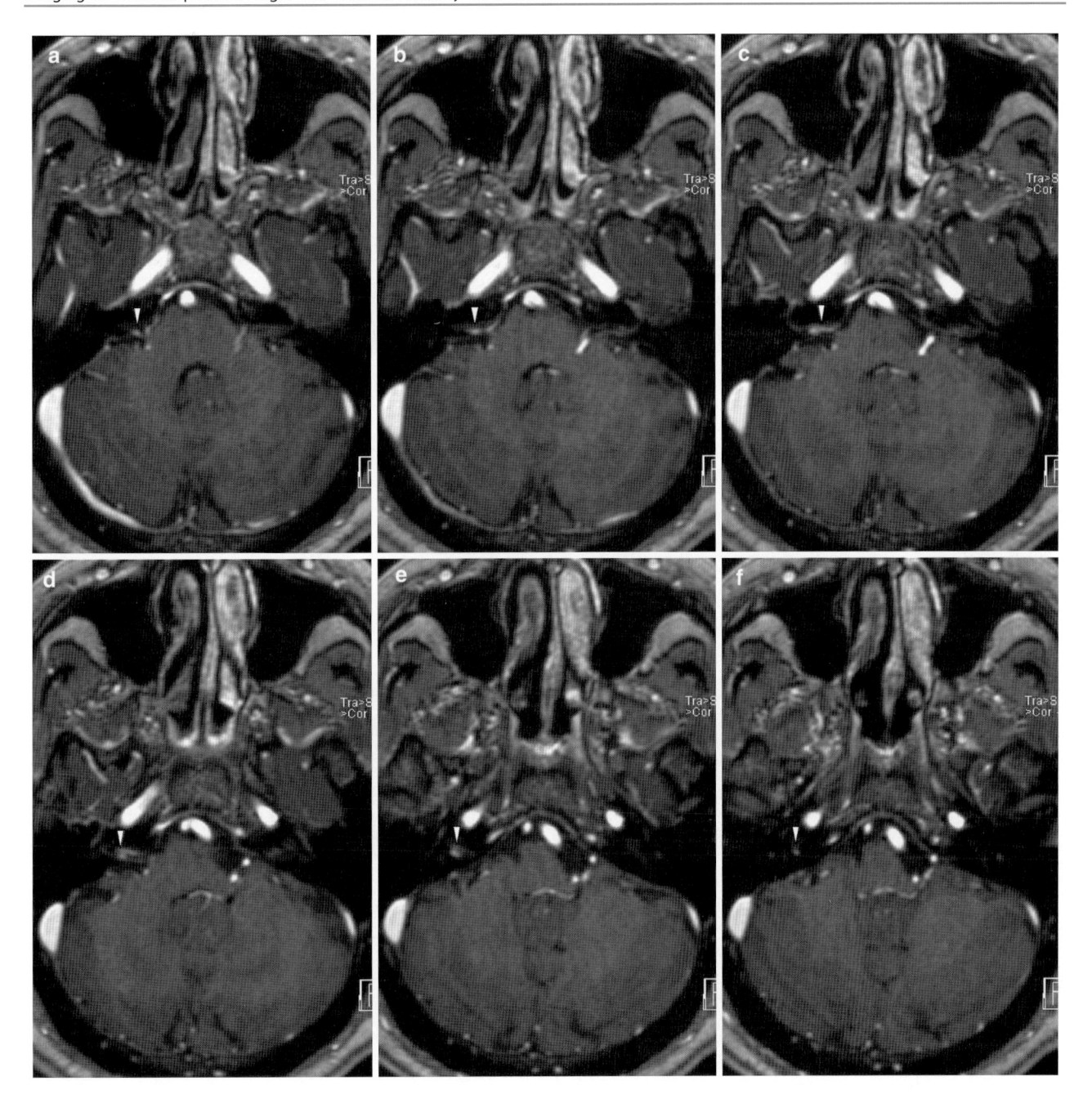

Fig. 55 64-year-old male investigated for deafness on the right side lasting for a least 15 years. Investigation was performed in a pre-cochlear implant setup. a–f Consecutive 1 mm thick gadolinium-enhanced 3D GRE T1-weighted images showing the presence of an enhancing vascular loop (*arrowheads*) entering the IAC reaching the fundus of IAC. Conclusion: Vascular loop entering the IAC reaching the fundus of the IAC. This patient had no documented history of tinnitus on the right side

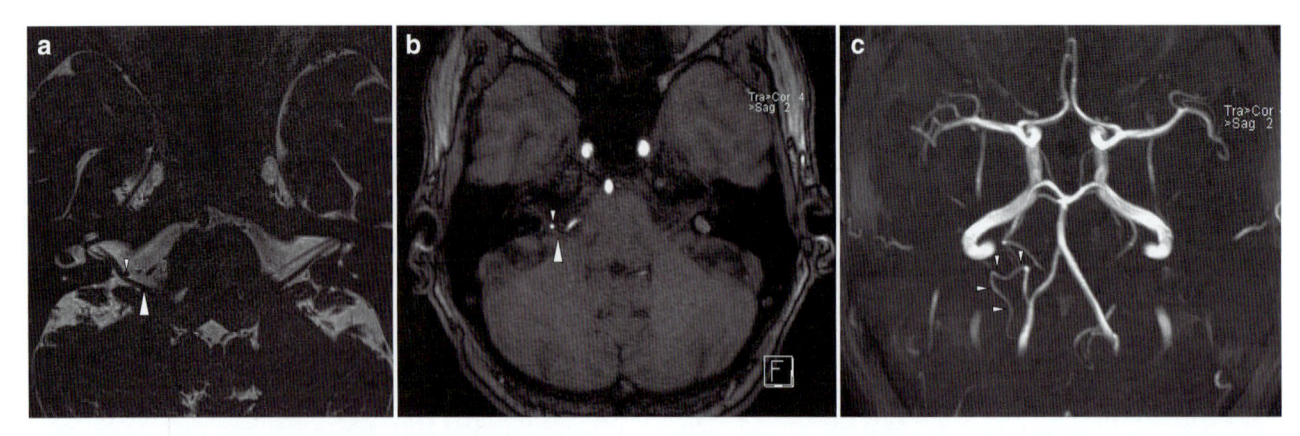

Fig. 56 61-year-old male investigated for right-sided pulsatile tinnitus. **a** Axial 0.4 mm 3D TSE T1-weighted through the IAC. The right vestibulocochlear nerve (*large arrowhead*) is posteriorly displaced by a rounded to ovoid zone of signal void, compatible with the PICA (*small arrowhead*). **b** Axial 1 mm unenhanced 3D TOF MR angio sequence (same level as Fig. 56a) at the level of the IAC showing the spontaneous hyperintense PICA (*small arrowhead*) displacing the vestibulocochlear nerve posteriorly (*large arrowhead*). **c** 3D TOF MR angio displaying the carotid and vertebrobasilar circulation as well as the large PICA (*arrowheads*) on the right side. Conclusion: Posterior displacement of the right vestibulocochlear nerve by the PICA possibly causing the pulsatile tinnitus in this patient. Decompressive surgery with Teflon interposition was proposed to the patient but refused by the patient as he spontaneously got rid of his tinnitus a few weeks after the MRI examination

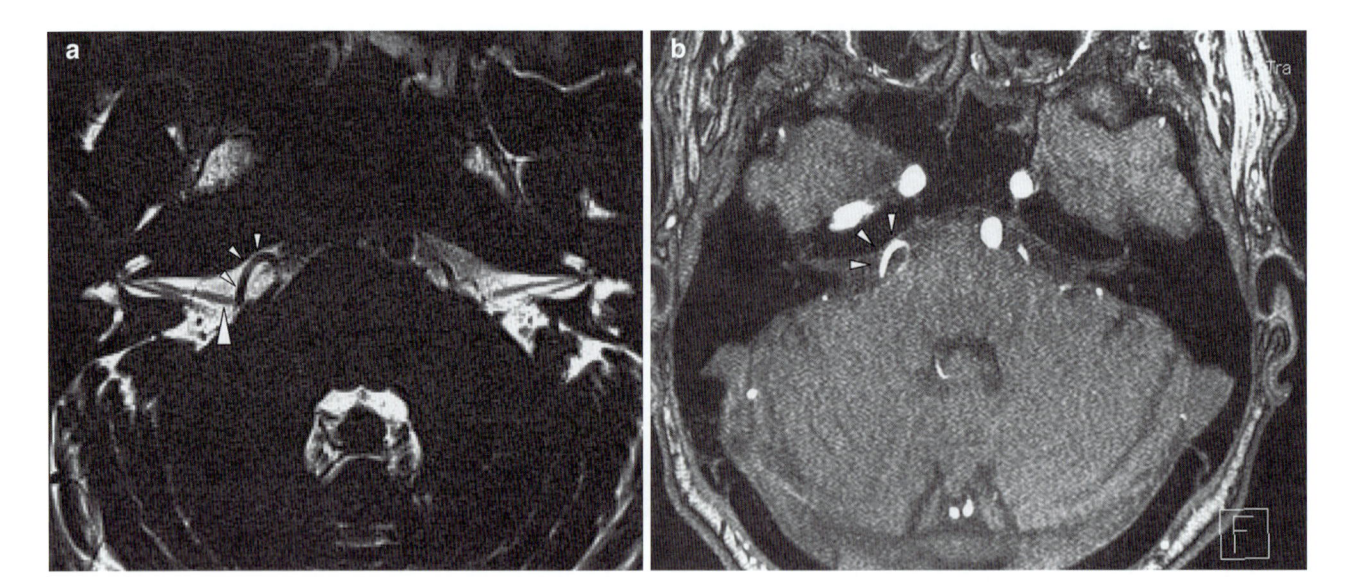

Fig. 57 42-year-old male with a clinical history of right-sided hemifacial spasms. **a** Axial 0.4 mm thick 3D TSE T2-weighted image through the IAC on both sides. Note the loop (*small arrowheads*) of a vascular structure running in the right CPA over the root entry zone of the facial nerve (*large arrowhead*). **b** Axial 1 mm thick unenhanced 3D TOF MR angio sequence demonstrating the vascular loop in the right-sided CPA (*small arrowheads*). In this case it was a loop of the anterior-inferior cerebellar artery. Conclusion: Patient with right-sided hemifacial spasm due to neurovascular conflict. Patient was treated by Teflon interposition and is free of disease

Fig. 58 36-year-old female with a straightforward clinical image of glossopharyngeus neuralgia (pain attacks in oropharynx and tongue). **a** Axial 0.4 mm thick 3D TSE T2-weighted image through the posterior fossa. The 9th, 10th and 11th nerve complex is seen running from posteromedial to anterolateral (*large arrowhead*). There is a small nodular vascular flow void visible lying against the anterior delineation of the nerve complex (*small arrowhead*). **b** Axial unenhanced 1 mm thick 3D TOF MR angio sequence through the posterior fossa (same level as Fig. 58a) displaying the PICA as two small high signal intensity dots (*arrowheads*). **c** Axial 0.4 mm thick 3D TSE T2-weighted image through the posterior fossa. There is a rectangular hypointense zone visible in the lower right cistern (*small arrowheads*), compatible with an interposed piece of Teflon. Conclusion: Neurovascular conflict of the PICA and the glossopharyngeal nerve treated by Teflon interposition. The patient was free of complaints after the intervention

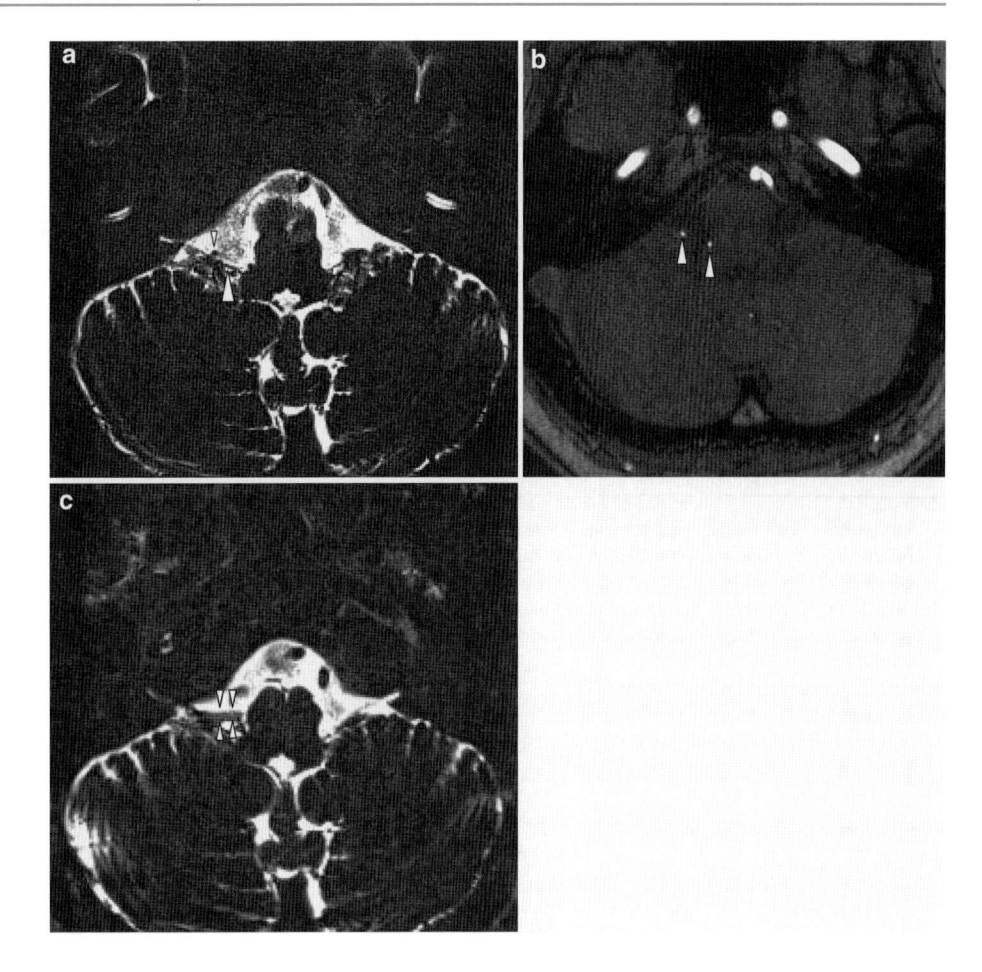

References

Aschenbach R, Heydel A, Eger C et al (2005) Aplasia of the n. cochlearis with retrocochlear deafness: the role of thin-slice 3D T2-weighted imaging. Eur Radiol 15:1768–1770

Ayache D, Trabalzini F, Bordure P et al (2006) Serous otitis media revealing temporal en plaque meningioma. Otol Neurootol 27: 992–998

Barath K, Schuknecht B, Monge Naldi A et al (2014) Detection and grading of endolymphatic hydrops in Meniere disease using MR imaging. Am J Neuroradiol (Feb 2013. Epub ahead of print)

Bonneville F, Savatovsky J, Chiras J (2007a) Imaging of cerebellopontine angle lesions: an update. Part 1: enhancing extra-axial lesions. Eur Radiol 17:2472–2482

Bonneville F, Savatovsky J, Chiras J (2007b) Imaging of cerebellopontine angle lesions: an update. Part 2: intra-axial lesions, skull base lesions that may invade the CPA region and non-enhancing extra-axial lesions. Eur Radiol 17:2908–2920

Borges A, Casselman J (2007) Imaging the cranial nerves: part II: primary and secondary neoplastic conditions and neurovascular conflicts. Eur Radiol 17:2332–2344

Casselman JW, Kuhweide R, Ampe W et al (1996) Inner ear malformations in patients with sensorineural hearing loss: detection with gradient-echo (3DFT-CISS) MRI. Neuroradiology 38: 278–286

Casselman JW, Offeciers FE, Govaerts PJ et al (1997) Aplasia and hypoplasia of the vestibulocochlear nerve: diagnosis with MR imaging. Radiology 202:773–781

Chadha NK, Weiner GM (2008) Vascular loops causing otological symptoms: a systematic review and meta-analysis. Clin Otolaryngol 33:5–11

de Ridder D, de Ridder L, Nowé V et al (2005) Pulsatile tinnitus and the intrameatal vascular loop: why do we not hear our carotids. Neurosurgery 57:1213–1217

de Foer B, Vercruysse JP, Spaepen M et al (2010) Diffusion-weighted magnetic resonance imaging of the temporal bone. Neuroradiology 52:785–807

Goebell E, Ries T, Kucinski T et al (2005) Screening for cerebellopontine angle tumors: is a CISS sufficient? Eur Radiol 15:286–291

Gultekin S, Celik H, Akpek S et al (2008) Vascular loops at the cerebellopontine angle: is there a correlation with tinnitus. Am J Neuroradiol 29:1746–1749

Hamilton BE, Salzman KL, Patel N et al (2006) Imaging and clinical characteristics of temporal bone meningioma. Am J Neuroradiol 27:2204–2209

Holman MA, Schmitt WR, Carslon ML et al (2013) Pediatric cerebellopontine angle and internal auditory canal tumors: clinical article. J Neurosurg Pediatr 12:317–324

Jackler RK (1996) Cost-effective screening for acoustic neuroma with unenhanced MR: a clinician's perspective. Am J Neuroradiol 17:1226–1228

Juliano AF, Ginat DT, Moonis G (2013) Imaging review of the temporal bone: part I. Anatomy and inflammatory and neoplastic processes. Radiology 269:17–33

Kano T, Ikota H, Kobayashi S et al (2010) Malignant transformation of an intracranial large epidermoid cyst with leptomeningeal carcinomatosis: case report. Neurol Med Chir 50:349–353

Kioumehr F, Dadsetan MR, Feldman N et al (1995) Postcontrast MRI of cranial meninges: leptomeningitis versus pachymeningitis. J Comput Assist Tomogr 19:713–720

Lakshmi M, Glastonbury CM (2009) Imaging of the cerebellopontine angle. Neuroimaging Clin N Am 19:393–406

Mohan S, Hoeffner E, Bigelow DC et al (2012) Applications of magnetic resonance imaging in adult temporal bone disorders. Magn Reson Imaging Clin N Am 20(545):572

Mukherjee P, Street I, Irving RM (2011) Intracranial lipomas affecting the cerebellopontine angle and internal auditory canal: a case series. Otol Neurotol 32:670–675

Pollock BE, Drisoll CL, Foote RL et al (2006) Patient outcomes after vestibular schwannoma management: a prospective comparison of microsurgical resection and stereotactic radiosurgery. Neurosurgery 59:77–85

Silk PS, Lane JI, Driscoll CL (2009) Surgical approaches to vestibular schwannomas: what the radiologist needs to know. Radiographics 29:1955–1970

Somers T, Casselman JW, de Ceulaer G et al (2001) Prognostic value of magnetic resonance imaging findings in hearing preservation surgery for vestibular schwannoma. Otol Neurotol 22:87–94

Van de Langenberg R, de Bondt BJ, Nelemans PJ et al (2009) Follow-up assessment of vestibular schwannomas: volume quantification versus two-dimensional measurements. Neuroradiology 51:517–524

Van der Steenstraten F, de Ru JA, Witkamp TD et al (2007) Is microvascular compression of the vestibulocochlear nerve a cause of unilateral hearing loss? Ann Otol Rhinol Laryngol 116:248–252

Verbist BM (2012) Imaging of sensorineural hearing loss: a pattern-based approach to disease of the inner ear and cerebellopontine angle. Insights Imaging 3:139–153

Warren FM, Shelton C, Wiggins RH 3rd et al (2008) Imaging characteristics of metastatic lesions of the cerebellopontine angle. Otol Neurotol 29:835–838

Wiggins RH 3rd, Harnsberger HR, Salzman KL et al (2006) The many faces of facial nerve schwannoma. Am J Neuroradiol 27:694–699

Yamazaki M, Naganawa S, Kawai H et al (2009) Increased signal intensity of the cochlea on pre- and post-contrast enhanced 3D-FLAIR in patients with vestibular schwannoma. Neuroradiology 51:855–863

Yamazaki M, Naganawa S, Kawai H et al (2010) Signal alteration of the cochlear perilymph on 3 different sequences after intratympanic Gd-DTPA administration at 3 Tesla: comparison of 3F-FLAIR, 3D-T1-weighted imaging, and 3D-CISS. Magn Reson Med Sci 9:65–71

Yamazaki M, Naganawa S, Tagaya M et al (2012) Comparison of contrast effect on the cochlear perilymph after intratympanic and intravenous gadolinium injection. Am J Neuroradiol 33:773–778

Inner Ear Pathology

Christoph Kenis, Bert De Foer, and Jan Walther Casselman

Contents

1 Introduction 219
2 **Labyrinthine Inflammation** 219
2.1 Pathogens and Modes of Spread 219
2.2 Imaging 221
2.3 Cogan's Syndrome 224
2.4 Sudden Sensorineural Hearing Loss 224
3 **Intralabyrinthine Hemorrhage** 225
4 **Intralabyrinthine Tumor** 225
4.1 Schwannoma 225
4.2 Non-schwannoma Tumors 228
5 **Endolymphatic Hydrops and Ménière's Disease** 230
6 **Superior Semicircular Canal Dehiscence** 231
References 233

Abstract

Imaging one of the smallest organs in the human body such as the inner ear frequently challenges the radiologist to depict millimetric changes in the labyrinth. Fortunately, the continuously increasing resolution of computed tomography (CT) as well as magnetic resonance imaging (MRI) makes it possible to see pathology in the labyrinth that was not detectable before. MRI is the technique of choice to image most of the acquired inner ear changes, but as in many parts of the body, CT will still be complementary in making the correct diagnosis. This chapter will try to focus on some characteristic features of the different pathologies and how to differentiate them from other lesions.

1 Introduction

This chapter will discuss the imaging features of acquired inner ear pathologies such as labyrinthine inflammation/hemorrhage, intralabyrinthine tumors, endolymphatic hydrops, and superior semicircular canal dehiscence. Anatomy, congenital inner ear pathology, and otodystrophies are discussed elsewhere in this book.

In the early 1990s, changes in the labyrinth became detectable with magnetic resonance imaging (MRI) (Seltzer and Mark 1991; Casselman et al. 1993; Mafee 1995). Three MRI sequences are conventionally used to diagnose intralabyrinthine pathology: heavily T2-weighted images (three-dimensional (3D) Fourier transformation constructive interference in steady state (3DFT-CISS), 3D turbo spin-echo (3D-TSE), 3D driven equilibrium radiofrequency reset pulse (3D-DRIVE), 3D fast imaging employing steady-state acquisition (3D-FIESTA), …), unenhanced T1-weighted images and gadolinium enhanced T1-weighted images. Close evaluation of the lesion characteristics on these three imaging sets will allow differentiation of inflammation,

C. Kenis (✉) · J.W. Casselman
Department of Radiology, AZ Sint Jan Hospital,
Ruddershove 10, 8000 Brugge, Belgium
e-mail: christophkenis@hotmail.com

B. De Foer · J.W. Casselman
Department of Radiology, GZA Sint Augustinus Hospital,
Oosterveldlaan 24, 2610 Wilrijk, Belgium

J.W. Casselman
Department of Radiology, University of Ghent, Gent, Belgium

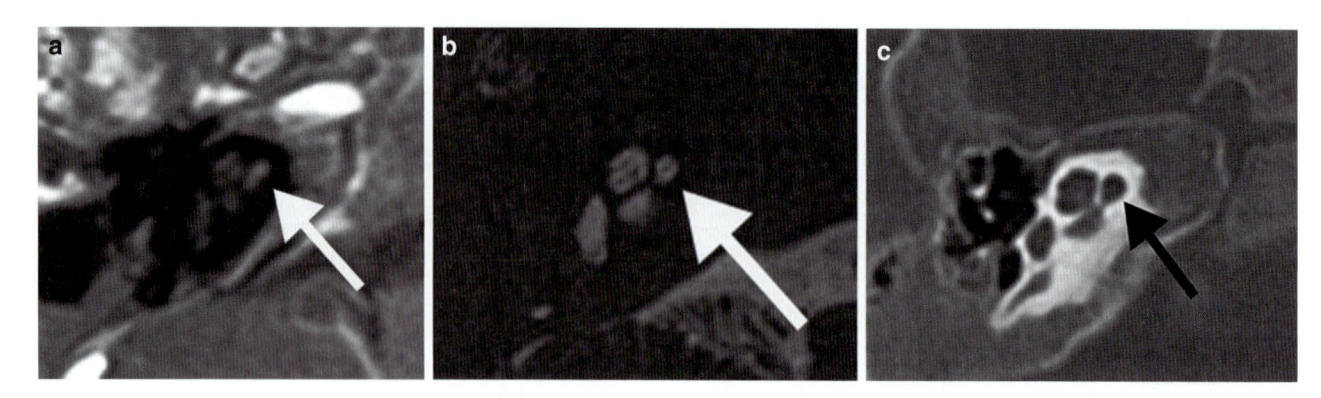

Fig. 1 A 3-month-old girl with a deaf *right* ear caused by a congenital cytomegalovirus infection. **a** Axial postcontrast T1-weighted MR image shows a hyperintense basal turn of the *right* cochlea (*arrow*) which can represent contrast enhancement, hemorrhage, or high protein content. No precontrast T1-weighted MR imaging was performed in this patient. **b** Axial 3D-TSE T2-weighted MR image of the *right* ear demonstrates no evidence of fibrosis as there is a normal fluid signal in the basal turn with a clear distinction of the scala vestibuli and tympani (*arrow*). **c** On the axial multidetector CT (MDCT) image of the *right* ear, there is no ossification visible in the basal turn, besides a normal dense osseous spiral lamina centrally (*arrow*). There was a normal cochlear nerve present (not shown), and the patient was successfully treated with a cochlear implant

tumor, or hemorrhage in most cases (Casselman et al. 1993; Mafee 1995; Dubrulle et al. 2010). Recently however, 3D-FLAIR images are of particular interest since they have been shown pathology such as inflammation or minor hemorrhage which could not be detected on conventional MRI sequences (Naganawa and Nakashima 2009; Tanigawa et al. 2010).

Furthermore, particular interest has increased for the evaluation of endolymphatic hydrops which has been associated with Ménière's disease. Three-dimensional fluid-attenuated inversion recovery (3D-FLAIR) and 3D inversion recovery turbo spin-echo (3D-IR-TSE) sequences are now able to demonstrate this entity after intratympanic or intravenous injection of gadolinium contrast (Nakashima et al. 2007, 2010).

2 Labyrinthine Inflammation

2.1 Pathogens and Modes of Spread

Inflammation of the labyrinth can be classified as infective or non-infective.

Infective causes of labyrinthitis can be viral, bacterial, protozoal, and fungal. Viral labyrinthitis can cause congenital or acquired hearing loss. Congenital cytomegalovirus has replaced rubella embryopathy as the most prevalent environmental cause of prelingual hearing loss in the USA (Fig. 1) (Morton and Nance 2006). Ramsay Hunt syndrome is believed to be caused by the reactivation of latent varicella zoster virus in the geniculate, spiral, and/or vestibular (Scarpa's) ganglia. It can cause inflammation of the external auditory canal, facial nerve, cochleovestibular nerve, and labyrinth (Fig. 2) and retrograde inflammation of the brain stem along the nerve sheaths (Kuhweide et al. 2002). Viral labyrinthitis is often preceded by an upper respiratory tract infection. The bacteria that cause labyrinthitis are the same that cause meningitis and otitis, and most frequently are Streptococcus pneumoniae, Haemophilus influenzae, and Neisseria meningitidis (Karanja et al. 2013). Syphilitic labyrinthitis, which is caused by the bacterium Treponema pallidum, is a rare manifestation of the disease (Smith and Anderson 2000). Bacterial labyrinthitis can be categorized as suppurative and serous. Suppurative labyrinthitis occurs when there is direct spread of bacteria into the labyrinth either intracranially or from the middle ear and mastoid. The term serous labyrinthitis is used when there is direct infiltration of the labyrinth by bacterial toxins and host inflammatory mediators such as cytokines, enzymes, and complement. These toxic substances penetrate through the round window, internal auditory canal (IAC), or cochlear aqueduct into the labyrinth, causing a sterile inflammatory reaction in the perilymph space (Jang et al. 2005).

Non-infective etiologies of labyrinthitis are various and include autoimmune diseases such as Cogan's syndrome, Wegener granulomatosis, relapsing polychondritis, polyarteritis nodosa, systemic lupus erythematosus, Sjögren's syndrome, ulcerative colitis, and Crohn's disease (Stone and Francis 2000; Teszler et al. 2008; Benson 2010; Weisert et al. 2012).

Another way to classify labyrinthitis is by cause or origin. Labyrinthitis can be tympanogenic, meningogenic, haematogenic, or traumatic in origin. Tympanogenic spread of infection occurs because of the passage of microorganisms, toxins, or pharmacological agents from the middle ear into the inner ear through the round or oval window (Swartz et al. 1985; Lemmerling et al. 2009). Labyrinthitis can also be due to labyrinthine fistulas which can occur after inflammatory or cholesteatomatous disease (Fig. 3) or postoperatively. Examples of the latter are prosthetic stapedotomy (Fig. 4) and surgery for,

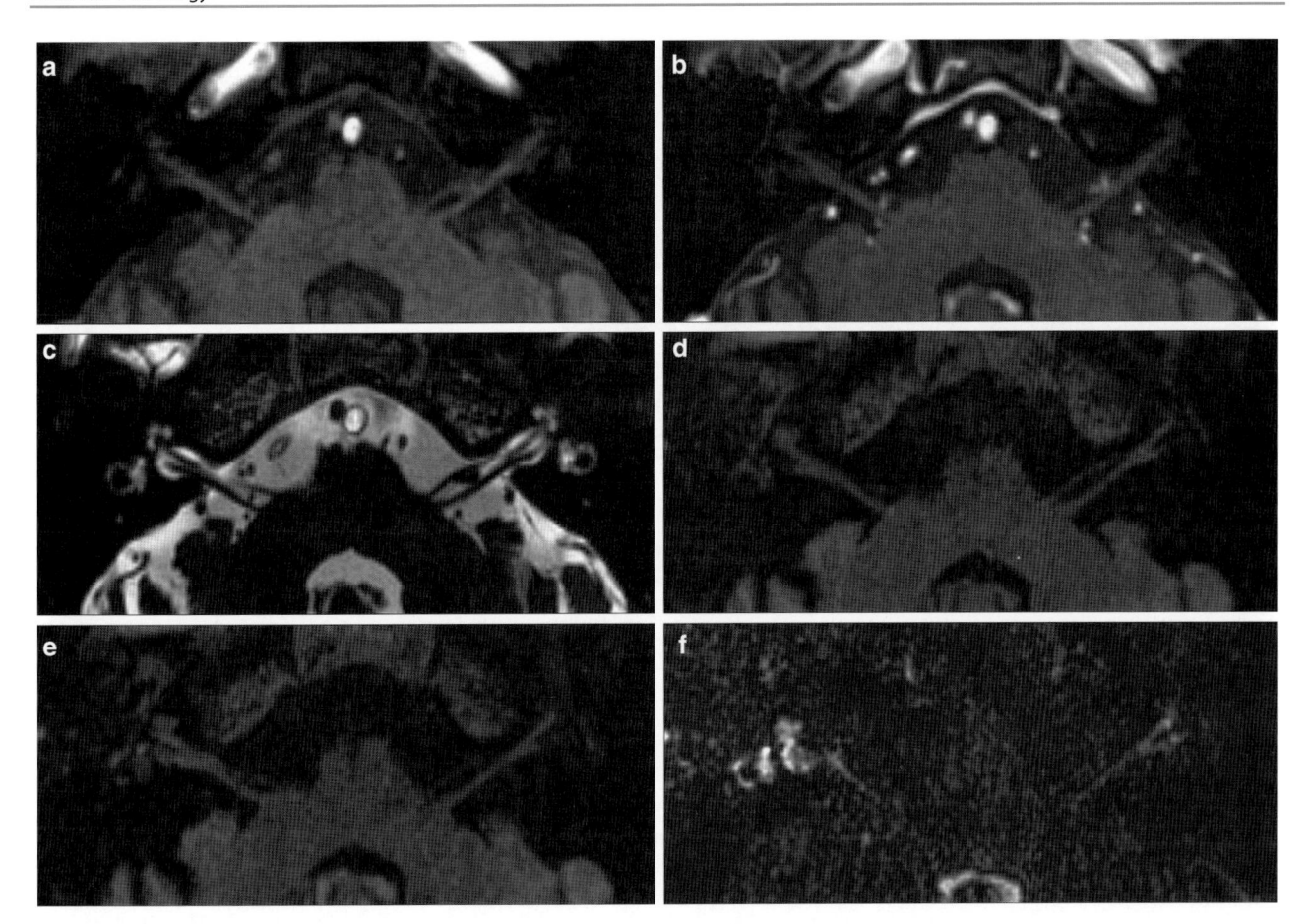

Fig. 2 An 81-year-old man with right-sided facial palsy (Ramsay Hunt syndrome). There were blisters in his *right* external auditory canal. MR images were obtained 1 week from onset of facial palsy. No significant signal increase of the *right* labyrinth is noted on the precontrast axial T1-weighted MR image (**a**) and postcontrast T1-weighted MR image (**b**). No signal alteration is seen on the axial 3D-CISS MR image (**c**). Slight signal increase of *right* labyrinth is visible on the precontrast axial 3D-FLAIR MR image (**d**), and further signal increase of *right* labyrinth is visible on the postcontrast axial 3D-FLAIR MR image (**e**). Remarkable signal increase of right labyrinth is seen on the postcontrast axial heavily T2-weighted 3D-FLAIR MR image (**f**), showing the extremely high sensitivity of the heavily T2-weighted 3D-FLAIR MR sequence (Courtesy of Shinji Naganawa, MD)

e.g., a vestibular schwannoma (Williams and Ayache 2004). Tympanogenic labyrinthitis is typically unilateral. Meningogenic labyrinthitis is usually bilateral (Fig. 5). The source of labyrinthine invasion is thought to be through the cochlear aqueduct or the lamina cribrosa in the vestibule (Hegarty et al. 2002). Bacterial meningitis typically occurs in children and is the most common cause of acquired childhood deafness (Fortnum and Davis 1993). Haematogenic labyrinthitis is the least commonly documented route of spread. Typical causative agents are mumps, measles, human immunodeficiency virus (HIV), cytomegalovirus, syphilis, and borreliosis.

2.2 Imaging

Histologically, the evolution of ossification following suppurative labyrinthitis can be classified into three stages: acute, fibrous, and ossification (de Souza et al. 1991; Xu et al. 2009). These stages have also been used in the radiological literature, and they have characteristic features on MRI and CT images (Table 1). In the acute stage, the fluid-filled spaces of the membranous labyrinth (ML) show a normal fluid signal on heavily T2-weighted images. Precontrast T1-weighted images and the more sensitive 3D-FLAIR sequence may show areas of high signal intensity, presumably representing inflammatory exsudate or minor hemorrhage (Casselman et al. 1994; Sugiura et al. 2007). After intravenous administration of gadolinium, T1-weighted images and 3D-FLAIR images demonstrate segmental or diffuse enhancement of the ML due to breakdown of the blood–labyrinth barrier with granulation tissue and angiogenesis (Figs. 1, 2, 3, 4 and 5). CT images will show no abnormality in this stage. When this acute stage of labyrinthitis persists, it progresses to a chronic stage with fibrous changes and later ossification. In the fibrous stage, fibrous strands replace the fluid in the ML, which is seen as a decrease of fluid signal on heavily T2-weighted images (Figs. 3, 5 and 6) (Casselman et al. 1993; Hegarty et al. 2002; Lemmerling et al. 2009; Dubrulle et al. 2010). This stage

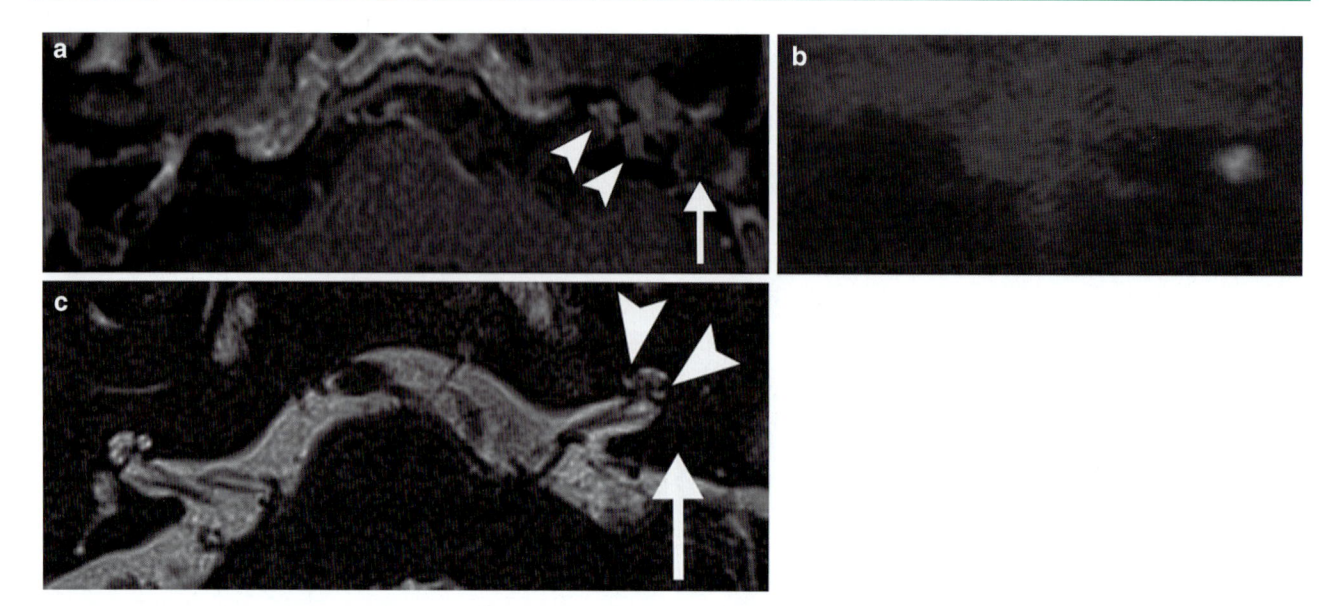

Fig. 3 A 61-year-old man patient with *left-sided* labyrinthitis caused by a cholesteatomatous fistula. **a** Axial postcontrast T1-weighted MR image demonstrates intense enhancement of the left labyrinth (*arrowheads*) and the presence of a cholesteatoma (*arrow*) in the middle ear and mastoid which is clearly diagnosed on the coronal b1000 DWI MR image as a nodular hyperintense lesion (**b**). **c** Axial 3D-TSE T2-weighted MR image shows decreased signal in the cochlea with absent signal in the scala vestibuli of the basal and middle turn (*arrowheads*) and absent signal in the vestibule (*arrow*). These findings are compatible with combined fibrous and ossified material, which was found during cochlear implantation, performed because the patient was already deaf on the contralateral side

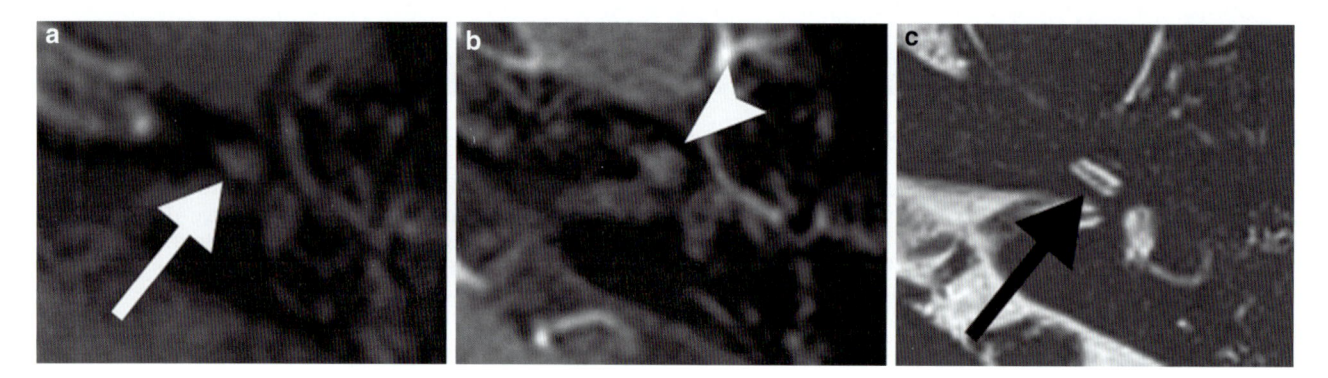

Fig. 4 A 47-year-old man with progressive tinnitus, vertigo, and progressive hearing loss 2 days after stapes surgery for *left-sided* otosclerosis. **a** Axial precontrast T1-weighted MR image shows a hyperintense focus (*arrow*) in the middle turn of the *left* cochlea compatible with minor hemorrhage or high protein content. **b** The cochlea enhances further on the postcontrast axial T1-weighted image (*arrowhead*). **c** Axial 3D-TSE T2-weighted image demonstrates a normal fluid signal in the middle turn (*arrow*). The imaging findings are characteristic of acute labyrinthitis

begins approximately 2 weeks after the onset of infection (de Souza et al. 1991; Xu et al. 2009). There may still be some hyperintense areas visible on pre- and postcontrast T1-weighted and 3D-FLAIR images as the presence of inflammatory exsudate and angiogenesis can persist, but contrast enhancement is less intense than in the acute stage. Differentiation with an intralabyrinthine schwannoma can be made as these tumors will show stronger contrast enhancement and a sharp delineation (Casselman et al. 1993; Dubrulle et al. 2010). CT may show a slight increase in density, but it is still of no use in this stage. The ossification stage is characterized by new bone formation. The evolution to ossification is most commonly a sequela from suppurative labyrinthitis following bacterial meningitis, but other causes are trauma, labyrinthine artery obstruction, autoimmune disease, otosclerosis, leukemia, and temporal bone tumors. In animals, osteoid deposition has been demonstrated as early as 3 days after bacterial infection (Tinling et al. 2004). The fluid-filled spaces of the ML are replaced by this new bone, and there will be no signal visible on heavily T2-weighted images. At this point, usually no abnormality will be seen on T1-weighted and 3D-FLAIR images before or after contrast administration. CT images demonstrate the presence of ossified portions of the labyrinth, and these images are crucial

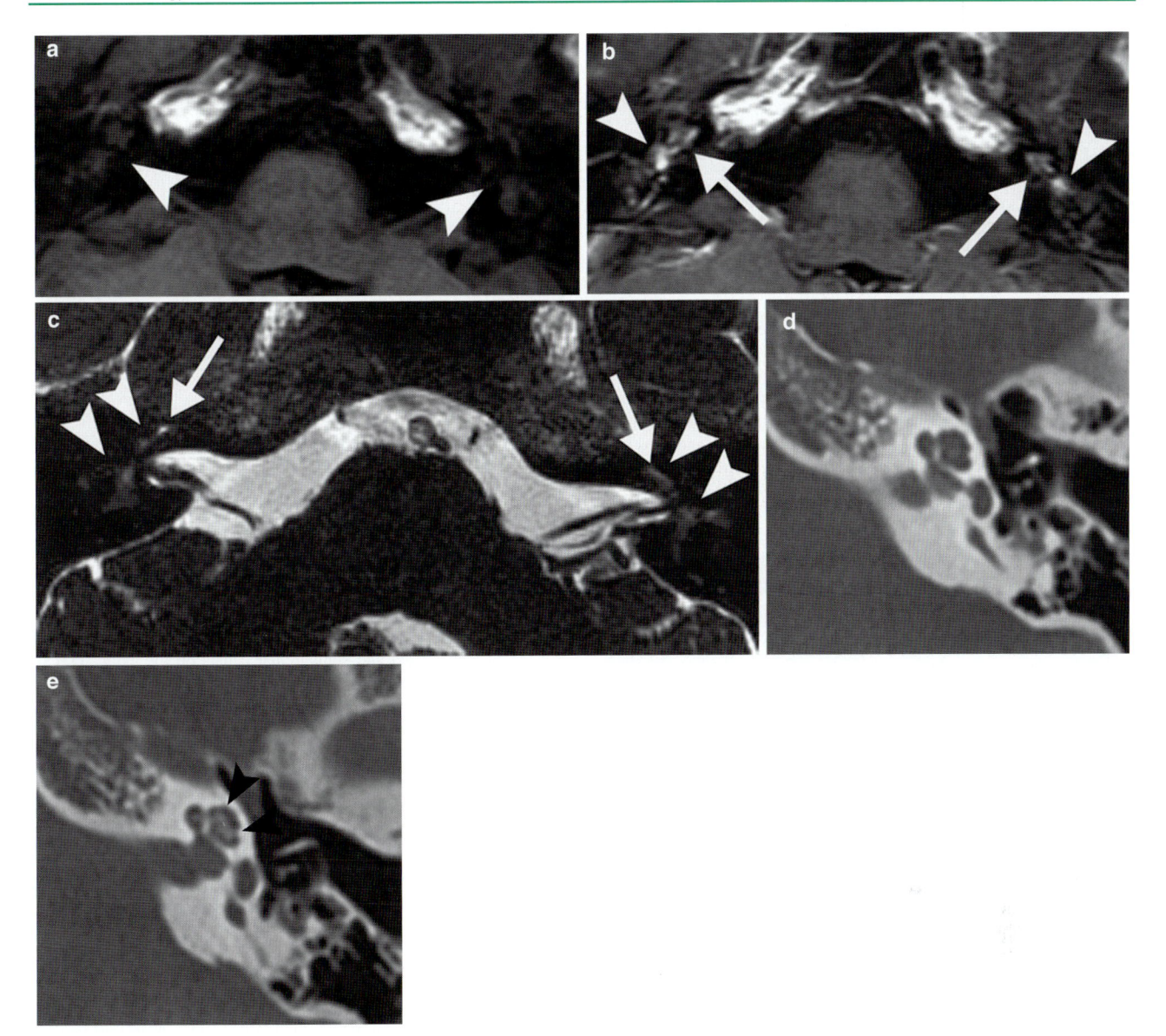

Fig. 5 A 45-year-old man with bilateral labyrinthitis and deafness after bacterial meningitis. **a** Axial precontrast T1-weighted MR image shows no abnormal signal in the labyrinth (*arrowheads*). **b** Axial postcontrast T1-weighted MR image demonstrates intense bilateral enhancement of the cochlea (*arrows*) and vestibule (*arrowheads*). **c** Axial CISS T2-weighted MR image shows decreased signal intensity of the labyrinth (*arrowheads*) with only faint fluid signal remaining in the middle turn of the cochlea (*arrows*). **d** Axial MDCT image of the *left* ear shows no calcification in the cochlea. The imaging findings are consistent with the fibrotic stage of labyrinthitis. **e** Axial MDCT image of the *left* ear 4 months later demonstrates extensive ossification of the *middle* and apical turn (*arrowheads*) of the cochlea compatible with the chronic stage of labyrinthitis with ossification

Table 1 MR and CT imaging features in the different stages of labyrinthitis

Stage	T1/3D FLAIR	T2	T1/3D FLAIR + Gd	CT
Acute	Normal or intense	Normal	Focal or diffuse enhancement	Normal
Fibrous	Normal or slightly intense	Decreased	No or slight enhancement	Normal or slightly increased density
Ossification	Normal	Absent	No enhancement	High density

in the precochlear implant evaluation (Figs. 5, 7 and 8). The combination of MRI and CT allows determination of in which scala and to what extent the ossification is present (Fig. 7). Overlap of the three stages can be present (Hegarty et al. 2002; Lemmerling et al. 2009; Xu et al. 2009; Berrettini et al. 2013).

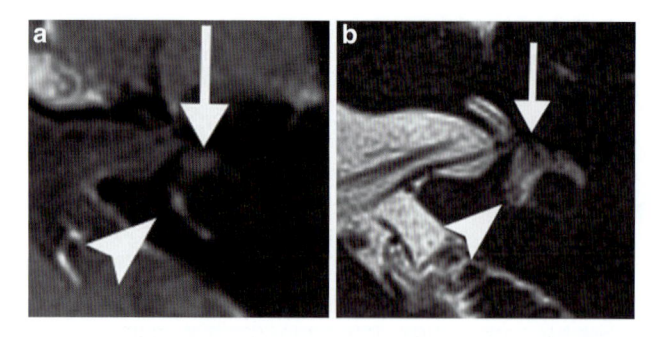

Fig. 6 A 23-year-old woman with progressive vertigo on the *left* since 3 weeks. **a** Axial postcontrast T1-weighted MR image of the left ear shows slight enhancement of the vestibule (*arrowhead*) and profound enhancement of the common crus (*arrowhead*) and posterior semicircular canal. **b** Axial DRIVE T2-weighted MR image demonstrates decreased signal intensity of the anterior (*arrow*) and posterior (*arrowhead*) parts of the vestibule. The imaging features are consistent with the chronic stage of labyrinthitis with fibrosis

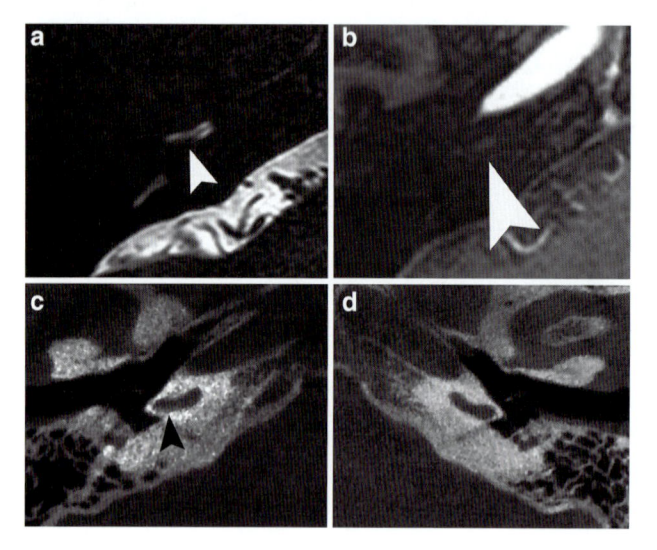

Fig. 7 A 45-year-old man who has been deaf bilaterally as a child after meningitis. **a** Axial DRIVE T2-weighted MR image of the *right* ear shows an absent signal in the scala tympani (*arrowhead*) posterior in the basal turn of the *right* cochlea. **b** Axial postcontrast T1-weighted MR image shows no enhancement at this level (*arrowhead*). **c** Axial cone-beam CT (CBCT) image of the *right* ear shows a string of ossification (*arrowhead*) posterior in the basal turn. **d** Axial CBCT image of the normal contralateral side for comparison. The imaging findings are compatible with the chronic stage of labyrinthitis with ossification

2.3 Cogan's Syndrome

Cogan's syndrome is a rare systemic disease characterized by non-syphilitic interstitial keratitis and audiovestibular symptoms which are similar to Ménière's disease (sudden onset of vertigo, tinnitus, nausea, vomiting, and gradual hearing loss). In about 70 % of the patients, there is associated systemic disease considered to be due to vasculitis, usually of the large- and medium-sized vessels. The aetiology and pathogenesis of Cogan's syndrome are unknown.

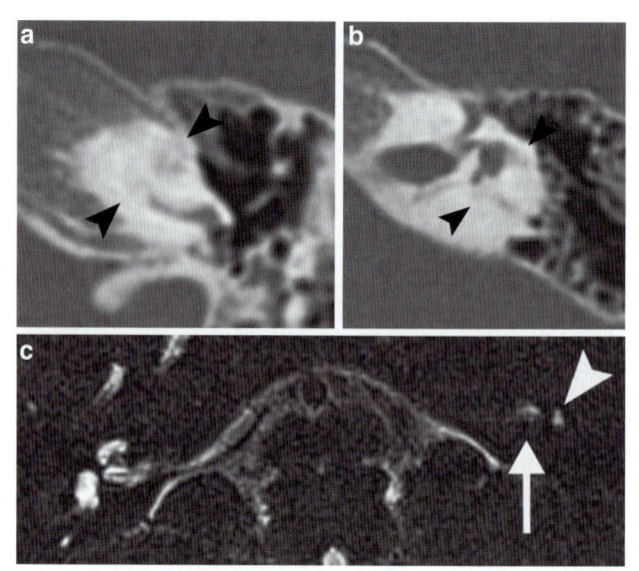

Fig. 8 A 5-year-old girl who is congenitally deaf on the left without a known cause. **a** Axial MDCT image reveals near-total ossification of the middle, apical and distal basal turn of the left cochlea (*arrowheads*). **b** Axial MDCT image shows near-total ossification of the semicircular canals (*arrowheads*) and part of the vestibule. **c** No fluid signal is detected in the cochlea and semicircular canals on the axial 3D TSE T2-weighted MR image. Only faint signal is visible in the vestibule (*arrowhead*) and the fundus of the internal auditory canal (*arrow*). Extreme example of the chronic stage of labyrinthitis with ossification

Initially, it was thought to be a disease caused by infection, with Chlamydia species being the mostly associated culprit. Nowadays, it is believed to be an autoimmune-mediated inflammatory disorder. A prodromen of an upper respiratory tract infection is often reported. The disease mostly affects young Caucasian adults, and there is no sex predilection (Mazlumzadeh and Matteson 2007; Greco et al. 2013). CT and MR imaging of Cogan's syndrome may be negative, but in most patients, the findings are similar to those of labyrinthitis. CT imaging fails to detect soft tissue changes in the fluid-filled spaces of the membranous labyrinth (ML), but it can detect calcific obliteration in the chronic stage. On MRI, there can be high signal in the ML on unenhanced T1-weighted and 3D-FLAIR images in some patients, which can be attributed to high protein content, but more likely due to hemorrhage as Cogan's syndrome is associated with vasculitis. Gadolinium enhancement can be seen in the acute stage of the disease and represents gadolinium leakage through the labyrinth membrane. On heavily T2-weighted images, the areas where the fluid-filled spaces of the ML are obliterated show low signal intensity (Fig. 9). The most frequently affected parts of the ML are the semicircular canals, followed by the basal turn of the cochlea and the vestibule (Casselman et al. 1994; Helmchen et al. 1998). Currently, there are no definitive therapeutic recommendations. Intravenous corticosteroids are the first-line agents of

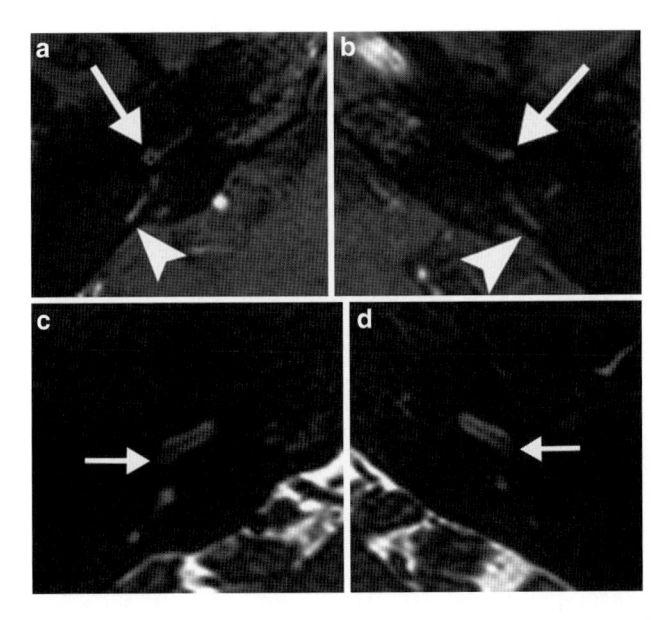

Fig. 9 A 28-year-old woman with recent progressive sensorineural hearing loss caused by Cogan's syndrome. **a, b** Axial postcontrast T1-weighted MR image of the *right* (**a**) and *left* (**b**) temporal bone shows faint bilateral contrast enhancement in the posterior part of the cochlear basal turn (*arrows*) and posterior semicircular canals (*arrowheads*). **c, d** Axial DRIVE T2-weighted MR image of the *right* (**c**) and *left* (**d**) temporal bone demonstrates a slightly decreased signal in the cochlea bilaterally, most evident in the posterior part of the basal turn (*arrows*) consistent with a mild degree of fibrosis

treatment, and immunosuppressants are used as second-line drugs (Mazlumzadeh and Matteson 2007; Greco et al. 2013). The hearing loss is generally bilateral and progresses to profound hearing loss in 60 % of cases. In the latter patient group, cochlear implantation remains the only treatment option and has been proven to be beneficial in many cases. In the preoperative evaluation, it is important that the radiologist reports in which scala of the cochlea there is fibrous or calcific obliteration present (Wang et al. 2010; Bovo et al. 2011).

2.4 Sudden Sensorineural Hearing Loss

Sudden sensorineural hearing loss (SSNHL) is defined as a sensorineural decrease in hearing of 30 dB or more, affecting at least three consecutive frequencies, occurring over a 72-h period. Up to 90 % of SSNHL is idiopathic at presentation, presumptively attributed to vascular, viral, or multiple etiologies (Stachler et al. 2012). Most MRI examinations performed because of SSNHL will show no inner ear abnormality, and the main purpose of referring patients for an MRI examination is to exclude an underlying tumor (Stokroos et al. 1998). MRI sequences such as 3D-FLAIR are now able to demonstrate labyrinthine fluid changes where the conventional heavily T2-weighted and pre- and postcontrast T1-weighted sequences fail to detect abnormalities (Otake et al. 2006; Tanigawa et al. 2010). In patients with SSNHL, the frequency of high signal found on precontrast 3D-FLAIR ranges from 25.8 to 64.6 % (Cadoni et al. 2006; Yoshida et al. 2008; Ryu et al. 2011; Lee et al. 2012; Berrettini et al. 2013). Of the 13/23 precontrast 3D-FLAIR-positive patients in one study, only three patients demonstrated a hypersignal on a conventional T1-weighted sequence (Berrettini et al. 2013). In two other studies, there was no abnormality visible on T1- and T2-weighted sequences in 31/48 and 12/35 3D-FLAIR-positive patients, respectively (Yoshida et al. 2008; Ryu et al. 2011). High signal intensities in the labyrinth on unenhanced 3D-FLAIR and T1-weighted images may reflect minor hemorrhage or increased protein concentration, and enhancement of the labyrinth and/or the vestibulocochlear nerve after contrast administration is a result of breakdown of the blood–labyrinth barrier (Figs. 10 and 11) (Lee et al. 2012; Berrettini et al. 2013). Most lesions detected on 3D-FLAIR images are isolated to the cochlea, followed by the involvement of the cochlea and the vestibule. Lesions isolated to the vestibule are rare. Vertigo can be present in up to 30 % of patients with SSNHL, and high signal intensities in the vestibule and/or semicircular canals are consistent with the occurrence of vertigo (Ryu et al. 2011; Berrettini et al. 2013). Gadolinium enhancement on 3D-FLAIR images is seen in about half of the cases that are positive on precontrast 3D-FLAIR images (Yoshida et al. 2008; Lee et al. 2012; Berrettini et al. 2013).

3 Intralabyrinthine Hemorrhage

Intralabyrinthine hemorrhage (ILH) is a rare entity. It has been reported in patients with coagulopathy, systemic lupus erythematosus, anemia, sickle cell disease, Cogan's syndrome, leukemia, trauma, superficial siderosis, cocaine consumption, leukemia, after vestibular schwannoma surgery, and after head and neck irradiation (Casselman et al. 1994; Whitehead et al. 1998; Nicoucar et al. 2005; Sugiura et al. 2006; Poh and Tan 2007; Salomone et al. 2008; Toyama et al. 2009; Dubrulle et al. 2010). SSNHL is the main symptom of ILH, and it can be accompanied by vertigo and tinnitus (Dubrulle et al. 2010). The diagnosis of ILH can be made with MRI where the areas of hemorrhage are spontaneously intense on unenhanced 3D-FLAIR and T1-weighted images (Figs. 11 and 12). These intensities are not well defined, and they do not have a nodular shape which allows differentiation with a lipoma or a schwannoma (Dubrulle et al. 2010). Furthermore, a lipoma will be saturated on fat-suppressed T1-weighted images (Dahlen et al. 2002). An intralabyrinthine schwannoma (ILS) is well defined on postcontrast T1-weighted and heavily T2-weighted images, and it is only slightly intense on unenhanced T1-weighted images compared to the high signal intensity of hemorrhage (Tieleman et al. 2008; De Foer et al. 2009; Lemmerling et al. 2009;

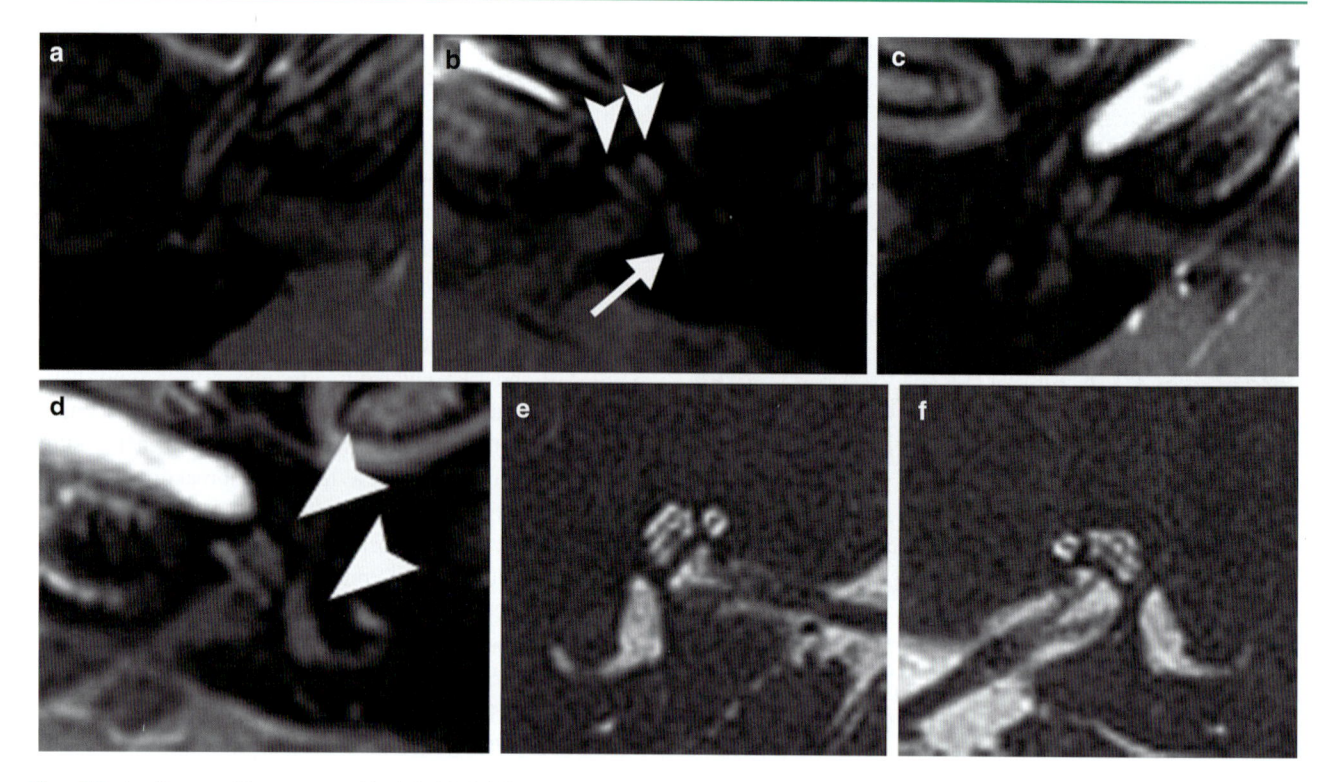

Fig. 10 A 40-year-old woman with left-sided idiopathic sudden sensorineural hearing loss. **a, b** Axial precontrast T1-weighted MR images of the *right* (**a**) and *left* (**b**) temporal bone show high signal intensities in the *left* cochlea (*arrowheads* in **b**) and vestibule (*arrow* in **b**) reflecting minor hemorrhage or high protein content. **c, d** Slight further enhancement is seen in the *left* labyrinth (*arrowheads* in **d**) on the postcontrast axial T1-weighted MR image. **e, f** There is no evidence of fibrotic changes on the axial 3D-TSE T2-weighted MR image

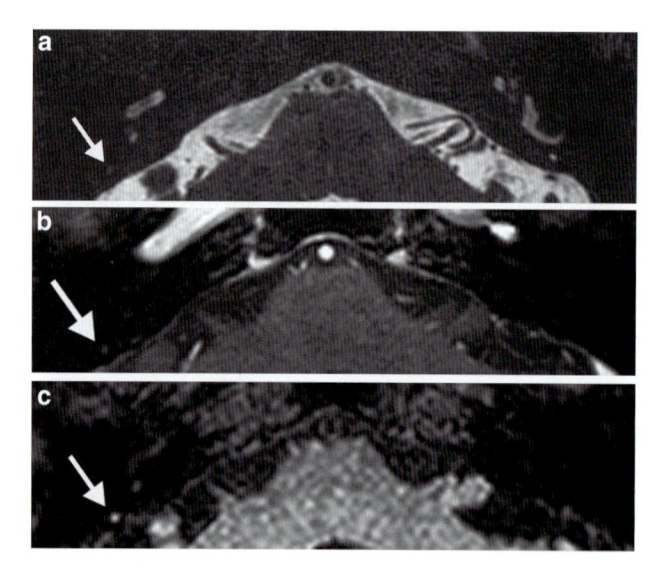

Fig. 11 A 77-year-old woman treated with anticoagulant medicine for cardiac disease presents with sudden sensorineural hearing loss, tinnitus, and vertigo. **a** Axial DRIVE T2-weighted MR image of the temporal bones demonstrates decreased signal in the posterior semicircular canal on the *right* (*arrow*) and slightly increased signal intensity on the postcontrast axial T1-weighted MR image (*arrow* in **b**). This high signal is more clearly depicted on the precontrast axial 3D-FLAIR MR image (*arrow* in **c**). The clinical diagnosis was compatible with intralabyrinthine hemorrhage. No lesions were detected in the cochlea

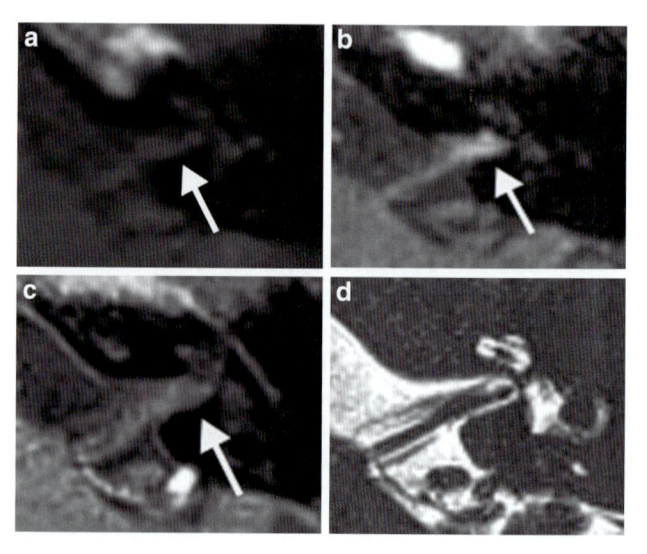

Fig. 12 A 33-year-old man with progressive tinnitus since 2 weeks after commotio cerebri. **a** Axial precontrast T1-weighted MR image demonstrates a faint hyperintensity (*arrow*) in the *left* IAC which is more clearly visible on the axial precontrast 3D-FLAIR MR image (*arrow* in **b**). **c** Axial postcontrast T1-weighted MR image shows subtle enhancement (*arrow*) of the *left* IAC. **d** Normal fluid intensity is present on the axial 3D-TSE T2-weighted MR image. These findings are consistent with posttraumatic hemorrhage in the IAC

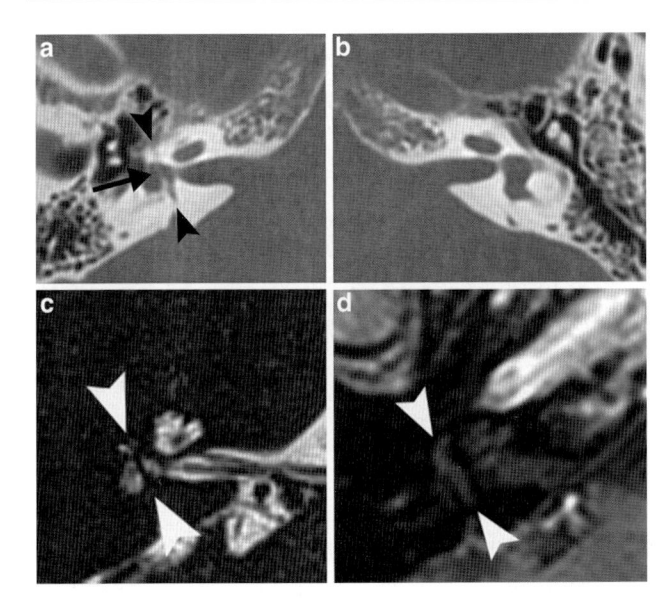

Fig. 13 A 49-year-old man with *right-sided* deafness after skull base trauma at the age of 6, now referred for precochlear implant evaluation. **a** Axial MDCT image of the *right* temporal bone shows a transverse fracture line through the vestibule (*arrowheads*) and a fine string of ossification (*arrow*) in the vestibule. **b** Axial MDCT image of the contralateral side for comparison. **c** Axial 3D-TSE T2-weighted MR image of the *right* temporal bone shows the absent signal of the string of ossification in the vestibule (*arrowheads*). There is decreased signal intensity in the vestibule, and no fluid is detected in the semicircular canals consistent with fibrosis. **d** This abnormal anatomy is also visible on the axial postcontrast T1-weighted MR image (*arrowheads*), but there is no contrast enhancement

Salzman et al. 2012). The high signal areas of ILH on unenhanced T1-weighted images can persist for over a year. After contrast administration, there can be additional diffuse enhancement of the membranous labyrinth. On heavily T2-weighted images, ILH shows a decreased signal of the normal fluid in the membranous labyrinth and these areas are also not well defined nor nodular, allowing differentiation with ILS. This hyposignal suggests the early development of fibrosis which can evolve into ossification (Fig. 13) (Dubrulle et al. 2010). High signal areas on unenhanced T1-weighted images can represent methemoglobin or high lipid content, and the differentiation is usually made based on the underlying condition (Casselman et al. 1994; Whitehead et al. 1998; Dubrulle et al. 2010). SSNHL in general may also be attributable to small amounts of hemorrhage, as discussed in the previous paragraph.

4 Intralabyrinthine Tumor

4.1 Schwannoma

Intralabyrinthine schwannomas (ILS) are benign tumors that spontaneously arise from the perineural Schwann cell sheath of the nerve branches in the cochlea, vestibule, semicircular canals, or a combination of these structures. They initially have no extension to the IAC (Neff et al. 2003). Intracochlear schwannomas develop on the intracochlear branches, and intravestibular schwannomas develop on the vestibular branches which can be the saccular nerve, utricular nerve, and lateral, superior, or posterior ampullary nerve. ILS are rare tumors with less than 200 cases described in the literature to date (Tieleman et al. 2008; Salzman et al. 2012; Bouchetemblé et al. 2013). However, due to the increasing resolution of MRI images, and conspicuity of the radiologist and the clinician, the prevalence of ILS will probably increase. They are reported in association with neurofibromatosis Type 2, but sporadic cases are more prevalent. Hearing loss is the main symptom which is present in practically all patients with ILS. Less common symptoms are tinnitus and vertigo (Tieleman et al. 2008; Salzman et al. 2012). ILS are most frequently located in the cochlea and are often located at the area between the basal and second turn. Most intracochlear schwannomas arise in the scala tympani (Fig. 14), and the remaining intracochlear lesions involve both scalae (Fig. 15). ILS does not appear to be found isolated in the scala vestibuli, and this is thought to be because of the proximity of the nerve to the scala tympani at the habenula perforate, which is the region where the nerve exits the osseous spiral lamina and runs toward the organ of Corti (Fig. 16). The lesions may grow from the scala tympani into the scala vestibuli. The scala tympani ends at the round window and has no connection with the vestibule. Therefore, it is presumed that lesions fill up the cochlea, grow into the scala vestibuli, and consequently grow into the vestibule through the continuous perilymphatic space around the saccule (Figs. 17 and 18). Vice versa, vestibular lesions can grow into the scala vestibuli through this space (Fig. 19) (Tieleman et al. 2008). Tieleman et al. (2008) found most ILS isolated in the vestibule to be in the anterior part with no lesion isolated in the posterior part. Isolated semicircular canal involvement in the non-neurofibromatosis patient seems to be very rare. The same study demonstrated that in only 11.1 % of patients, growth from the cochlea into the IAC could be noticed (Fig. 20). In this largest study on ILS published to date, overall growth rate of ILS was found to be 59.3 %. Serial MRI scan to document growth is therefore the most commonly used management. Hearing preservation is not possible when the ILS is removed, and surgery is considered when there is intractable vertigo and/or tinnitus, or tumor growth extending into the IAC or middle ear (Salzman et al. 2012; Bouchetemblé et al. 2013). Kennedy et al. (2004) proposed the following classification system for ILS: "intravestibular" when ILS is confined to the vestibule with or without involvement of the semicircular canals; "intracochlear" when ILS is confined to the cochlea; "intravestibulocochlear" when ILS is confined to both the cochlea and vestibule; "transmodiolar" when ILS extends

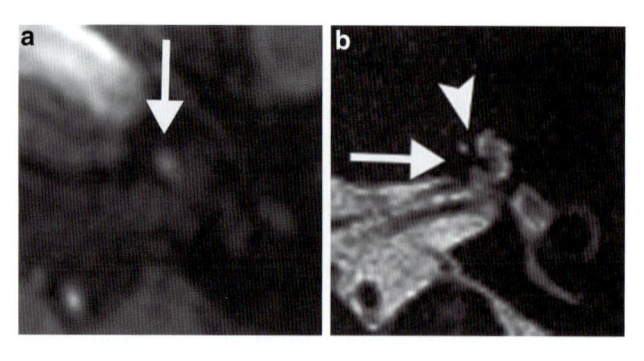

Fig. 14 A 67-year-old man with an intralabyrinthine schwannoma (ILS) isolated in the scala tympani. **a** Axial postcontrast T1-weighted MR image shows a tiny enhancing nodule (*arrow*) anterior in the basal turn of the left cochlea. **b** Axial 3D-TSE T2-weighted MR image locates the ILS in the scala tympani (*arrow*) where absent fluid signal is present. There is a normal fluid signal in the scala vestibuli located in between the ILS (*arrow*) and the medial interscalar septum (*arrowhead*). This ILS has been stable for the last 4 years

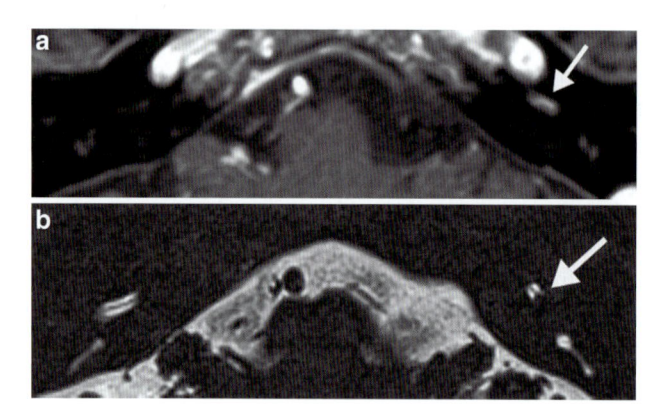

Fig. 15 A 60-year-old woman with an ILS in both scalae. **a** Axial postcontrast T1-weighted MR image displays a sharply delineated enhancing tumor (*arrow*) in the basal turn of the left cochlea. **b** Axial 3D-TSE T2-weighted MR image locates the tumor in both the scala tympani and scala vestibuli with a sharp anterior convex border (*arrow*). This ILS has not shown growth for 10 years

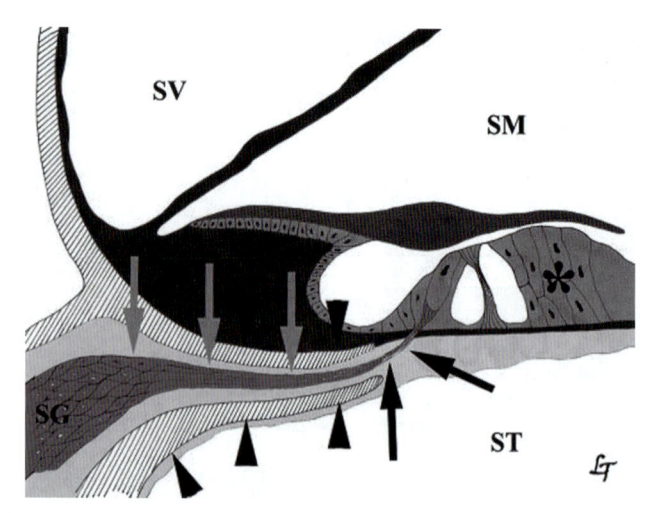

Fig. 16 Anatomical relationship between cochlear nerve and scala tympani (ST). Cochlear nerve (*gray* and *black arrows*), organ of Corti (*), and osseous spiral lamina (*black arrowheads*). SG indicates spiral ganglion; SM, endolymph in scala media; SV, perilymph in scala vestibule [from Tieleman in AJNR 29:898–905, 2008, © American Society of Neuroradiology, used with permission]

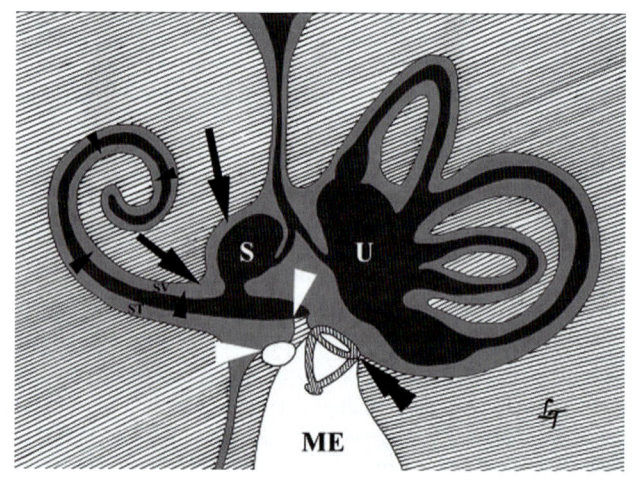

Fig. 17 Drawing of the intralabyrinthine perilymph (*light gray*) and endolymph (*dark gray*) spaces with indication of ILS extension routes. Intracochlear growth from scala tympani (ST) to scala vestibuli (SV; *black arrowheads*). ST ends at round window (*white arrowheads*). Growth from cochlea into vestibule and vice versa through the anatomical open connection between perilymph in ST and perilymphatic space around the saccule (*black arrows*). ME indicates middle ear cavity; S, endolymph in saccule, stapes (*double black arrowhead*); U, endolymph in utricle [from Tieleman in AJNR 29:898–905, 2008, © American Society of Neuroradiology, used with permission]

from the cochlea through the modiolus into the IAC; "transmacular" when ILS extends from the vestibule through the macula cribrosa into the IAC; "transotic" when ILS extends through the labyrinth into the IAC and middle ear; and "tympanolabyrinthine" when ILS extends through the labyrinth and middle ear.

Unlike IAC schwannomas, intravestibular schwannomas are not intimately located to the facial nerve. Stereotactic radiosurgery is therefore not used in the treatment of intravestibular schwannomas as surgical removal of these tumors will cause little risk of iatrogenic facial nerve injury compared to the risk of postradiation facial nerve palsy (Neff et al. 2003; Bouchetemblé et al. 2013).

4.1.1 Imaging

ILS is diagnosed with MRI, and its imaging characteristics are similar to those schwannomas arising in the IAC. On unenhanced T1-weighted images, ILS are slightly more intense than the intralabyrinthine fluid. After intravenous injection of gadolinium, the lesion presents as a sharply delineated, strongly and homogeneously enhancing region. On heavily T2-weighted images (3DFT-CISS, 3D-TSE,

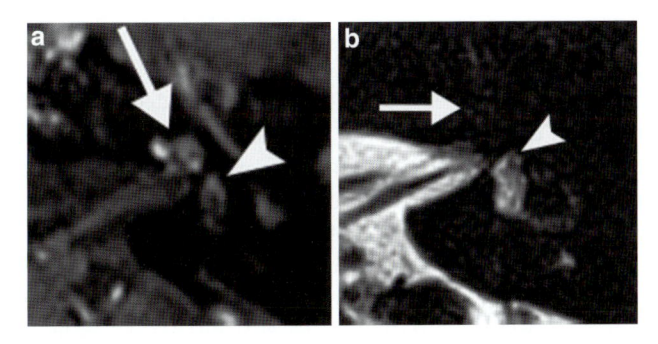

Fig. 18 A 63-year-old woman with a cochlear ILS extending into the vestibule. **a** Axial postcontrast T1-weighted MR image demonstrates enhancement of the entire cochlea (*arrow*) with a small extension into the vestibule (*arrowhead*). **b** Axial 3D-TSE T2-weighted MR image shows replacement of the fluid signal in the cochlea (*arrow*) by the ILS and subtle extension into the vestibule (*arrowhead*)

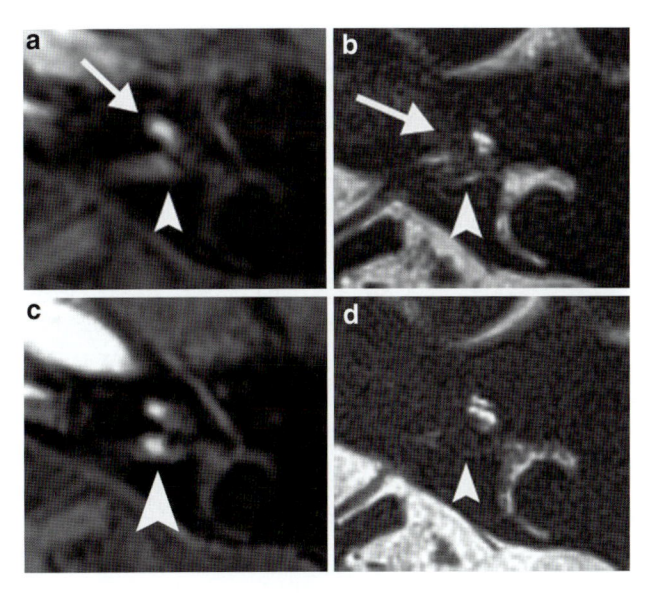

Fig. 20 An 81-year-old man with a cochlear ILS extending into the IAC. **a, b** Axial postcontrast T1-weighted MR image (**a**) and axial 3D-TSE T2-weighted MR image (**b**) show the ILS in the anterior part of the middle cochlear turn (*arrow*) on the *left side* and the extension in the fundus of the IAC (*arrowhead*). **c, d** Axial postcontrast T1-weighted MR image (**c**) and axial 3D-TSE T2-weighted MR image (**d**) performed 4 years later show subtle growth of the ILS in the IAC (*arrowhead*)

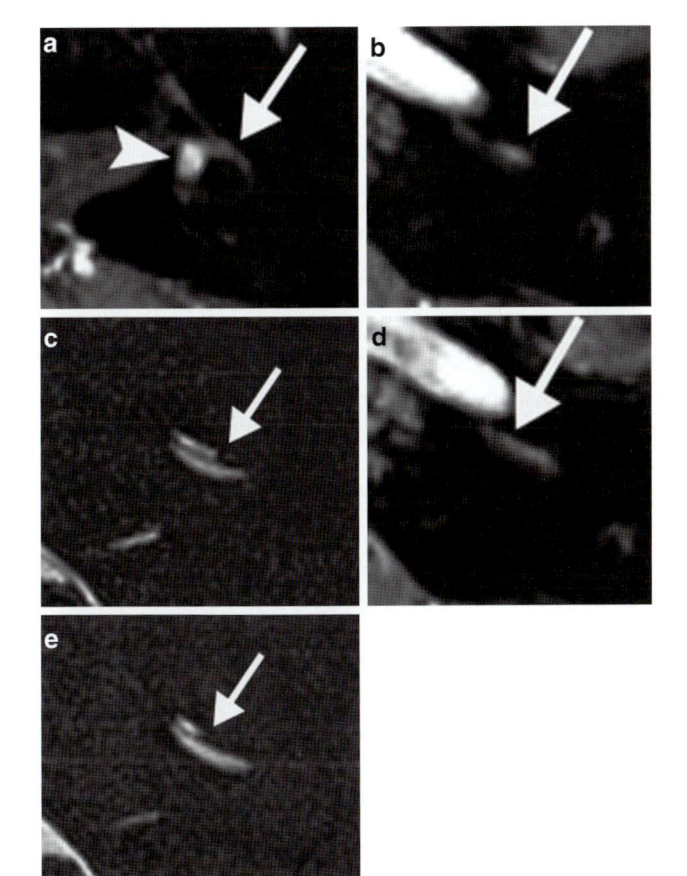

Fig. 19 A 35-year-old woman with a vestibular ILS growing into the scala vestibuli. **a, b** Axial postcontrast T1-weighted MR images of the *left* temporal bone show complete enhancement of the *left* vestibule (*arrowhead*) and the anterior (ampullary) part of the lateral semicircular canal (*arrow* in **a**). The ILS has grown into the basal turn of the cochlea (*arrow* in **b**). **c** Axial 3D-TSE T2-weighted MR image locates the ILS in the scala vestibuli of the cochlea (*arrow*). **d, e** Axial postcontrast T1-weighted MR image (**d**) and axial 3D-TSE T2-weighted MR image (**e**) 2 years later demonstrate subtle growth of the ILS in the scala vestibuli toward anterior (*arrow*)

3D-DRIVE, 3D-FIESTA, etc), the corresponding region will show replacement of the normal high signal intensity of the intralabyrinthine fluid. These T2-weighted sequences can determine in which scala the schwannoma is located (Figs. 14, 15, 18, 19 and 20). These images also allow differentiation with acute labyrinthitis where the intralabyrinthine fluid remains visible. In the ossific stage of labyrinthitis, the labyrinthine fluid will be replaced by ossified material and this is nicely demonstrated on CT images, differentiating it from an ILS. Furthermore, on postcontrast T1-weighted images, acute labyrinthitis generally is less sharply delineated than a schwannoma (Fig. 4), and in labyrinthitis ossificans, contrast enhancement will be absent. Differentiation between intralabyrinthine hemorrhage and lipoma can be made on unenhanced T1-weighted images as high signal intensities compared to the slightly intense schwannomas (Tieleman et al. 2008; De Foer et al. 2009; Lemmerling et al. 2009; Salzman et al. 2012).

4.2 Non-schwannoma Tumors

Tumors in the labyrinth other than schwannomas are rare.

Intravestibular lipomas are often associated with lipoma in the cerebellopontine angle, and they can result in sensorineural hearing loss. On precontrast T1-weighted images, lipomas are sharply delineated homogeneous hyperintense

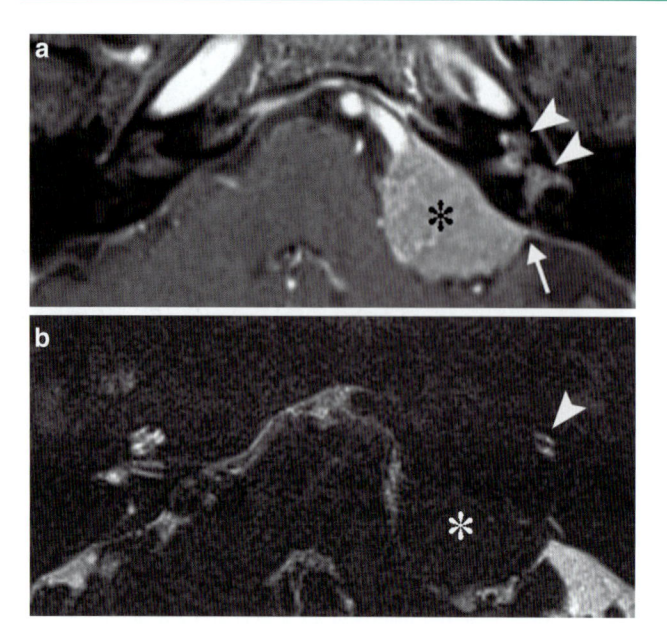

Fig. 21 An 80-year-old man with a meningioma extending into the labyrinth. **a** Axial postcontrast T1-weighted MR image shows a homogeneously enhancing tumor (*asterisk*) in the left cerebellopontine angle (CPA) with a broad base against the posterior temporal bone wall and an obtuse angle (*arrow*). There is near-total enhancement of the labyrinth (*arrowheads*). **b** Axial 3D-TSE T2-weighted MR image shows the CPA tumor (*asterisk*) and the little remaining fluid signal in the middle turn of the *left* cochlea (*arrowhead*)

masses. After contrast administration, lipomas do not enhance. Lipomas can easily be differentiated from other spontaneous hyperintensities on T1-weighted images such as hemorrhage and proteinaceous fluid because the signal of lipomas is suppressed on fat-saturated images (Dahlen et al. 2002).

The inner ear can be affected by meningioma expanding from other locations such as the temporal bone, geniculate ganglion, or IAC (Fig. 21). Primary meningioma of the inner ear is very rare. Its imaging features are the same as for meningiomas found elsewhere: isointense on T1-weighted images, iso- to hypointense on T2-weighted images, and homogeneous enhancement after contrast administration. Meningiomas can demonstrate internal ossification and remodeling of the surrounding bone (Aho et al. 2003). Other tumors that can occur in the cerebellopontine angle and internal auditory canal with involvement of the labyrinth are primary melanoma and leptomeningeal metastases (Whinney et al. 2001).

Intratemporal hemangioma is a rare tumor, and it most commonly involves the geniculate ganglion and the internal auditory canal, presumably because of the rich vascular network at these sites. Features that can aid to the diagnosis are blurred tumor margins and intratumoral bone spicules and calcification (Fierek et al. 2004).

Inflammatory pseudotumor is extremely rare in the temporal bone. However, some typical features of the tumor have been described. On CT images, a widening of the labyrinth can be present with variable destruction of middle ear structures. On MRI, a homogeneous contrast-enhancing mass is seen in the otic capsule with variable extension into the middle ear. On T2-weighted images, the tumor appears iso- to hypointense relative to brain due to its fibrous nature (Curry et al. 2010).

Congenital cholesteatoma can develop in the petrous bone and invade the membranous labyrinth. The lesion is sharply delineated, does not enhance, and demonstrates high signal intensity on b1000 DWI images, which allows differentiation with other tumors. Other tumors that may invade the labyrinth are hematogenous metastases, squamous cell carcinoma, lymphoma, Langerhans cell histiocytosis, and the various bone and soft tissue tumors that can arise in the petrous bone (De Foer et al. 2009).

5 Endolymphatic Hydrops and Ménière's Disease

Endolymphatic hydrops (EH) is defined as a condition of disordered fluid homeostasis in the inner ear which correlates with distension of Reissner's membrane in the cochlea (scala media) and/or distension of the endolymphatic compartment in the labyrinth. There is strong evidence that EH is the underlying cause of Ménière's disease (MD) which develops in middle-aged patients, presumably in combination with vascular disease (Foster and Breeze 2013). The 1995 American Academy of Otolaryngology–Head and Neck Surgery (AAO-HNS 1995) criteria for the diagnosis of MD use the presence of vertigo, sensorineural hearing loss, tinnitus or aural fullness, histopathology, and the absence of other causative disease to categorize patients into possible, probable, definite, or certain MD.

MRI is able to demonstrate the presence of EH. Nearly all authors working on the subject have used 3T MRI imaging to demonstrate EH because of the higher spatial resolution needed to visualize the very small endolymphatic spaces, especially the scala media of the cochlea. It is only recently reported that EH can be documented on 1.5T MRI after intravenous (Naganawa et al. 2013) and intratympanic (Grieve et al. 2012) administration of gadolinium, but the diagnostic accuracy of the two field strengths is not yet directly compared. Conventional MRI sequences at 3T can also demonstrate distorted membranous labyrinth architecture in patients with Ménière's disease (Carfrae et al. 2008). The two most commonly used sequences are 3D-FLAIR (Nakashima et al. 2007; Naganawa et al. 2008; Claes et al. 2012) and 3D-IR-TSE (Naganawa et al. 2008; Gürkov et al. 2012).

Table 2 Grading of endolymphatic hydrops on MRI (Nakashima et al. 2009)

Grade of hydrops	Vestibule (area ratio[a]) (%)	Cochlea
None	≤33.3	No displacement of Reissner's membrane
Mild	>33.3, ≤50	Displacement of Reissner's membrane; area of cochlear duct ≤ area of the scala vestibuli
Significant	>50	Area of the cochlear duct exceeds the area of the scala vestibuli

[a] Ratio of the area of the endolymphatic space to that of the fluid space (sum of the endolymphatic and perilymphatic spaces) in the vestibule measured on tracings of images

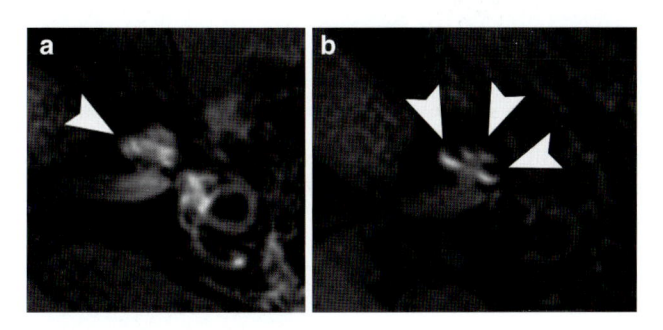

Fig. 22 Two patients with definite Ménière's disease. **a** Axial 3D-FLAIR MR image of the left temporal bone in a 46-year-old man obtained 24 h after intratympanic injection of gadolinium. There is good contrast distribution throughout the entire labyrinthine perilymphatic space without distension of the scala media (*arrowhead*) (grading: no hydrops). **b** Axial 3D-FLAIR MR image of the left temporal bone in a 40-year-old woman 24 h after intratympanic injection of gadolinium shows marked distension of the scala media (*arrowheads*) (grading: significant hydrops) (Courtesy of Luc van den Hauwe, MD)

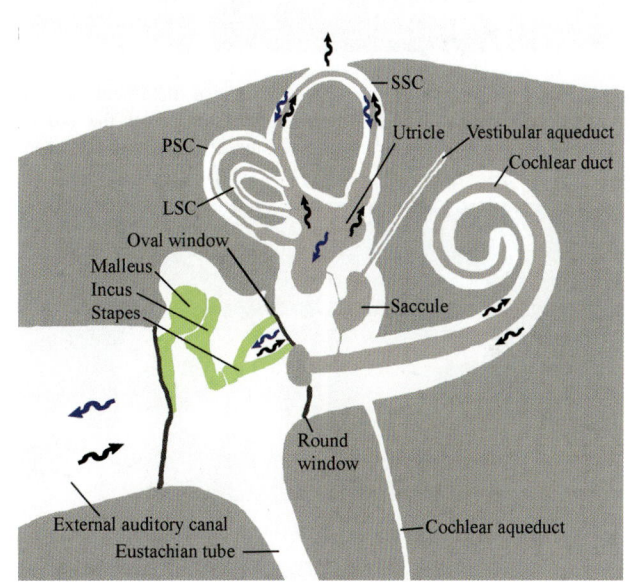

Fig. 23 Drawing of superior semicircular canal dehiscence. Positive pressure in the external auditory canal (e.g., loud noise) causes distention of the membranous canal and outward movement at the area of dehiscence. In the same way, acoustic energy can escape through the dehiscence (*black arrows*). Negative pressure in the external auditory canal causes inward movement at the area of dehiscence and distension of the membranous canal (*blue arrows*)

When intratympanic administration of gadolinium is used, after the injection, the patient's head is turned 30° off the sagittal line to the contralateral side when in a supine position. The patient should then remain supine for 60 min with the head 60° off the sagittal line toward the other ear. For optimal visualization of the cochlea and vestibule, MRI scanning should best be done after 24 h (Nakashima et al. 2007).

After intravenous gadolinium administration, grading of EH may be feasible within 3.5–4.5 h (Naganawa et al. 2012). Nakashima et al. (2009) proposed a classification for grading the severity of EH (Table 2), which is also used in many subsequent studies (Fig. 22). There is a positive correlation between the degree of EH and the degree of cochlear impairment and saccular function, implying that EH plays a crucial role in the progression of sensory deficits (Gürkov et al. 2012).

6 Superior Semicircular Canal Dehiscence

The fluid in the labyrinth is contained in the otic capsule by the surrounding bone and two mobile windows: the round and oval windows. Semicircular canal dehiscence can have different etiologies and may involve the superior, lateral, and posterior canals. The clinical presentation may be similar, but dehiscence of the superior semicircular canal (SSC) is most commonly encountered (Chien et al. 2011). Imaging for SSC dehiscence is being performed more frequently during the last decade as the syndrome was first described in 1998 (Minor et al. 1998). Dehiscence of the SSC creates a "third mobile window" (the round and oval windows being the other two) which allows the canal to be responsive to pressure and sound stimuli (Minor et al. 1998; Minor 2005). This abnormal communication between the SSC and the brain can result in vertigo and eye movements evoked by loud sounds (Tullio phenomenon), by pressure changes in the external auditory canal (Hennebert's sign) or by Valsalva maneuvers (Fig. 23) (Minor 2005; Chien et al. 2011). Beside vestibular symptoms, patients can present with auditory symptoms such as autophony, hearing their own eye movements, or their own pulse. The "third window" can result in the loss of the acoustic energy transmitted to the labyrinth from the ossicular chain and the oval window, appearing as a conductive hearing loss (Chien et al. 2011).

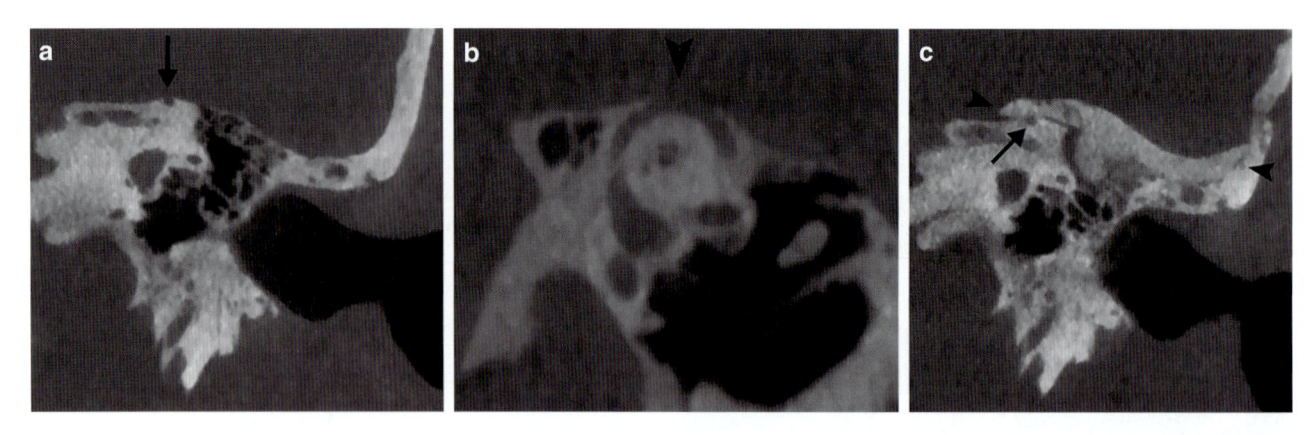

Fig. 24 A 46-year-old-man with a *left-sided* dehiscent superior semicircular canal (SSC). **a** Coronal CBCT image of the *left* ear demonstrates an absent bony covering of the SSC (*arrow*). **b** Plane of Pöschl's CBCT reformat demonstrates the full length of the dehiscence (*arrowhead*). **c** Coronal CBCT image after resurfacing of the SSC (*arrow*) and tegmen with a bone graft (*arrowheads*)

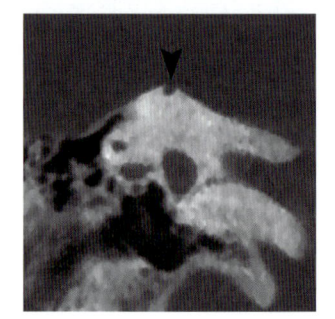

Fig. 25 A 75-year-old man with a *left-sided* dehiscent SCC. **a, b** Coronal CBCT image shows a SCC on the *left* (*arrowhead* in **b**) that is completely embedded in the intracranial soft tissues without bony covering. Compare with the normal bony covering of the SCC on the *right* (*arrowhead* in **a**)

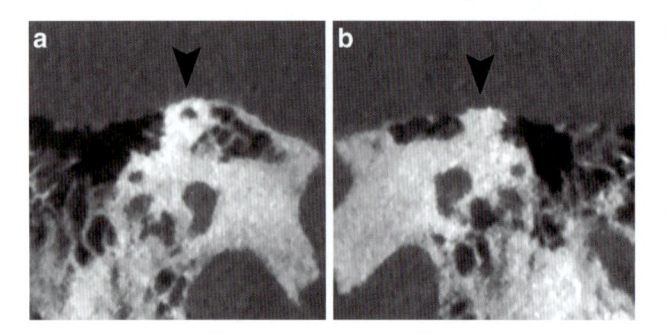

Fig. 26 A 56-year-old man with a clinical suspicion for a *right-sided* dehiscent SCC. Coronal CBCT image of the *right* temporal bone demonstrates no bony covering of the SCC (*arrowhead*). At surgery however, no bony defect was found

Therefore, when CT imaging is performed for the clinical question of otosclerosis, the radiologist should be aware of the possibility of canal dehiscence. A clinical test that is used to assess for SSC dehiscence is vestibular-evoked myogenic potentials (VEMP), recording the response from auditory clicks or tone bursts, either on the ipsilateral sternocleidomastoid muscle (cervical) or below the eye (ocular). These responses arise in the utricle and saccule (vestibular end organs), and the threshold for eliciting a response is lower in ears with dehiscence (Chien et al. 2011). The exact etiology of a SSC dehiscence remains unclear. A congenital thin bony layer associated with factors that produce a negative balance of the labyrinthine osseous metabolism helps explain the adult onset of symptoms (Brandolini et al. 2014).

On CT imaging, standard axial images and coronal reformats can be supported by additional reformatted planes along the SSC to evaluate for dehiscence (coronal: Stenver's plane; sagittal: Pöschl's plane) (Branstetter et al. 2006). A recent radioanatomical study found a 3.6 % incidence of radiological SSC dehiscence versus 0.5 % anatomical dehiscence with a 0.5-mm collimation compared to an older study that found 9 % incidence of radiological dehiscence using 1.0-mm collimation (Crovetto et al. 2010). Therefore, making the diagnosis of SSCC dehiscence on CT imaging is not always straightforward. Underestimating the possible thin bony layer on CT images is due to partial volume effects, and increasing scan resolution is needed to approach the true anatomical incidence of SSC dehiscence. In our institutions, we use cone-beam CT (CBCT) for scanning most of the temporal bones, because of the reduced dose and the thinner slice thickness of 0.15 mm compared with our multidetector scanner (MDCT) slice thickness of 0.625 mm (Figs. 24 and 25) (Peltonen et al. 2007; Miracle and Mukherji 2009; Penninger et al. 2011). Even with CBCT, we have encountered a case where no bony covering of the SSC was visible on the images and a thin bony covering was found during surgery (Fig. 26). However, patients with a near dehiscence may be identified clinically with an air–bone gap and using VEMP testing (Ward et al. 2013).

Surgical repair techniques of SSC dehiscence include plugging, resurfacing, and capping. The plugging technique uses bone dust to compress the membranous labyrinth, and the defect is then covered with bone or hydroxyapatite cement. This procedure can be made via a transmastoid (Beyea et al. 2012) or middle fossa approach (Ward et al. 2012). When the transmastoid approach is used, openings at the ampullated and non-ampullated side of the SSC are drilled and bone dust is used for occlusion (Fig. 27). For resurfacing the SSC, the

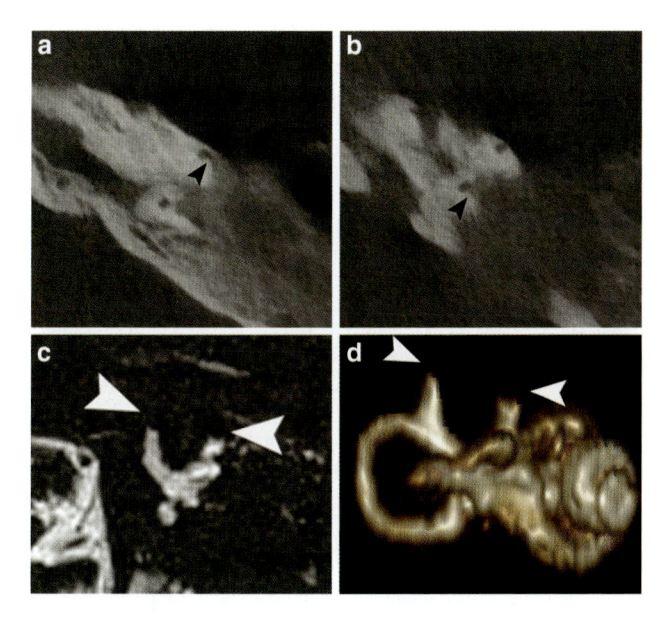

Fig. 27 Postoperative findings after SCC plugging. **a, b** Axial CBCT images of the *left* temporal bone demonstrate the access route to the anterior (ampullary) part (*arrowhead* in **a**) and a bit more cranial to the posterior part (*arrowhead* in **b**) of the SCC. **c, d** Plane of Pöschl's 3D-TSE T2-weighted MR image (**c**) and volume-rendered image (**d**) reveals the abrupt ending of the fluid signal in the SCC (*arrowheads*) at the sites of plugging, compatible with a satisfactory postoperative result

dehiscent canal is covered with bone, cartilage or fascia via a transmastoid (Amoodi et al. 2011) or middle fossa approach (Minor 2005) (Fig. 24). This bony graft may absorb and dislocate; therefore, this technique has become less favorable (Mueller et al. 2014). Capping is a modified technique of resurfacing and restores the bony defect with hydroxyapatite cement. This cement is not absorbed, and dislocation is less probable than with a bone graft (Mueller et al. 2014). Which technique to be used is dependent on the institution's experience. A recent meta-analysis showed higher success rates for canal plugging and capping over the resurfacing technique (Vlastarakos et al. 2009).

Lateral semicircular canal dehiscence is typically caused by erosion of the bony covering by cholesteatoma or granulomatous tissue in the setting of chronic otitis media. Dehiscence of the posterior semicircular canal is rare and has been associated with a high-riding jugular bulb and fibrous dysplasia (Chien et al. 2011).

References

Aho TR, Daspit CP, Dean BL, Wallace RC (2003) Intralabyrinthine meningioma. AJNR Am J Neuroradiol 24:1642–1645
American Academy of Otolaryngology-Head and Neck Foundation, Inc. (1995) Committee on hearing and equilibrium guidelines for the diagnosis and evaluation of therapy in Menière's disease. Otolaryngol Head Neck Surg 113:181–185
Amoodi HA, Makki FM, McNeil M, Bance M (2011) Transmastoid resurfacing of superior semicircular canal dehiscence. Laryngoscope 121:1117–1123
Benson AG (2010) Labyrinthitis ossificans secondary to autoimmune inner ear disease: a previously unreported condition. Otolaryngol Head Neck Surg 142:772–773
Berrettini S, Seccia V, Fortunato S, Forli F, Bruschini L, Piaggi P, Canapicchi R (2013) Analysis of the 3-dimensional fluid-attenuated inversion-recovery (3D-FLAIR) sequence in idiopathic sudden sensorineural hearing loss. JAMA Otolaryngol Head Neck Surg 139:456–464
Beyea JA, Agrawal SK, Parnes LS (2012) Transmastoid semicircular canal occlusion: a safe and highly effective treatment for benign paroxysmal positional vertigo and superior canal dehiscence. Laryngoscope 122:1862–1866
Bouchetemblé P, Heathcote K, Tollard E, Choussy O, Dehesdin D, Marie JP (2013) Intralabyrinthine schwannomas: a case series with discussion of the diagnosis and management. Otol Neurotol 34:944–951
Bovo R, Ciorba A, Trevisi P, Aimoni C, Cappiello L, Castiglione A, Govoni M, Martini A (2011) Cochlear implant in Cogan syndrome. Acta Otolaryngol 131:494–497
Brandolini C, Modugno GC, Pirodda A (2014) Dehiscence of the superior semicircular canal: a review of the literature on its possible pathogenic explanations. Eur Arch Otorhinolaryngol 271:435–437
Branstetter BF 4th, Harrigal C, Escott EJ, Hirsch BE (2006) Superior semicircular canal dehiscence: oblique reformatted CT images for diagnosis. Radiology 238:938–942
Cadoni G, Cianfoni A, Agostino S, Scipione S, Tartaglione T, Galli J, Colosimo C (2006) Magnetic resonance imaging findings in sudden sensorineural hearing loss. J Otolaryngol 35:310–316
Carfrae MJ, Holtzman A, Eames F, Parnes SM, Lupinetti A (2008) 3 Tesla delayed contrast magnetic resonance imaging evaluation of Menière's disease. Laryngoscope 118:501–505
Casselman JW, Kuhweide R, Ampe W, Meeus L, Steyaert L (1993) Pathology of the membranous labyrinth: comparison of T1- and T2-weighted and gadolinium-enhanced spin-echo and 3DFT-CISS imaging. AJNR Am J Neuroradiol 14:59–69
Casselman JW, Majoor MH, Albers FW (1994) MR of the inner ear in patients with Cogan syndrome. AJNR Am J Neuroradiol 15:131–138
Chien WW, Carey JP, Minor LB (2011) Canal dehiscence. Curr Opin Neurol 24:25–31
Claes G, Van den Hauwe L, Wuyts F, Van de Heyning P (2012) Does intratympanic gadolinium injection predict efficacy of gentamicin partial chemolabyrinthectomy in Menière's disease patients? Eur Arch Otorhinolaryngol 269:413–418
Crovetto M, Whyte J, Rodriguez OM, Lecumberri I, Martinez C, Eléxpuru J (2010) Anatomo-radiological study of the superior semicircular canal dehiscence radiological considerations of superior and posterior semicircular canals. Eur J Radiol 76:167–172
Curry JM, King N, O'Reilly RC, Corao D (2010) Inflammatory pseudotumor of the inner ear: are computed tomography changes pathognomonic? Laryngoscope 120:1252–1255
Dahlen RT, Johnson CE, Harnsberger HR, Biediger CP, Syms CA, Fischbein NJ, Schwartz JM (2002) CT and MR imaging characteristics of intravestibular lipoma. AJNR Am J Neuroradiol 23:1413–1417
De Foer B, Kenis C, Vercruysse JP, Somers T, Pouillon M, Offeciers E, Casselman JW (2009) Imaging of temporal bone tumors. Neuroimaging Clin N Am 19:339–366
de Souza C, Paparella MM, Schachern P, Yoon TH (1991) Pathology of labyrinthine ossification. J Laryngol Otol 105:621–624
Dubrulle F, Kohler R, Vincent C, Puech P, Ernst O (2010) Differential diagnosis and prognosis of T1-weighted post-gadolinium intralabyrinthine hyperintensities. Eur Radiol 20:2628–2636

Fierek O, Laskawi R, Kunze E (2004) Large intraosseous hemangioma of the temporal bone in a child. Ann Otol Rhinol Laryngol 113:394–398

Fortnum H, Davis A (1993) Hearing impairment in children after bacterial meningitis: incidence and resource implications. Br J Audiol 27:43–52

Foster CA, Breeze RE (2013) Endolymphatic hydrops in Ménière's disease: cause, consequence, or epiphenomenon? Otol Neurotol 34:1210–1214

Greco A, Gallo A, Fusconi M, Magliulo G, Turchetta R, Marinelli C, Macri GF, De Virgilio A, de Vincentiis M (2013) Cogan's syndrome: an autoimmune inner ear disease. Autoimmun Rev 12:396–400

Grieve SM, Obholzer R, Malitz N, Gibson WP, Parker GD (2012) Imaging of endolymphatic hydrops in Meniere's disease at 1.5 T using phase-sensitive inversion recovery: (1) demonstration of feasibility and (2) overcoming the limitations of variable gadolinium absorption. Eur J Radiol 81:331–338

Gürkov R, Flatz W, Louza J, Strupp M, Ertl-Wagner B, Krause E (2012) In vivo visualized endolymphatic hydrops and inner ear functions in patients with electrocochleographically confirmed Ménière's disease. Otol Neurotol 33:1040–1045

Hegarty JL, Patel S, Fischbein N, Jackler RK, Lalwani AK (2002) The value of enhanced magnetic resonance imaging in the evaluation of endocochlear disease. Laryngoscope 112:8–17

Helmchen C, Jäger L, Büttner U, Reiser M, Brandt T (1998) Cogan's syndrome. High resolution MRI indicators of activity. J Vestib Res 8:155–167

Jang CH, Park SY, Wang PC (2005) A case of tympanogenic labyrinthitis complicated by acute otitis media. Yonsei Med J 46:161–165

Karanja BW, Oburra HO, Masinde P, Wamalwa D (2013) Risk factors for hearing loss in children following bacterial meningitis in a tertiary referral hospital. Int J Otolaryngol 2013:354725

Kennedy RJ, Shelton C, Salzman KL, Davidson HC, Harnsberger HR (2004) Intralabyrinthine schwannomas: diagnosis, management, and a new classification system. Otol Neurotol 25:160–167

Kuhweide R, Van de Steene V, Vlaminck S, Casselman JW (2002) Ramsay Hunt syndrome: pathophysiology of cochleovestibular symptoms. J Laryngol Otol 116:844–848

Lee HY, Jung SY, Park MS, Yeo SG, Lee SY, Lee SK (2012) Feasibility of three-dimensional fluid-attenuated inversion recovery magnetic resonance imaging as a prognostic factor in patients with sudden hearing loss. Eur Arch Otorhinolaryngol 269:1885–1891

Lemmerling MM, De Foer B, Verbist BM, VandeVyver V (2009) Imaging of inflammatory and infectious diseases in the temporal bone. Neuroimaging Clin N Am 19:321–337

Mafee MF (1995) MR imaging of intralabyrinthine schwannoma, labyrinthitis and other labyrinthine pathology. Otolaryngol Clin N Am 28:407–430

Mazlumzadeh M, Matteson EL (2007) Cogan's syndrome: an audio-vestibular, ocular, and systemic autoimmune disease. Rheum Dis Clin North Am 33:855–874

Minor LB, Solomon D, Zinreich JS, Zee DS (1998) Sound- and/or pressure-induced vertigo due to bone dehiscence of the superior semicircular canal. Arch Otolaryngol Head Neck Surg 124:249–258

Minor LB (2005) Clinical manifestations of superior semicircular canal dehiscence. Laryngoscope 115:1717–1727

Miracle AC, Mukherji SK (2009) Conebeam CT of the head and neck, part 2: clinical applications. AJNR Am J Neuroradiol 30:1285–1292

Morton CC, Nance WE (2006) Newborn hearing screening—a silent revolution. N Engl J Med 354:2151–2164

Mueller SA, Vibert D, Haeusler R, Raabe A, Caversaccio M (2014) Surgical capping of superior semicircular canal dehiscence. Eur Arch Otorhinolaryngol 271:1369–1374

Naganawa S, Satake H, Kawamura M, Fukatsu H, Sone M, Nakashima T (2008) Separate visualization of endolymphatic space, perilymphatic space and bone by a single pulse sequence; 3D-inversion recovery imaging utilizing real reconstruction after intratympanic Gd-DTPA administration at 3 Tesla. Eur Radiol 18:920–924

Naganawa S, Nakashima T (2009) Cutting edge of inner ear MRI. Acta Otolaryngol Suppl 560:15–21

Naganawa S, Yamazaki M, Kawai H, Bokura K, Sone M, Nakashima T (2012) Visualization of endolymphatic hydrops in Ménière's disease after single-dose intravenous gadolinium-based contrast medium: timing of optimal enhancement. Magn Reson Med Sci 11:43–51

Naganawa S, Yamazaki M, Kawai H, Bokura K, Sone M, Nakashima T (2013) Visualization of endolymphatic hydrops in Ménière's disease after intravenous administration of single-dose gadodiamide at 1.5 T. Magn Reson Med Sci 12:137–139

Nakashima T, Naganawa S, Sugiura M, Teranishi M, Sone M, Hayashi H, Nakata S, Katayama N, Ishida IM (2007) Visualization of endolymphatic hydrops in patients with Meniere's disease. Laryngoscope 117:415–420

Nakashima T, Naganawa S, Pyykko I, Gibson WP, Sone M, Nakata S, Teranishi M (2009) Grading of endolymphatic hydrops using magnetic resonance imaging. Acta Otolaryngol Suppl 560:5–8

Nakashima T, Naganawa S, Teranishi M, Tagaya M, Nakata S, Sone M, Otake H, Kato K, Iwata T, Nishio N (2010) Endolymphatic hydrops revealed by intravenous gadolinium injection in patients with Ménière's disease. Acta Otolaryngol 130:338–343

Neff BA, Willcox TO Jr, Sataloff RT (2003) Intralabyrinthine schwannomas. Otol Neurotol 24:299–307

Nicoucar K, Sakbani K, Vukanovic S, Guyot JP (2005) Intralabyrinthine haemorrhage following cocaine consumption. Acta Otolaryngol 125:899–901

Otake H, Sugiura M, Naganawa S, Nakashima T (2006) 3D-FLAIR magnetic resonance imaging in the evaluation of mumps deafness. Int J Pediatr Otorhinolaryngol 70:2115–2117

Peltonen LI, Aarnisalo AA, Kortesniemi MK, Suomalainen A, Jero J, Robinson S (2007) Limited cone-beam computed tomography imaging of the middle ear: a comparison with multislice helical computed tomography. Acta Radiol 48:207–212

Penninger RT, Tavassolie TS, Carey JP (2011) Cone-beam volumetric tomography for applications in the temporal bone. Otol Neurotol 32:453–460

Poh AC, Tan TY (2007) Sudden deafness due to intralabyrinthine haemorrhage: a possible rare late complication of head and neck irradiation. Ann Acad Med Singapore 36:78–82

Ryu IS, Yoon TH, Ahn JH, Kang WS, Choi BS, Lee JH, Shim MJ (2011) Three-dimensional fluid-attenuated inversion recovery magnetic resonance imaging in sudden sensorineural hearing loss: correlations with audiologic and vestibular testing. Otol Neurotol 32:1205–1209

Salomone R, Abu TA, Chaves AG, Bocalini MC, Ade OV, Riskalla PE (2008) Sudden hearing loss caused by labyrinthine hemorrhage. Braz J Otorhinolaryngol 74:776–779

Salzman KL, Childs AM, Davidson HC, Kennedy RJ, Shelton C, Harnsberger HR (2012) Intralabyrinthine schwannomas: imaging diagnosis and classification. AJNR Am J Neuroradiol 33:104–109

Seltzer S, Mark AS (1991) Contrast enhancement of the labyrinth on MR scans in patients with sudden hearing loss and vertigo: evidence of labyrinthine disease. AJNR Am J Neuroradiol 12:13–16

Smith MM, Anderson JC (2000) Neurosyphilis as a cause of facial and vestibulocochlear nerve dysfunction: MR imaging features. AJNR Am J Neuroradiol 21:1673–1675

Stachler RJ, Chandrasekhar SS, Archer SM, Rosenfeld RM, Schwartz SR, Barrs DM, Brown SR, Fife TD, Ford P, Ganiats TG, Hollingsworth DB, Lewandowski CA, Montano JJ, Saunders JE,

Tucci DL, Valente M, Warren BE, Yaremchuk KL, Robertson PJ, American Academy of Otolaryngology-Head and Neck Surgery (2012) Clinical practice guideline: sudden hearing loss. Otolaryngol Head Neck Surg 146(3 Suppl):S1–S35

Stokroos RJ, Albers FW, Krikke AP, Casselman JW (1998) Magnetic resonance imaging of the inner ear in patients with idiopathic sudden sensorineural hearing loss. Eur Arch Otorhinolaryngol 255:433–436

Stone JH, Francis HW (2000) Immune-mediated inner ear disease. Curr Opin Rheumatol 12:32–40

Sugiura M, Naganawa S, Teranishi M, Sato E, Kojima S, Nakashima T (2006) Inner ear hemorrhage in systemic lupus erythematosus. Laryngoscope 116:826–828

Sugiura M, Naganawa S, Nakata S, Kojima S, Nakashima T (2007) 3D-FLAIR MRI findings in a patient with Ramsay Hunt syndrome. Acta Otolaryngol 127:547–549

Swartz JD, Mandell DM, Faerber EN, Popky GL, Ardito JM, Steinberg SB, Rojer CL (1985) Labyrinthine ossification: etiologies and CT findings. Radiology 157:395–398

Tanigawa T, Tanaka H, Sato T, Nakao Y, Katahira N, Tsuchiya Y, Nonoyama H, Ueda H (2010) 3D-FLAIR MRI findings in patients with low-tone sudden deafness. Acta Otolaryngol 130:1324–1328

Teszler CB, Williams MT, Belange G, Ayache D (2008) Labyrinthitis related to Wegener granulomatosis: magnetic resonance imaging findings. Otol Neurotol 29:721–722

Tieleman A, Casselman JW, Somers T, Delanote J, Kuhweide R, Ghekiere J, De Foer B, Offeciers EF (2008) Imaging of intralabyrinthine schwannomas: a retrospective study of 52 cases with emphasis on lesion growth. AJNR Am J Neuroradiol 29:898–905

Tinling SP, Colton J, Brodie HA (2004) Location and timing of initial osteoid deposition in postmeningitic labyrinthitis ossificans determined by multiple fluorescent labels. Laryngoscope 114:675–680

Toyama C, da Silva CJ, Braga FT, Brito R (2009) Intralabyrinthine hemorrhage associated with superficial siderosis of the central nervous system. Otol Neurotol 30:121–122

Vlastarakos PV, Proikas K, Tavoulari E, Kikidis D, Maragoudakis P, Nikolopoulos TP (2009) Efficacy assessment and complications of surgical management for superior semicircular canal dehiscence: a meta-analysis of published interventional studies. Eur Arch Otorhinolaryngol 266:177–186

Wang JR, Yuen HW, Shipp DB, Stewart S, Lin VY, Chen JM, Nedzelski JM (2010) Cochlear implantation in patients with autoimmune inner ear disease including Cogan syndrome: a comparison with age- and sex-matched controls. Laryngoscope 120:2478–2483

Ward BK, Agrawal Y, Nguyen E, Della Santina CC, Limb CJ, Francis HW, Minor LB, Carey JP (2012) Hearing outcomes after surgical plugging of the superior semicircular canal by a middle cranial fossa approach. Otol Neurotol 33:1386–1391

Ward BK, Wenzel A, Ritzl EK, Gutierrez-Hernandez S, Della Santina CC, Minor LB, Carey JP (2013) Near-dehiscence: clinical findings in patients with thin bone over the superior semicircular canal. Otol Neurotol 34:1421–1428

Weisert JU, Veraguth D, Probst R (2012) Bilateral deafness due to labyrinthitis in a patient with Crohn's disease. HNO 60:132–134

Whitehead RE, MacDonald CB, Melhem ER, McMahon L (1998) Spontaneous labyrinthine hemorrhage in sickle cell disease. AJNR Am J Neuroradiol 19:1437–1440

Williams MT, Ayache D (2004) Imaging of the postoperative middle ear. Eur Radiol 14:482–495

Whinney D, Kitchen N, Revesz T, Brookes G (2001) Primary malignant melanoma of the cerebellopontine angle. Otol Neurotol 22:218–222

Xu HX, Joglekar SS, Paparella MM (2009) Labyrinthitis ossificans. Otol Neurotol 30:579–580

Yoshida T, Sugiura M, Naganawa S, Teranishi M, Nakata S, Nakashima T (2008) Three-dimensional fluid-attenuated inversion recovery magnetic resonance imaging findings and prognosis in sudden sensorineural hearing loss. Laryngoscope 118:1433–1437

Imaging of Cochlear Implants

B. M. Verbist and J. H. M. Frijns

Contents

1 Introduction 237
2 Preoperative Assessment in Cochlear Implant Candidates 238
2.1 Imaging Modalities 239
2.2 Inner Ear Malformations 239
2.3 Labyrinthitis 239
2.4 Otosclerosis and Other Bony Dysplasia 240
2.5 Retrocochlear Disease 241
2.6 Anatomic Variations that May Influence Surgical Approach 242
3 Cochlear Implant Surgery 243
4 Postoperative Evaluation After Cochlear Implantation 244
4.1 Cochlear Coordinate Systems 244
4.2 Imaging Modalities 245
4.3 Complications 246
5 Conclusion 247
References 247

Abstract

Cochlear implantation has become a widely available tool for successful treatment of deafness or severe sensorineural hearing loss in patients who do not receive adequate benefit from hearing aids. Imaging plays an important role in the selection of suitable candidates and in the planning of the surgery. Therefore, preoperative assessment should provide optimal information on the anatomy of the ear with its normal variances and pathology of the temporal bone and auditory pathway. Postoperative imaging (mostly plain X-ray) is the standard of care in most centers to confirm correct intracochlear positioning of the array. Multislice CT-scanning or flat panel CT is done routinely in some centers, but is usually reserved for cochlear implant recipients with suspected complications after the surgery or malfunctioning of the implant. It is also applied in cochlear implant research to get better insights into the working of cochlear implants.

1 Introduction

Cochlear implants are a common, well-accepted treatment for profound hearing loss or deafness, nowadays, leading to high levels of word recognition, open set speech recognition, and even the ability to use the telephone in the average implant user. (FDA 1984; NIH Consensus Statement 1995; Wilson and Dorman 2008) Whereas conventional hearing aids merely amplify sound, cochlear implants directly stimulate the auditory nerve. This is the only way to restore hearing in those patients in whom damage to the (inner) ear is too large to produce a neural signal by amplification of sound waves.

A cochlear implant consists of an externally worn speech processor and a microphone and an implanted receiver and electrode array (Fig 1). The speech processor filters, analyzes, and converts the auditory signals captured by the

B. M. Verbist (✉)
Department of Radiology, Leiden University Medical Center, Leiden, The Netherlands
e-mail: B.M.Verbist@lumc.nl

B. M. Verbist
Department of Radiology, Radboud University Nijmegen Medical Center, Nijmegen, The Netherlands

J. H. M. Frijns
Department of Otolaryngology, Leiden University Medical Center, Leiden, The Netherlands

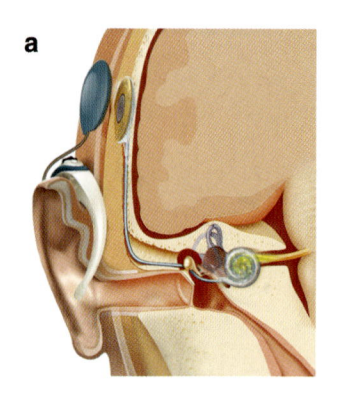

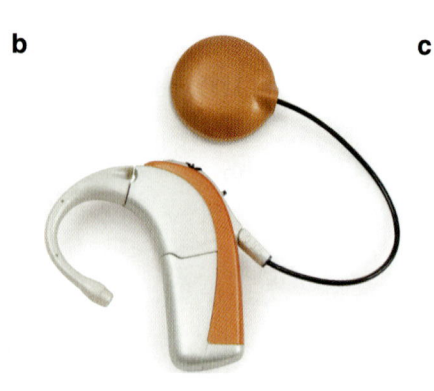

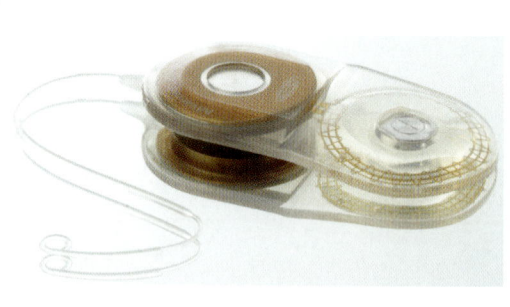

Fig. 1 **a** Schematic drawing of a cochlear implant showing the externally worn speech processor and microphone, which is magnetically attached to a subcutaneous implanted receiver. The receiver contains electronics to decode the signals and generate electrical stimuli. An electrode array is connected to this receiver and inserted into the scala tympani of the cochlea. The external (**b**) and internal (**c**) components of a cochlear implant (Advanced Bionics Hires 90K and Harmony speech processor) are shown. The behind the ear part (**b**) contains the speech processor and a built-in microphone. Alternatively, a body worn processor can be used. The internal components consist of the magnet, receiver, and electrode lead. Implants of other manufacturers have a slightly different appearance, but contain the same components

microphone to a digital code. Basically, the auditory signal is split into separate frequency bands, one for each channel of the cochlear implant. A channel consists of either one electrode contact combined with a distant reference electrode or a combination of multiple contacts. A so-called envelope extraction mechanism then usually determines the amplitudes of the various frequency bands. As such, the wide dynamic range of environmental sound (about 100 dB) is mapped into the narrow dynamic range of electrically evoked hearing (about 10 dB) at the expense of fine structure information within the frequency band. Such loss of fine structure information could degrade representation of speech sounds particularly in a noisy environment, tone patterns in tonal languages and musical sounds Wilson and Dorman 2008. A head piece containing a transmitting coil sends the signal from the speech processor to a subcutaneously implanted receiver to which it is magnetically attached. The receiver contains electronics to decode the signals and generate electrical stimuli. An electrode array is connected to this receiver and inserted into the cochlea, preferably into the scala tympani. In multichannel arrays, the electrode array contains several electrode contacts to ensure well-directed stimulation of the tonotopically organized cochlea. The number of electrode contacts and the geometry of the electrode array differ between manufacturers and electrode types. Standard electrode arrays of the four main manufacturers at present contain 12 (Med-EL GMBH of Innsbruck, Austria), 16 (Advanced Bionics Corp of Valencia, CA, USA), 20 (Neurelec, Vallauris Cédex, France), or 22 (Cochlear Ltd of Lane Cove, Australia) active electrode contacts. Electrodes designed for electro-acoustic stimulation (EAS) are used for electrical stimulation of high and middle frequencies, while sparing the natural sound perceptions from residual low frequency hearing and are therefore shorter than a standard electrode. Double electrodes consist of two short electrode arrays with different number of electrode contacts. These are used in partially ossified inner ears.

Whether a hearing impaired person is a suitable candidate who would benefit from cochlear implantation should be examined by a multidisciplinary team, based on medical history, clinical, audiological, and imaging findings as well as the social and psychological setting. Over the last years, criteria for cochlear implantation candidacy have expanded considerably. There has been a shift toward implantation at a younger age. Prelingual adults who have never had a hearing experience may receive implants. Malformed inner ears, be it nonsyndromic or syndromic, or ossified cochleae as a result of labyrinthitis are no longer considered contraindications for implantation. Since the success of implantations is, among other factors, determined by the physiology and anatomy of the inner ear and auditory pathway, imaging plays an important role in the assessment of cochlear implant candidates.

2 Preoperative Assessment in Cochlear Implant Candidates

There are many causes of sensorineural hearing loss. They include genetic conditions, infectious or inflammatory diseases, traumatic sequelae, ischemic events, and toxic agents. Imaging may establish the cause of deafness, but in many cases no structural abnormalities can be found.

Systematic analysis for developmental or obliterative inner ear disease, abnormalities of bone metabolism, retrocochlear pathology, and anatomic variants of the middle ear will render information on feasibility of the procedure, preferred surgical approach including operation side, and type of cochlear implant that should be chosen.

2.1 Imaging Modalities

Both computed tomography (CT) and magnetic resonance imaging (MRI) render complementary information in the preoperative assessment of cochlear implant candidates. CT is an excellent modality to identify anomalies of the bony labyrinth, vestibular aqueduct, otic capsule, and eventual concomitant middle ear anomalies or anatomic variations that may complicate surgery. MRI is superior in the assessment of the membranous labyrinth, internal auditory canal (IAC), cerebellopontine angle (CPA) cistern, and auditory pathway. Contrast administration will increase the detection of infectious, inflammatory, or autoimmune diseases of the inner ear and of meningeal pathology as a cause of hearing loss. These findings may directly impact patient management (Hegarty et al. 2002). If only one imaging modality is chosen, one should bear in mind that abnormalities detected with MRI are more likely to influence the implantation process (e.g., asymmetric nerve hypo- or aplasia, cochlear obstruction) (Parry et al. 2005).

2.2 Inner Ear Malformations

Congenital hearing loss or profound hearing loss in early childhood may be the result of developmental abnormalities of the cochleovestibular system. They may be part of a syndrome or due to sporadic chromosomal abnormalities, which may be linked to gestational infections or ototoxic drugs. As described in Congenital Malformations of the Temporal Bone, arrested or aberrant development of the labyrinth will lead to a myriad of malformations.

Labyrinthine or cochlear aplasias are absolute contraindications for CI. In other dysplasia CI may be considered, but decision-making should be taking into account the neural function of the auditory nerve and—particularly in syndromic cases—cognitive function. Prior documentation of hearing or proven auditory nerve function is considered beneficial. Surgery may be technically challenging, especially in syndromic cases with associated middle ear anomalies where normal anatomical landmarks such as the facial recess, stapes, or round window are distorted or absent. A precise description of the middle and inner ear status on imaging will render a roadmap for the surgeon. Moreover, imaging will identify anomalies which predispose to perilymph gusher or perilymph oozing. "Gushing" of cerebrospinal fluid (CSF) during cochleostomy is the result of perilymphatic hydrops due to a broad communication between the subarachnoid space and the perilymph in the cochlea as can be seen in X-linked hearing loss (Friedman et al. 1997). Preoperative perilymph oozing or slow, persistent flow of CSF may occur in patients with enlarged vestibular aqueducts and modiolar deficiency. In case of asymmetric developmental abnormalities, imaging might influence the choice of side of operation (Fig. 2).

2.3 Labyrinthitis

Labyrinthitis due to bacterial meningitis is the most common cause of postnatally acquired hearing loss. Other causes of labyrinthitis are viral infections, inflammatory conditions, trauma, and autoimmune diseases. (see also Inner Ear Pathology). In both infectious and noninfectious labyrinthitis, the labyrinth will become inflamed—leading to degeneration of sensory structures in the organ of Corti and of spiral ganglion cells. (Merchant and Gopen 1996; Rappaport et al. 1999; Klein et al. 2003). Eventually, labyrinthitis ossificans may develop with replacement of intralabyrinthine fluid by fibrous tissue or bone formation. This will increase the risk for complications during cochlear implantation or may even preclude implantation. Fibrous tissue may be removed preoperatively relatively easily with a little hook. Proximal bony obliteration may be drilled out increasing the surgical risk of damaging neural structures. Once the obliteration exceeds to the second half of the basal turn of the cochlea, surgical access to the scala tympani is precluded. In such cases, implantation of a double array may be considered. (Lenarz et al. 2001; Bredberg et al. 1997). If the ossificiation is limited to the scala tympani, a full insertion of the implant may be achieved into the scala vestibuli (Lin 2006) (Fig. 3e, f).

Labyrinthitis may progress rapidly to a fibro-osseous stage. Therefore, early audiometric testing and imaging are recommended and early intervention may be appropriate to improve the outcome in terms of hearing restoration. Bilateral implantation has been advocated by some groups. (Merkus et al. 2010).

Imaging findings will play a major role in treatment planning. Since MRI is sensitive to soft tissue changes in the early phase of labyrinthitis, it is the modality of choice in suspected acute labyrinthitis. In the acute phase of labyrinthitis, MRI will first show enhancement within the labyrinth without any signs of obliteration on T2 weighted images. As soon as fibroblastic proliferation occurs, T2 weighted images will show signal loss within the labyrinth. This fibrous tissue may or may not be enhancing. CT will frequently be normal in acute labyrinthitis or in case of purely fibrous replacement. Once neo-ossification occurs, CT will show osseous obliteration. The combination of MRI- and CT-findings will allow for differentiation between fibrous tissue and ossification (Fig 4).

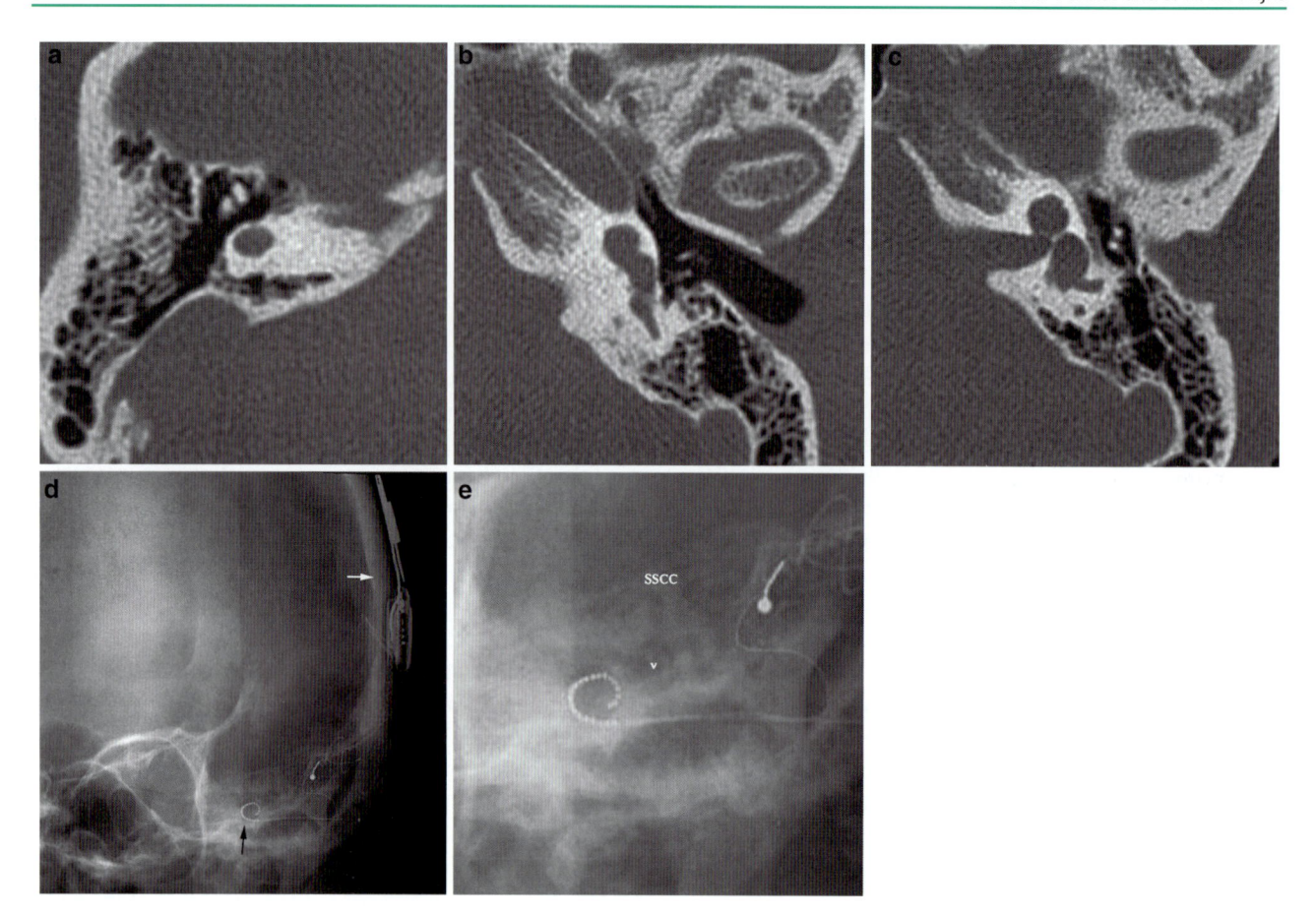

Fig. 2 Asymmetric congenital malformation determining side of operation: in this patient with congenital deafness on the right and profound sensorineural hearing loss on the left axial CT shows bilateral developmental abnormalities. On the *right* (**a**) labyrinthine aplasia precludes cochlear implantation. On the *left* (**b**, **c**) a small, cystic cochlea is present, which was successfully implanted. On a postoperative Stenvers view (**d**), the subcutaneously implanted receiver (*white arrow*) and the attached electrode lead with the cochlear implant (*black arrow*) is seen. On a magnified image **e** it is clearly seen that the electrode array projects medial to the promontory, which can be identified at the air-bone interface beneath the vestibulum (v) (*SSCC* superior semicircular canal)

The precise description of presence, location, and extent of obliteration of the cochlea will guide surgical planning as well as the choice of cochlear implant (single array, double array).

2.4 Otosclerosis and Other Bony Dysplasia

2.4.1 Otosclerosis

Otosclerosis usually causes mixed hearing loss and primary surgical treatment consists of stapes surgery. In advanced cases, however, cochlear implantation may be considered.

Otosclerosis is a disease of the otic capsule causing a cycle of bony changes leading to osteolytic foci and bone productive changes. The round window may become narrowed and sometimes abnormal bone formation to the cochlear lumen can be seen (Fig. 5). Ossification of the cochlea may also be seen as a complication after stapes surgery. Due to the altered, brittle bone, and anatomic distortions, the risk for complications during implant surgery increases (Rotteveel et al. 2004). Malpositioning of the cochlear implant may occur. Extensive osteolytic lesions or pathologic fractures due to manipulation may lead to CSF-leak. Postoperatively, the patients may experience stimulation of the facial nerve by sound. This is commonly thought to occur due to current spread toward the facial nerve through abnormal bone, but a recent study argued that rather than a decreased facial nerve threshold, increased levels for cochlear stimulation due to more current flowing out of the cochlea are responsible for this phenomenon. Fortunately, it is less frequently seen nowadays, as particularly perimodiolar designs with more shielding against lateral spread of current reduce the likelihood of facial nerve stimulation (Frijns et al. 2009).

Precise documentation of the extent and location, in particular in regard to round window stenosis and cochlear lesions should be given in the report.

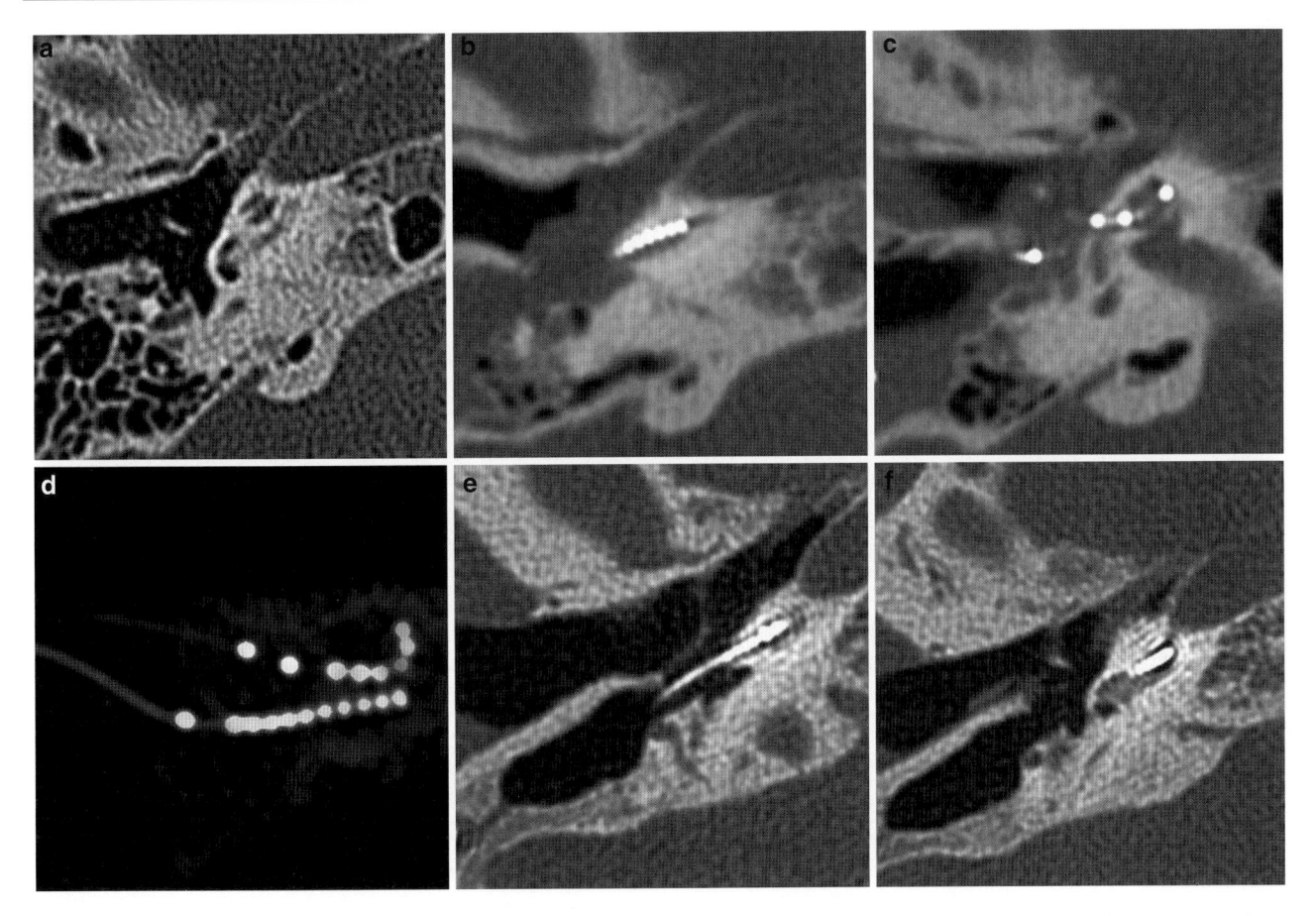

Fig. 3 Modified surgical approaches in labyrinthitis ossificans: Patient 1 (**a–d**) had a history of meningogenic labyrinthitis. Preoperative CT (**a**) shows extensive ossification in the basal turn of the cochlea, but a patent second and apical turn. **a** a double array was placed: the first array (**b**) is implanted into the proximal basal turn after drill-out. The second array (**c**) is directly inserted into the second turn of the cochlea through a second cochleostomy. Volume rendering image (**d**) illustrates the position of both arrays. In patient 2 (**e**, **f**) a scala vestibuli insertion was performed because of severe ossification of the scala tympani as seen in **f**

2.4.2 Other Bony Dysplasias

Bony disorders of the temporal bone such as fibrous dysplasia, Paget's disease, osteopetrosis, or osteogenesis imperfecta may suffer from profound hearing loss. (Fig. 6) This is often due to encroachment of the external auditory canal, middle ear, and internal auditory canal. In Sickle cell disease, hearing loss is thought to be the result of vascular compromise of the cochlea.

The value of cochlear implantation in these diseases is not yet clear.

2.5 Retrocochlear Disease

2.5.1 Cochleovestibular Nerve

Development of the cochleovestibular nerve is independent of the cochlea. If the cochlear nerve is absent, cochlear implantation is contraindicated. On CT, a narrow IAC (<2–3 mm) should raise the suspicion of cochlear nerve aplasia. Definitive diagnosis, however, can only be made with MRI.

Hypoplasia of the cochlear nerve has been correlated with poor outcomes of cochlear implantations. A strong positive correlation between the diameter of the cochlear, vestibular, and eighth cranial nerves with the total spiral ganglion cell has been reported (Nadol 1997), but the correlation between size and outcome still has to be established. Some have advocated the use of auditory brainstem implants (ABIs) in cochlear nerve hypoplasia (O'Driscoll 2011). In any case, the finding of cochlear nerve hypoplasia will influence patient counseling.

On CT, a small cochlear aperture may help to identify patients at risk for having a hypoplastic cochlear nerve (Fatterpekar et al. 2000) (Fig. 7). The nerve itself will be visualized on MR. Normally, the size of the cochlear nerve should be as large or larger than that of the facial nerve.

Infectious, inflammatory, or toxic conditions involving the cochlear nerve may cause irreversible hearing loss. In hemosiderosis, for instance, hemosiderine depositis due to recurrent subarachnoidal bleeding will cause neural damage to cranial nerves, in particular cranial nerves I and VIII, to the brain, and to the spinal cord. These patients develop

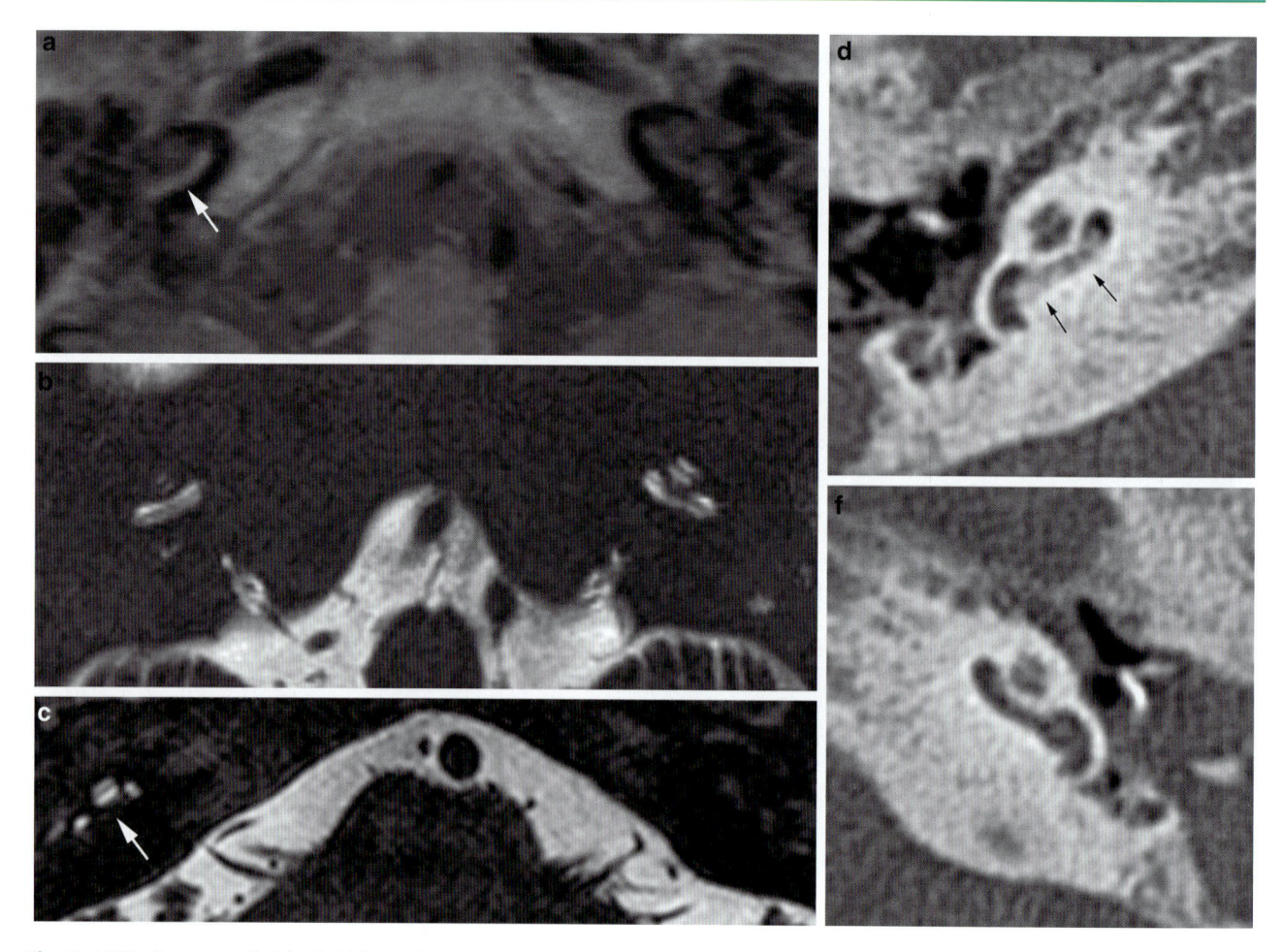

Fig. 4 MRI features of labyrinthitis ossificans: Patient 1 (**a, b**) developed hearing loss during meningitis. On contrast-enhanced T1 weighted MRI (**a**), enhancement of the basal turn of the cochlea is seen (*arrow*). A heavily T2 weighted image (**b**) shows normal signal intensity within the cochlea. This pattern indicates labyrinthitis in its acute stage whereinflammatory cells fill the perilymfatic spaces. This may rapidly progress to the obliterative stage, where fibroblastic proliferation and ossification will occur as seen in the second patient (**c–e**). T2 weighted MRI shows signal loss in the scala tympani on the right (*white arrow*) and complete signal loss of the membranous labyrinth on the left. On a corresponding axial CT-image, this is shown to be due to bone formation within the cochlea on the right (*black arrows* in **d**) and fibrosis on the left (**e**)

progressive sensorineural hearing loss and ataxia, pyramidal signs, and dementia. Occasionally, anosmia, visual loss or facial nerve paralysis may occur. The results of cochlear implantation are variable and patient counseling is important. (Dhooghe et al. 2002; Wood et al. 2008).

If a schwannoma is present in a cochlear implant candidate the contralateral ear will be implanted. In case of bilateral schwannomas associated with NF2, auditory brainstem implantation is preferred.

2.5.2 Auditory Pathway

Developmental, ischemic, post-traumatic, demyelinating, and tumoral lesions may be located in the auditory pathway and will influence patient management.

2.6 Anatomic Variations that May Influence Surgical Approach

The preoperative imaging report should contain anatomic variations that may influence surgical approach. The size and pneumatization of the mastoid and the presence of vascular anatomic variations such as a high riding jugular bulb, a dehiscent jugular bulb, or an anteriorly displaced sigmoid sinus will influence the surgical access. Rarely dehiscence of the carotid canal at the level of the basal turn of the cochlea is present. A large mastoid air cell inferior to the round window niche may be confused with the round window niche, and should be reported to the surgeon (Fig. 8).

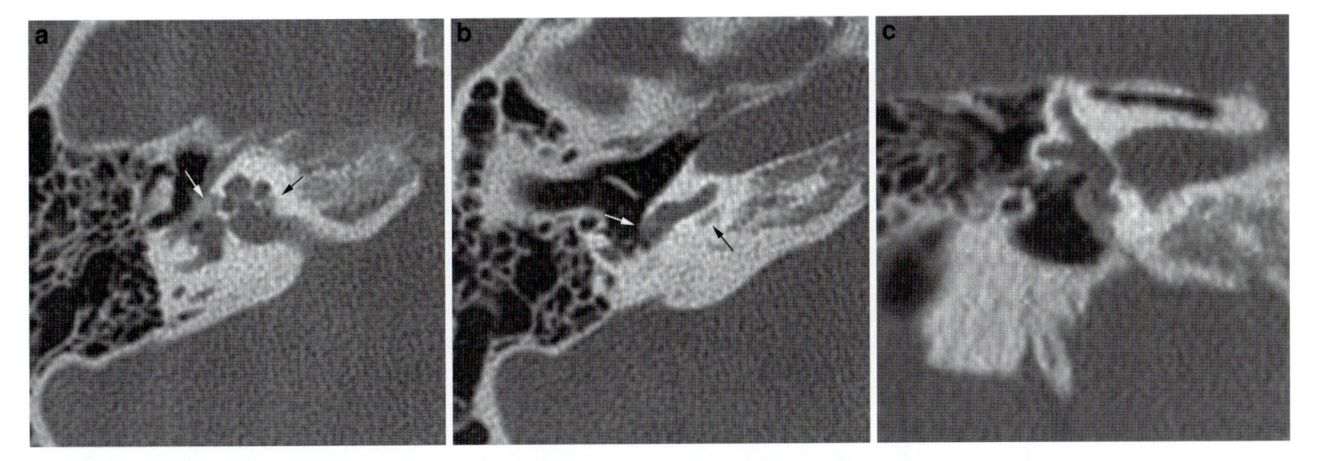

Fig. 5 Fenestral and retrofenestral otosclerosis with round window stenosis: on axial CT (**a**) an otospongiotic focus is seen at the fissula ante fenestram (*white arrow*) as well as posterior to the cochlea, extending into the internal auditory canal (*black arrow*). An axial image slightly more caudal to **a** shows narrowing of the round window niche due to an otospongiotic focus (*white arrow*), which obscures the surgical access route. Note also the lytic area posterior to the basal turn of the cochlea (*black arrow*). Coronal CT (**c**) shows the apposition of abnormal bone at the level of the fissula ante fenestram and round window

3 Cochlear Implant Surgery

Surgical techniques for cochlear implantation vary between devices and surgeons, but most commonly, the approach through the facial recess is used to reach the cochlea. First, a basic mastoidectomy is performed, with identification of the lateral semicircular canal and the incus. Then, while thinning the posterior canal wall, a posterior tympanotomy is carried out through the facial recess. This route is lateral to the mastoidal portion of the facial nerve, on which preferably a thin layer of bone is preserved, and medial to the chorda tympani, which can be spared in most cases. Through the posterior tympanotomy, the stapes and the round window niche can be visualized. Some surgeons prefer to uncover the round window membrane by drilling away the bony overhang (subiculum) and insert the electrode array through the (sometimes antero-inferiorly enlarged) round window, while others make a separate cochleostomy. The location of such a cochleostomy is crucial if one wants to insert the electrode reliably into the scala tympani, and recent research has demonstrated that the optimal placement of the cochleostomy is antero-inferior to the round window. The diameter of the cochleostomy depends on the electrode array and surgical preference, and is commonly between 0.8 and 1.2 mm. The way and depth the electrode is inserted differs between manufacturers.

An occasionally used alternative for the approach through the facial recess is the so-called suprameatal approach, in which a tunnel in the mastoid, postero-superior to the bony ear canal is drilled, through which the electrode is led to the middle ear, where it enters just lateral to the incus. In this approach, the tympanic membrane is elevated

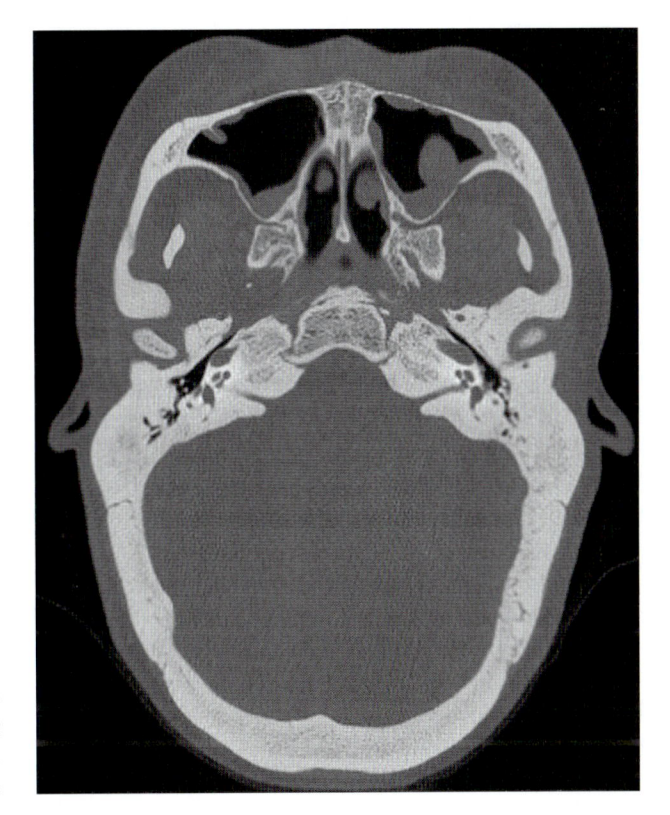

Fig. 6 Hearing loss due to bone dysplasia: in this patient with Robinow syndrome, a skeletal dysplasia characterized by dwarfism and craniofacial abnormalities, severe narrowing of the internal auditory canals is seen. The middle ear cavities were also encroached and the ossicles were thickened (not shown)

to drill a cochleostomy and insert the electrode in the cochlea through the ear canal.

Fig. 7 Cochlear nerve hypo- or aplasia: in this child with unilateral congenital hearing loss on the left a normal width of the bony fenestration at the base of the modiolus is seen in the right ear (**a**), whereas on the left a stenosis of the cochlear aperture is present, suggestive of cochlear nerve aplasia

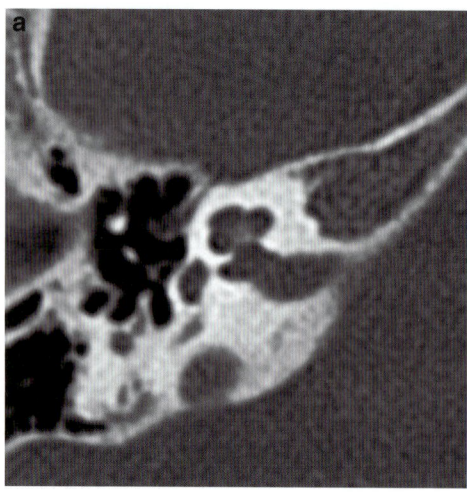

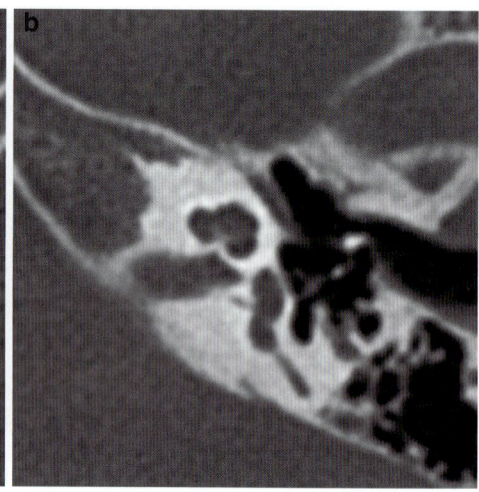

The receiver–stimulator package to which the electrode is connected, is placed on the skull, immediately posterior to the mastoidectomy and the pinna. Depending on the type of implant, many surgeons create a bony bed and a periosteal pocket in which the receiver-stimulator package is placed. Some surgeons additionally use tie-down sutures to further stabilize the implant, while others even do not drill a bony bed and fully rely on the periosteum to keep the implant in place. Depending on the surgeon's preference, the electrode lead can be led from the receiver-stimulator to the mastoid through a groove, which can be covered later with bone dust and/or fibrin glue or through a tunnel in the skull bone, which can help to keep the implant in place.

After skin closure, a pressure bandage is applied to prevent a hematoma. To prevent skin problems due to pressure of the magnet in the head coil, most cochlear implant centers wait 4–6 weeks before the external speech processor is fitted.

4 Postoperative Evaluation After Cochlear Implantation

Per- or post-operative imaging is performed to confirm intracochlear positioning of the cochlear implant and to report eventual breakage of the electrode lead or other complications like a flipped electrode lead within the cochlea. Electrophysical measurements are performed during the operation to test the function of the implant. Postoperative imaging will usually be done if malfunctioning or complications are suspected.

Postoperative imaging is also useful to provide feedback to the surgeon in challenging cases like congenital malformations and to evaluate the surgical result of new electrode designs such as a double array implant.

To get a better understanding of the differences in outcome of speech perception, research on frequency mapping is done. To relate the position of a contact to the perceived frequencies, precise information about the position of a contact within the tonotopically organized cochlea as well as information about the distance of a contact to the cochlear nerve is investigated in certain CI centers. The description of electrode positions and cochlear structures must be specified in a consistent manner.

4.1 Cochlear Coordinate Systems

To be able to assess and report cochlear anatomy and cochlear implant position in an objective and reproducible manner several cochlear frameworks have been introduced in the past decades. A histology-based framework (Stakhovskaya et al. 2007; Xu et al. 2000), both two dimensional and three dimensional imaging-based frameworks (Cohen 2000; Kos et al. 2005; Verbist et al. 2010a; Skinner et al. 2007) and a combined imaging and microscopic-based grid system (Verbist et al. 2010b) have been described and applied. These frameworks differ slightly in defining anatomical landmarks and a reference point for angular measurements of insertion depth, which makes comparisons of results obtained with different coordinates impossible or unreliable. Therefore, a universal cochlear coordinate system was defined by a consensus panel consisting of representatives of various subdisciplines involved in inner ear research. This cochlear coordinate system is a three dimensional, cylindrical coordinate system in which the basal turn of the cochlea serves as the plane of rotation and the modiolus provides the axis of rotation. The zero-reference angle is positioned at the center of the round window (Fig. 9). As such, every anatomic structure within the

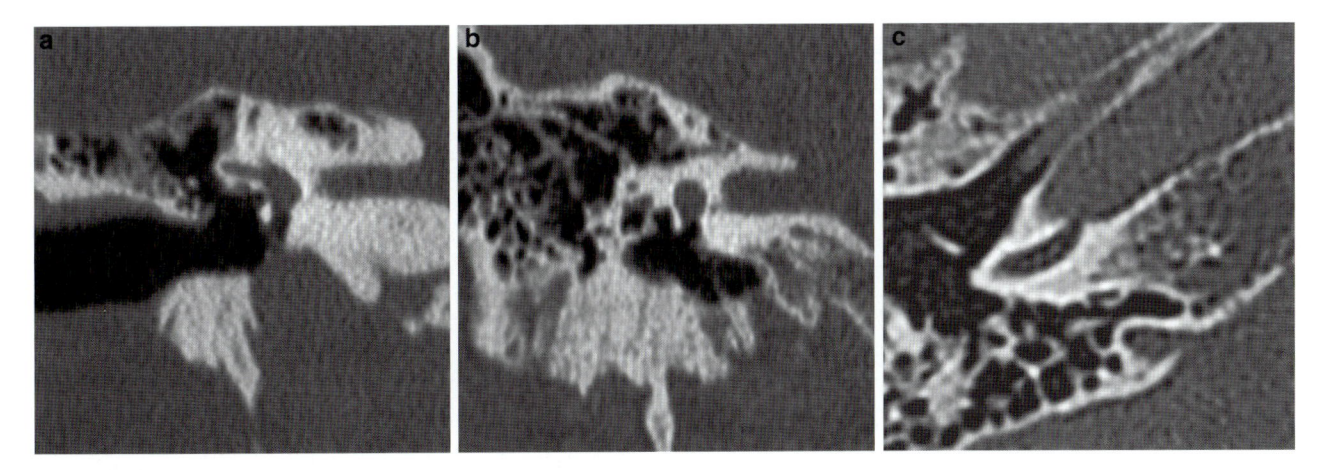

Fig. 8 Anatomical variants influencing surgical access: **a** a high riding and dehiscent jugular bulb abuts the round window niche. **b** A large, aerated mastoid cell inferior to the round window niche should be mentioned in the report. **c** Rarely dehiscence of the carotid canal toward the cochlea can be seen

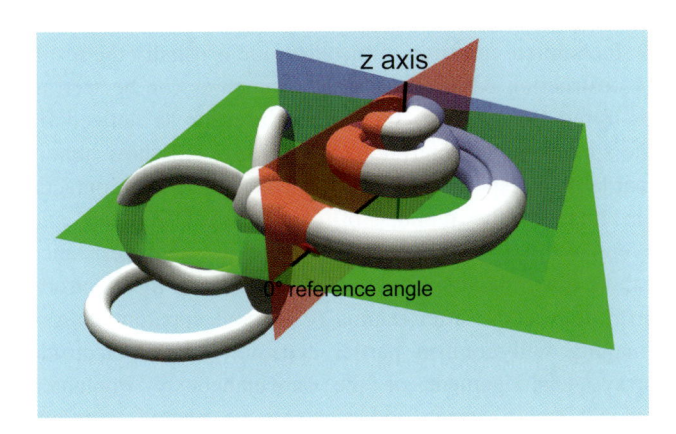

Fig. 9 Consensus coordinate system: a 3-dimensional coordinate system has been defined with the plane of rotation (*x*, *y* plane) through the basal turn of the cochlea (*green plane*) and the axis of rotation through the center of the modiolus (crossing of the *red* and *blue plane*), with its origin at the level of the helicotrema. The 0 reference angle is placed at the center of the round window (*red plane*). Measurements will be defined by rotational angle and distance to the modiolus

cochlea and every cochlear implant can be precisely located in relation to the basal end of the organ of Corti, which lies in close relationship to the round window. This provides a basis for reproducible assessment of angular insertion depths and more accurate assignment of frequency bands to stimulation sites in fitting individual implant users (Rebscher et al. 2008).

4.2 Imaging Modalities

4.2.1 X-ray

Postoperative imaging is usually done by conventional X-ray. It is a well-established, safe, and cheap technique to confirm that the implant has been placed intracochlearly and to assess integrity of the electrode array. An intraoperative portable plain radiograph may be obtained if the insertion was difficult or device malfunction is suspected on peroperative electrophysiological monitoring and repositioning might be needed. Several techniques have been used, such as Stenvers' view and intra orbital view. Xu et al. developed the *cochlear view*, a method of skull radiography to get an ideal picture of the intracochlear electrode array by directing the X-ray at the cochlea and parallel to the modiolus. This is achieved by a 50/0° posteroanterior oblique view with the midsagittal plane forming an angle of 50° with the plane of the film and the central ray 2 cm above and parallel to the infraorbitomeatal plane. (Marsh et al. 1993) On such images, certain anatomical landmarks can be well identified and help to evaluate the position of the implant. The cochlear promontory is located at the air–bone interface below the superior semicircular canal and vestibule. All electrode contacts medial to the promontory are assumed to be positioned within the cochlea. If the array follows a gentle, continuous curve with regular spacing of all electrode contacts, kinking or a rupture can be ruled out (Fig 2e) For measurements of angular insertion depths, a software package named CView©[1] is on the market. This program allows making measurements on pre- and post-operative cochlear view images that are independent of the size of the cochlea.

4.2.2 Computer Tomography and Cone Beam CT

Cross-sectional CT techniques, nowadays, provide detailed images of implanted ears without disturbing metal artifacts (Verbist et al. 2008). They can be extremely helpful in ears where normal anatomical landmarks are missing (e.g. congenital ear malformations, ossified vestibular system due to labyrinthitis) or to evaluate complicated electrode insertions and new electrode designs. CT provides high-resolution

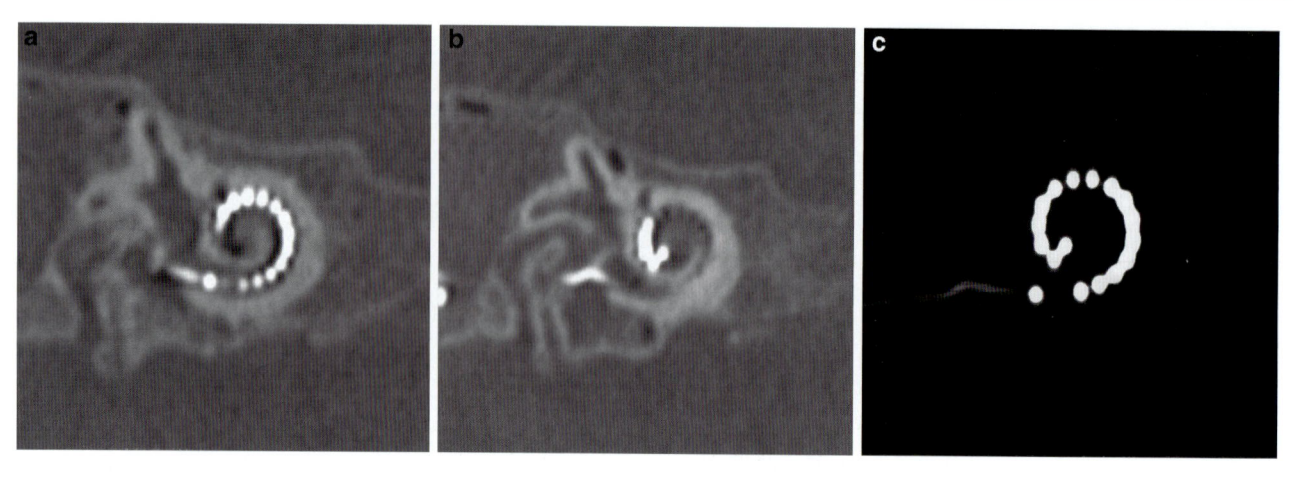

Fig. 10 Electrode kinking: multiplanar reconstructions (**a**, **b**) of a postoperative CT along the basal turn of the cochlea (W/L: 16000/6000) and a volume rendering image (**c**) show that 1 contact has flipped backward at the tip of the electrode array. This contact can be switched off to prevent complications during stimulation

images of the temporal bone on which anatomical landmarks, such as the round window niche, can be directly visualized. Visualization of individual contacts depends on the scanner's spatial resolution and the size and spacing of electrode contacts. Multiplanar reconstructions (MPRs) can be made within any desired plane. An oblique MPR parallel to the basal turn of the cochlea and perpendicular to the modiolus will render an optimal view on an implant. The volume scan also contains information of the height of the cochlea and thus enables evaluation of scala tympani versus scala vestibuli positioning of the device. Cone beam CT (Ruivo et al. 2009) may become a valuable alternative to CT because of its very high resolution and lower radiation dose, although comparative in vivo studies are still lacking.

In preoperative scans, localizations of anatomic structures can be related to the center of the round window. On postoperative scans, however, identification of the round window may be difficult due to surgical anatomical distortions and the presence of an implant. Angular measurements of insertion depths can, however, be related to the horizontal semicircular canal and then converted to the center of the round window using a correction angle of $34.6 \pm 0.4°$ (standard deviation) (Verbist et al 2010c).

4.3 Complications

Possible complications after cochlear implantation leading to dysfunction or failure of the implant are incomplete insertion, dislodgement, malpositioning, or breaks of the electrode lead.

In otosclerosis and developmental abnormalities of the ear, there is a risk of facial nerve stimulation, CSF-leaks, and meningitis during or after the procedure.

Incomplete insertion of the electrode is usually the result of obstruction within the cochlear lumen as can be seen in ossifying labyrinthitis. Incomplete insertion is noticed by the surgeon. Electrophysiolocigal testing will show abnormal/lack of response to the extracochlear electrode contacts. On imaging the number of extracochlear contacts and eventual flipping of the electrode tip at the site of resistance can be determined (Fig. 10). Dislodgement of the electrode array may occur after trauma or without apparent reason. Imaging will confirm partial extrusion of the electrode array. Dislodgement of the subcutaneously implanted magnet rarely occurs and seems to be related to minor trauma or exposure to magnetic fields, e.g. from magnetic toys. (Wild et al. 2010).

Malpositioning of the implant may occur if access to the round window is obscured. Cochlear implants have been described to be coiled in the middle ear and mastoid or misplaced in the cochlear aqueduct, Eustachian tube and carotid canal (Jain and Mukherji 2003; Nevoux 2010). In otosclerosis, bone apposition may distort the normal anatomy and the implant may perforate areas of altered bone density within the otic capsule (Fig. 11). In case of ossifying labyrinthitis, it may be necessary to drill-out part of the basal turn before implant insertion. In extensively ossified cases, a tunnel may be drilled out inadvertently outside the cochlea.

Facial nerve stimulation is the result of current spread from the device to the labyrinthine segment of the facial nerve usually through bone with low mineral density or may be due to electrode lead-nerve contact at the level of the mastoid. It will be treated by switching off those contacts that cause stimulation or by repositioning the electrode lead. CT can be helpful in localizing the source of facial nerve stimulation.

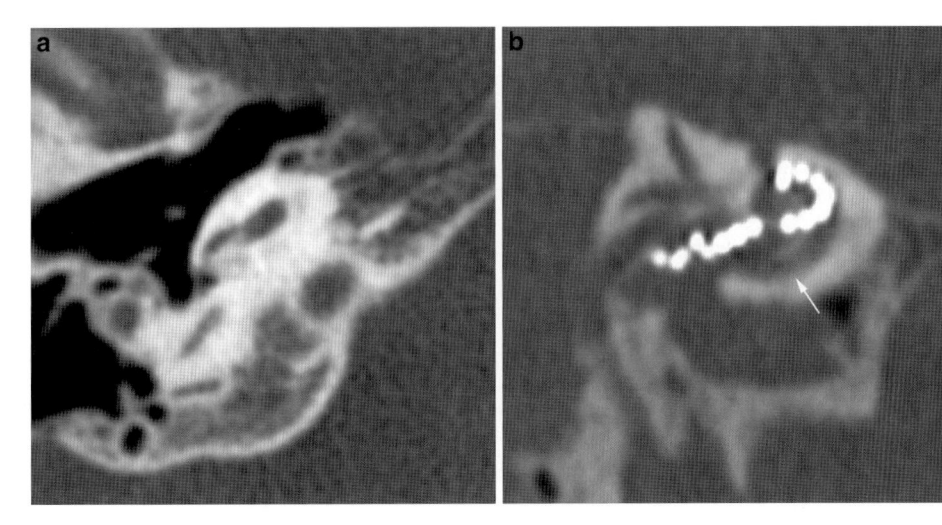

Fig. 11 Complications in otosclerosis: preoperative CT (**a**) shows an otospongiotic focus, narrowing the round window niche and extending posterior to the basal turn of the cochlea. **b** The anatomic distortion and altered appearance of the bone led to malpositioning (the cochleostomy was performed anterosuperior of the round window), incomplete insertion and kinking both in the proximal and distal segment of the implant, as seen on a postoperative MPR (*white arrow*: basal turn of the cochlea)

5 Conclusion

Cochlear implants are a well-accepted treatment for profound hearing loss or deafness. Preoperative imaging of cochlear implant candidates plays an important role in treatment planning. Anatomic variants and pathologic conditions might influence or even prevent surgical access and might influence outcome in terms of speech recognition. The report should include whether developmental or obliterative inner ear disease, abnormalities of bone metabolism, retrocochlear pathology, or anatomic variants of the middle ear and mastoid are present.

Postoperative imaging is usually done by means of conventional X-rays and allows for confirmation of intracochlear positioning and integrity of the implant. CT or conebeam CT is mainly used in case of complications, but will also provide useful information about the surgical results in developmental abnormalities and cochlear obstructive pathology.

References

Bredberg G, Lindström B, Löpponen H, Skarzynski H, Hyodo M, Sato H (1997) Electrodes for ossified cochleas. Am J Otol 18(6 Suppl):S42–S43

Cohen LT, Xu J, Tycocinski M, Saunders E, Raja D, Cowan R (2000) Evaluation of an X-ray analysis method: comparison of electrode position estimates with information from phase contrast X-ray and histology. In: 5th European symposium on paediatric cochlear implantation, Antwerp, Belgium

Dhooghe IJM, De Vel E, Urgell H et al (2002) Cochlear implantation in a patient with superficial siderosis of the central nervous system. Otol Neurotol 23:468–472

Fatterpekar GM, Mukherji SK, Alley J, Lin Y, Castillo M (2000) Hypoplasia of the bony canal for the cochlear nerve in patients with congenital sensorineural hearing loss: initial observations. Radiology 215(1):243–246

FDA (1984) Summary of safety and effectiveness data, 26 Nov 1984, PMA nr P830069

Friedman RA, Bykhovskaya Y, Tu G, Talbot JM, Wilson DF, Parnes LS, Fischel-Ghodsian N (1997) Molecular analysis of the POU3F4 gene in patients with clinical and radiographic evidence of X-linked mixed deafness with perilymphatic gusher. Ann Otol Rhinol Laryngol 106(4):320–325

Frijns JH, Kalkman RK, Briaire JJ (2009) Stimulation of the facial nerve by intracochlear electrodes in otosclerosis: a computer modeling study. Otol Neurotol 30(8):1168–1174

Hegarty JL, Patel S, Fischbein N, Jackler RK, Lalwani AK (2002) The value of enhanced magnetic resonance imaging in the evaluation of endocochlear disease. Laryngoscope 112(1):8–17

Jain R, Mukherji SK (2003) Cochlear implant failure: imaging evaluation of the electrode course. Clin Radiol 58(4):288–293

Klein M, Koedel U, Pfister HW, Kastenbauer S (2003) Morphological correlates of acute and permanent hearing loss during experimental pneumococcal meningitis. Brain Pathol 13:123–132

Kos MI, Boex C, Sigrist A, Guyot JP, Pelizzone M (2005) Measurements of electrode position inside the cochlea for different cochlear implant systems. Acta Otolaryngol 125:474–480

Lenarz T, Lesinski-Shiedat A, Weber BP et al (2001) The nucleus double array cochlear implant: a new concept for the obliterated cochlea. Otol Neurotol 22:24–32

Lin K, Marrinan MS, Waltzman SB et al (2006) Multichannel cochlear implantation in the scala vestibuli. Otol Neurotol 27:634–638

Marsh MA, Xu J, Blamey PJ et al (1993) Radiologic evaluation of multichannel intracochlear implant insertion depth. Am J Otol 14(4):386–391

Merchant SN, Gopen Q (1996) A human temporal bone study of acute bacterial meningogenic labyrinthitis. Am J Otol 17:375–385

Merkus P, Free RH, Mylanus EA, Stokroos R, Metselaar M, van Spronsen E, Grolman W, Frijns JH (2010) Dutch Cochlear Implant Group (CI-ON) consensus protocol on postmeningitis hearing evaluation and treatment. Otol Neurotol 31(8):1281–1286

Nadol JB Jr (1997) Patterns of neural degeneration in the human cochlea and auditory nerve: implications for cochlear implantation. Otolaryngol Head Neck Surg 117(3 Pt 1):220–228

Nevoux J, Loundon N, Leboulanger N, Roger G, Ducou Le Pointe H, Garabédian EN (2010) Cochlear implant in the carotid canal. Case report and literature review. Int J Pediatr Otorhinolaryngol 74(6):701–703

O'Driscoll M, El-Deredy W, Atas A, Sennaroglu G, Sennaroglu L, Ramsden RT (2011) Brain stem responses evoked by stimulation with an auditory brain stem implant in children with cochlear nerve aplasia or hypoplasia. Ear Hear 32(3):300–312

Parry DA, Booth T, Roland PS (2005) Advantages of MRI over CT in preoperative evaluation of cochlear implant candidates. Otol Neurotol 26(5):976–982

Rappaport JM, Bhatt SM, Kimura RS, Lauretano AM, Levine RA (1999) Electron microscopic temporal bone histopathology in experimental pneumococcal meningitis. Ann Otol Rhinol Laryngol 108:537–547

Rebscher SJ, Hetherington A, Bonham B, Wardrop P, Whinney D, Leake PA (2008) Considerations for design of future cochlear implant electrode arrays: electrode array stiffness, size, and depth of insertion. J Rehabil Res Dev 45:731–747

Rotteveel LJC, Proops DW, Ramsden RT et al (2004) Cochlear implantation in 53 patients with otosclerosis: demographics, computed tomographic scanning, surgery and complications. Otol Neurotol 25:943–952

Ruivo J, Mermuys K, Bacher K, Kuhweide R, Offeciers E, Casselman JW (2009) Cone beam computed tomography, a low-dose imaging technique in the postoperative assessment of cochlear implantation. Otol Neurotol 30:299–303

Skinner MW, Holden TA, Whiting BR et al (2007) In vivo estimates of the position of advanced bionics electrode arrays in the human cochlea. Ann Otol Rhinol Laryngol Suppl 197:2–24

Stakhovskaya O, Sridhar D, Bonham BH, Leake PA (2007) Frequency map for the human cochlear spiral ganglion: implications for cochlear implants. J Assoc Res Otolaryngol 8:220–233

NIH Consensus Statement (1995) Cochlear implants in adults and children, 2nd edn, vol 13, pp 1–3

Verbist BM, Joemai RM, Teeuwisse WM, Veldkamp WJ, Geleijns J, Frijns JH (2008) Evaluation of 4 multisection CT systems in postoperative imaging of a cochlear implant: a human cadaver and phantom study. AJNR Am J Neuroradiol 29(7):1382–1388

Verbist BM, Joemai RMS, Briaire JJ, Teeuwisse WM, Veldkamp JHM, Frijns JHM (2010a) Cochlear coordinates in regard to cochlear implantation: a clinically individually 3-dimensional CT-based method. Otol Neurotol 31(5):738–744

Verbist BM, Skinner MW, Cohen LT, Leake PA, James C, Boëx C, Holden TA, Finley CC, Roland PS, Roland T, Haller M, Patrick JF, Jolly CN, Faltys MA, Briaire JJ, Frijns JHM (2010b) Consensus panel on a cochlear coordinate system applicable in histological, physiological, radiological studies of the human cochlea. Otol Neurotol 31(5):722–730

Verbist BM, Joemai RMS, Briaire JJ, Teeuwisse WM, Veldkamp JHM, Frijns JHM (2010c) Cochlear coordinates in regard to cochlear implantation: a clinically individually 3-dimensional CT-based method. Otol Neurotol 31(5):738–744

Wild C, Allum J, Probst R, Abels D, Fischer C, Bodmer D (2010) Magnet displacement: a rare complication following cochlear implantation. Eur Arch Otorhinolaryngol 267(1):57–59

Wilson BS, Dorman MF (2008) Cochlear implants: current designs and future possibilities. J Rehabil Res Dev 45(5):695–730

Wood VH, Bird PA, Giles EC et al (2008) Unsuccessful cochlear implantation in two patients with superficial siderosis of the central nervous system. Otol Neurotol 29:622–625

Xu J, Xu SA, Cohen LT, Clark GM (2000) Cochlear view: postoperative radiography for cochlear implantation. Am J Otol 21:49–56

Petrous Apex Lesions

Marc Lemmerling

Contents

1 The Normal Petrous Apex 249
2 Lesions of the Petrous Apex 249
2.1 Don't Touch Lesions 250
2.2 True Petrous Apex Lesions 250

References 255

Abstract

The petrous apex is the most anterior and medial portion of the temporal bone, and rarely contains lesions. Imaging techniques in general, and MRI more specifically, are of great help to detect such lesions, and to differentiate them, in order to decide to leave them alone or to choose for therapeutic action.

1 The Normal Petrous Apex

The petrous apex is the most anterior and medial portion of the temporal bone, and articulates with the clivus at the petroclival junction. The petrous apex is pneumatized to a variable degree, and this degree of pneumatization or aeration correlates with the amount of pneumatized air cells in other parts of the temporal bone (Yetiser et al. 2002). Pneumatization of the petrous apex is present in 33 % of all temporal bones, and of these, all parts of the apex are pneumatized in only about 40 % of the cases (Hentona et al. 1994). The non-pneumatized portions of the temporal bone apex show a high signal on both T1- and T2-weighted MR images (Fig. 1). This is due to their fatty bone marrow content. The pneumatized portions in the normal petrous apex show no signal at all in normal conditions.

2 Lesions of the Petrous Apex

Petrous apex lesions are rare, and they are often noted incidentally, unrelated to the presenting clinical manifestation (Leonetti et al. 2001). However, in the presence of petrous apex lesions, a variety of clinical symptoms is noted, such as hearing loss, dizziness, headaches, and tinnitus (Muckle et al. 1998). Usually, these lesions can be precisely defined using imaging techniques such as CT and MR. Although MR-guided biopsies through a transsphenoidal access have been attempted in the petrous apex region (Bootz et al. 2001), such procedures are usually

M. Lemmerling (✉)
Department of Radiology, AZ St-Lucas Hospital,
Groenebriel 1, 9000 Gent, Belgium
e-mail: marc.lemmerling@azstlucas.be

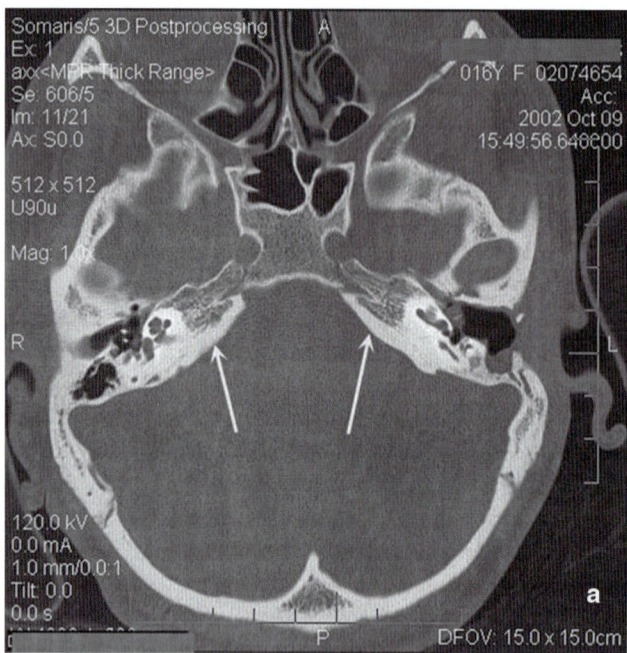

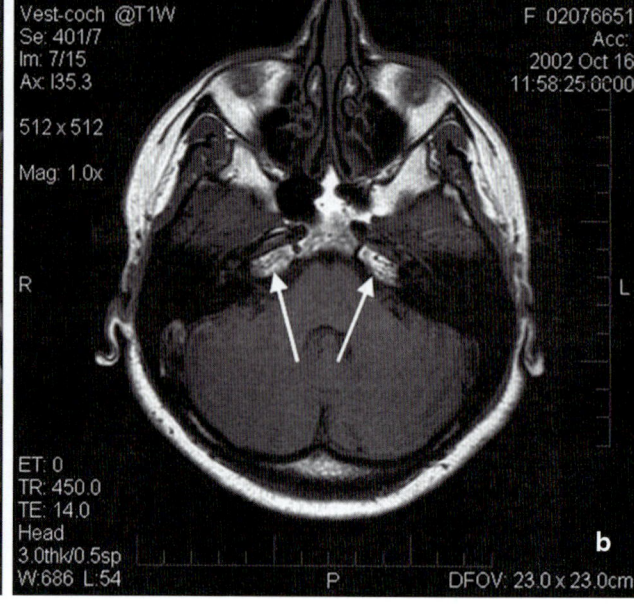

Fig. 1 The normal petrous apex as is it seen in most patients. On the CT images (**a**) the bone marrow in the petrous apex is obviously seen bilaterally (*arrows*). On the axial T1-weighted MR image (**b**) a hyperintense signal is noted bilaterally, lateral to the hyperintense clivus, indicating the presence of fatty bone marrow in the non-pneumatized apex (*arrows*)

unnecessary if an experienced radiologist studies the lesion. MR specifically plays an important role in the differentiation of petrous apex lesions, that can often be easily detected with CT, but where CT does not always permit to correctly differentiate the imaging finding (Pisanischi and Langer 2000). The importance of MR on this matter has been emphasized since the late 1980s and early 1990s (Griffin et al. 1987; Greenberg et al. 1988; Jackler and Parker 1992; Arriaga and Brackmann 1991). The study of the spontaneous signal intensities of these lesions on T1- and T2-weighted images and of the enhancement pattern of the internal matrix of the lesions often allows to provide a correct diagnosis with a very high degree of confidence (Curtin and Som 1995). Consequently, the radiologist plays an important role in the process of decision making, whether the area in question needs surgical therapy, and influences the process of deciding on the exact type of surgery that should be performed (Chang et al. 1998; Profant and Steno 2000; Brackmann and Toh 2002). MR scanning is helpful to evaluate for complete removal, complication, recurrence, or formation of complicating granulation tissue (Pisanischi and Langer 2000).

2.1 Don't Touch Lesions

On the basis of MR, two 'don't touch' entities in the petrous apex can be confused with pathologic lesions that need surgery: asymmetric presence of fatty marrow and trapped fluid in petrous air cells. Although both have specific imaging characteristics, radiologists do not always confidently define these two nonsurgical petrous apex lesions (Palacios et al. 2001; Moore et al. 1998).

2.1.1 Asymmetric Presence of Fatty Marrow

In case of asymmetric presence of fatty marrow, the radiologist should notice that the area with high signal in the petrous apex region has the same signal intensity as fat on all sequences (Roland et al. 1990; Moore et al. 1998) (Fig. 2). If still any doubt would remain, CT of the region can be performed and will show a less pneumatized petrous apex on the side that was considered suspicious on the MR examination. Fat-suppressed MR techniques can also give the solution.

2.1.2 Fluid-Filled Petrous Apex Air Cells

The petrous apex is aerated to a variable degree. It is believed that the degree of aeration as such is not responsible for the eventual presence of clinical symptoms (Yetiser et al. 2002). In some occasions, pneumatized petrous apex cells can be fluid-filled. Such cells have an intermediate or high signal on the T1-weighted images and a high signal on the T2-weighted images. Trapped fluid is mostly confused with cholesterol granuloma, but the latter does not enhance except for a thin rim, while trapped fluid will often enhance moderately. The presence of trapped fluid in other mastoid cells often accompanies the fluid trapping in the apex (Fig. 3). CT is also able to ensure the radiologist that the petrous apex is opacified in a non-expansile way in case of fluid trapping.

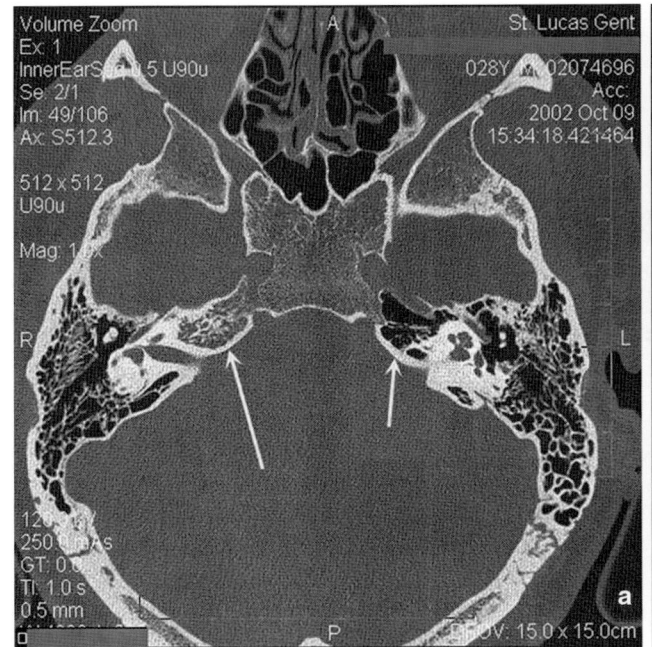

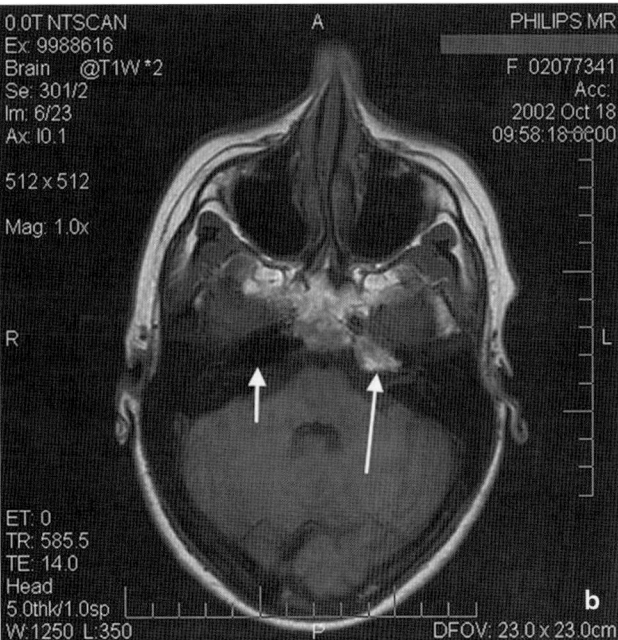

Fig. 2 Asymmetrical pneumatization of the petrous apex on CT (**a**), with pneumatization on the left side (*small arrow*) and non-pneumatization on the right side (*large arrow*). Note that on the T1-weighted MR image (**b**) a high signal is seen in the apex on the left side (*large arrow*), which should not be mistaken for tumor. The signal is identical to the one of fat in other locations (e.g., clivus, mandibular head, pterygopalatine fossa, etc.): normal fatty bone marrow in the non-pneumatized apex. The right petrous apex is pneumatized and shows no signal (*small arrow*)

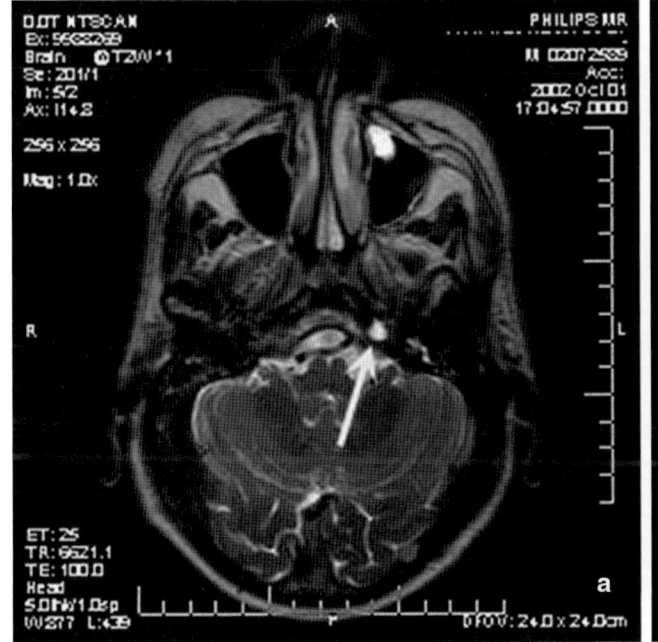

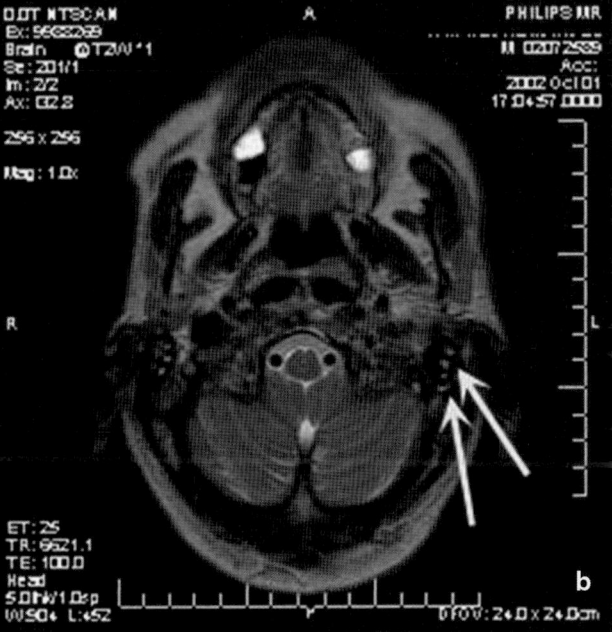

Fig. 3 Fluid trapping in pneumatized petrous apex cells show a high signal on the T2-weighted images (**a**) and are often accompanied by other mastoid cells that also contain trapped fluid (**b**)

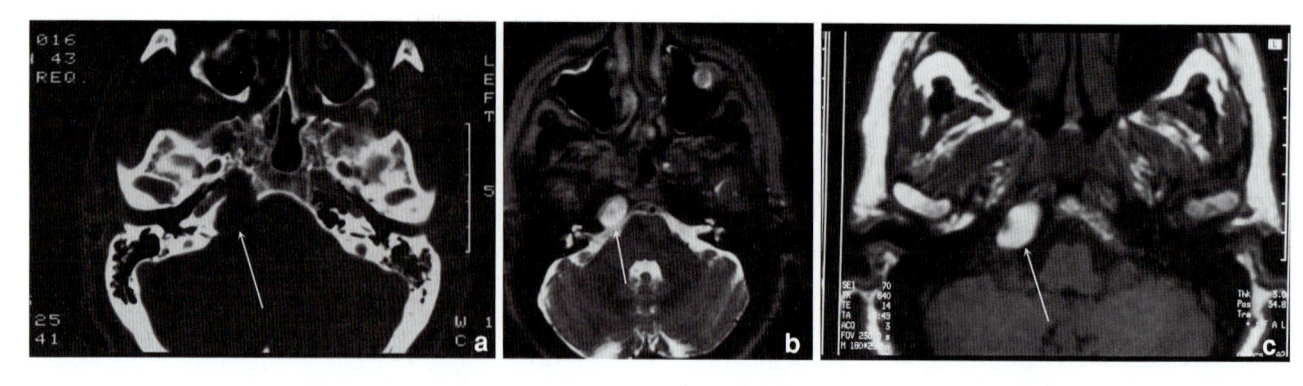

Fig. 4 Cholesterol cyst or cholesterol granuloma. CT (**a**) shows a round cystic lesion in the petrous apex on the right side. The finding is however aspecific. On MR, the well-defined mass is hyperintense on both the T2 (**b**)- and T1 (**c**)-weighted images. Note that the contralateral apex is partially pneumatized

2.2 True Petrous Apex Lesions

Petrous apex lesions have been classified in different ways by different authors. Where some divide the lesions in cystic and solid lesions, others distinguish destructive and nondestructive lesions. The two most frequent lesions in the petrous apex that need surgery are the cholesterol granuloma and cholesteatoma (Chang et al. 1998). Both are cystic and destructive/expansile lesions and account for respectively 60 and 9 % of all petrous apex lesions (Muckle et al. 1998). The differentiation between both is very important, because of their completely different therapeutic management. Cholesterol granuloma can be drained internally into the mastoid or middle ear, while cholesteatoma need a more aggressive removal, which often mandates the sacrifice of hearing (Chang et al. 1998; Profant and Steno 2000; Brackmann and Toh 2002). The experience of the surgeon is another important factor in the choice of the surgical approach (Haberkamp 1997).

2.2.1 Cholesterol Granuloma or Cyst

Cholesterol granuloma, also called cholesterol cyst or giant cholesterol cyst, is the most common primary lesion of the petrous apex, and accounts for 60 % of all lesions in that region (Muckle et al. 1998). They rarely occur bilaterally (Jaramillo and Winle-Taylor 2001). Cholesterol cysts contain a brownish liquid glistening with cholesterol crystals (Lo et al. 1984; Graham et al. 1985). Repetitive cycles of hemorrhage and granulomatous reaction—reason why such cysts are also referred to as granulomas—initiated by an obstruction of the ventilation outlet of the apex, are believed to cause cholesterol cysts (Nager and Vanderveen 1976).

Cholesterol cysts are most often seen in young adults and are treated surgically, by drainage of the petrous apex. The petrous apex can be achieved through different approaches, such as the transcanal infracochlear, transmastoid infralabyrinthine, middle fossa, translabyrinthine, and transotic ones. Determination of the best approach depends on the hearing status of the affected ear on the one hand, and the relationship between the petrous apex lesion and the surrounding neurovascular structures on the other hand. The translabyrinthine approach is useful in nonhearing ears, whereas the transcanal infracochlear approach with stenting is preferred in hearing individuals, if anatomy permits so (Brackmann and Toh 2002).

On MR, cholesterol cysts are hyperintense on both T1- and T2-weighted images (Fig. 4). Some have a hypointense rim on both T1- and T2-weighting (Greenberg et al. 1988). The contralateral apex is often pneumatized.

2.2.2 Primary Cholesteatoma or Epidermoid Cyst

Primary cholesteatoma of the petrous apex is also referred to as epidermoid cyst. The term 'cyst' is confusing since they contain desquamated keratin, which is a solid material. As already mentioned, epidermoid cysts are much rarer than the cholesterol cyst (Muckle et al. 1998).

Petrous apex cholesteatoma require surgical management and the removal is again done through different approaches, according to different parameters, such as the size of the cholesteatoma, the degree of hearing loss, and the remaining facial nerve function (Profant and Steno 2000).

On MR, epidermoid cysts are hyperintense on the T2-weighted and diffusion-weighted images, and are hypointense on the T1-weighted images. After injection of gadolinium, epidermoid cysts do not enhance or only their capsule is enhancing (Fig. 5) Mafee et al. (1994).

2.2.3 Other Petrous Apex Lesions

Petrous apicitis was a frequent occurrence in the past, but has become rare with the appropriate use of antibiotics in the treatment of middle ear disease. Inflammatory/infectious disease of the petrous apex is especially seen in the well-pneumatized apex and is treated by means of surgical

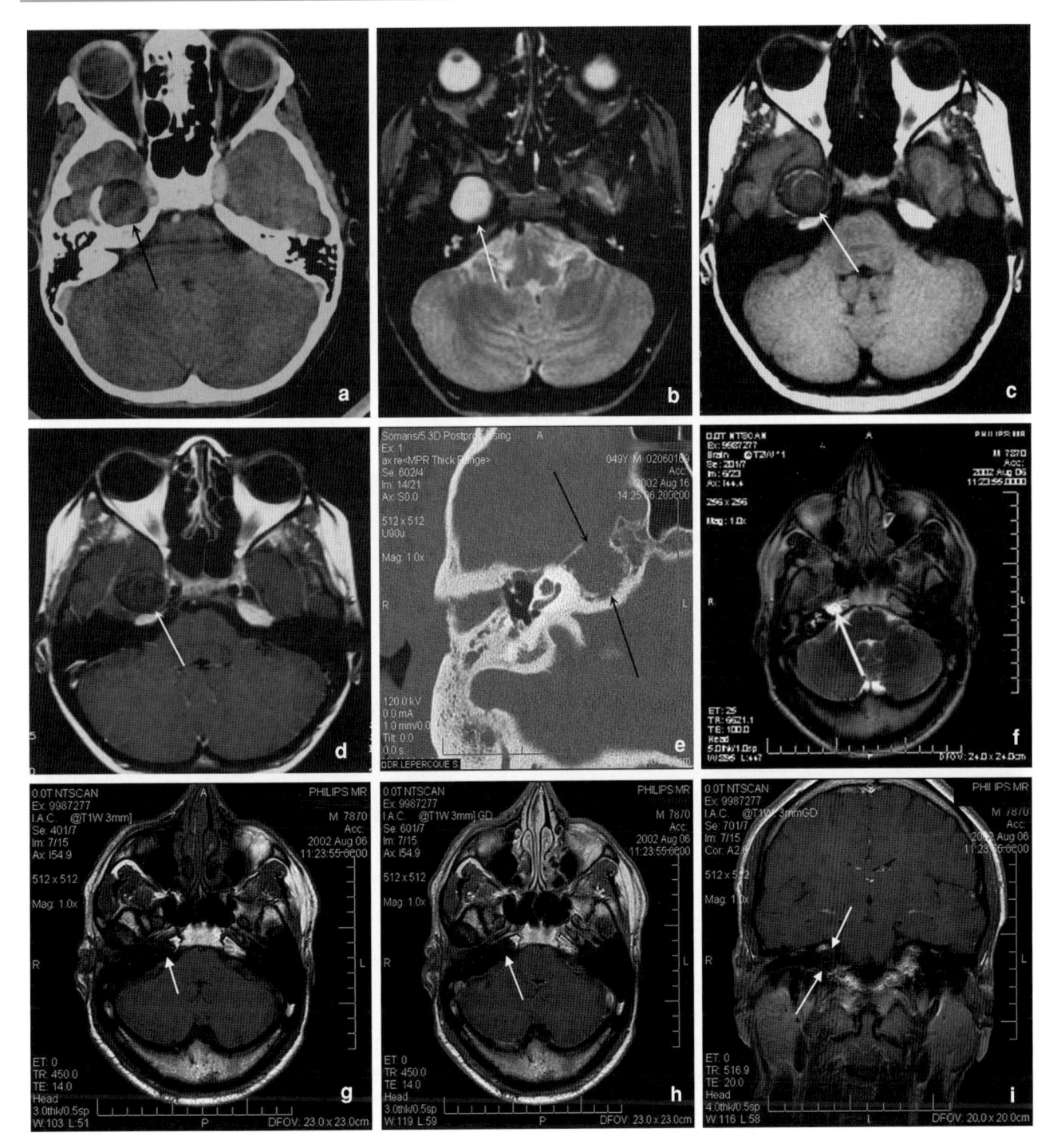

Fig. 5 Epidermoid cyst or congenital cholesteatoma. CT (**a**) shows an ovoid and destructive mass in the petrous apex on the right side in a child. CT is unable to differentiate. On MR, typical signs of an epidermoid cyst are noted: hyperintense signal on the T2-weighted images (**b**), hypointense signal on the T1-weighted images (**c**), and only capsular enhancement after intravenous injection of gadolinium (**d**), CT is also shown in another 49-year-old patient with a destructive lesion in the right petrous apex (**e**). Again CT is aspecific but MR proves that the lesion is an epidermoid: the mass is hyperintense on the T2-weighted images (**f**), hypointense on T1-weighting (**g**), and does show no enhancement at all on the axial (**h**) and coronal (**i**) T1-weighted images after intravenous injection of gadolinium

drainage. The petrous apex is heterogeneously hyperintense on the T2-weighted images, shows a heterogeneous and mixed signal on the T1-weighted images, and enhances heterogeneously after intravenous injection of gadolinium (Fig. 6). This enhancement pattern allows differentiation from cholesterol granuloma, which is a non-enhancing lesion. This inflammatory/infectious condition can become aggressive, leading to bone erosion and asymmetric clouding

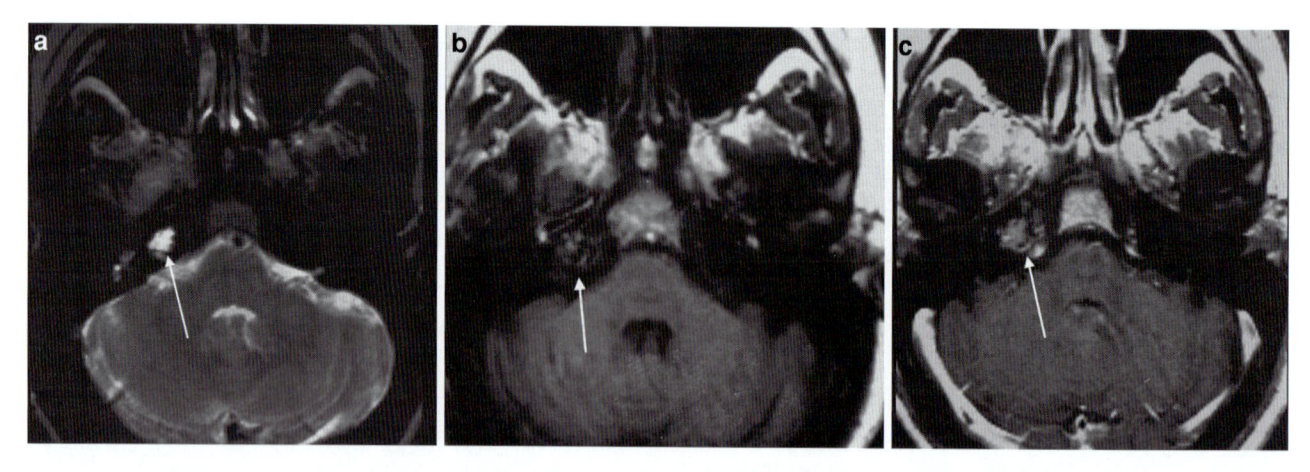

Fig. 6 In case of petrous apicitis, the petrous apex is heterogeneously hyperintense on the T2-weighted images (**a**), shows a heterogeneous and mixed signal on the T1-weighted images (**b**), and enhances heterogeneously after intravenous injection of gadolinium (**c**)

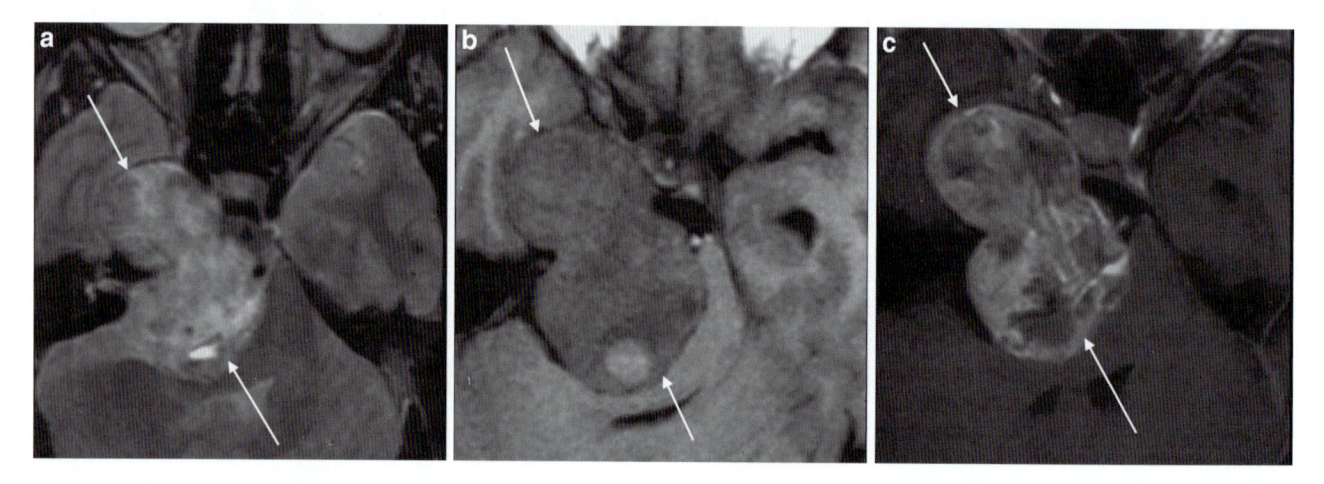

Fig. 7 Meningioma. A dumbbell-shaped tumor with heterogeneous high signal intensity on the T2-weighted images is growing around the petrous apex (**a**). The mass shows a heterogeneous low signal on the T1-weighted images (**b**) and enhances strongly and heterogeneously after intravenous injection of gadolinium (**c**)

of the petrous tip. This latter condition is best studied with CT (Chole and Donald 1983). In rare cases, petrous apicitis can become extremely aggressive and develop to nasopharyngeal abscess formation or cause facial nerve paralysis (Fitzgerald 2001). Extension into the neck has been reported in a child (Somers et al. 2001).

Primary mucoceles of the petrous apex are rare and their MR appearance varies depending on the degree of hydration or inspissation of the contents. They are best treated by an infralabyrinthine approach (Larson and Wong 1992). Their signal on the T1-weighted images increases with the increasing protein concentration. In some cases, it can be difficult to distinguish them from primary cholesteatoma.

Petrous apex arachnoid cysts are uncommon. They will rarely be symptomatic and are amenable to simple surgical drainage (Chang et al. 1998). Petrous apex cephaloceles are other uncommon lesions that are usually incidental, but that can rarely be symptomatic. They represent a protrusion of meninges and cerebrospinal fluid from the posterolateral portion of Meckel's cave into the petrous apex (Moore et al. 2001).

The petrous apex can be directly invaded by benign or malignant lesions arising from the meninges (Fig. 7), nasopharynx, temporal bone, or even parotid region (Fig. 8). Primary neoplasms arising from the bony or cartilaginous tissues of the petroclival junction are also found in the apex region, and are treated in another chapter.

Osseous sarcoidosis presenting as a destructive petrous bone lesion (Ng and Niparko 2002), as well as petrous apex blastomycosis (Blackledge and Newlands 2001) are other very rare petrous apex lesions that have been reported.

The interpretation of the signal intensities of the petrous apex can become confusing in patients who are of have recently been treated for hematologic diseases. The activated red bone marrow causes a decrease in signal intensity on both the T1- and T2-weighted images (Fig. 9).

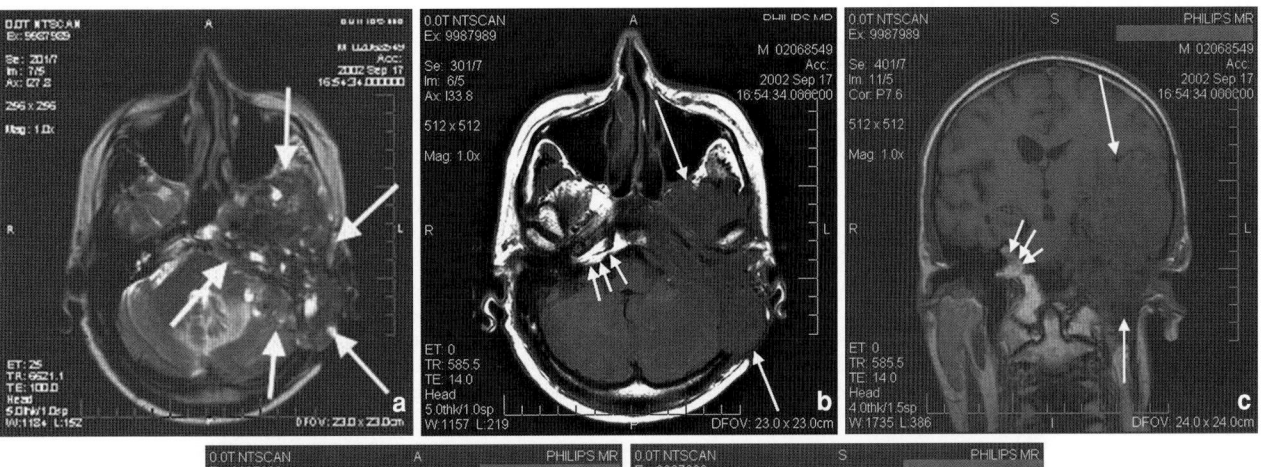

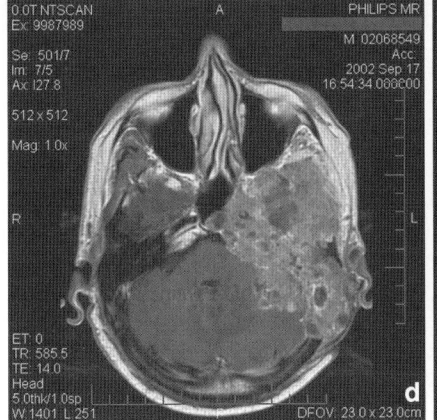

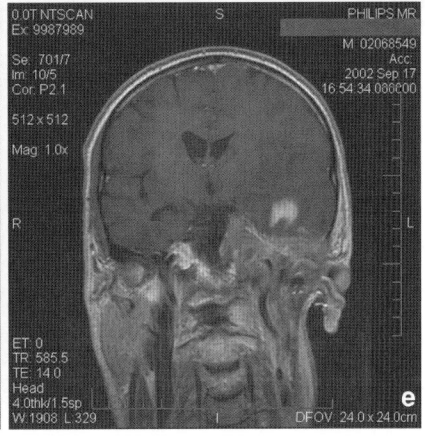

Fig. 8 The petrous apex can be directly invaded by neoplasms arising from other spaces in the neck, such as by this adenoid cystic carcinoma on the left side, extending to the apex, and initially growing in the parotid space. The huge tumor (arrows) shows a mixed signal on the T2-weighted images (**a**), and is isointense to cerebellar tissue on the axial (**b**) and coronal (**c**) T1-weighted images (between two large arrows). Note the normal hyperintense signal of the apex on the right side (three small arrows). After intravenous injection of gadolinium, heterogeneous enhancement is seen (**d** and **e**)

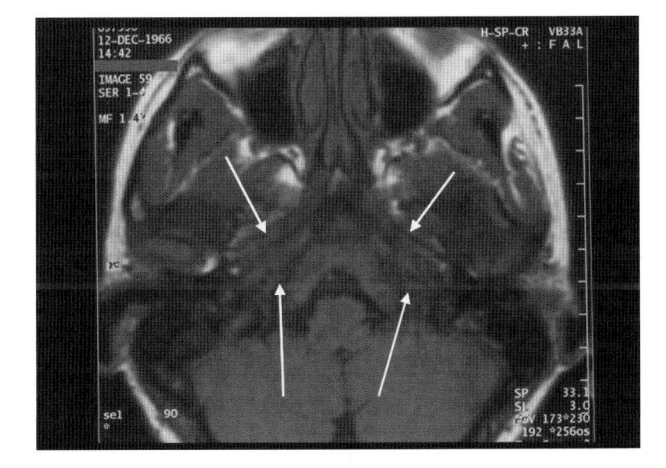

Fig. 9 The hyperintense signal intensity on the T1-weighted images that is normally seen in the non-pneumatized petrous apex, and that is caused by its fatty bone marrow content, is not present in this haematology patient. The normal soft tissue fat planes, such as those in the cheek and in the pterygopalatine fossa, still show their high signal. Note however that the high signal that is normally present in the bony structures in the clivus and the mandibular heads has also disappeared: the red bone marrow is activated due to therapy and has replaced the normal fatty bone marrow

References

Arriaga MA, Brackmann DE (1991) Differential diagnosis of primary petrous apex lesions. Am J Otol 12(6):470–474 Am J Otol May;13(3):297

Blackledge FA, Newlands SD (2001) Blastomyocosis of the petrous apex. AJNR Am J Neuroradiol 9(6):1205–1214

Bootz F, Keiner S, Schulz T, Scheffler B, Seifert V (2001) Magnetic resonance imaging–guided biopsies of the petrous apex and petroclival region. Otol Neurotol 22(3):383–388

Brackmann DE, Toh EH (2002) Surgical management of petrous apex cholesterol granulomas. Otol Neurotol 23(4):529–533

Chang P., Fagan PA, Atlas MD, Roche J (1998) Imaging destructive lesions of the petrous apex. Laryngoscope 108(4Pt1):599–604

Chole RA, Donald PJ (1983) Petrous apicitis. Clin Considerations. Ann Otol Rhinol Laryngol 92(6 pt 1):544–551

Curtin HD, Som PM (1995) The petrous apex. Otolaryngol Clin North Am 28(3):473–496

Fitzgerald DC (2001) Nasopharyngeal abscess and facial paralysis as complications of petrous apicitis: a case report. Ear Nose Throat J 80(5):305–307,310–312

Graham MD, Kemink JL, Latack JT, Kartush JM (1985) The giant cholesterol cyst of the petrous apex: a distinct clinical entity. Laryngoscope 95:1401–1406

Greenberg JJ, Oot RF, Wismer GL, Davis KR, Goodman ML, Weber AE, Montgomery WW (1988) Cholesterol granuloma of the petrous apex: MR and CT evaluation. AJNR Am J Neuroradiol 9(6):1205–1214

Griffin C, DeLaPaz R, Enzmann D (1987) MR and CT correlation of cholesterol cysts of the petrous bone. AJNR Am J Neuroradiol 8(5):825–829

Haberkamp TJ (1997) Surgical anatomy of the transtemporal approaches to the petrous apex. Am J Otol 18(4):501–506

Hentona H, Ohkudbo J, Tsutsumi T, Tanaka H, Komatsuzaki A (1994) Pneumatization of the petrous apex. Nippon Jibiinkoka Gakkai Kaiho 97(3):450–456

Jackler RK, Parker DA (1992) Radiographic differential diagnosis of petrous apex lesions. Am J Otol 13(6):561–574

Jaramillo M, Windle-Taylor PC (2001) Large cholesterol granuloma of the petrous apex treated via subcochlear drainage. J Laryngol Otol 115(12):1005–1009

Larson TL, Wong ML (1992) Primary mucocele of the petrous apex: MR appereance. AJNR Am J Neuroradiol 13(1):203–204

Leonetti JP, Shownkeen H, Marzo SJ (2001) Incidental petrous apex findings on magnetic resonance imaging. Ear Nose Throat J 80(4):200–202, 205–206

Lo WWM, Solti-Bohman LG, Brackmann DE, Gruskin P (1984) Cholesterol granuloma of the petrous apex: CT diagnosis. Radiol 153:705–711

Mafee MF, Kumar A, Heffner DK (1994) Epidermoid cyst (cholesteatoma) and cholesterol granuloma of the temporal bone and epidermoid cysts affecting the brain. Neuroimaging Clin N Am 4(3):561–578

Moore KR, Fischbein JN, Harnsberger HR, Shelton C, Glastonbury CM, White DK, Dillon WP (2001) Petrous apex cephaloceles. AJNR Am J Neuroradiol 22(10):1867–1871

Moore KR, Harnsberger HR, Shelton C, Davidson HC (1998) 'Leave me alone' lesions of the petrous apex. AJNR Am J Neuroradiol 19(4):733–738

Muckle RP, De la Cruz A, Lo WM (1998) Petrous apex lesions. Am J Otol 19(2):219–225

Nager CT, Vanderveen TS (1976) Cholesterol granuloma involving the temporal bone. Laryngoscope 85:204–209

Ng M, Niparko JK (2002) Osseous sarcoidosis presenting as a destructive petrous apex lesion. Am J Otolaryngol 23(4):241–245

Palacios E, Valvassori G, D'Antonio M (2001) 'Don't touch me' lesions of the petrous apex. Ear Nose Throat J 80(3):140

Pisaneschi MJ, Langer B (2000) Congenital cholesteatoma and cholesterol granuloma of the temporal bone: role of magnetic resonance imaging. Top Magn Reson Imaging 11(2):87–97

Profan M, Steno J (2000) Petrous apex cholesteatoma. Acta Otorhinolaryngol 120(2):164–167

Roland PS, Meyerhoff WL, Judge LO, Mickey BE (1990) Asymmetric pneumatization of the petrous apex. Otolaryngol Head Neck Surg 103(1):80–88

Somers TJ, De Foer B, Govaerts P, Pouillon M, Offeciers E (2001) Chronic petrous apicitis with pericarotid extension into the neck in a child. Ann Otol Rhinol Laryngol 110(10):988–991

Yetiser S, Kertmen M, Taser M (2002) Abnormal petrous apex aeration. Review of 12 cases. Acta Otorhinolaryngol Belg 56(1):65–71

Pathology of the Facial Nerve

Alexandra Borges

Contents

1 Introduction 258
2 Anatomy and Physiology 258
3 Clinical Topognostic Testing 261
4 Imaging Technique and Tailored Imaging Approach 262
5 Pathology 264
6 Congenital and Pediatric Facial Nerve Paralysis 289
7 Bilateral Facial Nerve Paralysis 302
References 302

Abstract

The facial nerve is the most common paralyzed nerve of the human body. It is responsible for facial mimic, lacrimation, salivation, and taste with dysfunction of this nerve having a tremendous negative impact on patient's lives. Its long and tortuous course within the densest bone of the human body and its fragile vascular supply make it particularly vulnerable to injury and difficult to rehabilitate functionally. As it is not amenable to direct clinical inspection, imaging plays a pivotal role in the diagnosis, management, and follow-up of patients with facial nerve dysfunction. The increasing resolution of imaging studies has lead to an increasing number of recognizable causes of facial nerve palsy improving the diagnostic yield and allowing for early treatment and functional rehabilitation. However, to keep high-resolution imaging within a reasonable time frame, it is advisable to tailor studies to the most likely location of a lesion along the course of the nerve. Clinically oriented topognostic testing is invaluable for this purpose. Appropriate imaging of the facial nerve requires detailed knowledge of its anatomy and physiology, mastering imaging technique, and recognition of the imaging features of the wide set of pathologic processes that may affect this nerve.

Abbreviations

FSE	Fast spin echo
DWI	Diffusion weighted imaging
GRE	Gradient echo
3DFT-CISS	Tridimensional Fourier transform constructive interference in the steady state
DRIVE	Driven equilibrium (optimized contrast using flip angle evolution)
FIESTA	Fast imaging employing steady-state acquisition
GRE-SSFP	Gradient echo steady-state free precessing

A. Borges (✉)
Radiology Department, Instituto Português de Oncologia Francisco Gentil- Centro de Lisboa, R. Prof. Lima Basto, 1099-023, Lisbon, Portugal
e-mail: borgalexandra@gmail.com

True-FISP	True fast imaging with steady-state precession
bFFE	Balanced fast-field echo
SPACE	Sampling perfection with application of optimized contrast
3D TOF MRA	Tridimensional time-of-flight magnetic resonance angiography
3D-FISP	Fast imaging with steady-state precession
3D-FLASH	Fast low-angle shot
3D CE-FAST	Contrast-enhanced Fourier-acquired steady state
SPGR	Spoiled gradient echo
MPRAGE	Magnetized prepared rapid gradient echo
VIBE	Volume interpolation breath hold enhancement
SENSE	Sensitivity encoding
SWI	Susceptibility weighted images

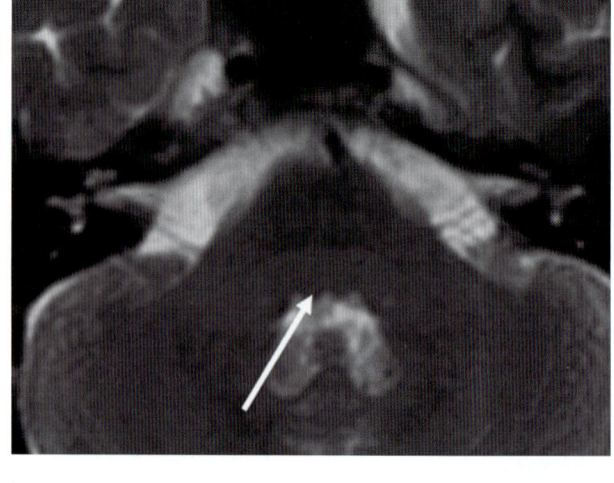

Fig. 1 Axial FSE T2 W image showing the nuclear projection of the facial nerve in the pontine tegmentum and the facial colliculi (*white arrow*)—two symmetrical prominences at the floor of the IVth ventricle—produced by the fascicular segment of the motor fibers looping posteriorly around the nucleus of the abducens nerve

1 Introduction

The facial nerve (cranial nerve VII) is the most commonly paralyzed nerve of the human body (Borges 2005; Benecke 2002; Rainsbury and Aldren 2007; Roob et al. 1999; Syed and Bhutta 2008). It provides motor innervation to the muscles of facial expression, parasympathetic secretomotor fibers to the lacrimal, submandibular, and sublingual glands and it receives special afferent fibers for taste sensation from the anterior two thirds of the tongue (Borges and Casselman 2007; Phillips and Bubash 2002; Raghavan et al. 2009; Finsterer 2008). Its long and tortuous course across the temporal bone and its terminal blood supply make it particularly vulnerable to injury, difficult to treat, and to rehabilitate functionally (Borges 2005; Borges and Casselman 2007; Jager and Reiser 2001; Veillon et al. 2010). As other cranial nerves, the facial nerve is occult to clinical inspection and its direct visualization can only be achieved by cross-sectional imaging. Neurological examination and electrophysiology testing are the mainstays to assess the functional integrity of the facial nerve (Sittel and Stennert 2001; Valls-Sole 2007). Moreover they are an important aid in localizing lesions along the course of the nerve and in tailoring imaging studies accordingly. Few impairments have such dramatic impact on patient's lives; therefore, clinical presentation usually calls for immediate action and patient's reassurance (Yeong and Tassone 2011). Potential causes of facial nerve palsy span a wide gamut and vary over the course of the nerve highlighting the importance of a segmental approach (Borges 2005; Borges and Casselman 2007; Veillon et al. 2008; Peitersen 2002). Of uttermost importance is the distinction between central and peripheral facial palsy, each carrying quite different causes and diagnostic approaches. Even though the most common cause of facial nerve palsy (FNP), Bell's palsy, often has a benign self-limited course, imaging plays an important role in predicting the patient's prognosis and in identifying potentially treatable causes of nerve palsy aiming for early functional recovery, before axonal degeneration ensues. Detailed knowledge of the anatomy, physiology, and pathology of the facial nerve and adequate tailoring of the imaging technique are the major requirements to master the radiologic management of the facial nerve.

2 Anatomy and Physiology

To understand the pathophysiology of facial nerve dysfunction and for a topognostic imaging approach to the nerve, detailed knowledge of facial nerve anatomy is crucial. The nerve comprises supra and infranuclear components, the latter divided into four main segments: brainstem, cisternal, intratemporal, and intraparotid segments. The long and tortuous temporal segment is further subdivided into intracanalicular, labyrinthine, tympanic, and mastoid segments (Borges 2005; Borges and Casselman 2007; Phillips and Bubash 2002; Raghavan et al. 2009; Al-Noury and Lotfy 2011).

1. Supranuclear segment:

    The upper motor neuron, responsible for voluntary facial movement is located in the motor cortex at the level of the pre- and post-central gyri. Output from these neurons is carried out, via the corticobulbar tract, through the posterior limb of the internal capsule and ventral aspect

Fig. 2 a Axial CISS image through the IAC shows the cisternal and intracanalicular segments of the facial nerve (1), the superior vestibular nerve (2), and the entrance to the IAC or porus acusticus (3). b Sagittal oblique section perpendicular to the fundus of the IAC as the reference white line in (a) demonstrates the facial nerve (1) in the superior and anterior quadrant of the IAC, above the cochlear nerve (2) and the superior (3) and inferior (4) vestibular nerves lying posteriorly (*Courtesy of Prof. F. Veillon*)

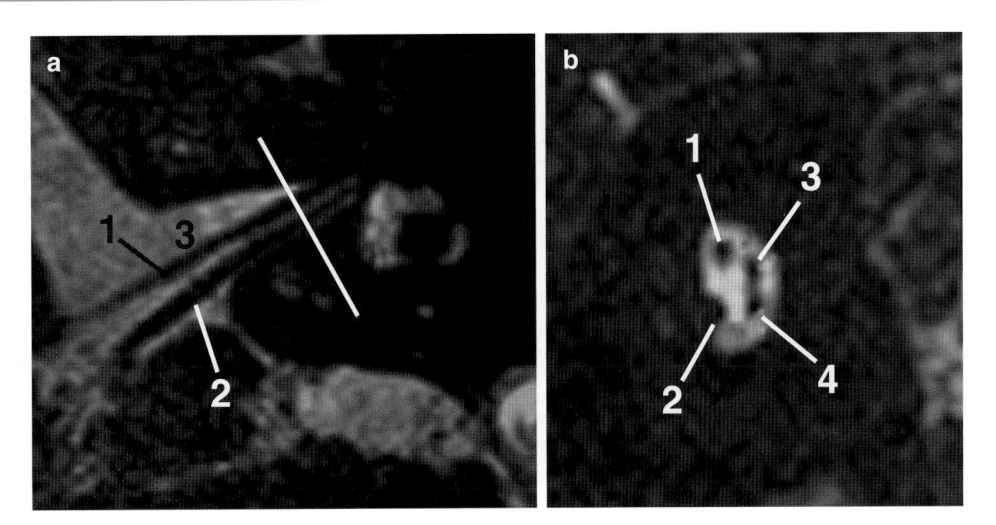

of the cerebral peduncles, to the motor facial nerve nuclei located in the pontine tegmentum. Whereas motor fibers supplying the forehead decussate only partially, those supplying the lower face decussate completely. This anatomical arrangement has important clinical implications: supranuclear lesions lead to central facial nerve palsy (CFNP), characterized by a spastic paralysis of the contralateral face, sparing the muscles of the forehead due to its bilateral nerve supply; infranuclear lesions cause flaccid peripheral facial nerve palsy (PFNP) affecting both the upper and lower face of the ipsilateral side.

2. Brainstem segment:

   This segment is composed by three different nuclei of the facial nerve located in the pontine tegmentum. The motor nucleus, the most ventral and medial, provides the motor fibers supplying the muscles of facial expression and the stapedius muscle. These fibers have a recurrent posterior course looping around the nucleus of the abducens nerve, producing a bulge at the floor of the IVth ventricle known as the facial *colliculus* (Fig. 1). Then the fibers course ventrolaterally in between the motor nucleus and the spinal trigeminal nucleus and tract. The lacrimal or superior salivatory nucleus located slightly more dorsolaterally provides parasympathetic secretomotor fibers to the lacrimal, submandibular, and sublingual glands. Finally, the gustatory or nucleus *solitarius*, receives special afferent fibers carrying taste sensation from the two anterior thirds of the tongue and somatic sensitive fibers from the pinna and external auditory canal. Fibers from the lacrimal and gustatory nuclei join together to form the intermediate nerve of Wrisberg and, just before exiting the brainstem through the pontomedullary sulcus, join with the motor fibers.

3. Cisternal segment:

   Upon exiting the brainstem, the facial nerve enters the cerebello-pontine angle cistern (CPA) where it joins the vestibulocochlear nerve and travels anterior and laterally toward the porus acusticus, the entrance of the internal auditory canal (IAC).

4. Intracanalicular segment:

   Within the IAC, the facial nerve moves anteriorly and superiorly so that it reaches the fundus at the anterior and superior quadrant of the IAC (Fig. 2), divided by a transverse bony ridge, the crista falciformis and by a vertical and incomplete fibrous ridge, known as Bill's bar.

5. Labyrinthine segment:

   At the fundus of the IAC the nerve enters its bony canal, also known as the fallopian canal, at its narrowest point—the facial meatus. From there it travels anterior and laterally making an angle of approximately 125° with the IAC and ends at the geniculate ganglion housed in the geniculate ganglion fossa in the anteromedial aspect of the petrous bone and partially covered by the dura of the medial cranial fossa (Fig. 3). The geniculate ganglion gives off the greater superficial petrosal nerve (GSPN), the first branch of the facial nerve which supplies visceromotor fibers to the lacrimal and salivary glands. The main trunk of the facial nerve then turns posteriorly at an acute angle called the anterior or first genu entering the tympanic cavity.

6. Tympanic segment:

   The tympanic segment of the nerve travels posterior–inferiorly along the medial wall of the middle ear cavity, passing slightly above the cochlear promontory and

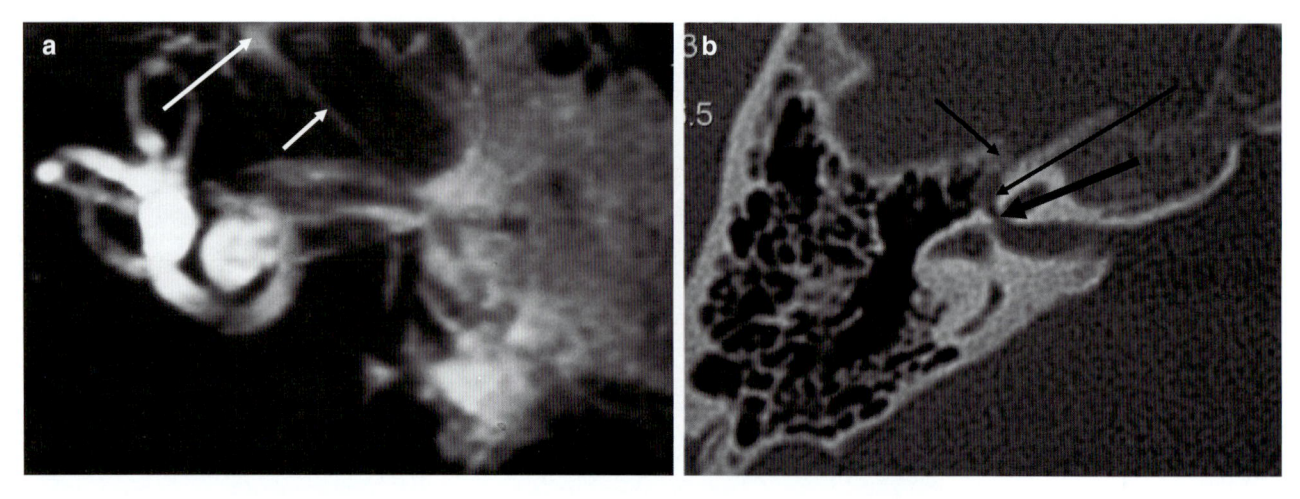

Fig. 3 a Maximal intensity projection (MIP) reconstruction from a CISS image shows the labyrinthine course of the facial nerve (*short white arrow*) and the geniculate ganglion fossa (*long white arrow*). **b** Axial CT image (bone algorithm) at the most superior level of the IAC shows the facial meatus (*thick arrow*), the labyrinthine segment of the facial nerve curving anteriorly (*long thin arrow*), and the geniculate ganglion fossa (*short arrow*)

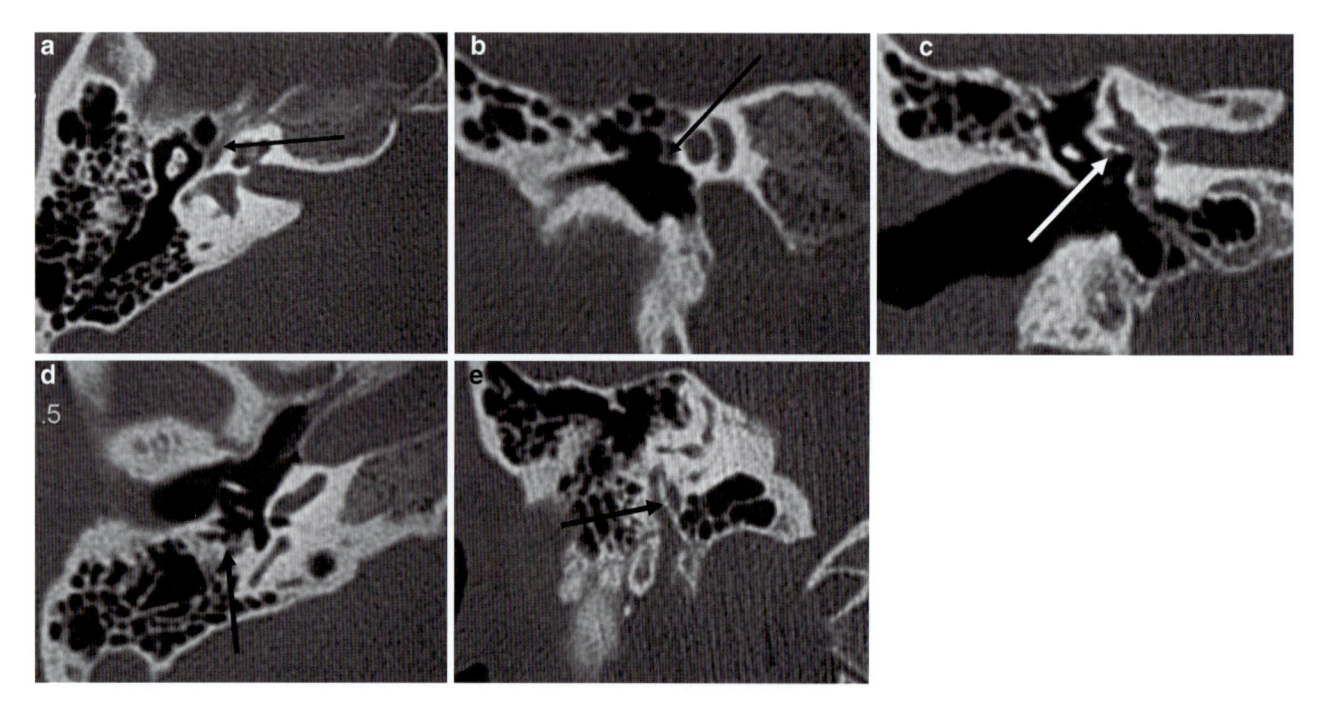

Fig. 4 CT images (bone algorithm). Axial (**a**) and coronal (**b**) images showing the proximal tympanic segment of the facial nerve at the level of the cochlear promontory (*black arrows*). **c** Coronal image showing the tympanic segment of the facial nerve coursing posteriorly immediately underneath the horizontal semicircular canal (*white arrow*). **d** Axial image showing the distal tympanic segment at the posterior wall of the tympanic cavity lying just lateral to the pyramidal eminence (*black arrow*). **e** Coronal section demonstrating the vertical mastoid segment of the facial nerve descending at the medial and anterior aspect of the mastoid (*black arrow*) and exiting the temporal bone through the stylomastoid foramen

below the lateral semi-circular canal (Fig. 4). When the Fallopian canal is dehiscent, the facial nerve can be exposed within the tympanic cavity, hanging over the oval window, which is an important finding to the ENT surgeon. The nerve then reaches the posterior wall of the tympanic cavity at the facial nerve recess, immediately lateral to the pyramidal eminence. Here it gives off its second branch supplying motor innervation to the neighboring stapedius muscle, responsible for the stapedius or sound dampening reflex. From here, the nerve makes a second turn at a 90° angle—the posterior genu and starts its vertical descending course.

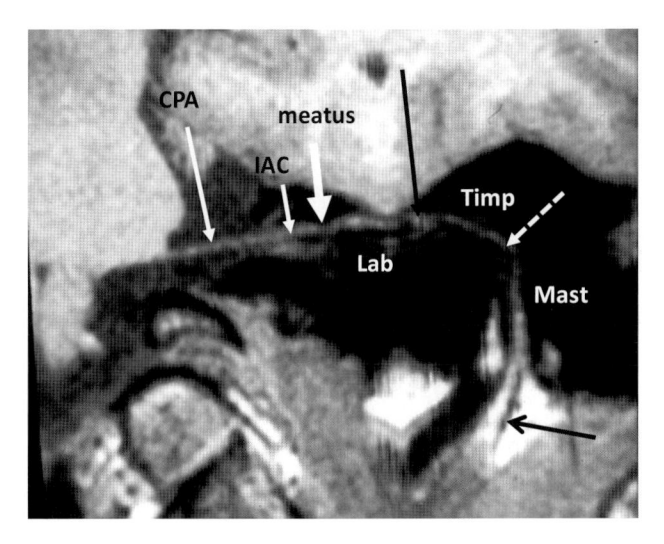

Fig. 5 Curved reconstruction from a high-resolution volumetric T1 W image showing the entire intracranial course of the facial nerve: the cisternal segment (*long white arrow*), the intracanalicular segment (*short white arrow*), the facial nerve meatus—the entrance to the facial bone canal—shown as a smooth stricture of the facial nerve (*thick white arrow*), the labyrinthine segment (Lab), the anterior genu (*long black arrow*), the tympanic segment (Timp), the vertical descending mastoid segment (Mast), the posterior genu (*short dotted arrow*), and the proximal parotid segment (*short black arrow*) (*Courtesy of Prof. J. Casselman*)

7. Mastoid segment:

   This segment of the facial nerve descends vertically within its bony canal in the anterior aspect of the mastoid bone, just posterior to the EAC (Fig. 4). Before exiting the temporal bone through the stylomastoid foramen it receives the chorda tympani, carrying afferent taste fibers from the two anterior thirds of the tongue.

8. Parotid segment:

   After exiting the temporal bone, the facial nerve travels anterior and laterally around the lateral aspect of the styloid process and styloid muscles to penetrate the parotid gland where it lays lateral to the retromandibular vein and to the branches of the external carotid artery (Fig. 5). The plane of the facial nerve divides the parotid gland into superficial and deep lobes and constitutes a major surgical landmark. Within the parotid gland it gives off its terminal branches (temporal, zygomatic, buccal, mandibular, and cervical nerves) providing motor innervation to the muscles of facial expression.

3 Clinical Topognostic Testing

Any patient presenting with facial nerve palsy should undergo neurological examination including long tract assessment, evaluation of other cranial nerves, and thorough evaluation of the motor and special functions of the facial nerve, including lacrimation, salivation, stapedius reflex, and taste (Borges 2005; Borges and Casselman 2007; Finsterer 2008; Linder et al. 2010; Lorch and Teach 2010). Evaluation of the motor facial nerve is crucial to differentiate central from peripheral facial nerve palsy. Patients with CFNP (contralateral spastic paralysis sparing the upper face) often present with other neurological deficits including long tract dysfunction. In this circumstance, the lesion should be searched for in the motor cortex or along the corticobulbar tract. Patients presenting with PFNP (flaccid paralysis of the ipsilateral upper and lower face) should undergo a detailed neurological exam of other cranial nerves to attempt to further localize the injury (Borges 2005; Borges and Casselman 2007; Finsterer 2008; Linder et al. 2010). Concurrent CN VI palsy points out the lesion at the pontine tegmentum/floor of the IVth ventricle where the abducens nucleus and the fascicular segment of the facial nerve lay close together. Associated vestibulochoclear dysfunction places the lesion at the CPA cistern or IAC. To further localize a lesion within the temporal bone it is helpful to evaluate the special facial nerve functions. Sparing of tearing and salivation locates the lesion distal to the geniculate ganglion where the GSPN originates; sparing of the stapedius reflex places the lesion distal to the tympanic segment of the nerve where this branch comes off and finally, sparing of taste in the two anterior thirds of the tongue places the lesion distal to the chorda tympani (Borges 2005; Borges and Casselman 2007; Finsterer 2008; Veillon et al. 2008; Linder et al. 2010). However, it should be kept in mind that topognostic testing although valuable when dealing with a complete nerve section may not be useful in localizing other lesions such as nerve sheath tumors. Lesions growing along the nerve sheath without direct involvement of nerve fibers may spare the functions of the facial nerve even when proximal to the facial nerve branch responsible for that function. The presence of conductive hearing loss pinpoints the lesion to the middle ear cavity. Involvement of the trigeminal nerve mandates evaluation of the brainstem, where the facial nuclei are in close vicinity with the spinal nucleus and tract as well as the geniculate ganglion fossa which lies close to Meckel's cave. The presence of hemifacial spasm or twitch is a sign of nerve irritation and altered nerve conduction often secondary to vascular lesions affecting the cisternal segment of the nerve at the root exit zone (REZ) where the nerve is more vulnerable to compression (see neurovascular conflict) (Borges and Casselman 2007; Finsterer 2008; Veillon et al. 2008).

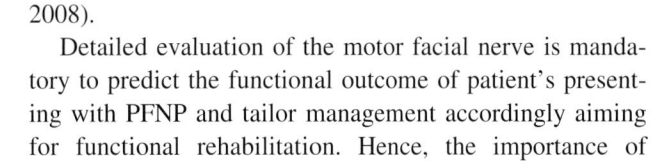

Detailed evaluation of the motor facial nerve is mandatory to predict the functional outcome of patient's presenting with PFNP and tailor management accordingly aiming for functional rehabilitation. Hence, the importance of

Table 1 Tailored imaging approach based on topognostic testing of the facial nerve

Topognostic location	Imaging modality	Imaging protocol
Brain and brainstem	MRI	Ax and Sag T1, PD, FSE T2, GRE T2* or SWI, DWI, post-gad 3DFT MPRAGE
CPA	MRI	Ax and Cor T1, 3DFT CISS, 3DFT FISP turbo MRA, post gad 3DFT MPRAGE
IAC	MRI/MDCT	Ax and Cor T1, 3DFT CISS, post gad 3DFT MPRAGE
Intratemporal segments	CT/MRI	Volumetric acq., HR bone algorithm, ax, cor, and sag reconstruct as needed
Parotid gland	MRI	Ax, and Sag T1, T2, STIR, and FATSAT T1 after gad

Table 2 MRI protocol

MR	FSE T2	SE T1 Pre and post-gad	3DFT CISS	3DFT MPRAGE	3DFT-FISP Turbo-MRA
TR (ms)	4000	684	12.25	11.6	35
TE (ms)	99	20	5.9	4.9	6.4
FA (°)	180°	90°	70°	12°	15°
Acq. Time (min)	3	5.31	7.14	10.51	4.8
Slice thick (mm)	4	2	0.7	1	0.75
Matrix	242 × 512	160 × 256	192 × 256	192 × 256	320 × 512
FOV (cm)	300	230	95	240	200
Pixel size (mm)	0.62 × 0.59	0.90 × 0.90	0.49 × 0.37	0.94 × 0.94	0.94 × 0.39

applying standardized outcome measures to patients presenting with FNP (Linder et al. 2010). Although the most common cause of PFNP is Bell's palsy and around 80 % of patients recover uneventfully, early recognition of those who will have a worse outcome is crucial to adequately select patients for more aggressive medical or surgical management before nerve degeneration occurs (Borges 2005; Borges and Casselman 2007; Peitersen 2002; Linder et al. 2010). Clinical outcome measures include the House-Brackmann grading system, the most commonly used in clinical practice, facial nerve paralysis recovery profile (FNPRP), and facial nerve paralysis recovery index (FNPRI) (Finsterer 2008; Sittel and Stennert 2001; Valls-Sole 2007; Linder et al. 2010).

Electrophysiologic testing can also be used as a prognostic indicator. These tests usually rely on percutaneous stimulation of the facial nerve distal to stylomastoid foramen (unless when performed intra-operatively) and only show significant abnormalities 72 h after nerve degeneration has ensued. Several measures have been used with variable correlation with the patient's outcome: minimum nerve excitability test, maximum stimulation test (MST), and electroneurography (ENOG); the latter measuring compound muscle action potentials (CMAP) which provides an estimate of the number of normal excitable axons when compared to the normal contralateral side (Sittel and Stennert 2001; Valls-Sole 2007).

MR imaging outcome measurements have also been extensively investigated with variable results. These have included several measures and indexes of T1 signal intensity and of contrast enhancement along the different segments of the facial nerve compared to the normal contralateral side (Kumar et al. 2000; Kinoshita et al. 2001; Iwai et al. 2000). Currently, there is still no consensus on the prognostic value of MRI which is, therefore, not routinely recommended in patients presenting with acute PFNP.

4 Imaging Technique and Tailored Imaging Approach

CT and MRI are the imaging techniques used to evaluate patients with facial nerve palsy. MRI is the modality of choice in most circumstances and is preferred to evaluate the supranuclear component, brainstem, cisternal, intracanalicular, and intraparotid segments of the facial nerve (Tables 1 and 2) (Borges 2005; Borges and Casselman 2007; Veillon et al. 2010; Burmeister et al. 2010; Ishibashi et al. 2010; Qin et al. 2011; Shelton 2000; Tada et al. 2000). To assess the intratemporal segments CT and MRI are often used complementarily (Borges and Casselman 2007; Jager and Reiser 2001; Veillon et al. 2010; Burmeister et al. 2009). MR is preferred in the case of suspected inflammatory or neoplastic involvement of the nerve whereas MDCT, particularly using high-resolution bone algorithm, is the modality of choice to evaluate the temporal bone in cases of trauma, suspected osteodystrophies, or bone dysplasias, in patients with history of middle ear infection, and whenever surgery is considered (Borges and Casselman 2007; Jager and Reiser 2001; Burmeister et al. 2010). Henceforth, a detailed clinical history and neurological examination are very useful to tailor the imaging approach. MDCT protocol

Table 3 Causes of FNP

1. Central Facial nerve palsy

Any cortical lesion affecting the cortical motor area or corticospinal tract:

Stroke, neoplasm, white matter disease, infection, vascular malformation, etc

2. Peripheral facial nerve palsy

(a) Brainstem (nuclear lesions):

Vascular: Infarct, AVM, cavernous angioma

Trauma: Duret's hemorrhages

Inflammatory disease: MS, ADEM, PML, neurosarcoidosis, Whipple's, primary and secondary vasculitis (Lupus, PAN, Wegener's, Behcet's, etc.), Bickerstaff's and brainstem encephalitis (Guillain Barré's variant)

Infectious rhombencephalitis (Listeria, HIV)

Neoplasm: Brainstem glioma, metastases, hemangioblastoma, infiltration by hematologic diseases (lymphoma, leukemia, Langerhan's, and non-Langerhan's cell histiocytosis, Rosai Dorfman, Erdheim–Chester)

(b) Cisternal and intratemporal segments:

Infectious/inflammatory: Bell's palsy or herpetic facial nerve palsy, Ramsay Hunt (VZV or HZV palsy), otitis media (acute, chronic, and cholesteatoma), MOE (malignant or necrotizing otitis externa), Lyme's disease, HIV, Miller Fisher syndrome, basilar meningitis (bacterial, tuberculous, fungal, sarcoid, and other inflammatory noninfectious leptomeningitis, hypertrophic pachymeningitis, Merkelson–Rosenthal syndrome.

Trauma: Accidental (temporal bone fractures), iatrogenic (middle ear, mastoid, and parotid surgery)

Neoplasm: Primary (schwannoma, hemangioma, choristoma, paraganglioma, neuroma, meningioma, epineurial pseudocyst); secondary (PNS of parotid and other head and neck malignancies, lepomeningeal carcinomatosis, leptomeningeal infiltration by hematologic malignancies and histiocytic proliferations or direct invasion from neighboring neoplasm (meningiomas, vestibular schwannomas, and skull base, petrous bone or temporomandibular neoplasm)

Neurovascular conflict (vascular loops, vertebrobasilar dolichoectasia, dural AVF, aneurysms)

Bone dysplasias: Fibrous dysplasia, osteogenesis imperfecta, osteopetrosis, otosclerosis, etc.

(c) Congenital lesions: Birth trauma, Mobius syndrome, craniofacial malformations affecting the first and second branchial arches (Hemifacial microssomia, CHARGE, fascioscapulohumeral muscular dystrophy, velocardial syndrome, teratogens)

should include volumetric acquisition of the temporal bone and parotid gland and multiplanar reconstructions in the axial, coronal, and sagittal planes as needed (Borges and Casselman 2007; Veillon et al. 2010; Burmeister et al. 2010). Images of the temporal bone should be acquired using high-resolution bone algorithm with 0.5 mm slice thickness and 0.1 mm table increment. Intravenous contrast is only used in patients with contraindications for complementary MR.

Patients presenting with CFNP require a regular brain protocol including DWI and contrast administration when needed. Evaluation of the brainstem segment requires high resolution imaging. FSE T2 W images, DWI and GRE T2* images are particularly useful to rule out the most common causes of PFNP affecting this segment of the nerve: infarct, cavernous angiomas and demyelinating diseases. 3D heavily T2 weighted MR sequences (3DFT CISS, DRIVE, FIESTA, GRE-SSFP, True-FISP, bFFE, DRIVE, and SPACE) are particularly useful to demonstrate the cisternal and intracanalicular segments of the nerve (Borges 2005; Veillon et al. 2010; Iwai et al. 2000; Shelton 2000). In these sequences the facial nerve can be clearly depicted as a dark linear structure against the bright CSF and multiplanar, curved (fig. 5) as well as 3D navigation reconstructions can be obtained. In patients presenting with hemifacial spasm or facial twitch additional 3D TOF MRA (3D-FISP turbo, 3D-FLASH, 3D CE-FAST) or CE-MRA should be performed to rule out a neurovascular conflict (Iwai et al. 2000; Burmeister et al. 2010). When contraindicated, MR can be replaced by CT angiography. To depict inflammatory and neoplastic involvement of the nerve, post-gadolinium high-resolution 3D T1 W images are required (such as 3D-SPGR, MPRAGE or VIBE) (Kinoshita et al. 2001; Iwai et al. 2000; Lim et al. 2012). The use of parallel imaging with surface coils and SENSE also allows for high-resolution imaging of the peripheral segments and branches of the facial nerve. For the intraparotid segment, contrast-enhanced fat-suppressed T1 W images are ideal to depict parotid gland neoplasms and perineural spread of disease (Kinoshita et al. 2001; Ishibashi et al. 2010; Qin et al. 2011).

The major imaging challenge when using MRI is to perform a high resolution study, covering the right anatomic area within a reasonable time frame. The use of high field MR scanners (1.5 to 3T), diffusion tensor imaging, parallel imaging, surface coils, thin slices, small FOV, and high matrix size contribute to increasing image resolution and have increased the diagnostic yield and the number of recognizable causes of FNP in the last decades (Veillon

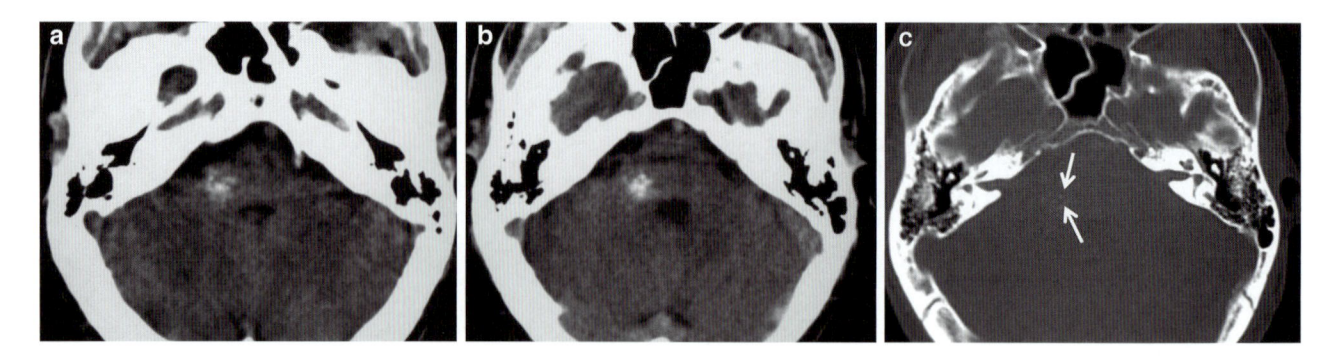

Fig. 6 Axial CT sections before (**a**) and after (**b**) intravenous contrast administration, show a lobulated lesion involving the pontine tegmentum and inner aspect of the middle cerebellar peduncle, close to the facial colliculus and along the course of the fascicular segment of the facial nerve. The lesion is spontaneously hyperdense due to recent hemmorrhage and due to presence of subtle microcalcifications (*white arrows*) best appreciated on the bone window (**c**). The lesion shows centripetal, cotton-like enhancement after intravenous contrast administration. Presumptive diagnosis: Cavernous angioma

et al. 2010; Iwai et al. 2000; Ishibashi et al. 2010; Burmeister et al. 2009; Gerganov et al. 2011; Roundy et al. 2012). Volumetric multidetector CT scanners (using up to 64 detector rows) have also enhanced the diagnostic yield of CT allowing for multiplanar and curved reconstructions and virtual endoscopic images. To maximize resolution and decrease examination time, adequate tailoring oriented by a detailed topognostic clinical examination is the key.

5 Pathology

Causes of facial nerve palsy are numerous and varied (Table 3) (Borges 2005, 2010; Veillon et al. 2008; Borges and Casselman 2007). The most common are by far infectious/inflammatory conditions, followed by trauma, neoplasms, and vascular anomalies. Studies including large series of patients with facial neuropathy show that infection accounts for 70 % of all cases of FNP (Bell's palsy comprising 60 %, Ramsay-Hunt syndrome 7 % and other infections 3 %), followed by trauma (17 %), neurovascular conflicts (4 %), congenital lesions (3 %), CNS disease (1 %), and other causes (7 %). The challenge is to recognize treatable causes of FNP and promote early functional recovery. Clinical history and serologic testing are helpful in the diagnosis of specific causes of FNP such as Lyme's disease, HIV infection, otomastoiditis, diabetes, sarcoidosis and trauma. For diagnostic imaging purposes, a segmental approach to facial nerve pathology is desirable.

1. Supranuclear segment:

The supranuclear segment of the facial nerve can be affected by any brain lesion involving the motor cortex or corticobulbar tract and FNP is rarely the single or the most relevant neurologic symptom. Stroke is by far the most common central cause of FNP but demyelinating disease, infection, neoplasm, and vascular malformations may all affect the central component of the facial nerve.

2. Brainstem segment:

Brainstem lesions affecting the nuclei and/or the fascicular segment of the facial nerve comprise stroke, trauma, vascular malformations, infectious and inflammatory disease, such as MS and rhombencephalitis and primary and secondary neoplasms (see Table 3) (Borges 2005; Borges and Casselman 2007; Burmeister et al. 2010). FNP palsy is rarely the most striking or the presenting symptom, but in rare cases this may occur.

Vascular pontine lesions are responsible for only 1 % of facial nerve palsies (Sherman and Thompson 2005; Agarwal et al. 2011; Novy et al. 2008; Roh et al. 1999; Thomke et al. 2002; Arnaout et al. 2009; Mathai 2009; Parizel et al. 2002). Facial weakness is a component of the AICA **stroke** syndrome which also includes ataxia, vertigo, and ipsilateral deafness. When the lesion affects the medial longitudinal fasciculus (MLF), abducens nerve and the paramedian pontine reticular formation patients present with the so-called "one-and-a-half syndrome" characterized by conjugate horizontal gaze palsy in one direction and internuclear opthalmoplegia in the other (Sherman and Thompson 2005; Agarwal et al. 2011; Novy et al. 2008; Roh et al. 1999) and when the facial nerve is additionally affected they present with the "eight-and-a-half syndrome." It is the second most common brainstem stroke following that of PICA. Due to the variable origin of the AICA (from caudal to middle pons) infarcts in this territory are highly variable. Acute facial nerve palsy, mimicking Bell's palsy, may however result from a lacunar infarct in the lower pontine tegmentum (Agarwal et al. 2011; Novy et al. 2008). In fact, pontine infarcts comprise around 7 % of all ischemic strokes and 15 % of posterior circulation infarcts, affecting basilar perforators and having hypertension as the major risk factor

(Agarwal et al. 2011). Diffusion weighted MRI is the modality of choice, depicting ischemic strokes as soon as 1 h after the ictus, although false negative results have been described in small lacunar infarcts affecting the posterior circulation within the first 24 h (Oppenheim et al. 2000), justifying a repeated scan when clinical suspicion remains.

Pontine hemorrhages are not uncommon particularly in the setting of hypertension, diabetes, vascular malformations, and trauma (Duret's hemorrhage). Depending on the exact location, different cranial nerve deficits may accompany long tract symptoms. Facial nerve palsy often courses with abducens nerve dysfunction and is exceedingly rare as an isolated symptom (Sherman and Thompson 2005; Roh et al. 1999; Thomke et al. 2002). Pre-contrast T1 W, GRE T2*, and SWI are the best imaging tools to depict this condition although CT can also identify a pontine hemorrhage as an ill-defined area of high attenuation particularly when using adequate windowing settings to look for blood (40–50 HU).

Although more commonly seen in the supratentorial compartment, **cavernous angiomas** are not infrequent in the brainstem and may lead to cranial nerve deficits including facial palsy (Arnaout et al. 2009; Braga et al. 2006; Giliberto et al. 2010; Duckworth 2010; Zausinger et al. 2006). These lesions have been increasingly recognized since the routine use of GRE T2* and, most recently, SWI in the imaging protocol of the brain. These sequences enhance the susceptibility effect of blood degradation products presenting as low signal intensity or a signal void often with a "blooming" effect. The typical imaging appearance is that of a lobulated (popcorn like) lesion, with variable signal intensity on both T1 and T2 W images depending on the age of blood degradation products and on the presence of recent hemorrhage (Giliberto et al. 2010; Zausinger et al. 2006). Contrast administration may disclose an associated developmental venous anomaly shown as a radial tangle of small enhancing venules (*caput medusa*) connected to a larger draining vein heading to the pial surface or to a dural sinus (Zausinger et al. 2006). CT also plays a role in the diagnosis as calcifications are seen in as many as 33 % of all cavernous angiomas (Fig. 6). They maybe sporadic or familial and may also be secondary to brain irradiation, particularly during childhood (Borges 2005).

Brainstem **AVMs** are much less common. Whereas pial lesions are typically supplied by the SCA or AICA and may be completely excised, those that are intraparenchymal are supplied by perforating arteries and cannot be safely removed in most cases (Arnaout et al. 2009). Cranial nerves dysfunction in this setting may result from direct compression by the vascular nidus, from stealing phenomenon or from hemorrhage. A thorough description of the imaging features of AVMs is beyond the scope of this chapter.

Pontine bleeding secondary to **head trauma** can result from major brain injury leading to increased intracranial pressure, descending brainstem herniation, and disruption of brainstem perforators (Duret's hemorrhages) or from a milder and isolated injury to the brainstem due to direct inertial impact against the petrous apex, clivus, or tentorium or from diffuse axonal injury and microbleeds related to acceleration-deceleration inertial forces (Mathai 2009; Parizel et al. 2002). The etiopathogeny and amount of blood are the main prognosticators with the former having a dismal prognosis and the latter often baring a benign course. Reversible long tract motor deficits and facial palsy have been reported in association with isolated traumatic lesions to the brainstem involving the pons and mesencephalon (Roh et al. 1999; Mathai 2009).

Demyelinating diseases such as **multiple sclerosis (MS)** and acute disseminated encephalomyelitis (ADEM) may course with facial nerve palsy but again this symptom is not usually isolated (Critchley 2004; Carter et al. 1950; Fukazawa et al. 1997; Schnorpfeil and Braune 1997; Telischi et al. 1991; Haacke et al. 2009; Grabner et al. 2011). Facial nerve palsy is present in around 20 % of patients with MS although in autopsy series the incidence of facial nerve involvement is much higher, reaching over 50 % (Carter et al. 1950). As the presenting symptom, FNP has only been reported in 1 to 5 % of cases (Critchley 2004; Fukazawa et al. 1997; Schnorpfeil and Braune 1997). This incidence is probably underestimated as FNP, as the inaugural symptom of MS, is likely to be misinterpreted as Bell's palsy. The degree of palsy is variable but predominantly mild (Fukazawa et al. 1997). Hemifacial spasm has also been reported in association to multiple sclerosis (Telischi et al. 1991). MR imaging discloses demyelinating lesions involving the nuclei and/or the fascicular segment of the facial nerve (Figs. 7 and 8). In the acute inflammatory phase, lesions are hyperintense on PD, T2, and FLAIR, may show enhancement after gadolinium administration, due to a transient breakdown of the BBB, and restricted water diffusion on DWI. In the chronic phase they become hypointense on T1, no longer enhance and show increased water diffusivity. SWI is being increasingly used in the detection and characterization of MS lesions, featuring their iron content and microangioarchitecture (Haacke et al. 2009; Grabner et al. 2011). Tumefactive MS plaques may be a diagnostic imaging challenge specially when isolated.

Other inflammatory diseases coursing with FNP include progressive multifocal leucoencephalopathy (PML), HIV encephalitis, neurosarcoidosis, autoimmune conditions (Miller Fisher and Bickerstaff brainstem encephalitis), connective tissue disorders, and vasculitis (Davies and Burgin 1996; Alper et al. 1996; Mori et al. 2008; Nicolao et al. 2011; Chataway et al. 2001). Several viral, bacterial,

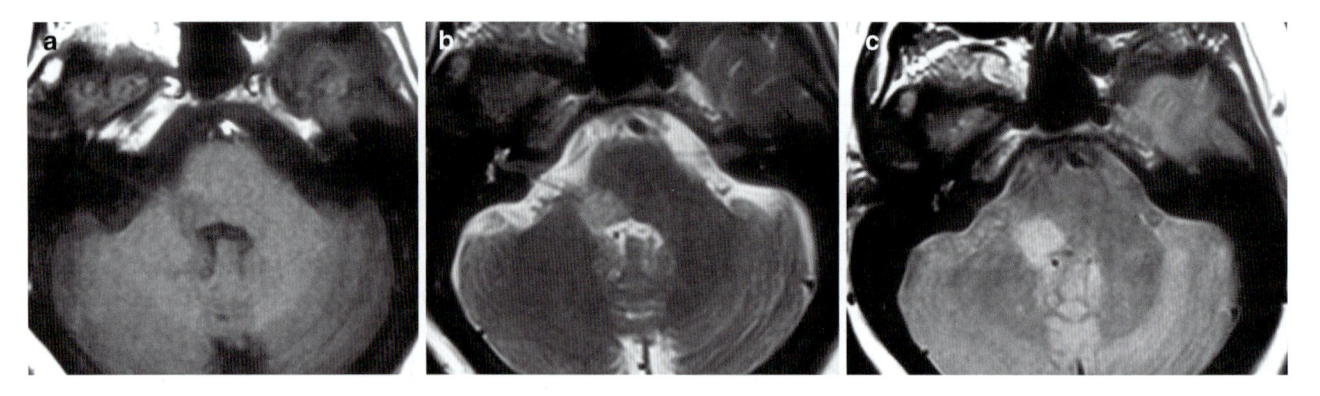

Fig. 7 Axial T1 W (**a**), T2 W (**b**), and PD (**c**) images show a rounded area of low signal intensity on T1 W and high signal intensity on PD and T2 W images in the pontine tegmentum, just anterior and lateral to the floor of the IVth ventricle affecting the nuclear and fascicular projection of the facial nerve as well as the restiform body in a patient with multiple sclerosis presenting with SNHL and facial weakness. The lesion bulges slightly the floor of the IVth ventricle in the region of the facial colliculus. Diagnosis: Tumefactive MS lesion

Fig. 8 Sagittal (**a**) and axial (**b**) T2 W images show a small rounded T2 hyperintense lesion in the pontine tegmentum. Similar lesions were noted in the high cervical spinal cord. Diagnosis: Multiple sclerosis

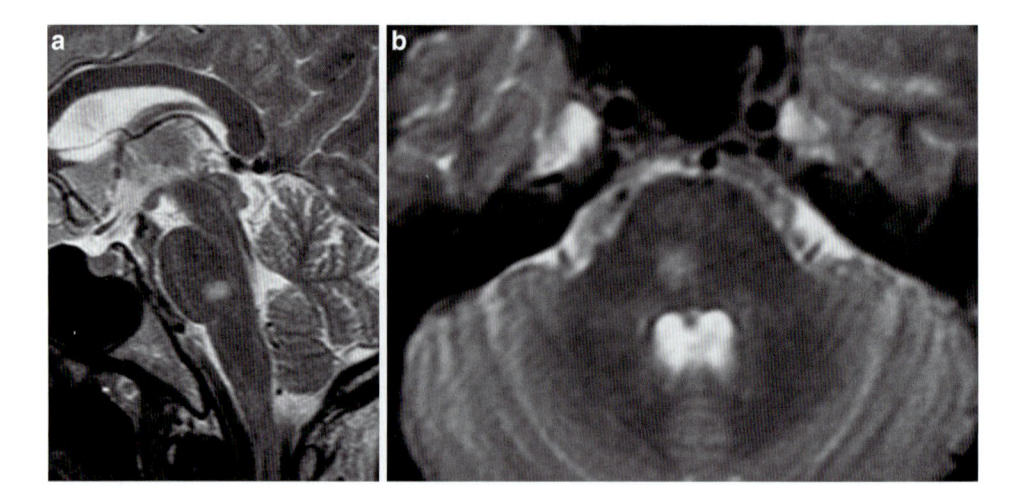

fungal, and parasitic infections may affect the brainstem as part of a diffuse encephalitic process or as a local abscess. Of particular note is **Listeria monocytogenes rhomboencephalitis** which, as the name implies, affects predominantly or exclusively the rhombencephalon and courses with variable associations of cerebellar dysfunction, cranial nerve deficits, and long tract signs depending on the exact location of the encephalitic lesions (Davies and Burgin 1996; Alper et al. 1996). MR discloses PD, T2, and FLAIR hyperintense, patchy, ill-defined lesions of variable size which may enhance after gadolinium administration, located in the brainstem and cerebellum (Davies and Burgin 1996). Associated meningitis and/or abscess may also be seen. Differential diagnosis is vast, namely with viral encephalitis, vasculitic diseases (Lupus and Behcet's), neurosarcoidosis, tuberculosis, MS, ADEM, and lymphoma (Alper et al. 1996). Timely diagnosis is important as early treatment is mandatory to decrease the morbidity and mortality associated to this infection. Pathogen isolation in the blood or CSF and imaging findings associated to a high degree of clinical suspicion are mandatory to establish the appropriate diagnosis (Davies and Burgin 1996; Alper et al. 1996). Although most commonly seen in immunocompromised patients, this infection can also occur in the general population in specific endemic contexts.

Bickerstaff's brainstem encephalitis is a rare inflammatory disorder with overlapping features with both Guillain–Barré's and Miller Fisher syndromes characterized clinically by ataxia and ophthalmoplegia although other symptoms such as limb and facial weakness may also be present (Mori et al. 2008; Nicolao et al. 2011). Etiopathogeny is varied including infection, post-infectious autoimmune injury, and lymphoma. Anti-CQ1b antibodies are found in two-thirds of patients with this condition and are common to Miller Fisher (Chataway et al. 2001). Imaging findings are nonspecific and comprise ill-defined PD, T2,

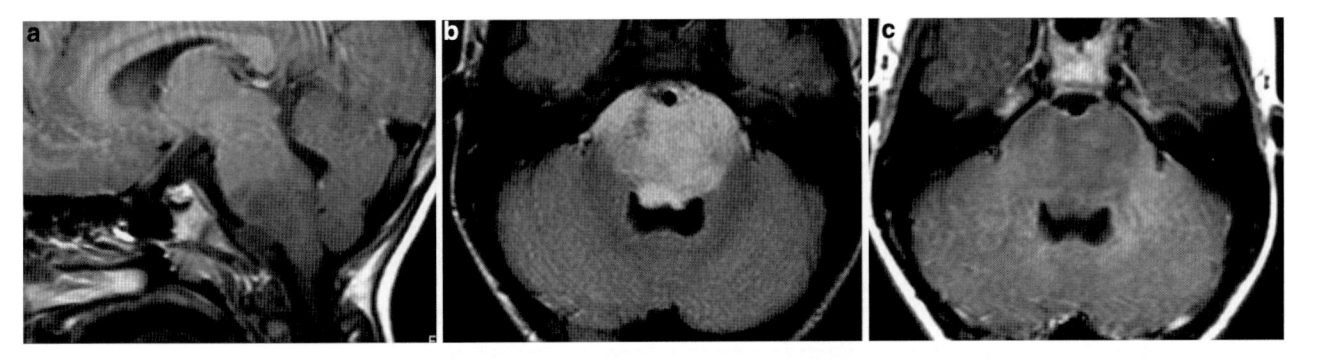

Fig. 9 Sagittal T1 W (**a**), axial T2 W (**b**), and gadolinium-enhanced T1 W images (**c**) demonstrate an infiltrative lesion expanding the brainstem affecting the pontine tegmentum, facial coliculli and nuclear projections of the facial nerve. Diagnosis: Brainstem glioma in a child

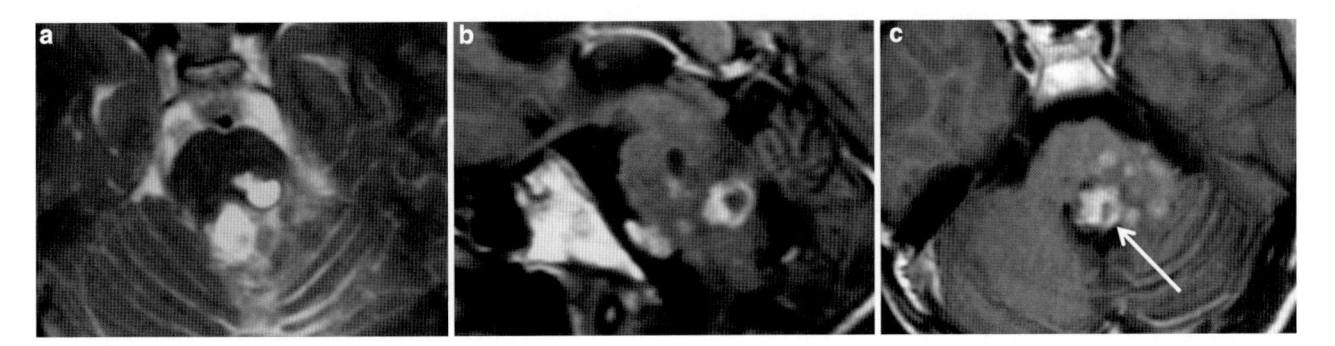

Fig. 10 Axial T2 W (**a**) and gadolinium-enhanced sagittal (**b**) and axial (**c**) T1 W images shown a diffuse, infiltrative, partially necrotic neoplasm involving the brainstem at the level of the nuclear projection of the facial nerve. Note the exophytic enhancing component affecting the region of the facial coliculi (*white arrow*). Diagnosis: Recurrent pontine glioma

and FLAIR hyperintense lesions in the brainstem, affecting predominantly the pons, midbrain, and medulla (Chataway et al. 2001).

Primary and secondary **brainstem neoplasms** are another source of nuclear and fascicular injury to the facial nerve. Brainstem glioma is the most common primary tumor with a higher prevalence in the pediatric age group (Laigle-Donadey et al. 2008; Boop 2011; Leach et al. 2008). Hemangioblastomas, either sporadic or associated to Von Hippel–Lindau disease, may also affect the brainstem. Secondary involvement may result from hematogenous metastasis (most commonly form lung, breast, melanoma, and kidney) or direct invasion by neighboring neoplams such as PNETs of the posterior fossa. Diffuse brainstem infiltration by hematologic malignancies (lymphoma and leukemia) and by histiocytic infiltrations (Langerhan's and non-Langerhan's cell histiocytosis including Erdheim-Chester and Rosai-Dorfman disease) are rare causes of FNP.

Brainstem glioma accounts for 10 % of pediatric brain tumors with 75 % of cases diagnosed under age 20 and a peak incidence seen between 5 and 10 years of age (Laigle-Donadey et al. 2008). Genetic factors appear to play a role in the pathogenesis as many genetic syndromes are associated with an increased incidence of this neoplasm, including tuberous sclerosis, neurofibromatosis type 1, Li-Fraumeni, Turcot, and basal nevus carcinoma syndromes (Boop 2011; Leach et al. 2008). Diffuse glioma is by far the most common subtype characterized by an infiltrating growth throughout the brainstem, mesencephalon, and medulla oblongata (Leach et al. 2008). Focal gliomas account for only 20 % of cases, are confined to a sub-region of the brainstem, most often the midbrain and medulla oblongata, and may show an exophytic growth being more amenable to surgical resection (Laigle-Donadey et al. 2008). Clinical presentation is often by cranial nerve deficits and long tract signs but some cases present with increased intracranial pressure from obstructive hydrocephalus secondary to compression of the IVth ventricle. Imaging discloses expansion and signal abnormality of the brainstem (hypointense on T1 and hyperintense on T2/FLAIR with no enhancement after gadolinium administration) with effacement of the surrounding cisterns and/or IVth ventricle (Fig. 9). Pontine gliomas (the most common) tend to efface the prepontine cistern and encase the basilar artery. More rostral lesions, involving the pontine tegmentum, are more likely to compress the IVth ventricle and lead to noncommunicating hydrocephalus. Moreover, they are the most likely to present with facial and abducens nerve palsies. Focal forms tend to present as a mass lesion with an exophytic growth. Most cases are histologically low-grade

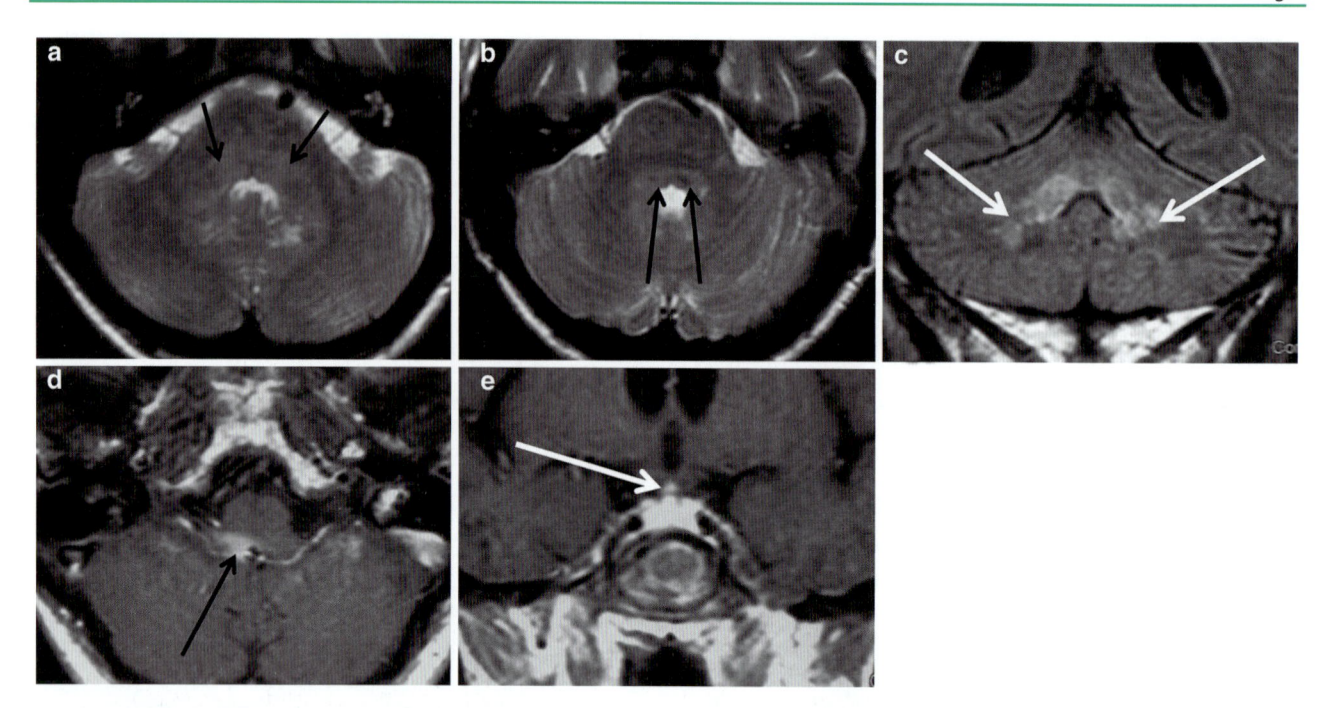

Fig. 11 Axial T2 W (a and b), coronal FLAIR (c), and gadolinium-enhanced axial (d) and coronal (e) T1 W images. a, b, and c show patchy areas of T2 and FLAIR hyperintensity involving the pons, the middle cerebellar peduncles, and the dentate nuclei bilaterally (*white arrows in* c). Note the involvement of the pontine tegmentum and facial coliculli (*black arrows in* a and b). d Shows vivid enhancement of one of the lesions involving the right restiform body (*black arrow*). e Shows thickening of the pituitary stalk (*white arrow*) Diagnosis: Erdheim–Chester disease in a patient presenting with progressive cerebellar dysfunction, diabetes insipidus, and multiple cranial nerve deficits including facial weakness and NSHL

tumors with insidious growth. Recurrent lesions have a more aggressive imaging and histological appearance, showing focal or patchy areas of contrast enhancement and even necrosis (Fig. 10).

Erdheim Chester disease is a non-Langerhan's cell histiocytosis also known as polyostotic sclerosing histiocytosis (Sedrak et al. 2011). It is a multissystemic disease involving long bones, lung, skin, kidneys, and cardiovascular system with CNS involvement seen in 50 % of patients. There is a high propensity for involvement of the posterior fossa including the brainstem and cerebellum which accounts for the clinical presentation with *diabetes insipida* and cerebellar syndrome (Sedrak et al. 2011). On MR imaging symmetrical and often tumefactive lesions affecting the brainstem, cerebellum and/or pituitary stalk, hypertintense on T2/FLAIR and with persisting gadolinium enhancement over the course of several days are the hallmark of this condition (Fig. 11). Extra-axial masses may also be seen. Main differential diagnosis is with other histiocytoses, multiple sclerosis, granulomatous, and metabolic diseases.

3. Cisternal segment:

The cisternal segment of the facial nerve is most often affected by extrinsic causes, namely compression by neighboring tumors or vascular variants and by meningeal diseases. The root exit zone (REZ) corresponding to a transition zone between central (oligodendroglia) and peripheral (Schwann cell) myelination, where the myelin sheath covering the nerve is usually thinner, is particularly prone to nerve irritation and disturbed electrical conductance manifesting clinically as hemifacial spasm or hyperkinesis (Borges 2005; Borges and Casselman 2007; Phillips and Bubash 2002; Raghavan et al. 2009; Veillon et al. 2008; Chavin 2003). Hemifacial spasm is slightly more prevalent in women and is characterized by intermittent, involuntary, unilateral clonic jerking movements of the facial muscles, usually beginning in the upper face (orbicularis oculi) and spreading downward to other facial muscles.

Neurovascular conflict is the most common cause of this condition, where a vascular loop, an aneurysm or an AVM, impinge upon the nerve at the REZ. Less often, causes other then vascular variants or malformations may cause this symptom including neighboring neoplasm arising from the CPA or the IAC and, more rarely, Bell's palsy (Borges 2005; Borges and Casselman 2007; Phillips and Bubash 2002; Raghavan et al. 2009; Veillon et al. 2008; Chavin 2003). Chronic nerve compression at the REZ leads to focal demyelination prompting the axons to electrical misfiring causing repeated involuntary contraction of the facial muscles. EMG with nerve conduction velocity testing is useful to confirm the diagnosis and MRI is essentially

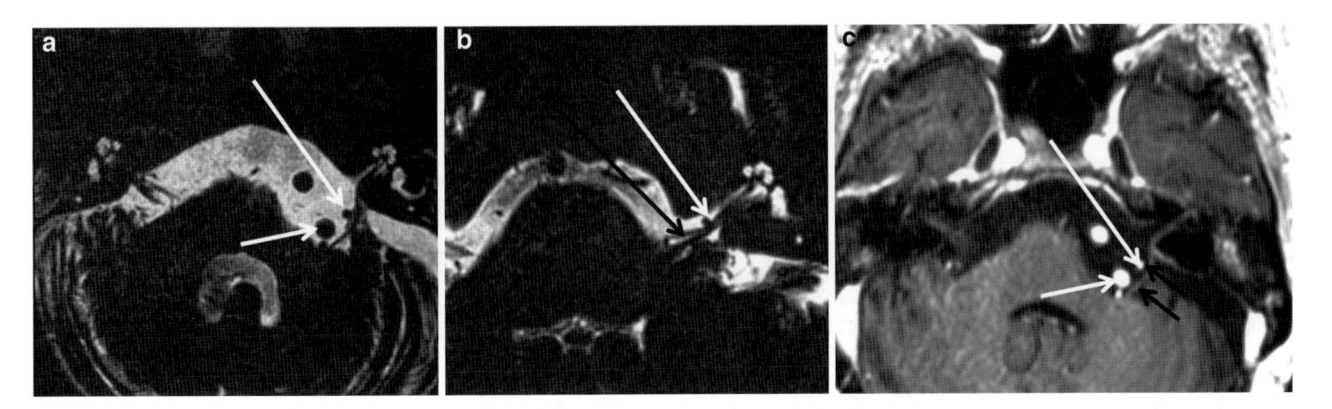

Fig. 12 Axial reconstructions from a volumetric CISS acquisition (**a** and **b**) and axial post-gadolinium T1 W image show a loop of the basilar artery (*short white arrows*) and of the AICA (*long white arrows*) impinging upon the REZ of the statoacustic nerve bundle with posterior displacement and kinking of the facial (*short black arrows*) and cochlear (*long black arrow*) nerves on the left side. Diagnosis: neurovascular conflict with vascular loops of the basilar artery and AICA. (*Courtesy from Prof. B. de Foer*)

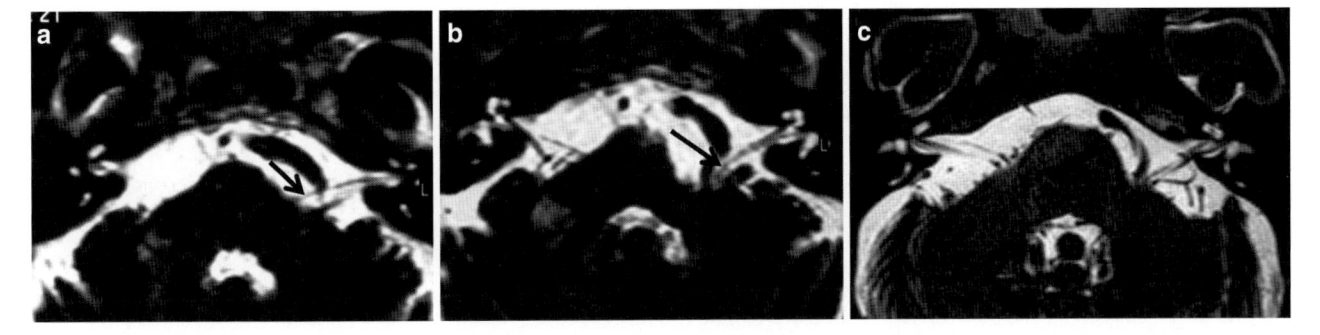

Fig. 13 Axial 3D CISS MR images show a tortuous course of the basilar artery flow void which loops laterally to the left side impinging upon the cisternal segment of the facial (*black arrow in* **a**) and cochlear (*black arrow in* **b**) nerves at the REZ in a patient with hemifacial spasm. **c** Axial CISS image on another patient with left-sided hemifacial spasm, showing a vascular loop of the basilar artery impinging upon the REZ of the statoacustic bundle. Diagnosis: Neurovascular conflict due to vertebro-basilar dolichoectasia

performed to determine the cause of compression (Sittel and Stennert 2001; Valls-Sole 2007). As neurovascular contacts are quite common in asymptomatic individuals, clinical correlation is mandatory and strict diagnostic imaging criteria have emerged (Borges and Casselman 2007; Chang et al. 2002; Chung et al. 2000; Fukuda et al. 2003; Leal et al. 2009, 2010). According to these criteria, the offending vessel has to be an artery, it must cross the nerve perpendicularly at the REZ (which for the facial nerve means between 5 and 7 mm after exiting the brainstem) and cause deviation or indentation of the nerve. However, NVC by aberrant veins or by encasement between an artery and a vein have been reported in the literature (Veillon et al. 2008; Borges and Casselman 2007). The AICA is the most common vessel implicated in NVC with the facial nerve (Fig. 12), followed by PICA, vertebral artery, and vertebrobasilar dolichoectasia (Fig. 13). It has also been shown that the presence of a small CPA cistern may be a predisposing factor. High-resolution MRA and 3D CISS imaging as well as CTA may identify the site of impingement and the offending vessel(s). Recently, loss of anisotropy depicted by diffusion tensor imaging (DTI) and anisotropy maps have been shown in patients with trigeminal neuralgia which potentially may be used to monitor and follow-up patients after decompression surgery (Lutz et al. 2011; Leal et al. 2011). Conservative therapies include anticonvulsant drugs, muscle relaxants, and botulinic toxin (Botox) injections. Surgical placement of a Teflon sponge between the offending vessel and the nerve is performed upon failure of conservative measures (Chang et al. 2002; Chung et al. 2000; Leal et al. 2010, 2011; Bonneville et al. 2007).

Extrinsic compression of this segment of the nerve can be secondary to a wide range of tumors, most often arising from the CPA cistern (vestibular schwannomas, meningiomas, epidermoid and arachnoid cysts), but also by petroclival and central skull base tumors (Fig. 14) (Bonneville et al. 2007). These lesions may impinge the nerve directly or displace it against another structure such as a vessel, dural leaflet or bone.

Schwannomas of the CPA and IAC most common origin is the inferior vestibular nerve by far (Fig. 15), followed by the facial nerve, which comprises only 3 % of all CPA tumors (Ishikura et al. 2010). Distinction between the two may be challenging as they both present with

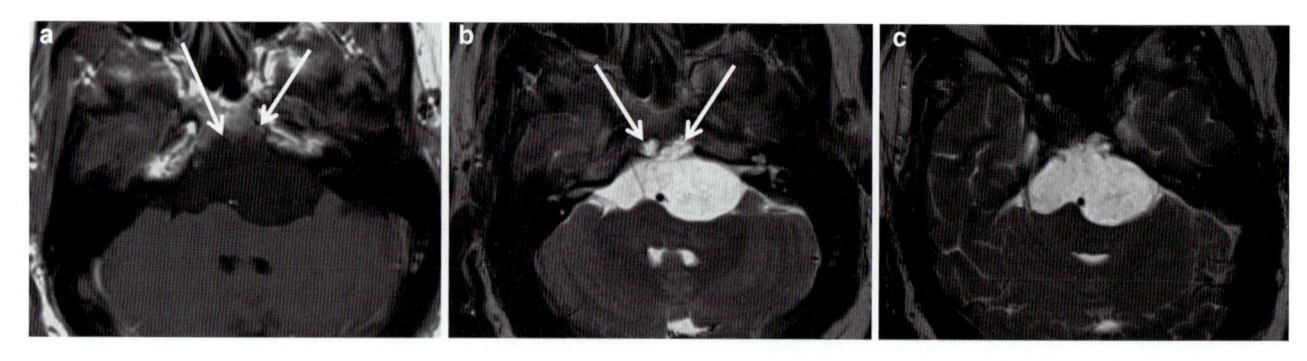

Fig. 14 Axial T1 W (**a**) and T2 W images (**b** and **c**) show an expansive multilobulated lesion in the pre-pontine and CPA cisterns impinging upon the brainstem and left middle cerebellar peduncle. The lesion displaces the cisternal segment of several cranial nerves: the trigeminal nerve and statoacustic bundle on the right which cannot be recognized on these images, probably displaced by the lesion. Note the involvement of the clivus accounting for its origin from notochordal remnants (*white arrows*). Although the MR imaging features resemble those of epidermoid cyst, contrast enhancement (not shown) and bone invasion suggest a more aggressive tumor. Diagnosis: Clival chordoma (*Courtesy from Prof. B. de Foer*)

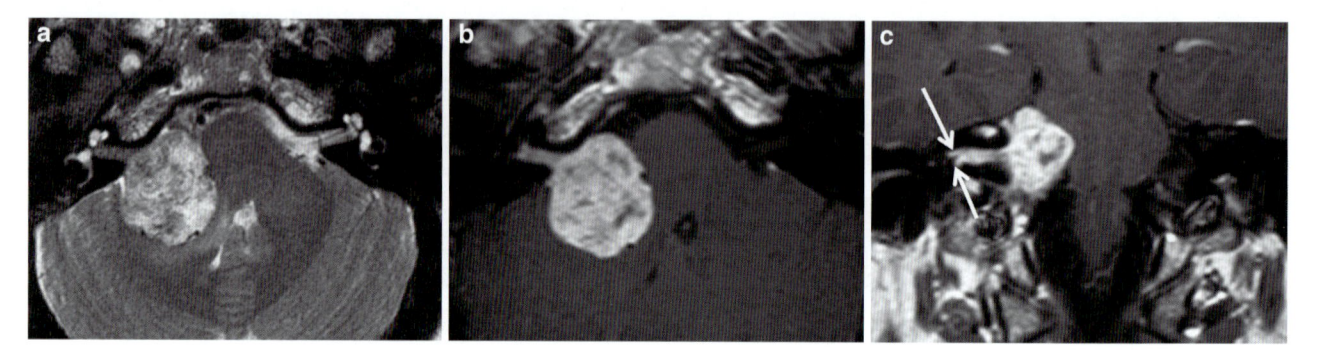

Fig. 15 Axial T2 W (**a**) and gadolinium-enhanced axial and coronal T1 W images (**b** and **c**) demonstrate a mass lesion centered at the porus acusticus of the right IAC, with a larger component filling and expanding the CPA cistern and a smaller component filling and expanding the IAC from the porus to the fundus with no remaining T2 W hyperintense CSF seen in the IAC. Normal fluid signal intensity remains within the labyrinthine structures. Severe compression of the middle cerebellar peduncle and anterior cerebellum is seen with a thin rim of surrounding edema, and slight leftward tilting of the pons. After gadolinium administration there is intense but heterogeneous enhancement, which extends along both the superior and inferior divisions of the vestibular nerve best seen on the coronal image (*white arrows on* **c**). Diagnosis: Vestibular nerve schwannoma

vestibulocochlear symptoms and signs accounting for the higher vulnerability of the tightly packed, thinly myelinated fibers of the vestibulochoclear nerve to compression and hypoperfusion (Ishikura et al. 2010). Volumetric heavily T2 W MR sequences (3D CISS) or volumetric T1 W images after gadolinium administration in a parasagittal plane, perpendicular to the fundus of the IAC, may be useful to determine the true origin of the tumor when it is small (Veillon et al. 2008; Ishikura et al. 2010). Location in the anterior and superior quadrant along with the identification of the other nerve branches suggests the diagnosis of a facial nerve schwannoma (Veillon et al. 2008; Borges 2010; Borges and Casselman 2007; Roche and Regis 2005). Moreover, tumor extent anteriorly along the labyrinthine segment of the nerve or the presence of a second tumor component in the geniculate ganglion fossa points out the correct diagnosis (see facial nerve schwannoma).

CPA meningiomas are dural-based hemispheric lesions facing the petrous bone, most often the petrous ridge, and protruding into the CPA cistern (Fig. 16) (Roche and Regis 2005; Roser et al. 2005; Iwai et al. 2001). They enhance vividly, often with a dural tail, and tend to follow the signal intensity of gray matter on all MR pulse sequences. Facial nerve dysfunction is present in 16 % of cases and the site of dural attachment determines the direction in which the facial/vestibulocochlear bundle is displaced (Iwai et al. 2001). The sites of dural origin are in decreasing order of frequency anterior (26 %), posterior (21 %), superior (18 %), and inferior (16 %) to the IAC (Roche and Regis 2005). Origin within the IAC is seen in 10 % of cases where these tumors may be difficult to distinguish from a vestibulochoclear schwannoma (Roser et al. 2005). Facial nerve dysfunction is the most common microsurgical complication (Nakamura et al. 2005).

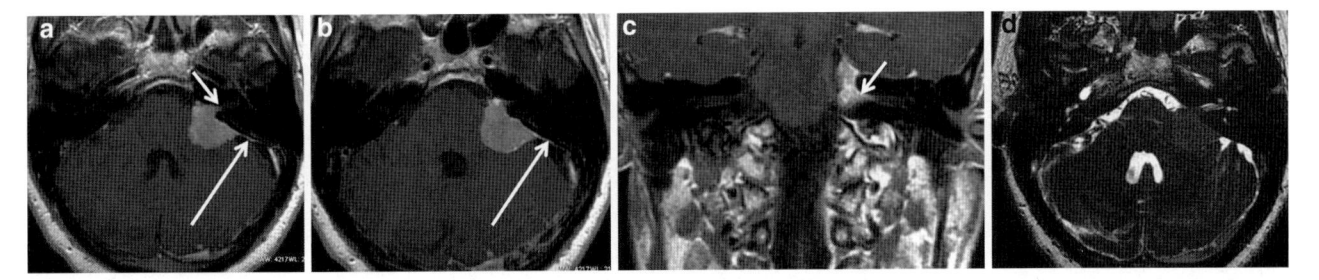

Fig. 16 Gadolinium–enhanced axial (**a** and **b**) and coronal (**c**) T1 W images and axial CISS images (**d**) through the IAC show a well-marginated dural-based hemispheric lesion in the left CPA cistern growing into the IAC (*short white arrows*) through a slightly enlarged porus acusticus. Vivid homogeneous contrast enhancement is seen as well as a thin dural tail along the tentorium (*long white arrows*). The CISS image clearly shows obliteration of the porus acusticus although CSF signal remains within the distal IAC and in the membranous labyrinth (*dashed white arrow*). The center of the mass is eccentric regarding the IAC lying slightly posterior to it. Diagnosis: CPA meningioma

Fig. 17 Gadolinium-enhanced axial (**a**) and coronal (**b**) T1 W images, axial T2 W image (**c**) and DWI image ($b = 1000$) (**d**) show a lobulated lesion in the left CPA cistern extending into the prepontine and peribulbar cisterns, impinging upon the left cerebellar hemisphere and brainstem and displacing the stato-acoustic bundle superiorly (*white arrow*). The lesion shows intermediate signal intensity on T1 W and is hyperintense on T2 W with a few internal septations. Restricted diffusion is also noted on the DWI image (**d**). Diagnosis: Epidermoid cyst

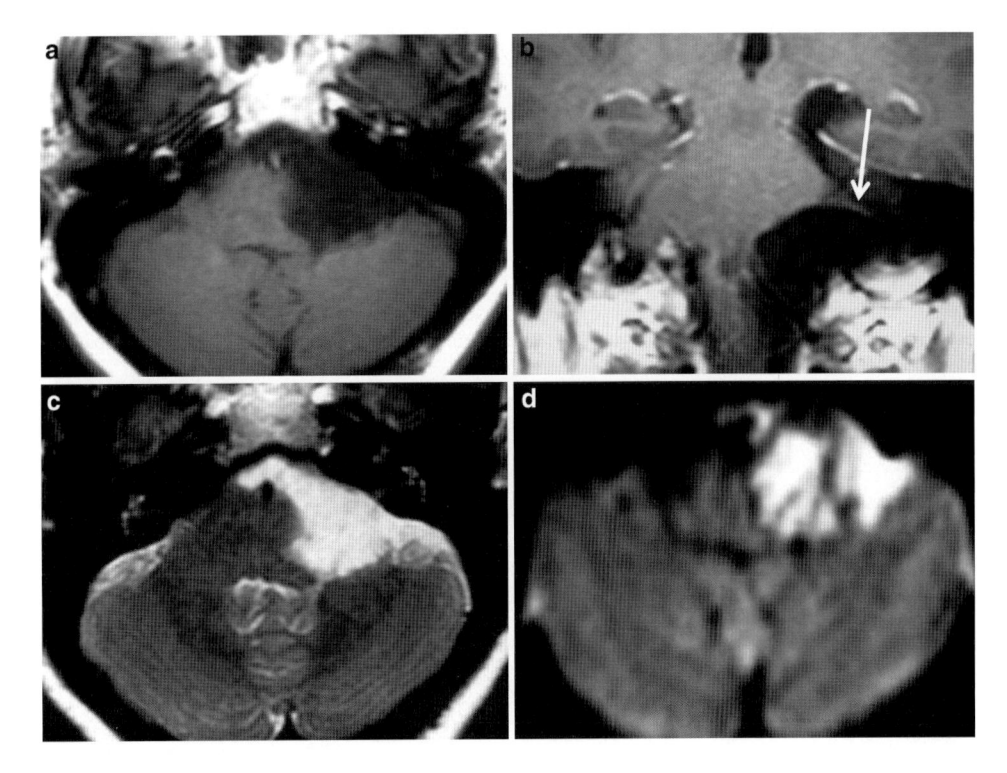

Cystic lesions affecting the CPA cistern, such as **arachnoid** and **epidermoid cysts** may impinge upon the cisternal segment of the facial nerve (Revuelta-Gutierrez et al. 2009; Akhavan-Sigari et al. 2007; Alaani et al. 2005). These cystic lesions can be accurately differentiated by using DWI: arachnoid cysts follow the signal intensity of CSF in all pulse sequences, whereas epidermoid cysts (Fig. 17) tend to have higher signal intensity then CSF on PD and FLAIR images and, due to their keratin content, show restricted diffusion (Nguyen et al. 2004). Other distinguishing features include the presence of thin intracystic septa and the lobulated contour of epidermoid cysts which tend to invaginate into the crevices and furrows of adjacent structures making them quite cumbersome to excise completely.

Meningeal diseases such as hypertrophic pachymeningitis, infectious/inflammatory meningitis, and primary and secondary meningeal neoplasms may all affect the cisternal segment of the FN (Borges and Casselman 2007; Bohne et al. 2010).

Hypertrophic pachymeningitis is a rare disorder characterized by localized or diffuse dural thickening due to a chronic sclerosing inflammatory process (Caldas et al. 2012; Yamashita et al. 2012; Vale et al. 2013; Christakis et al. 2012). It has been associated with several disorders such as rheumatoid arthritis, Wegener's granulomatosis, syphilis, tuberculosis and cancer, although the causative role of these entities has not been yet elucidated (Caldas et al. 2012; Yamashita et al. 2012; Vale et al. 2013; Christakis et al. 2012). The idiopathic form is a diagnosis of

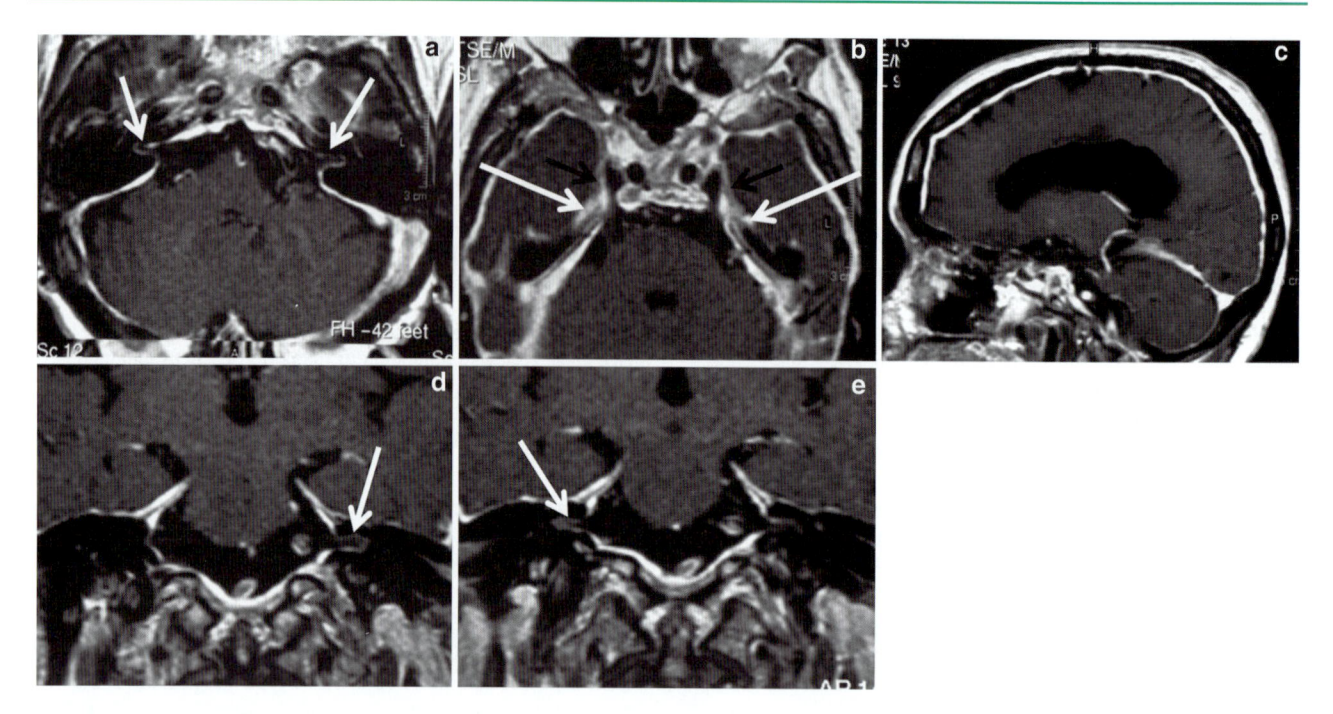

Fig. 18 Gadolinium-enhanced T1 W images in the axial (**a** and **b**), sagittal (**d**) and coronal (**e**) planes demonstrate diffuse, thick, smooth dural enhancement over the cerebral and cerebellar convexities, along the basilar cisterns and cranial nerves as they enter their bony and dural foramina. Note the enhancement along the IAC (*white arrows*), encircling Meckel's cave bilaterally (*short white arrows*) and over the petrous bone involving the geniculate ganglion fossa (*long white arrows*). Diagnosis: Idiopathic hypertrophic pachymeningitis

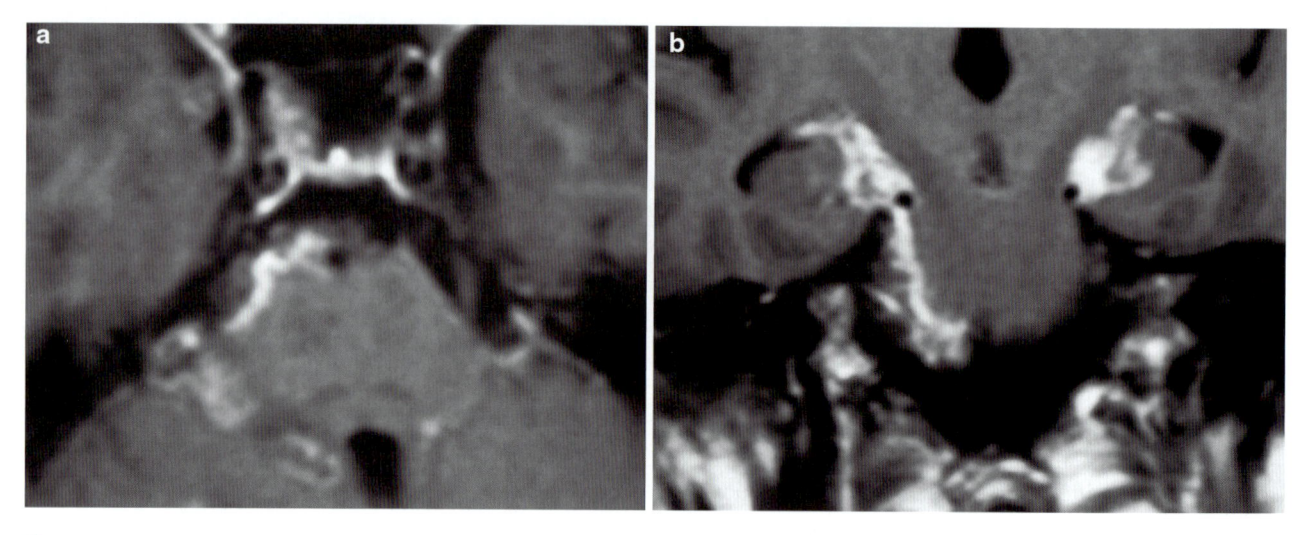

Fig. 19 Post-gadolinium axial (**a**) and coronal (**b**) T1 W images show thick, irregular leptomeningeal enhancement coating the surface of the brainstem and choroidal fissures, involving the cisternal course of the cranial nerves while crossing through the basilar and perimesencephalic cisterns, in a patient with history of breast cancer presenting with multiple cranial nerves deficits. Diagnosis (confirmed by cytopathological analysis of the CSF): Leptomeningeal carcinomatosis

exclusion when no associated disease can be found. Chronic headache, multiple cranial nerve deficits, ataxia, and seizures are the most common presenting symptoms. Cranial nerve dysfunction is secondary to nerve encasement by dense fibrous tissue leading to ischemic compression of cranial nerves. Dural thickening of the CPA cistern and petrous ridge may affect the facial nerve and manifest as facial weakness (Fig. 18), although facial nerve dysfunction is not usually a prominent feature of this condition (Pai et al. 2007; Lee et al. 2003; Friedman and Flanders 1997).

Leptomeningeal diseases with a propensity for the basilar meninges tend to course with cranial neuropathies. These include infectious and inflammatory basilar meningitis (tuberculous and fungal meningitis, sarcoidosis and Wegener's granulomatosis, to mention the most common) and primary and secondary neoplastic processes such as

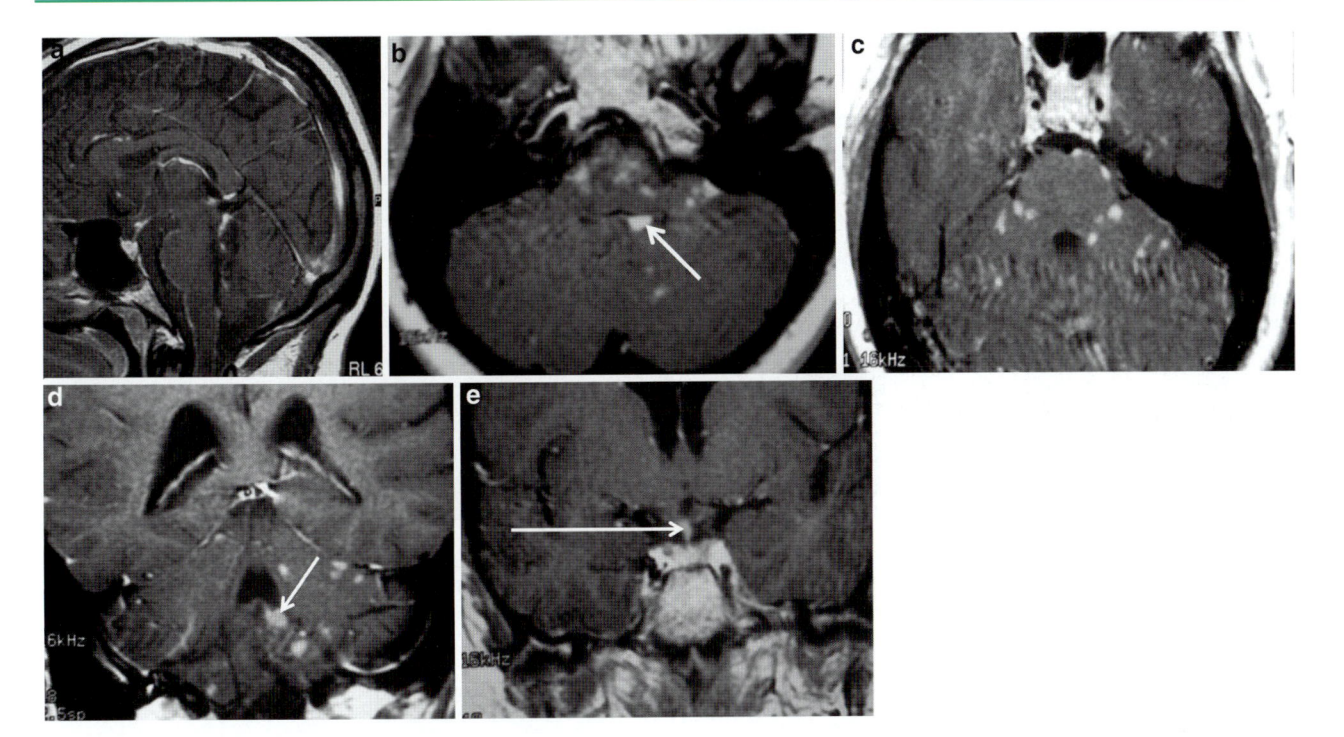

Fig. 20 Post-gadolinium sagittal (**a**), axial (**b** and **c**), and coronal (**d** and **e**) T1 W images demonstrates thick linear and nodular leptomeningeal enhancement, more striking in the basilar cisterns, coating the surface of the brainstem and involving the basilar, perimesencephalic and suprasellar cisterns. Note the abnormal enhancement in the floor of the IVth ventricle (*short white arrows*) and thickening of the pituitary stalk (*long white arrow*) in this patient presenting with diabetes insipidus and facial nerve palsy on the left side. Diagnosis: Neurosarcoidosis

leptomeningeal carcinomatosis (Fig. 19), leptomeningeal involvement by hematologic malignancies, and by histiocytic proliferations (such as Langerhan's cell histicocytosis in pediatric patients) (Borges 2005; Borges and Casselman 2007). Cranial nerve deficits are the most common presenting feature of patients with neurosarcoidosis and the facial nerve is involved in 50 % of cases (Fig. 20) (Spiegel et al. 2012; Nozaki and Judson 2012; Loor et al. 2012). Facial nerve involvement maybe secondary to basilar meningitis or parotid gland involvement as part of the Heerfordt syndrome, a triad of facial nerve paralysis, uveitis and parotid gland enlargement.

4. Temporal bone segments:

Bell's palsy is the most common cause of acute facial nerve paralysis accounting for over 60 % of all cases, with a reported annual incidence of 0.15 % to 0.4 % (Borges and Casselman 2007; Peitersen 2002; De Diego-Sastre et al. 2005). Increased incidence has been reported in patients with a positive family history and in diabetics. It is a benign, usually self limited disease, first described by Sir Charles Bell in 1821, as an "isolated, sudden, unilateral facial nerve paralysis of unknown etiology." Since then, increasing evidence was gathered for a viral induced neuronitis as the cause of this condition and HSV pointed out as the most frequently implicated agent (Borges and Casselman 2007;

Table 4 Atypical presentations and bad prognostic signs that should prompt imaging studies, particularly MRI

(a) Subacute onset
(b) Recurrent episodes
(c) Associated neurological symptoms
(d) Facial spasm, twitch or hyperkinesia
(e) Prolonged course (>3 months)
(f) High House Brackmann grade from onset (>5)
(g) Signs of denervation on early electrophysiologic testing

Yetiser et al. 2003). The virus is thought to be lodged in the geniculate ganglion in a dormant state and can be reactivated by a nonspecific triggering event such as cold, stress, or superinfection by a heterotopic virus. The induced inflammatory response, characterized by mononuclear cell infiltration and nerve edema, leads to nerve compression against the rigid walls of the fallopian canal and to a final common pathway of ischemia and axonal degeneration (Borges 2005; Borges and Casselman 2007; Veillon et al. 2008). The labyrinthine segment and meatal foramen are the narrowest segments of the facial bone canal and, in terms of blood supply, constitute a watershed zone between the vertebral and carotid artery systems, which make them the most susceptible to injury (Benecke 2002; Roob et al. 1999; Jager and Reiser 2001). Clinically, the most striking

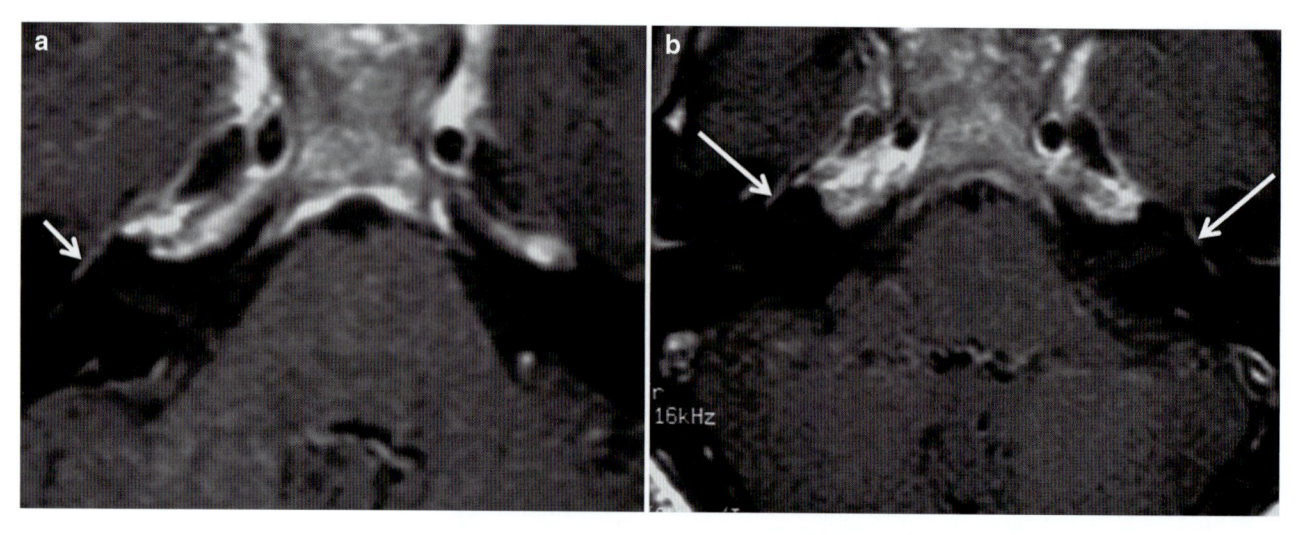

Fig. 21 Gadolinium-enhanced T1 W images in two different patients with no facial nerve related symptoms show **a** unilateral enhancement of the proximal tympanic segment of the facial nerve on the right side and **b** bilateral faint enhancement along the tympanic segment of the facial nerve representing normal enhancement along the perineural venous plexus

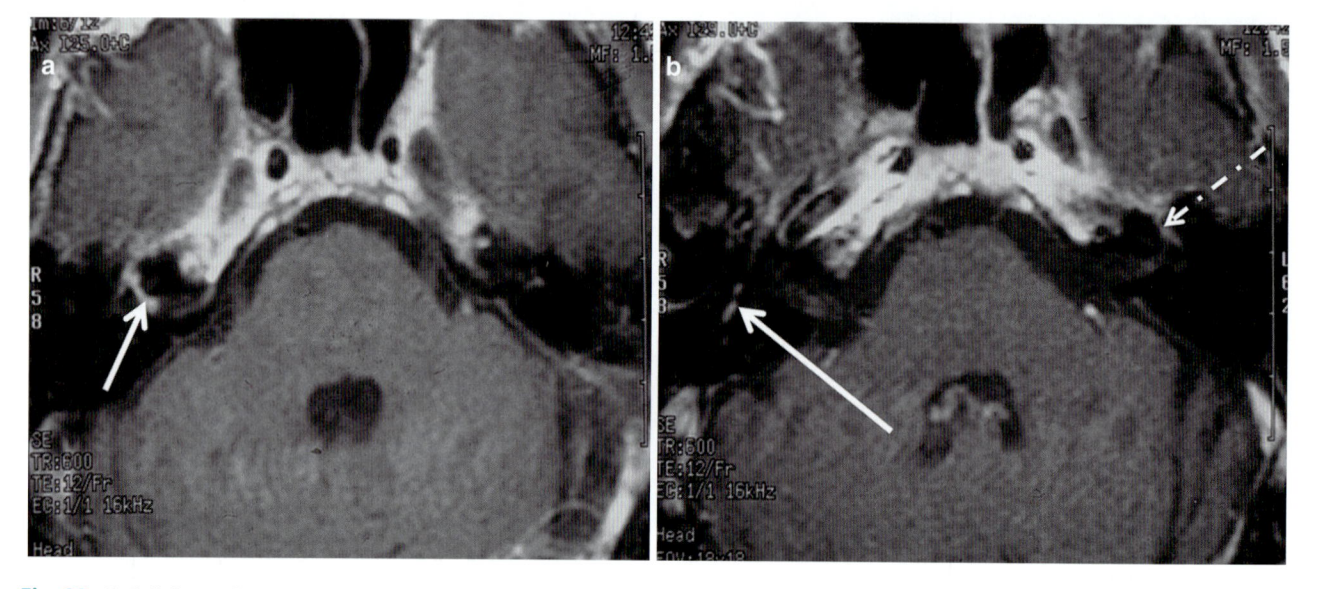

Fig. 22 Gadolinium-enhanced axial T1 W images show smooth linear enhancement along the facial nerve meatus, labyrinthine segment (*white arrow*) and geniculate ganglion fossa (**a**) and along the proximal tympanic segment (*long white arrow*) of the facial nerve (**b**) in a patient with acute onset of right sided facial nerve palsy (Bell's palsy). Also note faint enhancement at the geniculate ganglion and proximal tympanic segment of the facial nerve in the contralateral asymptomatic side (*dashed white arrow*). Diagnosis: Bell's palsy (viral neuronitis)

symptom is the acute onset of facial weakness of variable intensity affecting the upper and lower face, often associated with hyperacusis (14 %), dysgeusia (34 %), and disordered lacrimation and salivation (67 %) (Roob et al. 1999; Peitersen 2002). A viral prodrome can precede the onset of facial palsy and tinnitus, fever and post-auricular pain (50 %) are common accompanying symptoms (Roob et al. 1999; Peitersen 2002; Han 2010). The natural history of this condition is that of spontaneous recovery in 80 % of patients, recurrent disease in 10 % and progressive, unremitting disease in the remainder 4–10 % (Peitersen 2002).

Routine imaging of patients with acute FNP is still a matter of debate as most cases are due to Bell's palsy, and this condition evolves to spontaneous functional recovery in 80 % of cases (Peitersen 2002). In these circumstances, the role of imaging would be to predict which patients are prone to an unfavorable outcome and to depict other potentially treatable cause of FNP before axonal damage ensues, aiming for differential treatment and early functional rehabilitation (Borges 2005; Borges and Casselman 2007; Veillon et al. 2008; Kress et al. 2002, 2004; Mantsopoulos et al. 2011). It should be kept in mind that primary and

Fig. 23 Patient presenting with acute FNP, SNHL, vertigo, and a vesicular eruption in the right auricle. Axial gadolinium-enhanced T1 W images show **a** abnormal enhancement in the geniculate ganglion (1), labyrinthine segment (2), and facial nerve meatus (3) **b** Gadolinium-enhanced coronal T1 W image demonstrates abnormal cochlear enhancement (*white arrow*). Diagnosis: Ramsay-Hunt syndrome

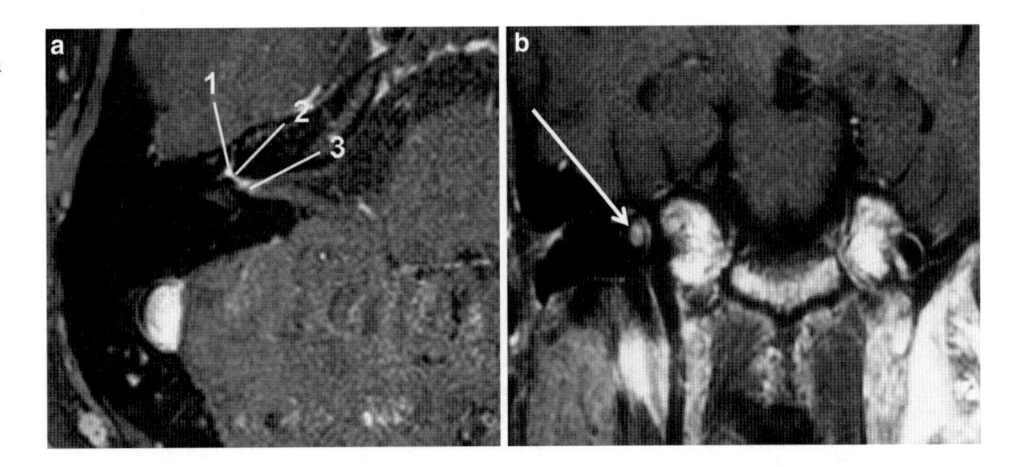

secondary neoplasms of the facial nerve may seldom present by acute FNP, mimicking Bell's palsy. This may occur due to sudden increase in tumor size secondary to tumor necrosis or hemorrhage or whenever the degree of axonal compression by the tumor overcomes vascular pressure and neural ischemia ensues. Imaging is mandatory in the case of atypical presentations, when other diagnostic possibilities are in question or in the presence of unfavorable prognostic signs which may be an indication for surgical decompression (Table 4) (Borges 2005; Borges and Casselman 2007). These include a high House Brackmann grade of facial palsy from onset of the disease and the presence of early signs of denervation depicted on electrophysiologic testing. Unfortunately, even the best and most reliable prognostic electrophysiological test in PFNP- measurement of compound action potentials- has limited prognostic value: it will only show abnormalities 72 h after the onset of axonal degeneration and no early then 7 days after the onset of facial palsy (Sittel and Stennert 2001; Valls-Sole 2007). Therefore, a lot of effort has been put on the use of MRI as a potential prognostic predictor in patients with FNP. The imaging hallmark of inflammatory conditions of the facial nerve is the presence of linear contrast enhancement along segments of the nerve that do not normally enhance and which is thought to be due to disruption of the blood-nerve barrier (Kuzma and Goodman 1997). The presence of a perineural vascular plexus accounts for the enhancement along the segments of the facial nerve where this plexus is most prominent and where the facial bone canal is wider: usually the tympanic and mastoid segments. Henceforth, enhancement along these segments can be seen uni- or bilaterally in asymptomatic patients, is usually faint and tends not to involve entire segments of the nerve (Fig. 21). Enhancement of the pre-geniculate segments of the facial nerve is the most specific feature for Bell's palsy (Fig. 22). Several attempts have been made to correlate the degree and extent of facial nerve enhancement with the severity and outcome of patients with FNP with conflicting results (Burmeister et al. 2011). While some studies found no correlation between the degree and extent of facial nerve enhancement and the severity and outcome of FNP; others describe a shift of the enhancing segments of the nerve over time from central to peripheral and still others argue that in the acute edematous phase no enhancement is seen due to reduced gadolinium supply to the ischemic compressed segments of the nerve. More recently, MR indexes based on quantitative measurements of signal intensity on post-contrast T1 W images, along the five different segments of the facial nerve, have been correlated with patient's outcome showing significantly higher indexes in patients with unremitting palsy compared to those with an uneventful recovery (Kress et al. 2002, 2004; Kondo et al. 2012; Kaylie et al. 2003; Song et al. 2008). Signal intensity in the intracanalicular segment of the nerve showed the best performance separating patients with an uncomplicated course from those with unfavorable outcome with 100 % sensitivity and 97 % specificity (Kress et al. 2004). Moreover they agreed and were able to predict electrophysiologic data (CMAP- compound muscle action potentials) obtained in the same patients. A recent study using a 3T MR scanner (Burmeister et al. 2011) has compared signal intensity increase percentage (SIIP) between pre- and post gadolinium T1 W images in the normal and affected side with patients outcome. Whereas higher signal intensity was shown in the pre-meatal segments of the facial nerve on the affected side, both on pre- and post-gadolinium T1 W images, no correlation was found between signal intensity measurements, clinical findings or patient's recovery. In short, evidence gathered up to this date does not justify the routine use of MRI in patients with typical clinical picture of Bell's palsy.

Early steroid treatment (within 72 h after symptoms onset) has been proven useful but not the routine use of antiviral drugs (acyclovir) (Hato et al. 2003; Sullivan et al. 2007; Fishman 2011; Oczkowski 2008).

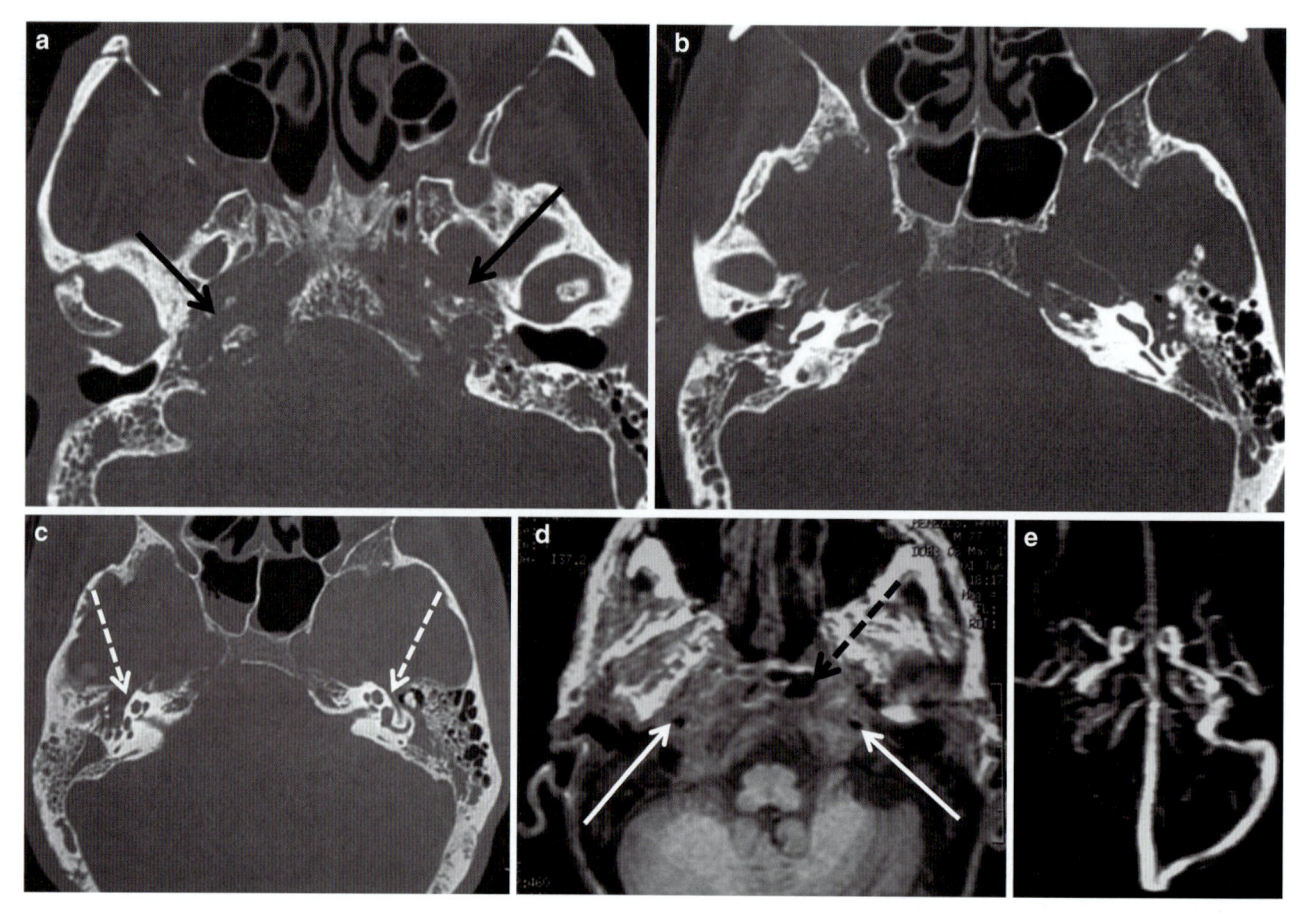

Fig. 24 Axial CT sections through the temporal bone (**a**, **b**, and **c**) show bilateral filling of the middle ear cavities and extensive bone changes with a permeative pattern involving the mastoid and petrous temporal bone and the central skull base. Note the involvement of the petrous carotid canals (*black arrows*) with encasement of the petrous carotid arteries best appreciated on the axial T1 W MR image (**d**) (*white arrows*). Also note the involvement of the geniculate ganglion fossa at the anterior aspect of the petrous bone (*dashed white arrows*) and along the intratemporal segments of the facial nerve. Extensive central skull base osteomyelitis is seen with inflammatory tissue replacing the central skull base and an abscess pocket/necrotic bone in the region of the clivus (*doted black arrow*). MRV on the same patient disclosed thrombosis of the transverse and sigmoid sinuses on the right side (**e**). Diagnosis: Necrotizing otitis externa in a diabetic patient

Ramsay-Hunt syndrome is another neurotropic viral infection characterized by acute FNP, sensorineural hearing loss, vertigo, facial pain, and vesicular eruptions over the face, eardrum and neck caused by a herpes zoster infection also known as herpes zoster *oticu*s or herpes zoster *cephalicus*. The infection affects most commonly cranial nerves V, VII, and VIII accounting for the clinical symptoms. Serologic testing both in blood and CSF may disclose an increase in VZV antibody titers. Facial nerve palsy is often more severe than that seen in Bell's palsy and bares a worse outcome with only 10 % of total remissions and 66 % of partial recoveries. The imaging hallmark is again abnormal enhancement along the course of affected nerves, which is usually more intense than that seen in Bell's palsy and may last as long as 13 months after disease onset (Jager and Reiser 2001). The presence of associated labyrinthine enhancement is useful to distinguish this condition from Bell's palsy secondary to herpes simplex virus (HSV) infection (Fig. 23). So far, no correlation has been found between the degree of contrast enhancement or electroneurographic results with patient's outcome. In this setting, antiviral therapy given within 3 days after onset, has proven helpful in terms of functional recovery (Gilchrist 2009; Kinishi et al. 2001).

Other viral infections, such as rubeolla, mumps, EBV, coxsackievirus, and HIV may lead to FNP but are less common.

Bacterial infections, most often tympanogenic or meningogenic may course with FNP. **Lyme's disease** or **Lyme's borreliosis** is a tick-borne spirochetal infection caused by the *Borrelia* species (Garcia-Monco 2002; Siwula and Mathieu 2002; Lipsker 2004; Larrosa et al. 1999). The disease is transmitted to humans by a tick bite and the main clinical symptoms include fever, headache, fatigue and a

Fig. 25 Pre (**a**) and post gadolinium axial T1 W images (**b, c,** and **d**) show a diffusely enhancing soft tissue mass filling in the left the middle ear cavity, extending into the petroclival region, Meckel's cave and cavernous sinus antero-medially, into the left parotid and masticator space inferior-laterally and into the jugular foramen posterior-inferiorly with encasement of the petrous carotid artery. The geniculate ganglion fossa, tympanic, and mastoid segments of the facial nerve are involved by this infiltrating mass. Permeative bone changes are noted in the central and posterior skull base, in the temporal bone and mandibular condyle.
Diagnosis: Necrotizing otitis externa

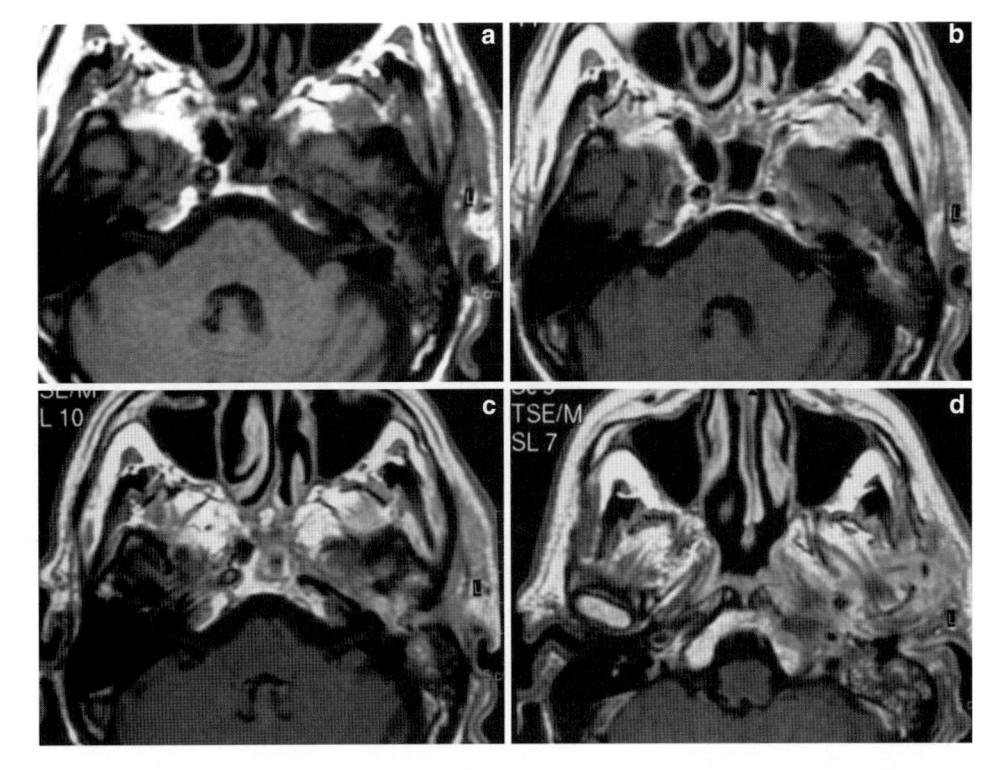

typical skin rash known as erythema *migrans* (Garcia-Monco 2002; Siwula and Mathieu 2002; Lipsker 2004; Larrosa et al. 1999). Involvement of the CNS is, together with joint and cardiac involvement, part of the late symptoms when the disease is left untreated (Djukic et al. 2011). Neuroborreliosis is characterized by a meningoneuritis with involvement of the facial nerve and FNP seen in 10 % of patients among which 25 % is bilateral (Djukic et al. 2011). In the USA, it is now the most common cause of FNP in the pediatric age group (see congenital and pediatric facial nerve palsy). The diagnosis is clinical and serologic (Makhani et al. 2011). On MRI leptomeningeal enhancement, enhancement along the course of the facial nerve(s) and white matter lesions, most likely secondary to vasculitis, may be disclosed (Abul-Kasim 2010). Antibiotic treatment with amoxycilin or doxycycline is effective at eradicating the disease.

Any **acute or chronic infection of the middle ear cavity (MEC)** such as acute or chronic otitis media, cholesteatoma, malignant or necrotizing otitis externa (MOE), petrous apicitis and cholesterol granuloma may involve the facial nerve and lead to PFNP (Borges 2005; Borges and Casselman 2007; Helms et al. 2003; Kristensen and Hahn 2012; Roberts et al. 2010). Facial palsy secondary to acute and chronic middle ear infection has markedly decreased in the post-antibiotic era so that at the present, the most common ear infection associated with FNP is **MOE** (Roberts et al. 2010). This condition, most often secondary to a *Pseudomonas aeruginosa* infection and affecting diabetic and other immunocompromised patients, starts at the external auditory canal and from there spreads inferiorly into the parotid space, medially into the middle ear cavity, petrous apex and central skull base and posteriorly into the jugular foramen and posterior cranial fossa (Borges and Casselman 2007; Roberts et al. 2010). Facial nerve involvement is seen in 38 % of patients and is an ominous sign predictive of poor survival. When the patient does survive the chance of functional recovery is 50 % (Borges and Casselman 2007; Veillon et al. 2008; Roberts et al. 2010). The nerve maybe involved by spread of infection through the stylomastoid foramen as well as by direct involvement of the facial bone canal at the mastoid or tympanic segments.

Imaging may suggest the diagnosis in the appropriate clinical setting, is crucial to determine the extent of infection, detect any drainable fluid collections and potential complications and is also used in the follow-up of treatment (Borges and Casselman 2007; Veillon et al. 2008; Roberts et al. 2010; Reiter et al. 1982). Whereas CT is useful to depict bone destructive changes, abscesses, and venous thrombosis, CE-MRI is the modality of choice to depict cranial nerves involvement, determine the extent of inflammatory soft tissue and to depict bone marrow involvement (Reiter et al. 1982). MRA and MRV may disclose involvement of the petrous and cavernous carotid artery and venous thrombosis, common complications of this aggressive infectious process (Figs. 24 and 25) (Borges and Casselman 2007; Reiter et al. 1982). When facial nerve

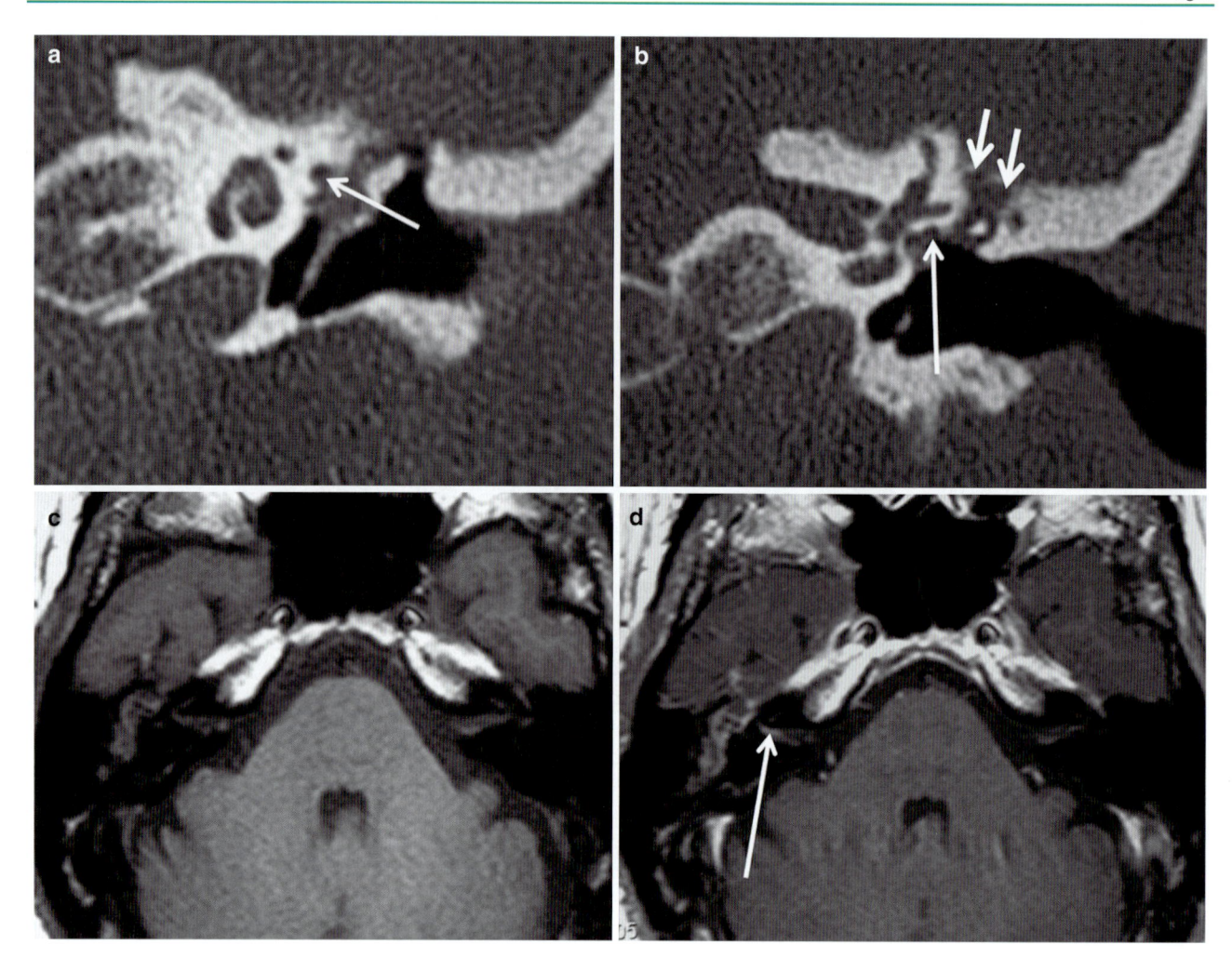

Fig. 26 Patient with chronic otitis media presenting with acute facial nerve palsy. Coronal CT sections through the tympanic cavity demonstrate a soft tissue mass filling Prussak's space and the eptympanum, amputation of the scutum and bony erosions in the roof of the middle ear (*short white arrows*). Erosion of the tympanic segment of the facial nerve canal is also noted in the region of the cochlear promontory- *white arrow* in (**a**)- and below the horizontal semicircular canal- *long white arrow* in (**b**). Plain (**a**) and gadolinium-enhanced (**b**) axial T1 W MR images on the same patient show a rim enhancing mass in the middle ear cavity and abnormal enhancement along the labyrinthine segment of the facial nerve- *white arrow* in (**d**). Diagnosis: Attical cholesteatoma with erosion of the fallopian canal and inflammation of the facial nerve with disruption of the blood-nerve barrier

paralysis is present, enhancement of the facial nerve and/or erosion of the facial bone canal are often depicted. Treatment is with long-term intravenous aminoglicosides, or third generation anti-pseudomonal penicillin/cephalosporin but surgical debridement is often needed.

Once the leading cause of infectious FNP, **acute otitis media** has currently a reported incidence of 0.16 % (Helms et al. 2003). The tympanic segment is the most commonly involved either through pre-existing bony dehiscences or through erosion of the fallopian canal that can be disclosed on high resolution CT scans using a bone algorithm (Borges 2005; Helms et al. 2003). Facial nerve edema, compression by granulation tissue, or an intrafallopian abscess may result leading to acute FNP. Paralysis persisting beyond 48 h is an indication for mastoidectomy and facial nerve decompression.

Chronic otitis media and **cholesteatoma** may also lead to progressive erosion of the bony facial canal and to gradual onset of facial nerve palsy (Borges 2005; Borges and Casselman 2007; Veillon et al. 2008). Diagnosis is usually straightforward showing abnormal soft tissue density within the MEC and demineralization or erosion of the ossicular chain and of the walls of the tympanic cavity (Fig. 26). In more aggressive cases, erosion of the geniculate fossa can be seen. Diffusion weighted MRI and delayed post-contrast T1 W sequences are ideal to differentiate these entities with cholesteatomas showing restricted diffusion and only marginal enhancement (Fig. 27) (Szymanski et al. 2012;

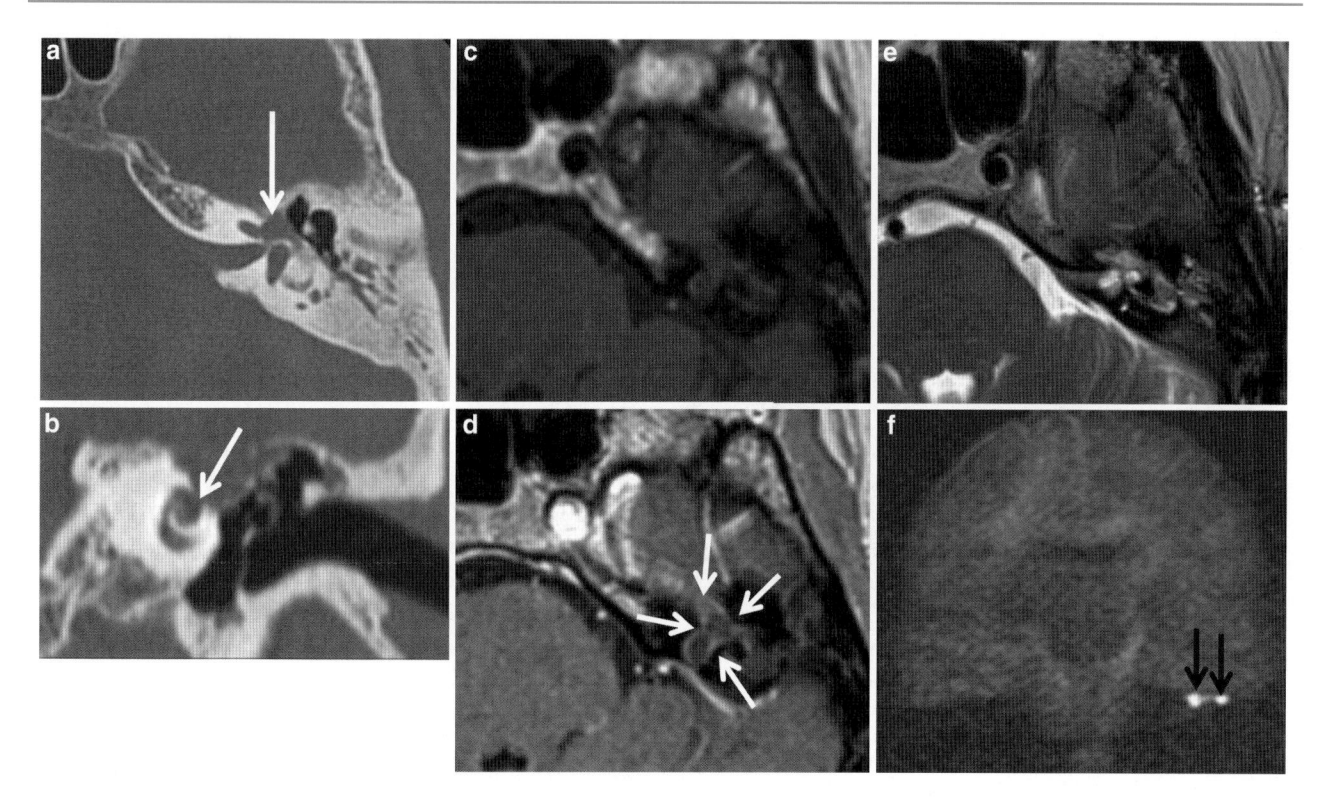

Fig. 27 Axial and coronal CT reconstructions from a MDCT acquisition show a soft tissue mass centered in the anterior petrous bone in the geniculate ganglion fossa eroding the labyrinthine segment of the facial nerve along the cochlear promontory (*white arrows* in **a** and **b**). On MR, pre- (**c**) and post-gadolinium (**d**) T1 W images and axial T2 W image (**e**) the lesion is hypointense on T1, slightly hyperintense on T2WI and shows faint marginal enhancement after gadolinium (*small white arrows*). Additional coronal non-EPI DWI, ($b = 1000$) the lesion demonstrates restricted diffusion (*black arrows* in **f**). Diagnosis: Congenital cholesteatoma in a 50 year old woman presenting with sudden FNP

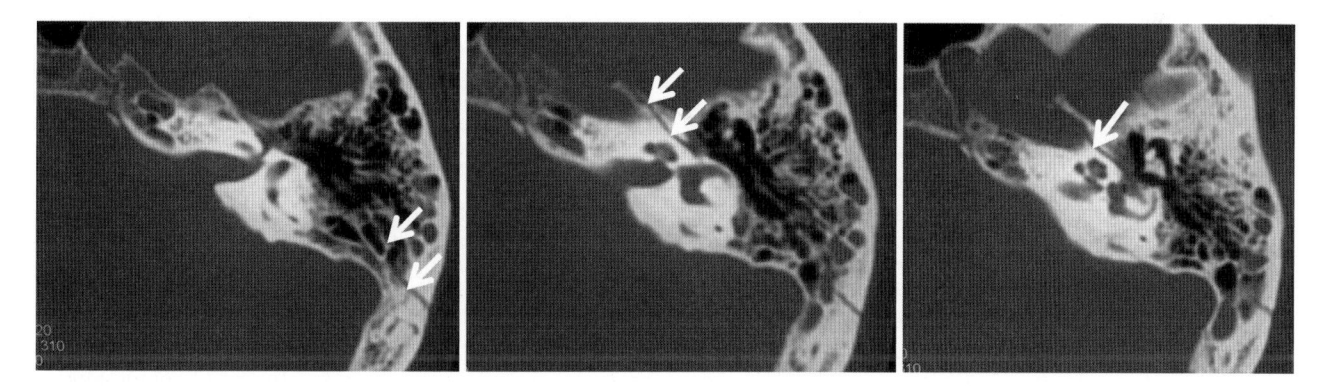

Fig. 28 Axial CT sections through the temporal bone show a longitudinally oriented fracture line crossing, from posterior to anterior (*short white arrows*), through the mastoid, middle ear cavity, and otic capsule parallel to the Eustachian tube ending at the geniculate ganglion fossa. Diagnosis: Longitudinal temporal bone fracture in a patient status post-motor vehicle accident with delayed facial nerve palsy

Hoa et al. 2013). Involvement of the facial nerve results in abnormal enhancement along the temporal segments of the nerve.

Cholesterol granuloma is a chronic inflammatory cystic lesion characterized by the presence of granulation tissue containing multinucleated giant cells, cholesterol crystals which account for the typical MR signal intensity of this lesion- hyperintense on both T1 and T2 W images- red blood cells and blood break down products (Hoa et al. 2012, 2013; Gore et al. 2011). Peripheral hemossiderin deposits may be present, shown on MR as a T1 and T2 hypointense rim. The presence of a connective tissue capsule with

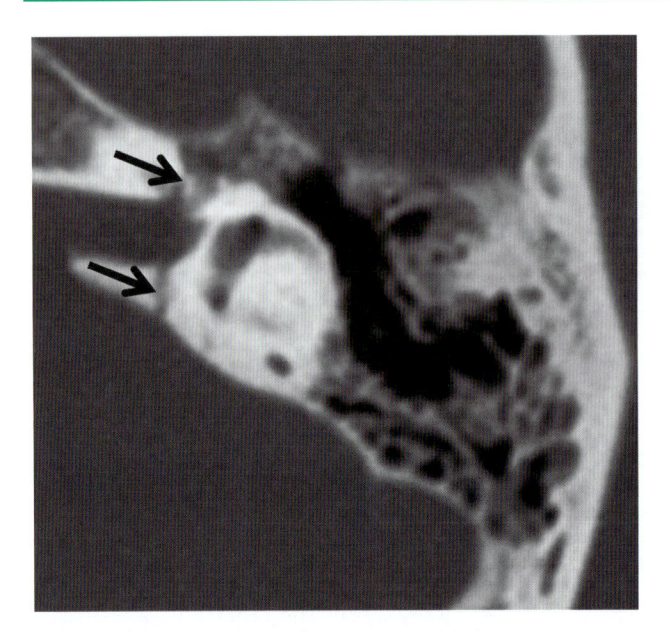

Fig. 29 Axial CT sections through the temporal bone show a fracture line crossing the temporal bone perpendicular to its long axis travelling through the fundus of the IAC and labyrinth affecting the labyrinthine segment of the facial nerve (*black arrows*). Diagnosis: Transverse temporal bone fracture in a patient status post-hit and run with immediate and complete facial nerve palsy

fragile blood supply is responsible for the faint peripheral enhancement of this lesion on post gadolinium T1 W images. The most common locations in the temporal bone are the mastoid air cells, followed by the tympanic cavity and the petrous apex. This expansive lesion may compress, remodel and erode adjacent bone and may affect the mastoid or tympanic segments of the facial nerve. When arising from the petrous apex, the geniculate fossa. Gradenigo's syndrome is a common clinical presentation characterized by a triad of suppurative otitis media, pain in the distribution of the trigeminal nerve and abducens nerve palsy (Hoa et al. 2012, 2013; Gore et al. 2011). Only rarely is FNP part of the clinical picture.

Trauma ranks second in the list of causes of PFNP and may be accidental or iatrogenic, during parotid or temporal bone surgery (Borges 2005; Hsu et al. 2008; Odebode and Ologe 2006; Rotondo et al. 2010). CN VII is the most commonly injured nerve in craniofacial trauma. Temporal bone fractures have a reported incidence of 5 % after blunt head trauma, increasing to 40 % when skull base fractures are present (Odebode and Ologe 2006). Fractures of the temporal bone can be longitudinal- accompanying the long axis- or transverse- perpendicular to the long axis of the petrous bone. The former are usually extra-labyrinthine, comprise 80 % of temporal bone fractures but only 10–20 % are associated to FNP (Figs. 28 and 29). When present FNP is often delayed and transient and results from injury of the geniculate ganglion or proximal tympanic segment by a shock wave leading to nerve traction, contusion or impingement by bony spicules (Pownder et al. 2010). Transverse fractures result in FNP in 30–50 % of cases which is usually immediate, complete, and irreversible. The mechanism of injury of these translabyrinthine fractures is nerve impingement or transection proximal to the geniculate ganglion affecting the labyrinthine segment of the nerve (Pownder et al. 2010; Barreau 2011). CT is the imaging modality of choice to depict the fracture lines whereas MR is reserved for FNP unexplained by CT findings (Barreau 2011). In these circumstances, MR may disclose a facial nerve hematoma or abnormal facial nerve enhancement due to disruption of the blood-nerve barrier which may persist as long as 2 years after trauma (Rotondo et al. 2010). Dural enhancement along the anterior petrous ridge may be the only sign of facial nerve trauma (Jager and Reiser 2001), Iatrogenic lesions of the facial nerve secondary to temporal bone surgery often affect the tympanic segment of the facial nerve, immediately above the oval window and below the lateral semi-circular canal, or at the level of the pyramidal eminence (Rinaldo et al. 2002; Safdar et al. 2006; Xu et al. 2011). More recently, with the introduction of cochlear implants, hemifacial spasm and hyperkinesis have been recognized as potential complications when electrodes are placed too close to the labyrinthine segment of the facial nerve, to the geniculate ganglion or to the cochlear promontory (Fig. 30) (Ciorba et al. 2012; Stoddart and Cooper 1999; Falcioni et al. 2003). CT is particularly useful to depict small post-surgical defects of the fallopian canal.

Facial nerve neoplasms may be primary or secondary. Primary facial nerve tumors are rare and most commonly affect the temporal segments of the facial nerve (Falcioni et al. 2003). Although they represent only 5 % of all causes of FNP, early recognition is mandatory if one aims for functional rehabilitation of the nerve (Roob et al. 1999; Veillon et al. 2008; Borges and Casselman 2007). A facial nerve neoplasm should be suspected in patients presenting with progressive, longstanding, recurrent episodes of FNP or in patients with associated facial twitches or spasm. However, one should keep in mind that 30 % of cases may present with sudden paralysis due to abrupt compromise of blood supply to the nerve, mimicking Bell's palsy. Topognostic testing is of little value as the nerve may suffer significant stretching before losing its functional integrity. Therefore, preservation of special functions of the facial nerve does not necessarily mean that the tumor is distal to the facial nerve branches responsible for that function (Borges 2005; Veillon et al. 2008; Borges and Casselman 2007). It is not uncommon that patients present with symptoms unrelated to the facial nerve making the diagnosis difficult. CT and MRI have a complementary role in the evaluation of facial nerve tumors: whereas CT may

Pathology of the Facial Nerve

Fig. 30 MDCT axial and coronal reconstructions in high resolution bone algorithm of the right (**a** and **b**) and left temporal bones (**c** and **d**) of a 16-year-old girl status post bilateral cochlear implants presenting with facial spasm and hyperkynesia on the right. On the *left side*, the electrodes are in normal position and do not touch the course of the facial nerve (**c** and **d**). On the *right side* (**a** and **b**), an electrode (*black arrows*) is seen in close proximity with the labyrinthine and proximal tympanic segments of the facial nerve, close to the cochlear promontory (*white arrows*)

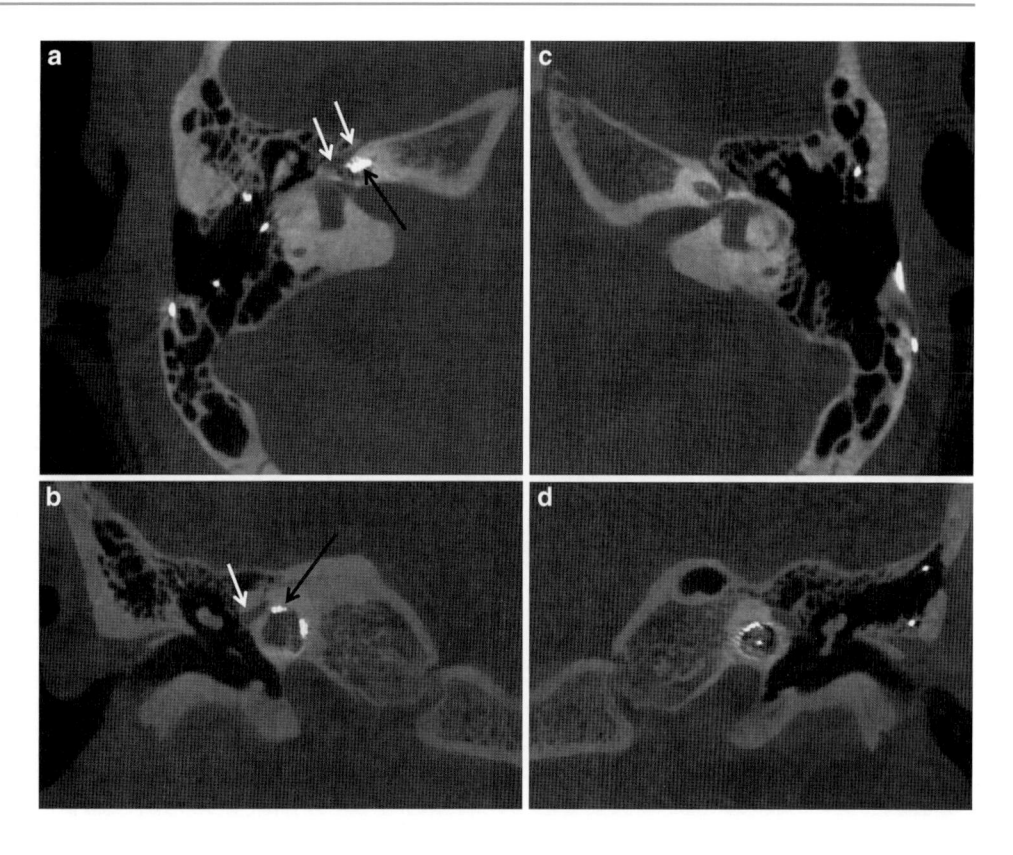

Fig. 31 Post-gadolinium axial and coronal T1 W images showing multiple supra and infratentorial meningiomas as well as multiple schwannomas affecting cranial nerves V (*dashed arrow*), VI (*short arrow*), VII (*long arrow*) and VIII (*dotted arrow*), in a patient with neurofibromatosis type 2

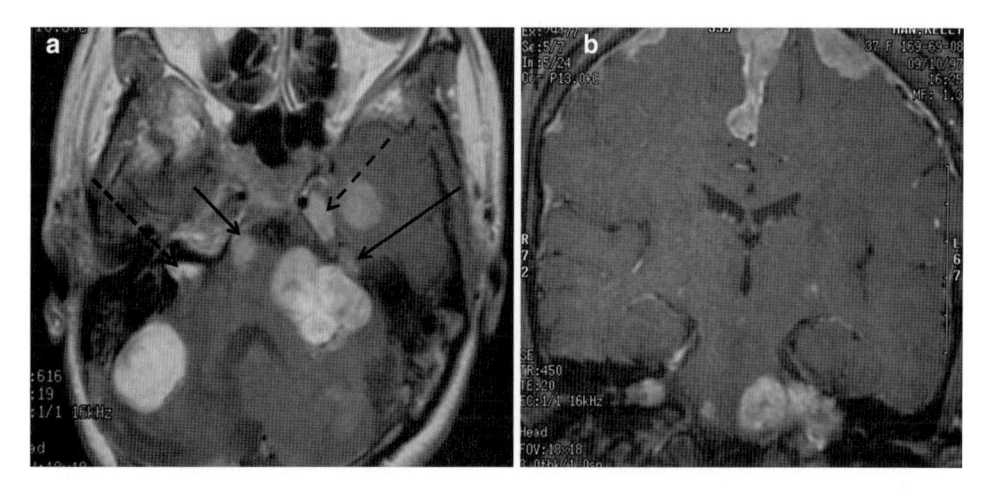

Fig. 32 Gadolinium-enhanced axial T1 W images (**a** and **b**) show an enhancing lesion along the labyrinthine segment of the facial nerve (*long white arrow*) with a more nodular component in the region of the geniculate ganglion slightly bulging into the middle cranial fossa (*short white arrows*). Diagnosis: Facial nerve schwannoma of the labyrinthine segment and geniculate ganglion

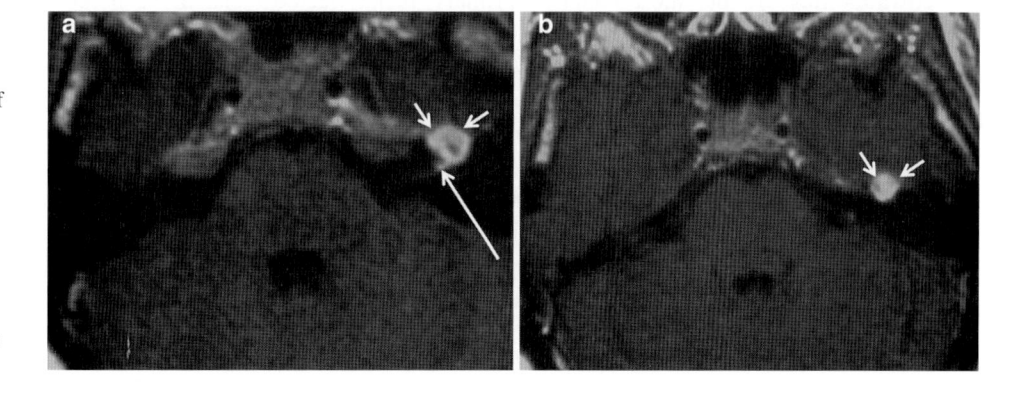

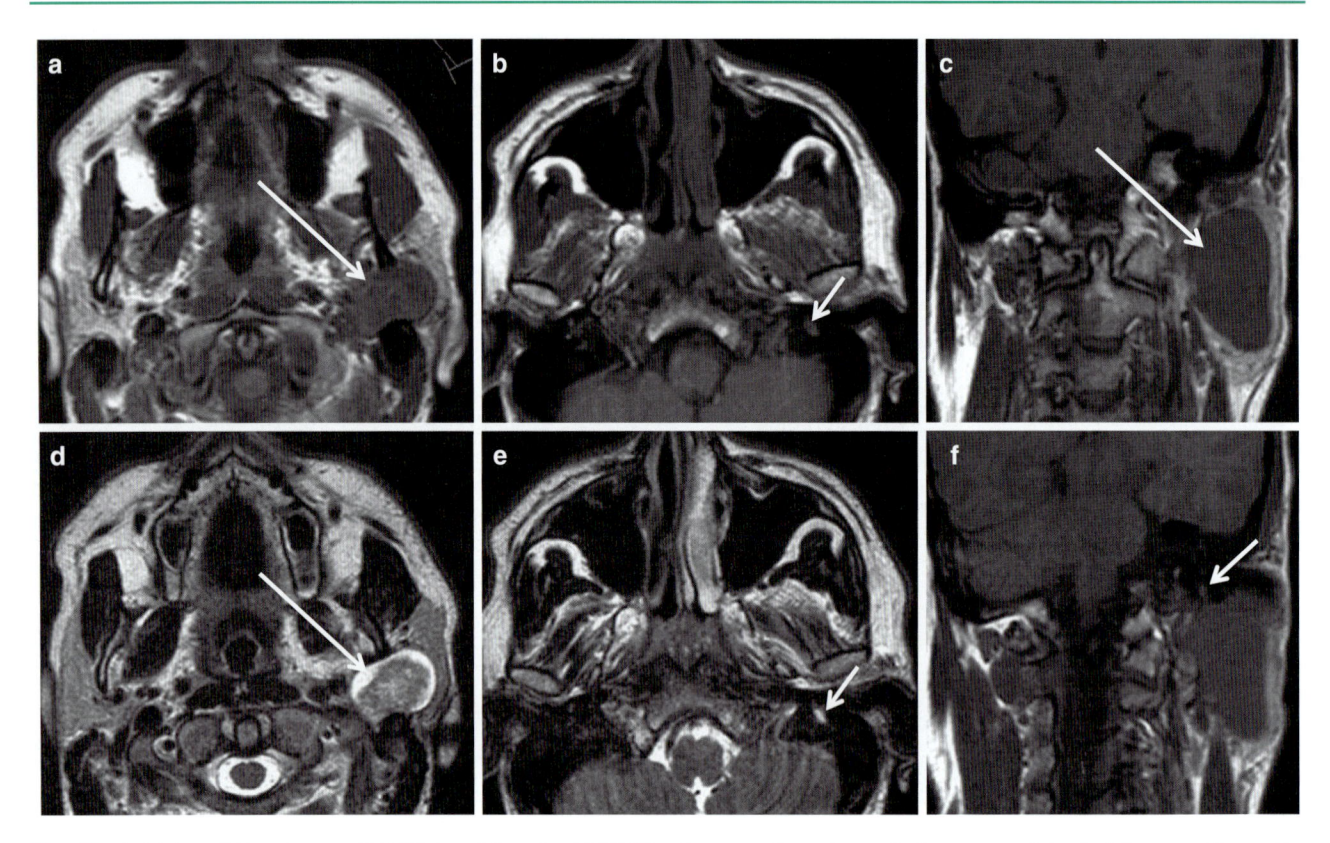

Fig. 33 Axial (**a** and **b**) and coronal T1 W (**c** and **f**) and axial T2 W (**d** and **e**) images demonstrate a well-defined soft tissue mass in the left parotid gland (*white arrows*) extending through the stylomastoid foramen along the vertical segment of the facial nerve (*short white arrows*). Diagnosis: Facial nerve schwannoma.

depict enlargement, remodeling or erosion of the facial nerve canal, MR depicts the tumor directly, offers better soft tissue characterization and detects tumors when they are too small to produce any bone changes (Burmeister et al. 2010).

The facial nerve is most commonly affected by direct invasion from neighboring tumors or by perineural spread of head and neck malignancies than by primary tumors. The latter include schwannomas, hemangiomas, choristomas, primary facial nerve meningiomas, epineurial pseudocysts, and paragangliomas some of which are quite rare with only few cases reported in the literature (Borges 2005; Veillon et al. 2008; Burmeister et al. 2010).

Schwannomas are the most common primary facial nerve tumors. These are nerve sheath tumors originating from Schwann cells and expanding the nerve eccentrically away from its axons. They can occur in isolation or as part of neurofibromatosis type 2 (Fig. 31) (Gerganov et al. 2011; Fabiano et al. 2010; Shimizu et al. 2005; Thompson et al. 2009). Clinical presentation depends on tumor location along the facial nerve as well as on tumor size. The region of the geniculate ganglion is the most commonly affected, followed by the mastoid, intracanalicular and labyrinthine, tympanic and extracranial segments (Borges and Casselman 2007; Fabiano et al. 2010). Tumors of the cisternal and intracanalicular segments present with vestibulocochlear dysfunction and may mimic vestibular schwannomas both clinically and on imaging grounds. Tumors of the geniculate ganglion may remain asymptomatic until they impinge upon the middle cranial fossa and Meckel's cave due to growth along the greater superficial petrosal nerve (Fig. 32) (Borges 2005; Veillon et al. 2008). In the tympanic segment, schwannomas manifest as conductive hearing loss due to mechanical interference with the ossicular chain. A retrotympanic mass may be disclosed on otoscopic examination. Inadvertent biopsy of such a lesion may lead to acute facial nerve palsy (Fabiano et al. 2010; Thompson et al. 2009). Schwannomas of the mastoid segment are those most commonly associated to acute or gradual onset of facial nerve palsy. When affecting the intraparotid segment, facial nerve schwannomas maybe indistinguishable from other commoner parotid masses (Shimizu et al. 2005). Even when there is associated enlargement of the stylomastoid foramen a parotid malignancy with perineural spread cannot be excluded on imaging grounds (Fig. 33). The presence of facial spasms or twitches should alert for causes of FNP other then Bell's palsy.

Fig. 34 Curved reconstruction from a 3D gadolinium-enhanced T1 W sequence shows a fusiform lesion along the labyrinthine and tympanic segments of the facial nerve (*white arrows*). Diagnosis: Facial nerve schwannoma (*Courtesy of Prof. Jan Casselman*)

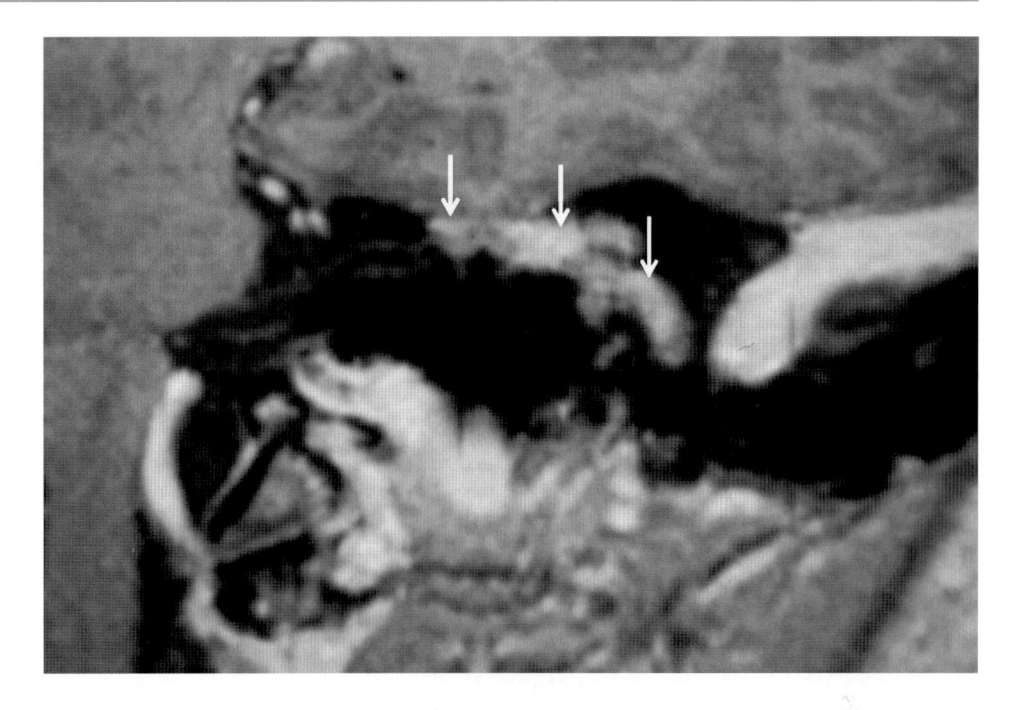

Fig. 35 Axial CT section and gadolinium-enhanced T1 W MR image show an expansive lesion involving the labyrinthine segment of the facial nerve (*black arrow*) and the geniculate ganglion (*white arrow*), with multiple bone trabecula within the lesion. The MR image clearly demonstrates the lobulated contour and the cotton-like pattern of enhancement. Diagnosis: Ossifying facial nerve hemangioma (*Courtesy of Prof. F. Veillon*)

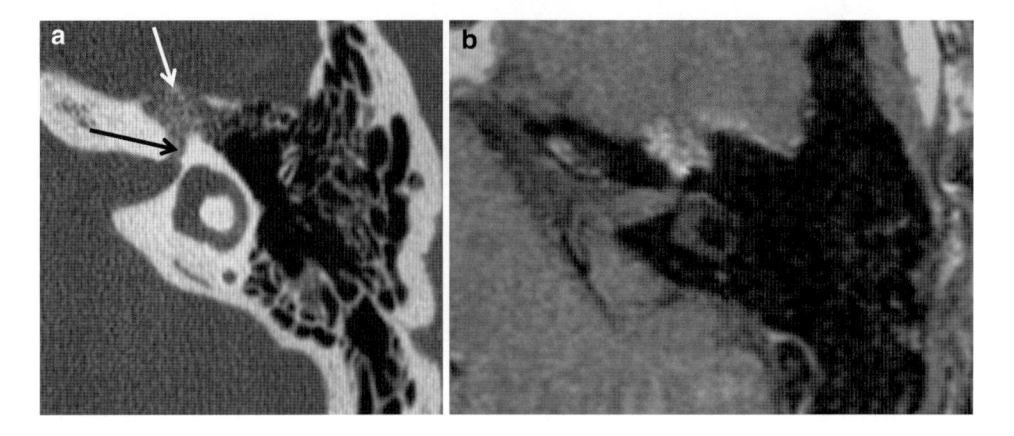

CT is very useful in the evaluation of tumors of the tympanic segment to establish the relationships with the ossicular chain and to look for erosions of the cochlear promontory and lateral semi-circular canal. In the mastoid segment, CT depicts the presence of erosions of the posterior wall of the external auditory canal and determines the relationship of the tumor with the tympanic membrane. One should also be aware of potential pitfalls such as an aberrant intra-tympanic course of the petrous carotid artery or a persistent stapedial artery which should not be mistaken for a facial nerve tumor.

On MR facial nerve schwannomas present as well-defined oval or fusiform-shaped masses following the expected course of the nerve, most often hypointense on T1 W and hyperintense on T2 W images, often with cystic areas and showing variable enhancement after gadolinium (Figs. 32, 33 and 34).

FN **hemangiomas** are most commonly seen in the region of the geniculate ganglion and extension into the labyrinthine segment is classic (Benoit et al. 2010; Gonzalez-Darder and Pesudo-Martinez 2007; Salib et al. 2001) (Fig. 35). FNP occurs early in the development of these tumors in spite of their small size (Veillon et al. 2008). CT is useful to demonstrate the presence of bony spicules of lamellar bone that are the hallmark of ossifying hemangiomas and allows the differential diagnosis with facial nerve schwannomas (Borges 2005; Veillon et al. 2008; Salib et al. 2001) (Fig. 35). The IAC is the second most common location. Here tumors tend to present with tinnitus and, on occasion, with hemifacial spasm, besides FNP. On MRI hemangiomas are lobulated, poorly defined lesions of variable signal intensity and variable enhancement, due to the presence of trabecular bone and possible blood degradation products (Borges 2005; Veillon et al. 2008;

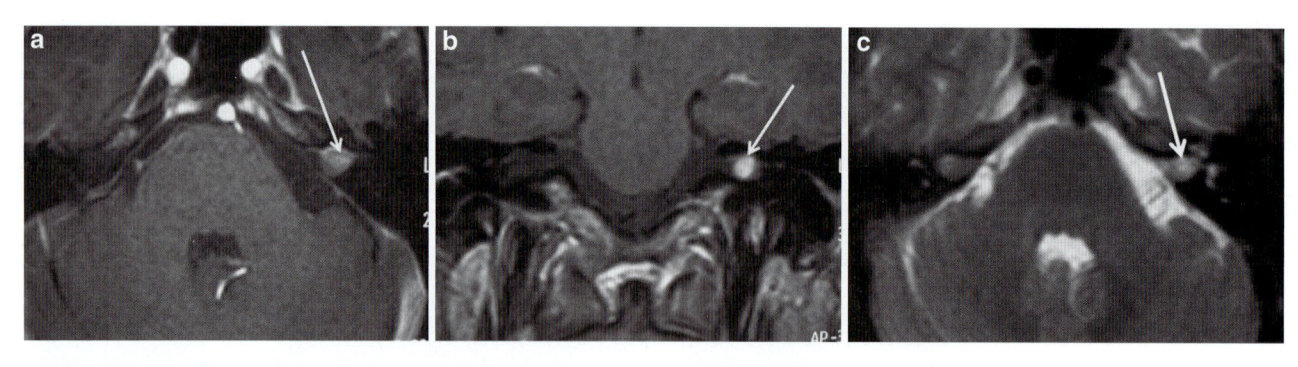

Fig. 36 Gadolinium-enhanced axial (**a**) and coronal (**b**) T1 W images and axial (**c**) T2 W images sections show expansion and abnormal globular enhancement within the anterior and superior aspect of the IAC along the labyrinthine segment of the facial nerve (*white arrows*). Note the globular hyperintensity on the T2 W image. Diagnosis: Facial nerve hemangioma (labyrinthine segment) in a patient presenting with tinnitus, facial nerve palsy and hemifacial spasm

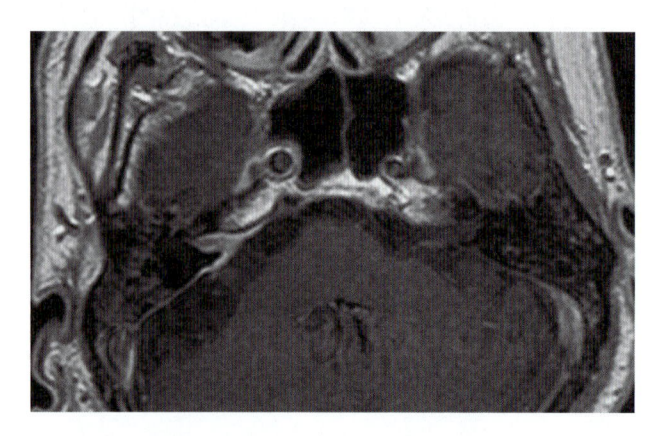

Fig. 37 Post-gadolinium axial T1 W image through the IAC shows thick dural enhancement along the dural sheath of the statoacoustic bundle and a dural tail along the posterior petrous ridge. Diagnosis: IAC Meningioma (*Courtesy of Prof. M. Lemmerling*)

Salib et al. 2001). Most show intermediate signal intensity on T1 W, are predominantly hyperintense on T2 W images and show vivid enhancement on late post contrast T1 W images (Borges 2005; Veillon et al. 2008; Salib et al. 2001) (Figs. 35 and 36). However, differential diagnosis with schwannoma can be difficult on imaging grounds, particularly in the absence of ossification and or hemmorrhage. Another tumor to include in the differential diagnosis is meningioma.

Meningiomas affecting the facial nerve tend to originate from the dural covering of the statoacoustic bundle at the IAC or from the dural covering of the geniculate fossa at the anterior petrous ridge but they rarely cause FNP (Veillon et al. 2008; Jabor et al. 2000; Namdar et al. 1995). These dural-based tumors, follow the signal intensity of gray matter in all sequences, show intense and homogeneous enhancement and a dural tail (tapering dural enhancement along the tumor borders) on MR (Fig 37). On CT lesions tend to be spontaneously hyperdense and expansion and remodeling of the petrous bone is the rule. Intratumoral calcifications may be seen as well, imposing differential diagnosis with hemangiomas (Fig. 38). **Primary meningiomas of the facial nerve canal** are exceedingly rare with most cases resulting from extension from neighboring tumors most often originating from the CPA cistern, parasellar or petroclival regions (Jabor et al. 2000). Although the dura terminates a few milimeters within the IAC, the arachnoid may further extend along the fallopian canal to the region of the geniculate ganglion and beyond to finally fuse with the epineurium of the facial nerve. Primary meningiomas of the facial nerve canal are thought to result from these ectopic arachnoid remnants which tend to cluster at the IAC, geniculate ganglion, and sulcus of the greater petrosal superficial nerve (Jabor et al. 2000). However, this diagnosis requires thorough exclusion of a potential intracranial origin, namely from the endocranium or from a neurovascular foramen, in this particular case from the dural attachment to the internal acoustic meatus. Meningiomas of the geniculate ganglion are the most common location and manifest as expansile lesions with associated bony sclerosis/hyperostosis (Fig. 38), sometimes with irregular margins, making it hard to differentiate from the most common ossifying hemangiomas (Jabor et al. 2000).

Choristomas are masses of normal tissues in aberrant locations and are regarded as self-limited developmental heterotopias (Namdar et al. 1995). The two most common types affecting the facial nerve are composed of smooth muscle cells and fibrous tissue, most often reported in the region of the geniculate ganglion and in the intracanalicular segment of the facial nerve, and heterotopic masses of salivary gland tissue, most often seen along the mastoid and tympanic segments, rarely associated with facial nerve dysfunction (Namdar et al. 1995). Imaging features are nonspecific showing benign appearing, soft tissue masses along the course of the facial nerve enlarging and remodeling the IAC or different segments of the fallopian canal (Fig. 39).

Fig. 38 MDCT of the temporal bone: axial (**a** and **b**) and coronal (**c** and **d**) reconstructions on high resolution bone algorithm shows an expansive lytic lesion at the geniculate ganglion fossa with extensive bone sclerosis/hyperostosis (*white arrows*) The fallopian canal at the level of the cochlear promontory appears intact (*black arrow*). Presumptive diagnosis: Meningioma of the geniculate ganglion (*Courtesy of Dr. Joana Ruivo*)

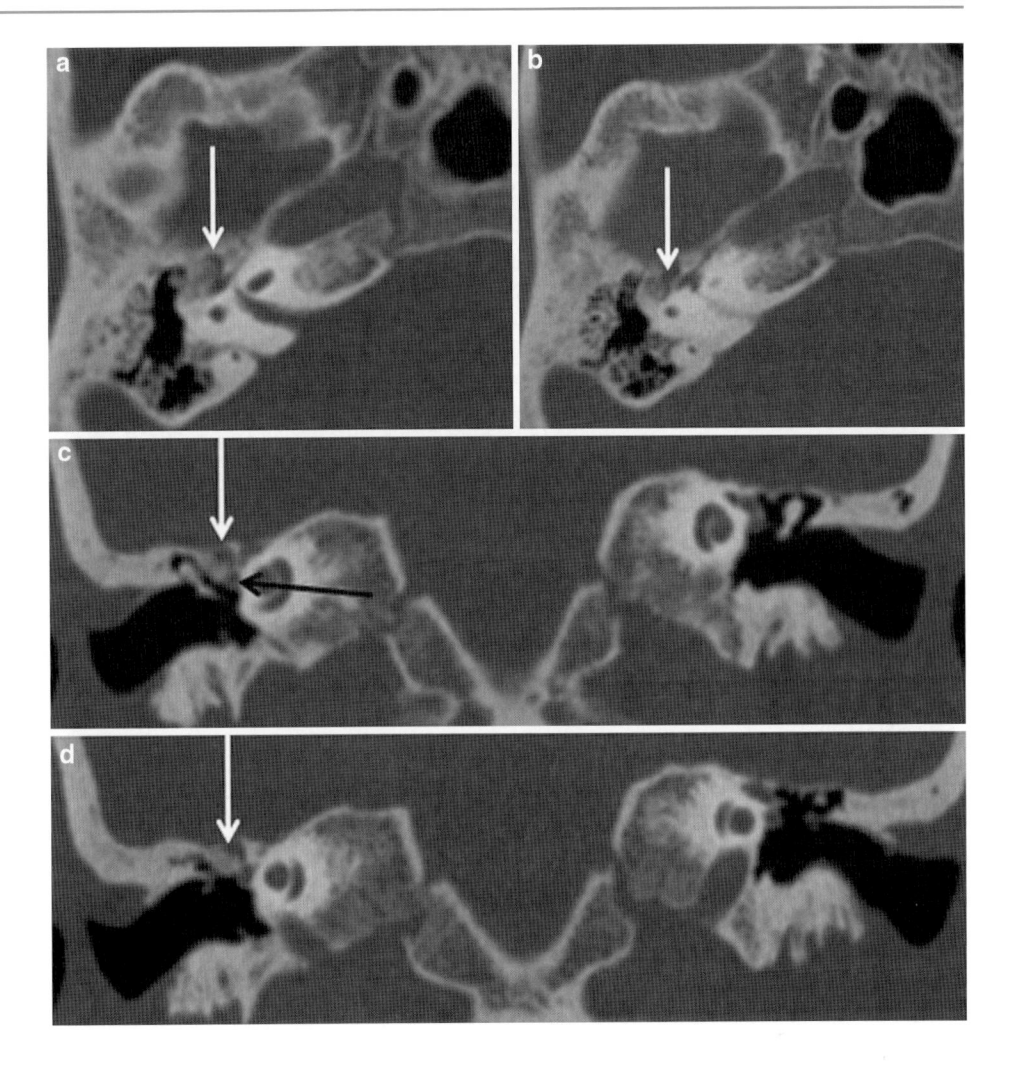

Epineurial pseudocysts are rare benign lesions of the facial nerve canal, exclusively reported in the mastoid segment of the nerve (Fig. 40) (Michalopoulos et al. 2008; Pertzborn et al. 2003). They can be incidental imaging findings but have been also found in association with facial nerve symptoms such as recurrent palsy or spasticity. They can mimic a cystic lesion on CT but on pathology they are composed of fibroadipose tissue in continuity with the epineurium of the facial nerve (Pertzborn et al. 2003).

Paragangliomas arising primarily from the facial nerve are a rare occurrence (Kunzel et al. 2012; Wippold et al. 2004; Petrus and Lo 1996). Most often the facial nerve is affected secondarily by paragangliomas originating from the jugular bulb, the tympanic branch of the glossopharyngeal nerve (Jacobsen's nerve), the auricular branch of the vagus nerve (Arnold's nerve) or from paraganglia in the region of the cochlear promontory (Figs. 41 and 42) (Noujaim et al. 2000). The mastoid and tympanic segments of the facial nerve are the most commonly involved. A few cases of paragangliomas arising primarily from the facial nerve have been reported in the literature most often from paraganglia located along the mastoid segment of the facial nerve (Kunzel et al. 2012; Wippold et al. 2004; Petrus and Lo 1996). Typically, these tumors enlarge the descending, vertical segment of the fallopian canal and may protrude through the stylomastoid foramen into the parotid gland mimicking perineural spread from a parotid neoplasm. The presence of permeative bone changes can be helpful in the differential diagnosis with other benign tumors affecting this segment of the nerve, namely schwannomas. Anterior growth into the fundus of the external auditory canal and into the region of the facial nerve recess has been reported, and is probably due to tumor growth along the chorda tympani. These hypervascular tumors show an arterial-like enhancement on dynamic contrast-enhanced studies (short time to peak and rapid wash out) accounting for the flow voids seen on MRI, responsible for the typical "salt and pepper" pattern, best seen in tumors over 2 cm in size (Van den Berg et al. 1999). Angiography demonstrates early arterial vascular blush, arteriovenous shunting, and early draining veins. Whereas most jugular paragangliomas are mainly supplied by the ascending pharyngeal artery, facial

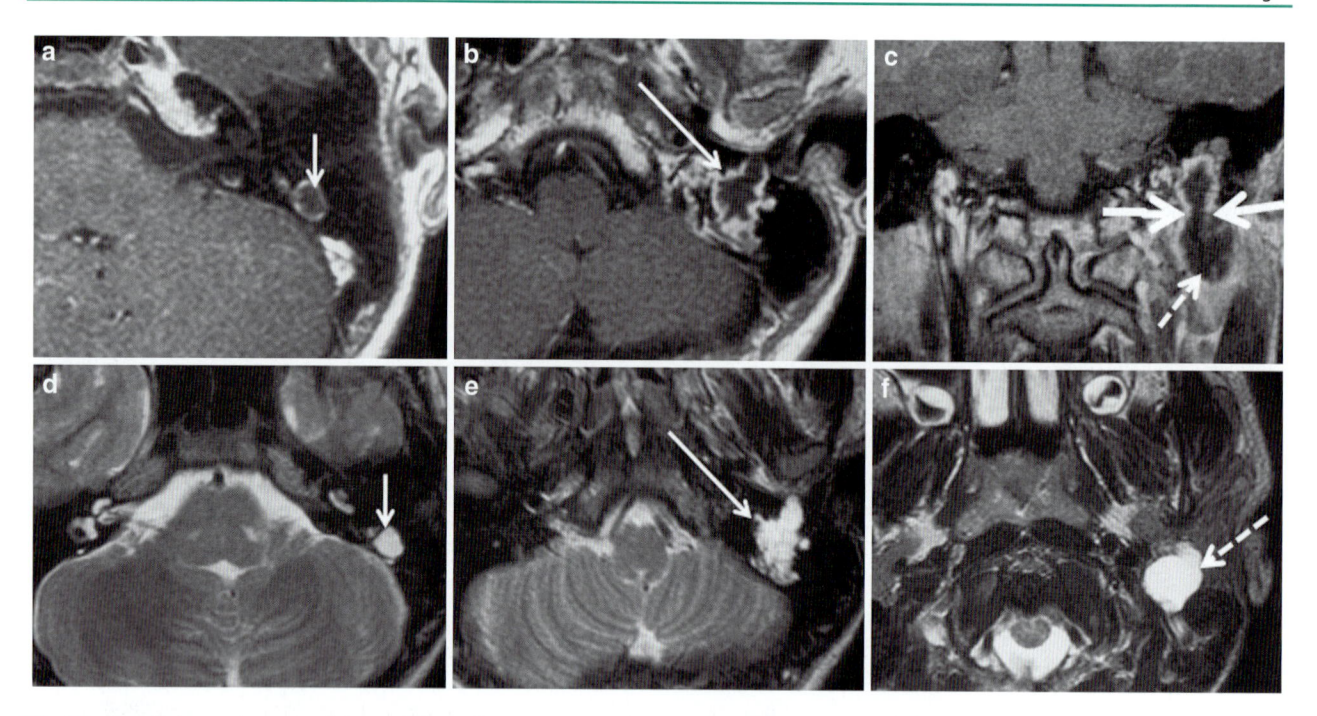

Fig. 39 Gadolinium-enhanced axial (**a** and **b**) and coronal (**c**) T1 W and axial T2 W (**d**, **e**, and **f**) MR images show an irregular, lobulated, and hourglass-shaped lesion along the distal tympanic (*long white arrows* in **b** and **e**), mastoid (*short white arrows* in **a** and **d**) and intraparotid (*dashed arrows* in **c** and **f**) segments of the facial nerve. A tumor waist is best seen on the coronal image (*thick arrows* in **c**) corresponding the exiting neuroforamina- the stylomastoid foramen. The lesion is very bright on T2 W images and shows only marginal enhancement after gadolinium. Diagnosis: Facial nerve choristoma (salivary gland type)

nerve paragangliomas arising from the mastoid segment derive their arterial supply from the posterior auricular and occipital arteries (Van den Berg et al. 1999).

Endolymphatic sac adenocarcinoma is another rare tumor that may involve the mastoid and posterior tympanic segments of the facial nerve and lead to facial nerve dysfunction (Martinez-Miravete et al. 2007; Malhotra et al. 2006). They may occur in isolation or as part of Von Hippel-Lindau disease and manifest, on imaging, as an expansive, destructive lesion in the region of the endolymphatic sac and duct in the posterior petrous bone, showing variable enhancement (Fig. 43) (Mukherji and Castillo 1996). On MR the tumor is often hyperintense on T1 W images and may show a hypointense rim accounting for the presence of intratumoral hemmorrhage. In patients with Von Hippel-Lindau disease associated hemangioblastomas and leptomeningeal angiomatosis may also be seen (Fig. 44) (Borges 2005).

In children presenting with a temporal bone mass and FNP one should think of histiocytosis, lymphoma, sarcoma, leukemic infiltrates, or metastasis (see pediatric FNP).

In adults **metastasis** affecting the temporal bone may occasionally present with FNP. The most common primaries are: breast (Fig. 45), lung (Fig. 46), kidney, stomach, pharynx, prostate, and liver (Veillon et al. 2010; Yildiz et al. 2011; Kundu et al. 2001). The petrous apex is most commonly involved and therefore the segments of the facial nerve most often involved are the intracanalicular and labyrinthine segments.

Perineural spread of head and neck malignancies may affect the facial nerve and its branches and may lead to facial nerve dysfunction (Borges 2005; Diamond et al. 2011; Jungehuelsing et al. 2000). The most common primaries are parotid gland neoplasms most often adenoid cystic and mucoepidermoid carcinomas. Whereas 12 to 35 % of patients with parotid malignancies have a partial or complete FNP at presentation, 50 % of patients with adenoid cystic carcinoma of the parotid gland show perineural tumor spread. Henceforth, quite often this spread is asymptomatic and can only be disclosed by imaging (Quesnel et al. 2010). MRI is the best imaging modality to depict perineural spread and should always be used in the staging of parotid malignancies to adapt surgical treatment and/or radiation ports. Tumor spread along the perineurium may be retrograde or anterograde and skip lesions are not uncommon, obliging to a complete scrutiny of the entire course of the nerve from the brainstem nuclei to its peripheral branches. Obliteration of foraminal fat pads is an important and early clue to the diagnosis that can be easily depicted both on CT and MR (Fig. 47). Abnormal enhancement of the facial nerve is best depicted on MRI and allows for a precise evaluation of the perineural spread (Ginsberg 2002, 2004). Enlargement and remodeling of the facial nerve canal seen on CT is a late indirect finding

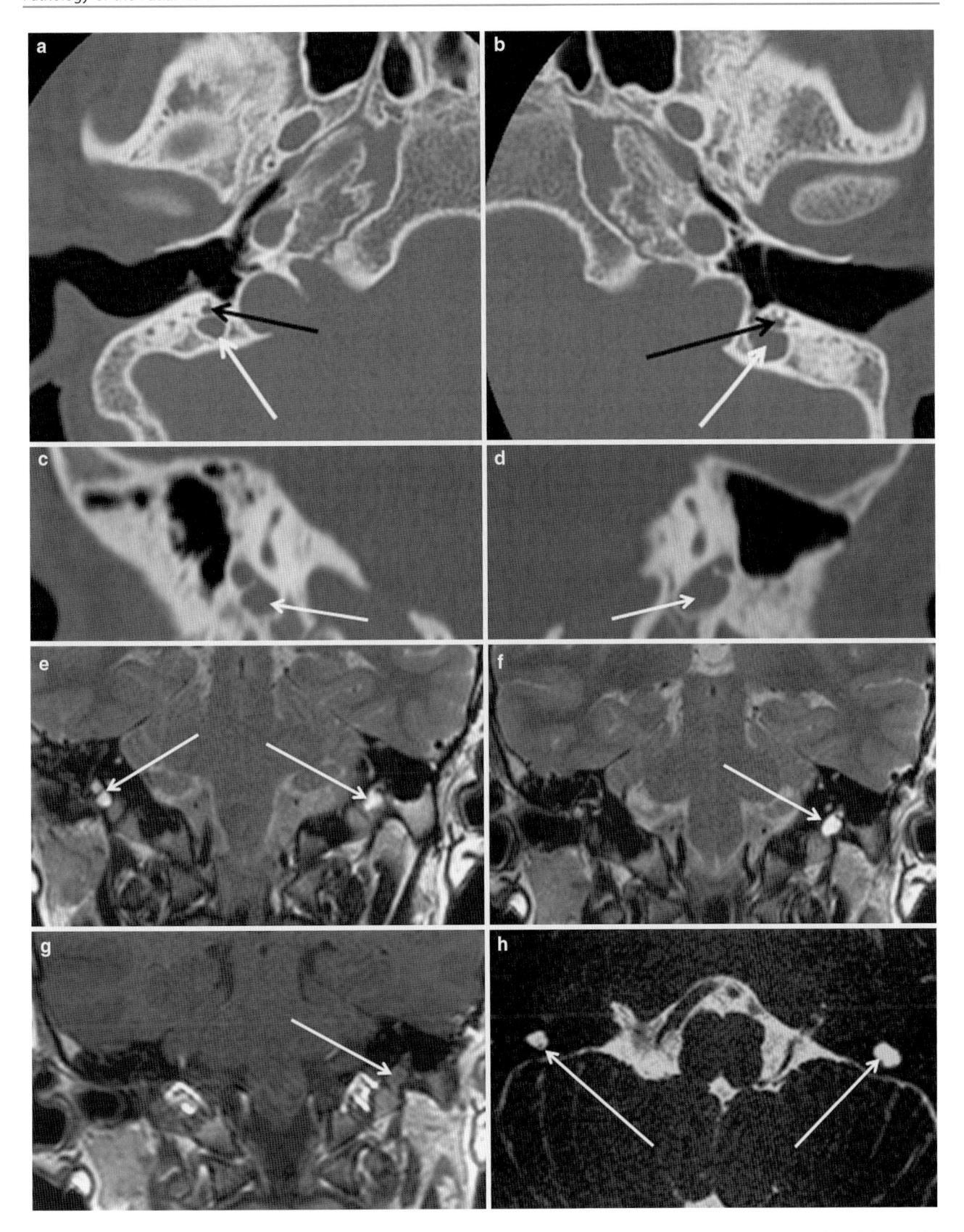

Fig. 40 MDCT of the temporal bone: Axial (**a** and **b**) and coronal (**c** and **d**) reconstructions in high resolution bone algorithm show bilateral and symmetrical lytic expansive lesions (*white arrows*) in the mastoid bone, immediately posterior to the mastoid segment of the facial nerve canal (*black arrows* in **a** and **b**). MR on the same patient coronal T2 W (**e** and **f**), post-gadolinium T1 W (**g**) and coronal CISS reconstruction (**h**) demonstrate the cystic nature of the lesions which are hyperintense on long TR images and show only faint linear peripheral enhancement (*white arrows*). Diagnosis: Bilateral epineural cysts in a 15-year-old girl status post-transmeatal resection of a right sided cholesteatoma (*Courtesy of Prof. B. de Foer*)

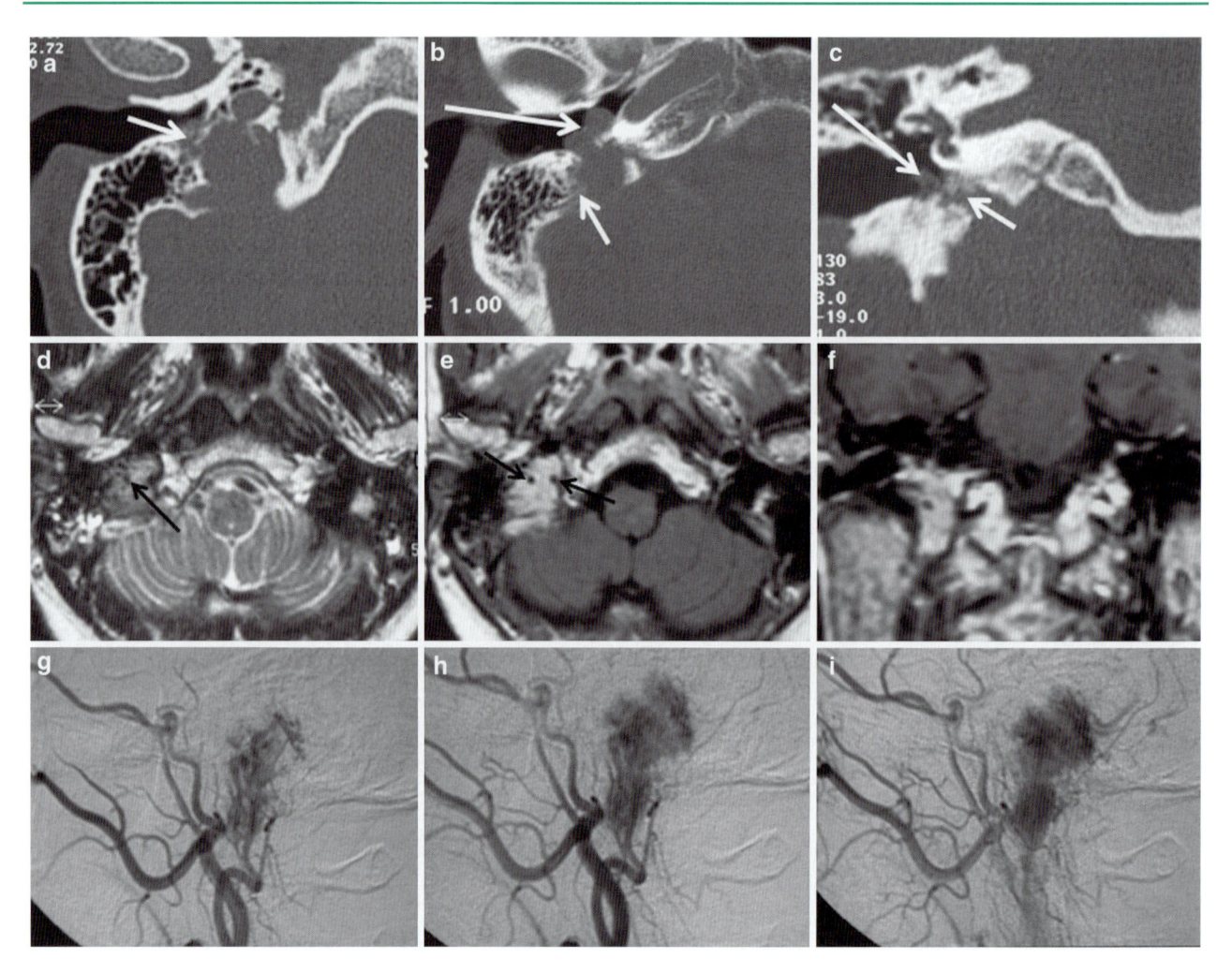

Fig. 41 Axial (**a** and **b**) and coronal (**c**) CT sections through the temporal bone show an expansive lesion enlarging the jugular foramen associated to permeative and destructive bone changes (*short white arrows*) in the adjacent mastoid bone, affecting the vertical mastoid segment of the facial nerve and protruding into the hypotympanum (*long white arrows*). Corresponding MR shows a "salt and pepper" pattern on the axial T2 W image (**d**) due to the presence of vascular flow voids within the lesion. After gadolinium administration (**e**) axial and (**f**) coronal T1 W images vivid enhancement is shown, again with flow voids seen within the tumor mass (*black arrows*). DS angiography images from an external carotid artery injection (**g**, **h**, and **i**) shows early arterial enhancement of the lesion (**g**) containing multiple tortuous vessels, intense vascular blush (**h**) and early venous drainage (**i**) due to the presence of arteriovenous shunting. Diagnosis: Glomus jugulo-tympanicum involving the jugular foramen and Arnold's nerve along the mastoid canaliculus into the MEC

implying a large tumor burden (Fig. 48). Another late indirect sign is the presence of denervation atrophy of the muscles supplied by the facial nerve, which as shown to be a good outcome predictor of facial nerve grafting (Kaylie et al. 2003).

The parotid gland should always be included on the imaging protocol for patients presenting with PFNP as this may be the first sign of a parotid malignancy. Besides salivary gland neoplasms, squamous cell carcinoma, melanoma, and lymphoma (Figs. 49 and 50) are among the malignancies more prone to this type of spread (Ginsberg 1999).

Any head and neck malignancy accessing the facial nerve or its branches, particularly the chorda tympani and greater superficial petrosal nerve, may show perineural spread (Ginsberg and Eicher 2000). Due to the large number of neural connections with other cranial nerves the facial nerve may also be affected by perineural tumor spread from remote head and neck neoplasms. Therefore, it is important to know the main neural connections between the facial and other cranial nerves (trigeminal, vestibulo-choclear, glossopharyngeal, and vagus nerves) to understand and to depict the full extent of this type of tumor spread (Diamond et al. 2011). Connections with the trigeminal nerve occur via the auriculotemporal, buccal, mental, lingual, infra-orbital and zygomatic branches as well as with branches of the ophthalmic division of the trigeminal nerve (Ozdogmus et al. 2004). Communications with the vestibular nerve are seen within the IAC and explain the vestibular disturbance

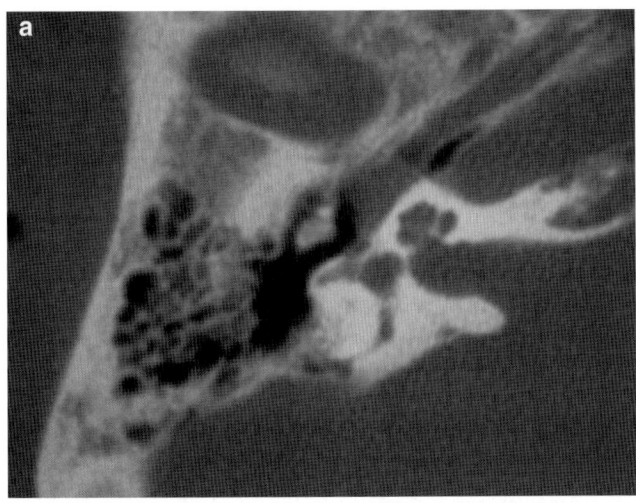

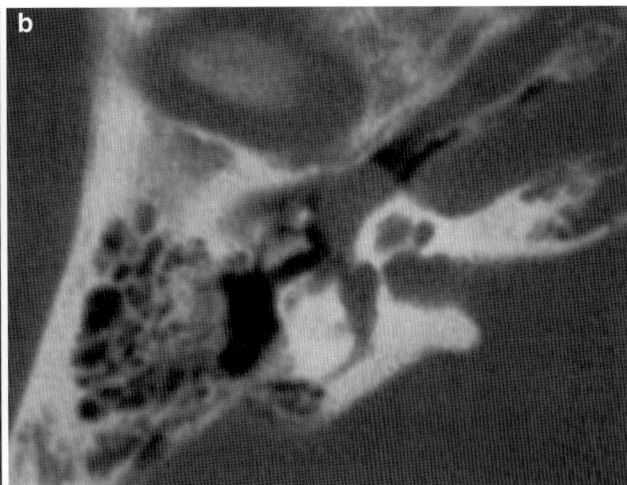

Fig. 42 Axial CT sections (**a** and **b**) through the temporal bone show a well-defined mass lesion over the cochlear promontory, involving the proximal tympanic segment of the facial nerve canal. The lesion impinges upon and displaces the head of the malleus leading to CHL. No permeative bone changes are seen associated to this small lesion. A retrotympanic vascular mass was disclosed on otoscopy. Diagnosis: Paraganglioma arising from paraganglionic cells over the cochlear promontory

seldom associated with facial nerve palsy. Neural connections with the glossopharyngeal nerve occur via the geniculate ganglion and the greater petrosal superficial nerve with the lesser petrosal nerve, between the facial nerve and the tympanic plexus as well as through the chorda tympani (Ozdogmus et al. 2004). The facial nerve also communicates with the auricular branch of the vagus nerve (Arnold's nerve) via its posterior auricular branch. Connections between sympathetic fibers include the vidian nerve, composed by the deep petrosal and greater superficial petrosal nerves (Veillon et al. 2010; Ozdogmus et al. 2004).

Bony dysplasias affecting the temporal bone may involve the facial nerve canal and lead to nerve dysfunction. These include otosclerosis, fibrous dysplasia, Paget's disease (Fig. 51), osteogenesis imperfecta, and osteoptrosis to mention the most common (Jethanamest and Roehm 2011; Zaytoun et al. 2008; Shonka and Kesser 2006). Temporal bone involvement by fibrous dysplasia is present in 24 % of cases although monostotic fibrous dysplasia of the temporal bone is exceedingly rare (Song et al. 2005). The most common clinical symptom is progressive conductive hearing loss (80 % of cases), secondary to stenosis or obliteration of the external auditory canal or ossicular chain dysfunction. FNP has been described in 10 % of patients as transient, recurrent or irreversible, most often due to direct compression or destruction of the bony canal by the dysplastic process but also secondary to otological complication of the disease such as cholesteatoma, keratosis obturans or abscess formation in the middle ear cavity (Jethanamest and Roehm 2011; Zaytoun et al. 2008; Shonka and Kesser 2006). Facial nerve palsy can also be a consequence of otosclerosis most commonly due to involvement of the facial nerve canal in the region of the choclear promontory or in the vicinity of the oval window immediately below the lateral semi-circular canal. The labyrinthine segment of the facial nerve can rarely be affected in patients with retrofenestral otosclerosis.

5. Parotid segment:

This segment of the nerve is most commonly affected by perineural spread of parotid malignancies. Any parotid neoplasm reaching the plane of the facial nerve (extending into the deep lobe of the parotid gland) may spread perineurally. Primary tumors affecting this segment are rare although a nerve sheath tumor should be included in the differential diagnosis of a benign appearing parotid mass, particularly when extending towards the stylomastoid foramen and mastoid segments of the facial nerve (Fig. 34). Parotid space infections seldom course with FNP (Kristensen and Hahn 2012; Noorizan et al. 2009).

Trauma to this segment is most often iatrogenic, during parotid surgery. Any parotid lesion extending into the deep lobe requires intra-operative monitoring of the facial nerve. Problems may arise with lesions that appear to arise from the parapharyngeal (Fig. 52) or submandibular spaces (Fig. 53) and are in fact originating from the deep lobe or inferior tail of the parotid gland, respectively.

6 Congenital and Pediatric Facial Nerve Paralysis

In pediatric patients facial nerve paralysis is 2 to 4 times less common than in adults and has some particular features both regarding clinical presentation and etiology (Finsterer 2008; Pavlou et al. 2011; Shargorodsky et al. 2010; Toelle and Boltshauser 2001). Similarly to adults, infection is the

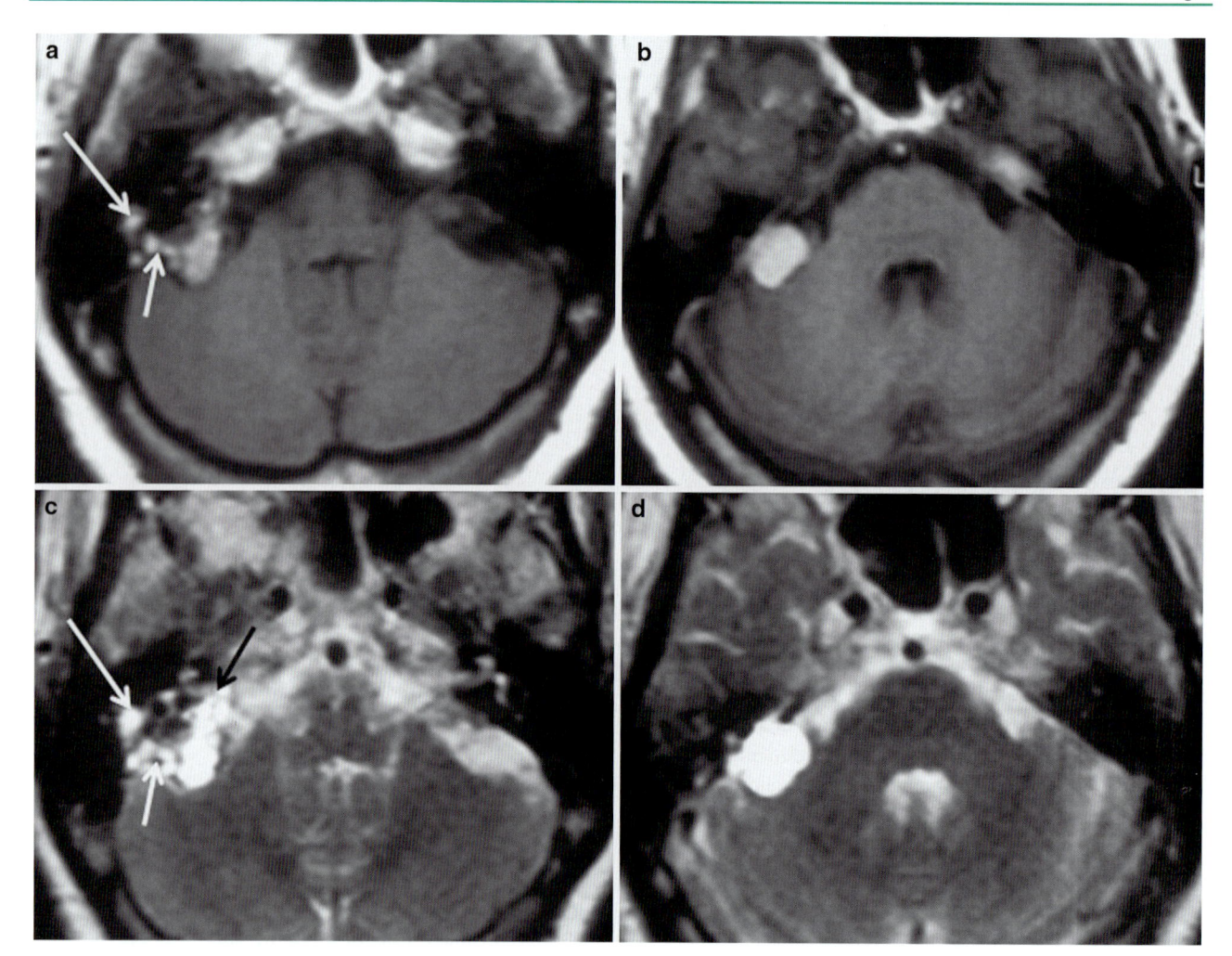

Fig. 43 Axial T1 W (**a** and **b**) and axial T2 W (**c** and **d**) MR images show a mass lesion at the posterior aspect of the petrous and mastoid bone centered in the region of the vestibular aqueduct and affecting the posterior tympanic (*long white arrows*) and mastoid segments (*short white arrows*) of the facial nerve canal. Impingement upon the posterior aspect of the porus acusticus and cisternal segment of the statoacustic bundle is also noted (*black arrow*). The lesion is heterogeneous in signal intensity, mostly hyperintense on both T1 W and T2 W images due to subacute hemmorrhage (intracellular metahemoglobin). Hypointense speckles best seen on T2, may reflect the presence of hemossiderin or bone fragments engulfed within the lesion. Diagnosis: Adenocarcinoma of the endolymphatic sac

leading cause of FNP however with a different prevalence of the various infectious agents. Children appear more susceptible to FNP secondary to viral and Borrelia infection (Lymes' disease) and, overall, show a more favorable outcome (Rizk et al. 2005; Burgio et al. 2000). Congenital causes rank second accounting for 8 to 14 % of all pediatric cases of facial nerve paralysis. Therefore, in this age group, one should always consider congenital abnormalities and be aware of normal variants that may mimic pathology. In neonates birth trauma is by far the leading cause, responsible for 88 % of all cases.

The most common anatomical variants of the facial nerve involve the temporal bone segments and include bony dehiscence of the fallopian canal, most often seen in the tympanic segment either in the region of the cochlear promontory or immediately below the lateral semi-circular canal, and anterior displacement of the mastoid segment of the facial nerve canal, laying immediately behind the posterior wall of the external auditory canal. These variants may occur in isolation but other associated abnormalities should be ruled out. They are particularly relevant whenever temporal bone surgery is being considered to avoid damage to the facial nerve. Facial nerve dehiscence at the level of the tympanic segment may lead to conductive hearing loss by impinging upon the stapes and oval window (Figs. 54 and 55).

In **newborns**, the diagnosis of facial nerve palsy is challenging and requires a high degree of suspicion. Not only are clinical signs nonspecific as they can be overshadowed by other defects, particularly when facial nerve palsy is part of a syndromic congenital malformation (Pavlou et al. 2011; Shargorodsky et al. 2010; Toelle and

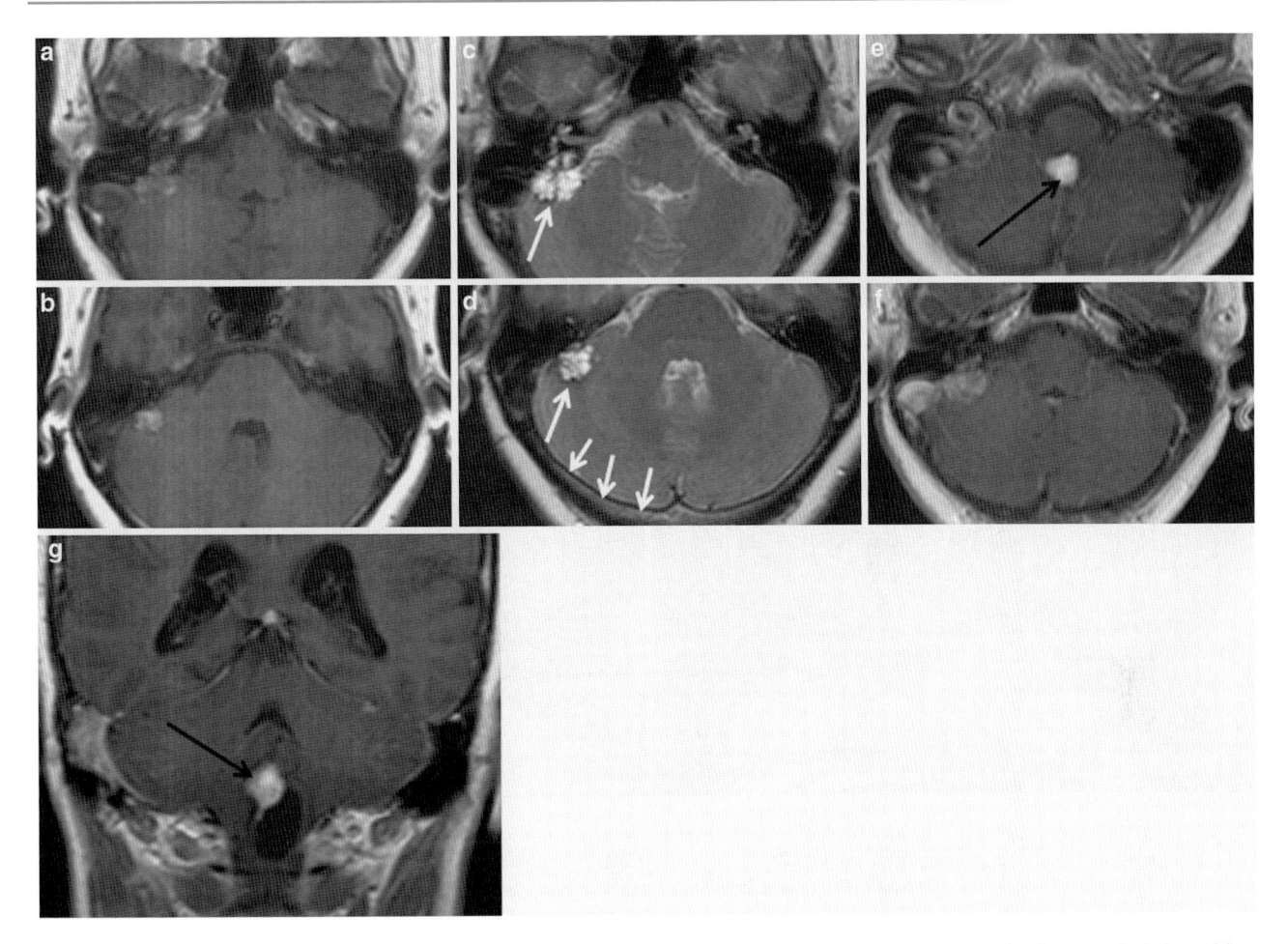

Fig. 44 Axial T1 W (**a** and **b**), T2 W (**c** and **d**) and gadolinium-enhanced axial (**e** and **f**) and coronal (**g**) T1 W images show a similar lesion (as in Fig. 43), spontaneously hyperintense on plain T1 W images, margined by an hypointense rim which can also be seen at the surface of the cerebellum reflecting the presence of hemossiderin and superficial siderosis (*white arrows* in **d**). A cystic lesion with an enhancing mural nodule is also depicted in the inferior vermis bulging into the IVth ventricle (*black arrows* in **e** and **g**). Diagnosis: Endolymphatic sac tumor and cerebellar hemangioblastoma in a patient with Von Hippel Lindau syndrome

Fig. 45 Post-gadolinium axial and coronal T1 W images demonstrate abnormal enhancement along the course of cranial nerves VII and VIII from the brainstem exit to the fundus of the IAC bilaterally (*white arrows*). Diagnosis: Bilateral breast cancer metastasis to the IAC in a 61 year old woman presenting with left FNP (*Courtesy of Prof. M. Lemmerling*)

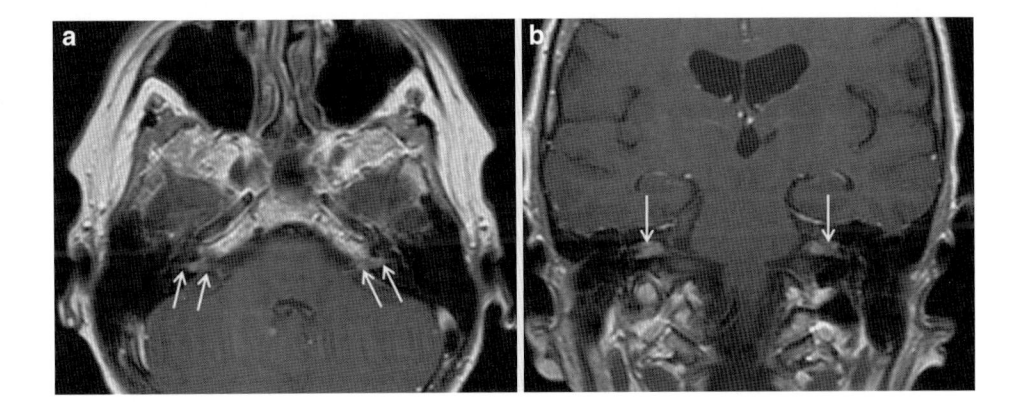

Boltshauser 2001). Asymmetric facial movements, difficulty feeding, and incomplete eye closure are the most striking findings in this age group and should raise the suspicion. Determining the etiology is of uttermost importance as treatment and prognosis differ widely depending on the underlying cause. Family and birth history, imaging studies, and neurophysiologic testing are the mainstays for etiologic diagnosis. Evidence of a difficult and prolonged labor due to cephalopelvic disproportion and the use of forceps suggest possible traumatic cause for the paralysis,

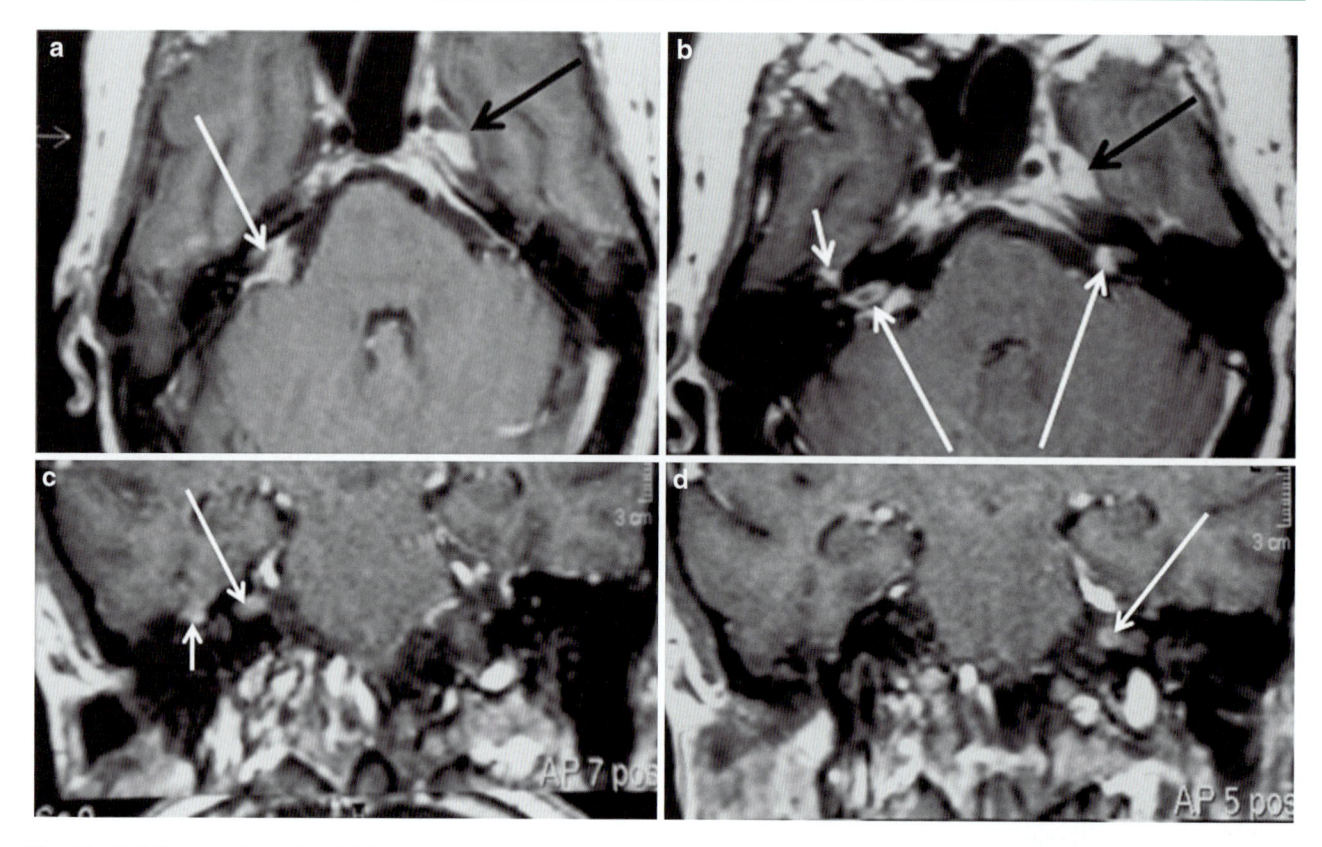

Fig. 46 Gadolinium-enhanced axial (**a** and **b**) and coronal (**c** and **d**) T1 W images show multiple nodular extra-axial enhancing lesions in the IAC bilaterally (*long white arrows*), in the right geniculate ganglion (*short white arrow*) and in Meckel's cave on the left (*black arrow*) in a patient presenting with multiple cranial nerve deficits and prior history of lung cancer. Diagnosis: Hematogenous metastasis

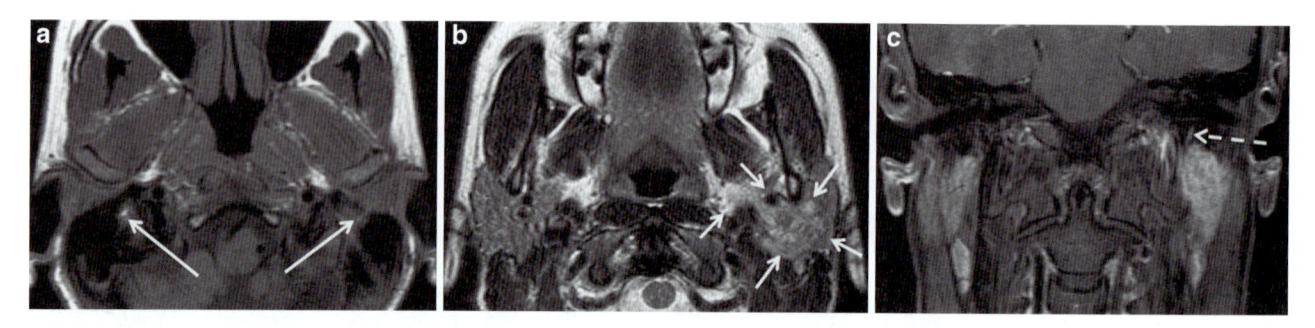

Fig. 47 Axial T1 (**a**) and T2 (**b**) and coronal post gadolinium T1 W MR images (**c**) show effacement of the stylomastoid neuroforaminal fat pad on the left side compared to the right (*long white arrows*), an ill-defined soft tissue mass within the right parotid gland extending into the deep lobe through the stylomandibular tunnel (*short white arrows*). After gadolinium administration, the lesion enhances heterogeneously and abnormal enhancement is also noted along the mastoid segment of the facial nerve (*dashed arrow*). Diagnosis: Perineural spread of adenoid cystic carcinoma in a 35-year-old woman with persistent left facial nerve palsy for 6 months. (*Courtesy of Prof. B. de Foer*)

whereas a positive family history of congenital malformations or of facial palsy in infancy or childhood raises the suspicion for a developmental cause (Al Tawil et al. 2010). Bilateral palsy is highly suggestive of a congenital defect and is exceedingly rare as a consequence of birth trauma. The latter is accompanied by other signs of trauma such as facial echymosis, hemotympanum and head deformity (Burgio et al. 2000; Al Tawil et al. 2010; Duval and Daniel 2009). A thorough neurological and general physical examination should be undertaken to exclude other cranial nerve palsies and neurological deficits as well as facial, ear, and limb malformations, the most commonly associated with congenital FNP (Pavlou et al. 2011; Toelle and Boltshauser 2001). Evaluation of the degree of paralysis is also important for patient's management and to predict functional rehabilitation.

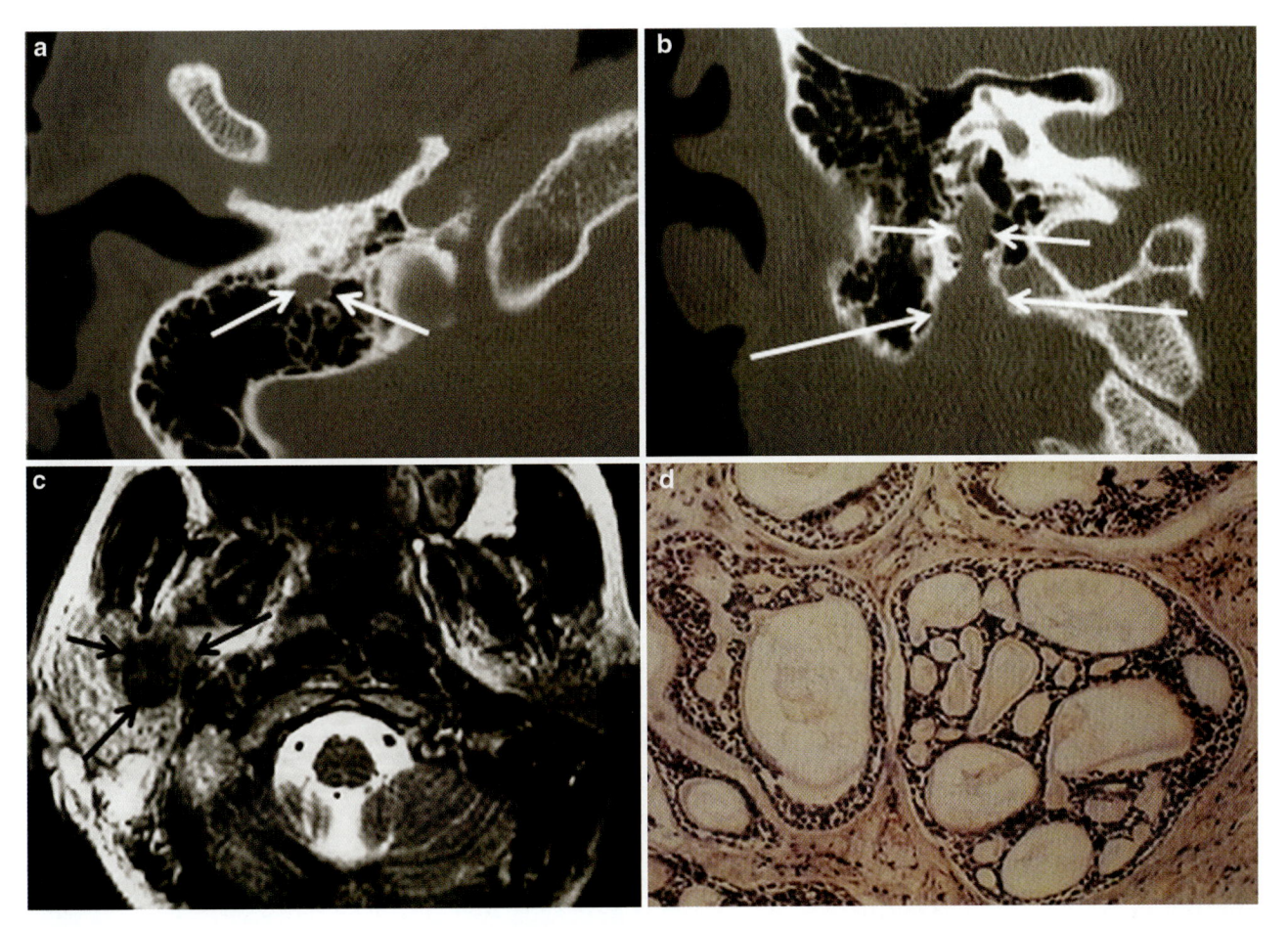

Fig. 48 Axial (**a**) and coronal (**b**) CT sections show widening of the styloid mastoid foramen (*long white arrows*) and an enlarged and remodeled facial nerve canal along the mastoid segment (*short white arrows*). Axial T2 W MR image (**c**) on the same patient demonstrates a parotid gland tumor widening the stylomandibular tunnel, laying at the presumed course of the facial nerve. The lesion is ill-defined and shows low signal intensity suggesting high cellularity (*black arrows*). Pathology specimen (HE magnification of 40Xs), shows nests of cells with neatly punched out spaces, which are not true ductal or glandular lumina but are in continuity with the supporting connective stroma. Diagnosis: Adenoid cystic carcinoma (cribiform type) with perineural spread along the facial nerve

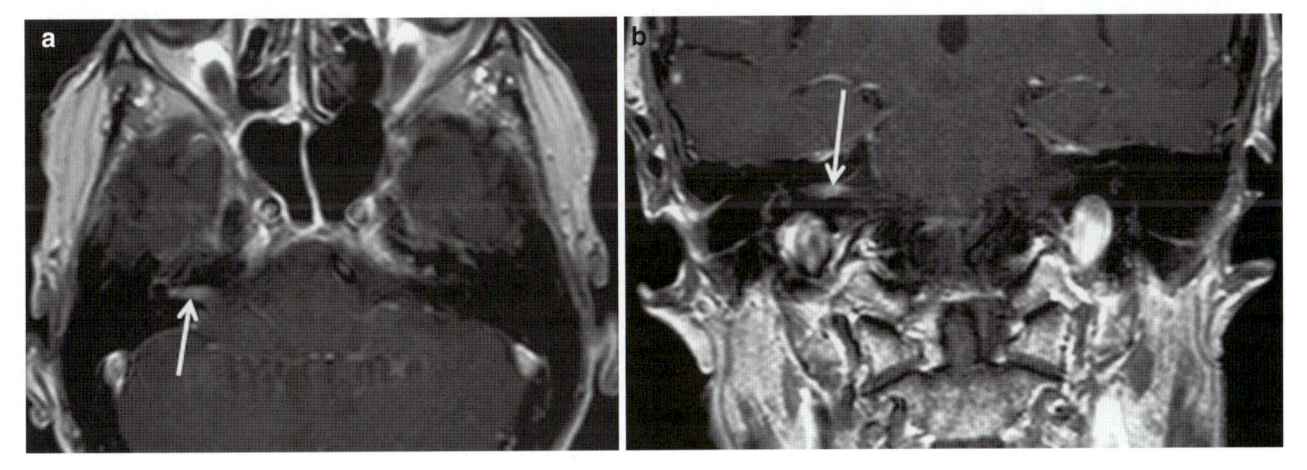

Fig. 49 Post-gadolinium axial (**a**) and coronal (**b**) MR images demonstrate abnormal enhancement along the IAC on the right side (*white arrows*) extending from the porus acusticus to the fundus. Diagnosis: Perineural spread of mantle cell lymphoma in a 79-year-old woman presenting with right facial nerve palsy. (*Courtesy of Prof. M. Lemmerling*)

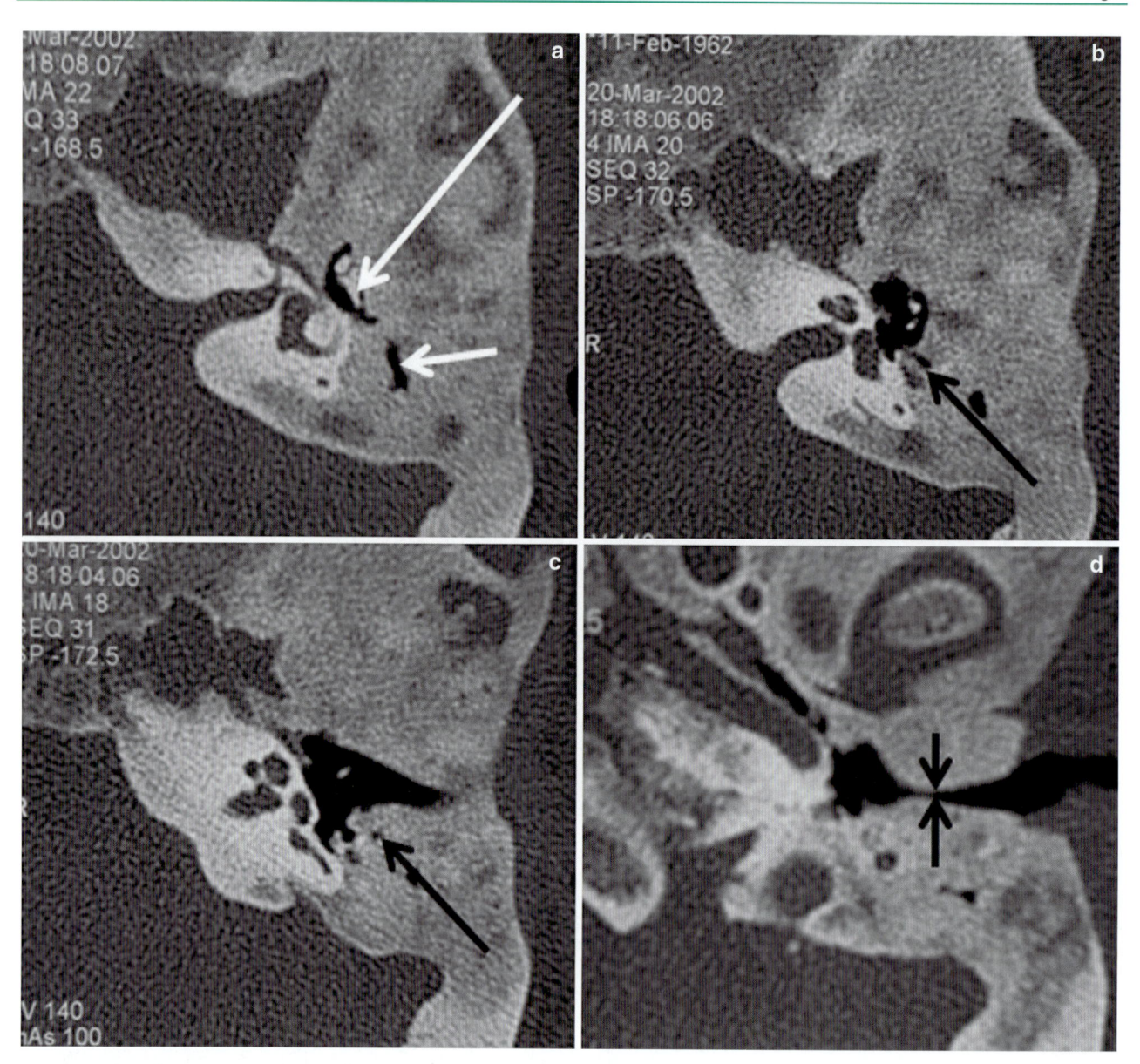

Fig. 50 Axial CT sections through the temporal bone (**a**, **b**, **c**, and **d**) show expansion and sclerosis of the temporal bone with a ground glass appearance, sparing the otic capsule. The bone expansion leads to obliteration of most mastoid air cells with a slit like tympanic cavity (*long white arrow*) and mastoid antrum (*short white arrow*). The facial nerve recess and mastoid facial nerve canal are stenotic (*black arrows*) leading to compressive ischemia of the nerve. Stenosis of the external auditory canal is also noted (*short black arrows*). Diagnosis: Fibrous dysplasia

The reported incidence of facial paralysis in live births is 8–20/10^4, among which 88 % are associated with a difficult labor (Shargorodsky et al. 2010; Al Tawil et al. 2010; Duval and Daniel 2009). **Birth trauma** is the most common cause of neonatal facial palsy with 67 to 90 % of cases resulting from forceps delivery (Duval and Daniel 2009). Additional risk factors include birth weight over 3,500 g and primiparity (Duval and Daniel 2009). Birth related FNP is typically unilateral, transient, and reversible in 90 % of cases, as complete transection of the facial nerve is rare. Neonates are particularly prone to pressure injury due to the underdevelopment of the mastoid and to the superficial course of the facial nerve after exiting the stylomastoid foramen. Pressure from the forceps blade upon the mastoid and parotid region can compress the vertical and/or the intraparotid segments of the nerve leading to transient ischemia (Pavlou et al. 2011; Al Tawil et al. 2010; Duval and Daniel 2009). Facial nerve trauma may also occur in utero, during difficult labor, from repeated pressure of the infant's face upon the sacral prominence.

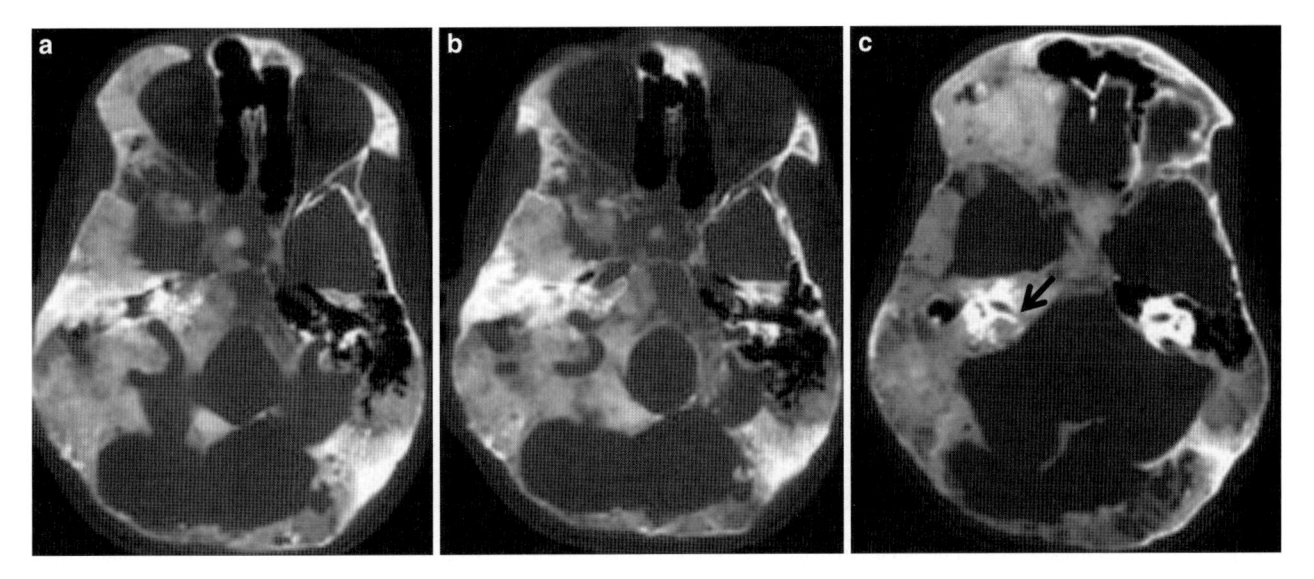

Fig. 51 Axial CT sections (**a**, **b**, and **c**) show expansion of the skull base, calvarium and temporal bone, more striking on the right side with a woven appearance of the trabecular bone. There is almost complete obliteration of the MEC on the right, severe stenosis of the IAC (*black arrow*) and stenosis of several skull base neurovascular foramina including all segments of the facial nerve canal. The otic capsule is partially spared. Diagnosis: Paget's disease

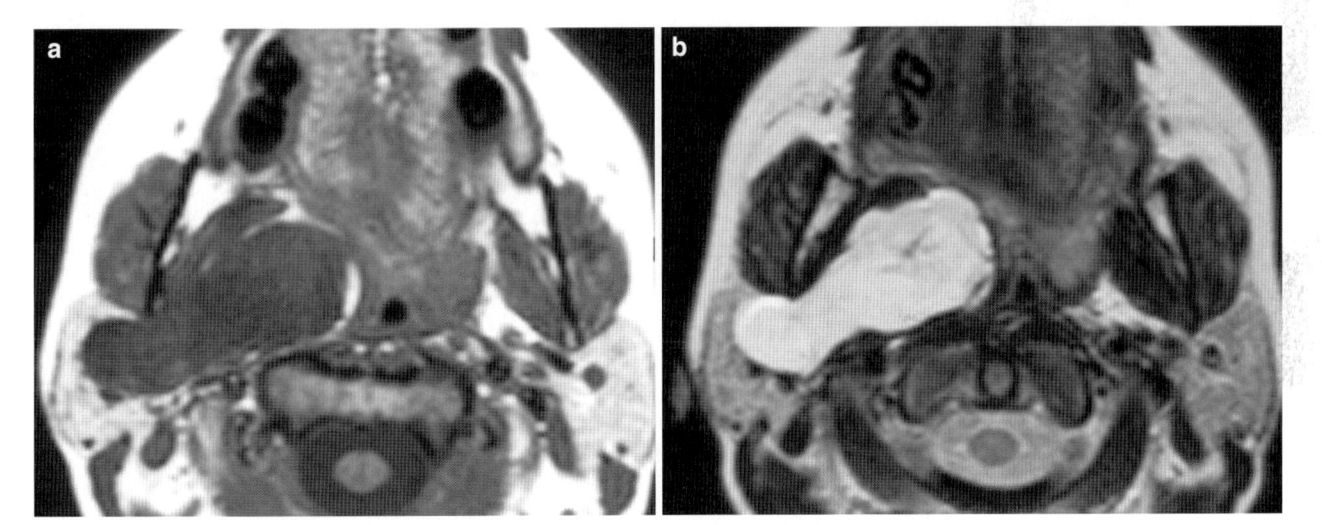

Fig. 52 Axial T1 and T2 W MR images show a large mass lesion involving the pre-styloid parapharyngeal space and deep lobe of the parotid gland enlarging the stylomandibular tunnel. In these circumstances it is difficult to assign the origin of the lesion and surgical resection requires facial nerve control. In this case the presence of a thin strip of fat surrounding the inner contour of the lesion suggests its origin from the deep lobe of the parotid gland. Diagnosis: Pleomorphic adenoma

Surgical management should be considered when the paralysis is complete and lasts over 3–5 days, when there is evidence of temporal bone trauma based on imaging and physical exam and when no improvement is noted by 5 weeks of age.

Developmental causes rank second in frequency and include those related to malformation syndromes and teratogens (Berker et al. 2004; Carvalho et al. 1999; Ferriby et al. 1998; Rahbar et al. 2001). These conditions bare a bad prognosis in terms of functional rehabilitation of the facial nerve. **Mobius syndrome** (oro-mandibular-limb hypogenesis) is the paradigm of developmental facial nerve paralysis with an incidence of $2–20/10^6$ births. It is characterized by bilateral facial nerve paralysis, uni- or bilateral paralysis of the abducens nerve and, on occasion, limb and chest wall abnormalities may also be present (Berker et al. 2004; Ferriby et al. 1998; Rahbar et al. 2001; Lima et al. 2009). Patients with this condition lack facial expression which can easily be mistaken for mental retardation (Lima et al. 2009). Although a few familial cases have been described, most cases are sporadic. Traumatic pregnancy and fetal exposure to drugs such as misoprostol, thalidomide, cocaine and ergotamine have been linked to this condition (Pavlou et al. 2011; Shargorodsky et al. 2010).

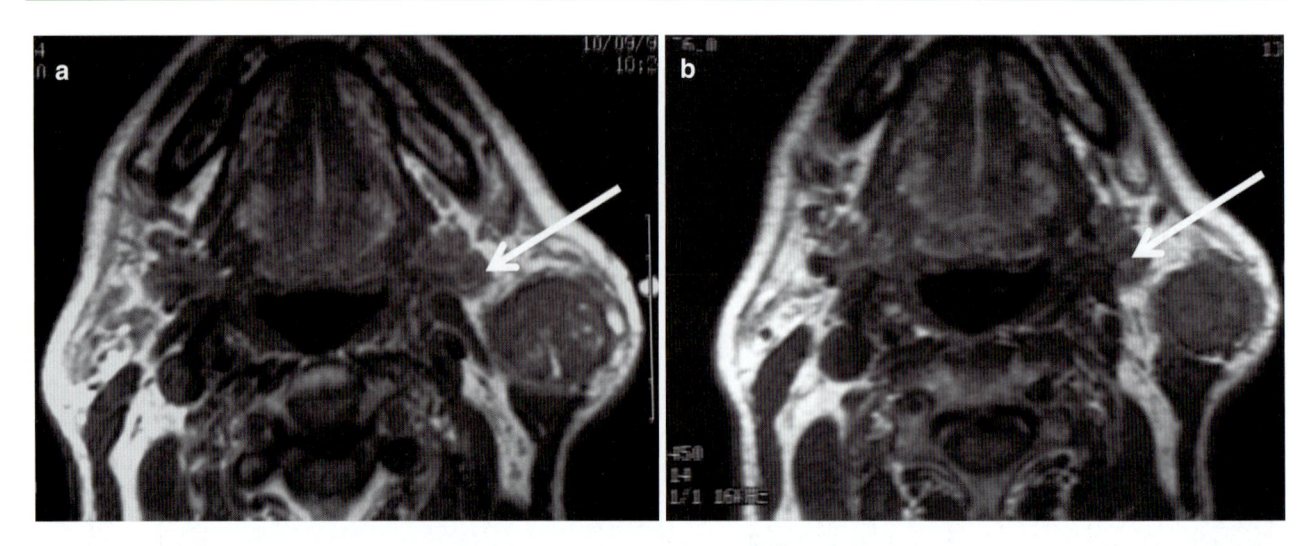

Fig. 53 Axial T1 W images through the submandibular space (**a** and **b**), show a rounded mass lesion below the angle of the mandible, in front of the anterior belly of the sternocleidomastoid muscle and behind and separated from the deep lobe of the submandibular gland (*white arrows*). The lesion is located in the parotid tail and surgical resection requires facial nerve control. Diagnosis: Mucoepidermoid carcinoma of the parotid gland

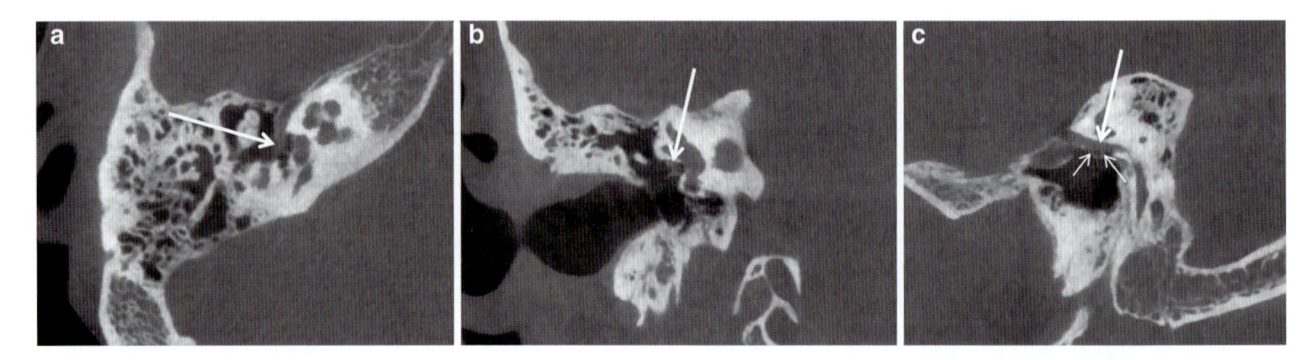

Fig. 54 MDCT of the right temporal bone: **a** Axial, **b** coronal, and **c** sagittal oblique sections in high resolution bone algorithm showing dehiscence of the tympanic segment of the facial nerve canal (*white arrows*), with inferior bulging of the nerve, impinging upon the crura of the stapes (*short white arrows*) and oval window in a 11-year-old boy with conductive hearing loss on the right

Fig. 55 MDCT axial and coronal sections through the right (**a** and **c**) and left (**b** and **d**) temporal bones show an abnormal course of the left facial nerve running beneath the oval window (*white arrows*). Note the normal course of the right facial nerve above the oval window and immediately below the lateral semi-circular canal (*black arrow*). Another associated abnormality, a monopodal stapes (*dashed white arrow*) is also noted which was responsible for the conductive hearing loss in this patient. Note the normal stapes with two crura on the right side (*short white arrows*). (Courtesy of Prof. B. de Foer)

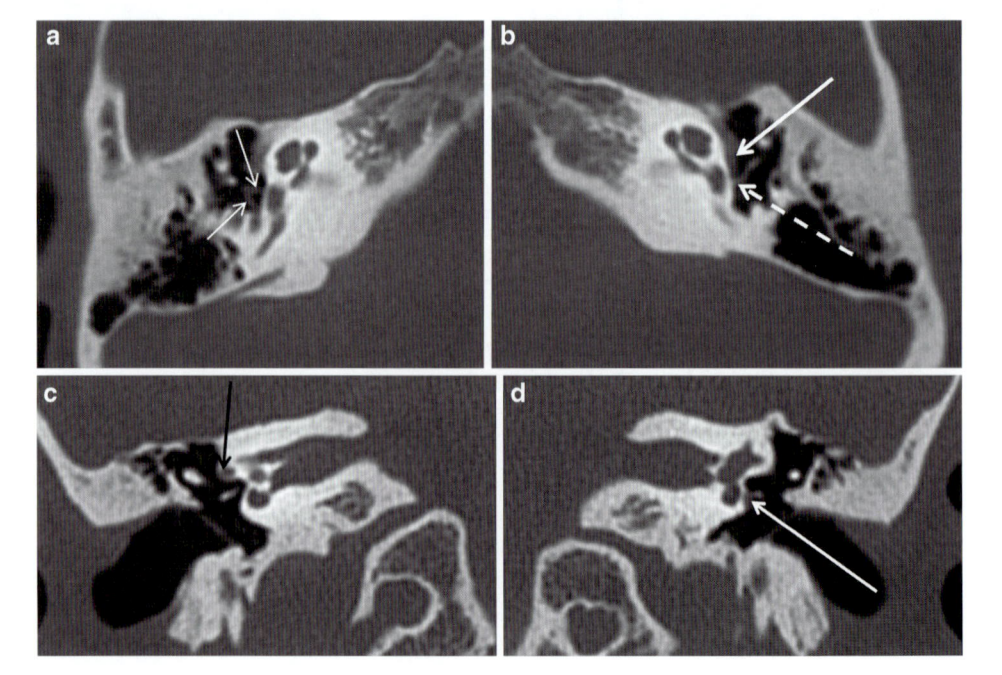

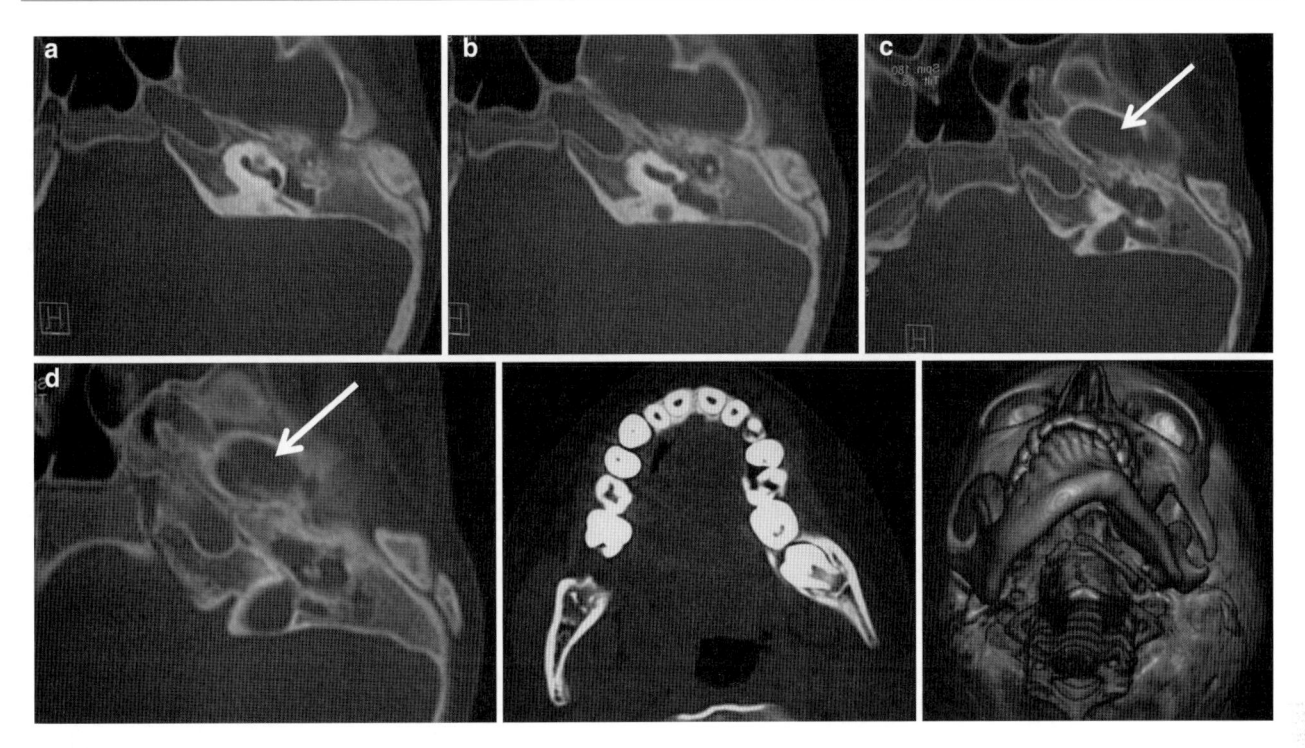

Fig. 56 Axial CT sections through the temporal bone (**a, b, c,** and **d**) show an hypoplastic and atretic MEC with underdeveloped, fused and malformed ossicles and an atretic oval window. A normal pyramidal eminence is not seen at the posterior wall of the tympanic cavity and the facial nerve recess is probably atretic. The tympanic and mastoid segments of the fallopian canal cannot be recognized either. Bony atresia of the EAC is also seen. Mastoid aeration is absent. There is an empty glenoid cavity due to condylar hypoplasia (*white arrows*). CT sections through the mandible show unilateral left sided mandibular hypoplasia leading to important facial asymmetry best seen on the 3D MIP reconstruction. Diagnosis: Hemifacial microsomia in a patient with CHL and facial nerve palsy

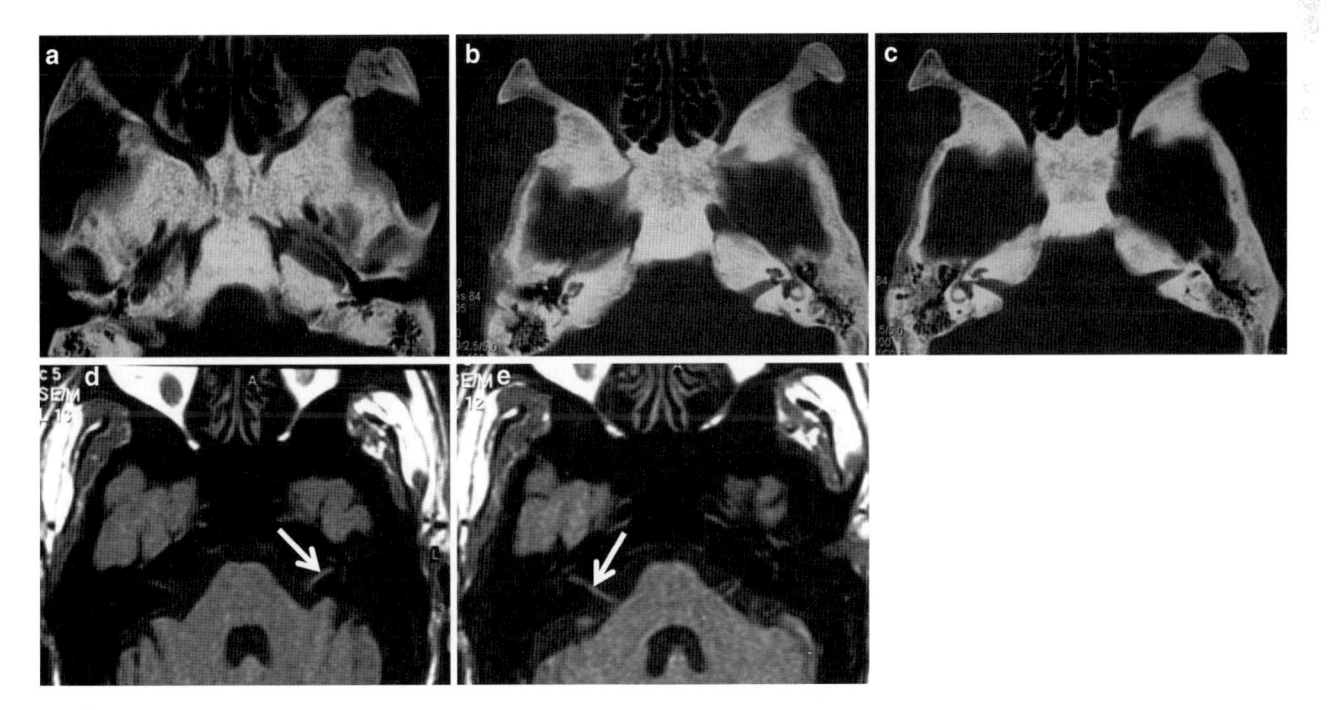

Fig. 57 Axial CT (**a, b,** and **c**) and axial T1 W MR sections (**d** and **e**) show severe sclerosis of the bony skull base and temporal bone with obliteration of the medullary cavity leading to loss of differentiation between spongiotic and cortical bone. On the MR images (**d** and **e**) stenosis of the IAC and stretching of the statoacustic bundle can be recognized (*white arrows*). The bone shows an homogeneous signal void with no recognizable bone marrow. Diagnosis: Ospeoptrosis (Albers-Schonberg disease)

Fig. 58 MDCT axial sections through the IAC in a 22 year-old woman with a known Mondini malformation (incomplete partition type 2) showing a congenital variant of the facial nerve canal, consisting on a separate bony canal anterior to the IAC seen bilaterally (*black arrows*)

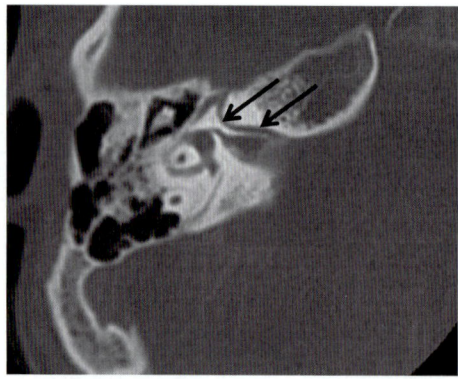

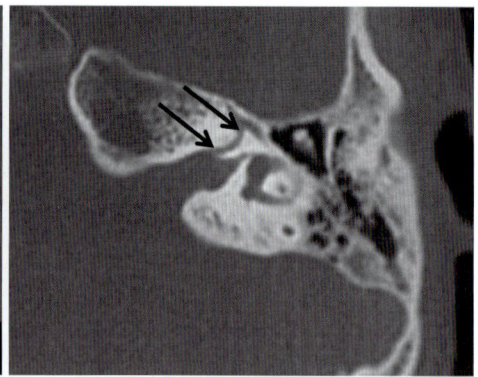

The pathophysiology of this syndrome is poorly understood and several theories have been proposed, all supported by autopsy findings: aplasia or hypoplasia of cranial nerve's nuclei, nuclear degeneration, peripheral nerve abnormality, primary myopathy and vascular disruption in the territory of the fetal subclavian artery (Lima et al. 2009; Dubrey et al. 2009). Neurophysiologic studies in patients with Mobius syndrome favor a nuclear or peripheral nerve dysfunction.

The hallmark of this disease on MR imaging is pontine hypoplasia, particularly involving the tegmentum, with effacement of the facial colliculi and a depressed floor of the IVth ventricle, secondary to aplasia or hypoplasia of the VI and VII cranial nerves nuclei and lower motor neurons (Fons-Estupina et al. 2007; Hillerer et al. 2007). Absence of the hypoglossal prominence can be seen in patients with CN XII hypoplasia and cerebellar hypoplasia has also been described. Moreover, structural facial abnormalities such as hypoglossia, micrognatia, cleft palate, and microtia are often disclosed.

Facioscapulohumeral muscular dystrophy is an autossomal dominant condition that can also present with facial diplegia at birth. As opposed to Mobius syndrome lateral gaze is intact and is characterized by a distal myopathy associated with facial weakness (de Greef et al. 2010).

A disorder commonly mistaken for unilateral facial nerve palsy in neonates is the congenital unilateral lower lip palsy (CULLP), a common disorder affecting 1 in 160 live births with no implications other then cosmesis, when isolated (Pratap et al. 2007). Pathophysiology of this disease is congenital absence or hypoplasia of the depressor anguli oris, the depressor of the inferior lip (Pratap et al. 2007; Kobayashi 1979). One should be aware that in 10 % of cases this condition is associated with other malformations, particularly heart defects, suggesting that this condition may be part of the spectrum of the velocardiofacial syndrome (Kobrynski and Sullivan 2007).

Velocardiofacial syndrome (DiGeorge syndrome) and cardiofacial syndrome are now known to be part of the 22q11.2 deletion syndrome and associate facial nerve palsy and congenital heart disease (Kobrynski and Sullivan 2007).

Hemifacial microsomia is another congenital condition that may course with facial nerve palsy and is part of the spectrum of oculo-auriculo-vertebral disorders secondary to developmental anomalies related to the first and second branchial arches (Berker et al. 2004; Ferriby et al. 1998; Rahbar et al. 2001). This condition is characterized mainly by conductive hearing loss due to external and middle ear abnormalities but sensorineural hearing loss and facial nerve dysfunction are often underappreciated although the latter has been reported in over 25 % of patients with this condition (Berker et al. 2004; Ferriby et al. 1998; Rahbar et al. 2001). Facial nerve abnormalities include abnormal course of the facial nerve canal, most often anterior displacement of the mastoid segment (Fig. 56), as well as segmental atresia of the facial nerve canal which cannot be identified in some patients (Rahbar et al. 2001).

Osteopetrosis, Albers-Schönberg or marble bone disease is a rare cause of facial nerve palsy that may present in the neonatal period or later in childhood. It is characterized by the presence of dense, brittle bones due to osteoclast dysfunction and failure of bone remodeling (Cure et al. 2000). Bone expansion can lead to cranial nerves compression, ischemia, and dysfunction (Fig. 57).

CHARGE syndrome, an acronym for coloboma, heart disease, choanal atresia, retarded growth, genitals hypoplasia, and ear anomalies, is associated with cranial nerves dysfunction in 75 % of cases with the facial nerve involved in 43 % (Abadie et al. 2000).

Most common teratogens associated with facial nerve paralysis include thalidomide and misoprostol (Lima et al. 2009; Dubrey et al. 2009). Thalidomide was widely used in the late 1950s as an antiemetic in pregnant women to treat morning sickness. Teratogenic effects included phacomelia, ear malformations and paralysis of the facial and abducens nerves. Misoprostol, a synthetic prostaglandin used to induce uterine contractions as an abortive drug, was also associated to the development of Mobius syndrome secondary to vascular disruption of the subclavian artery at the 4–6 week of pregnancy, leading to an ischemic brain event (Lima et al. 2009; Dubrey et al. 2009).

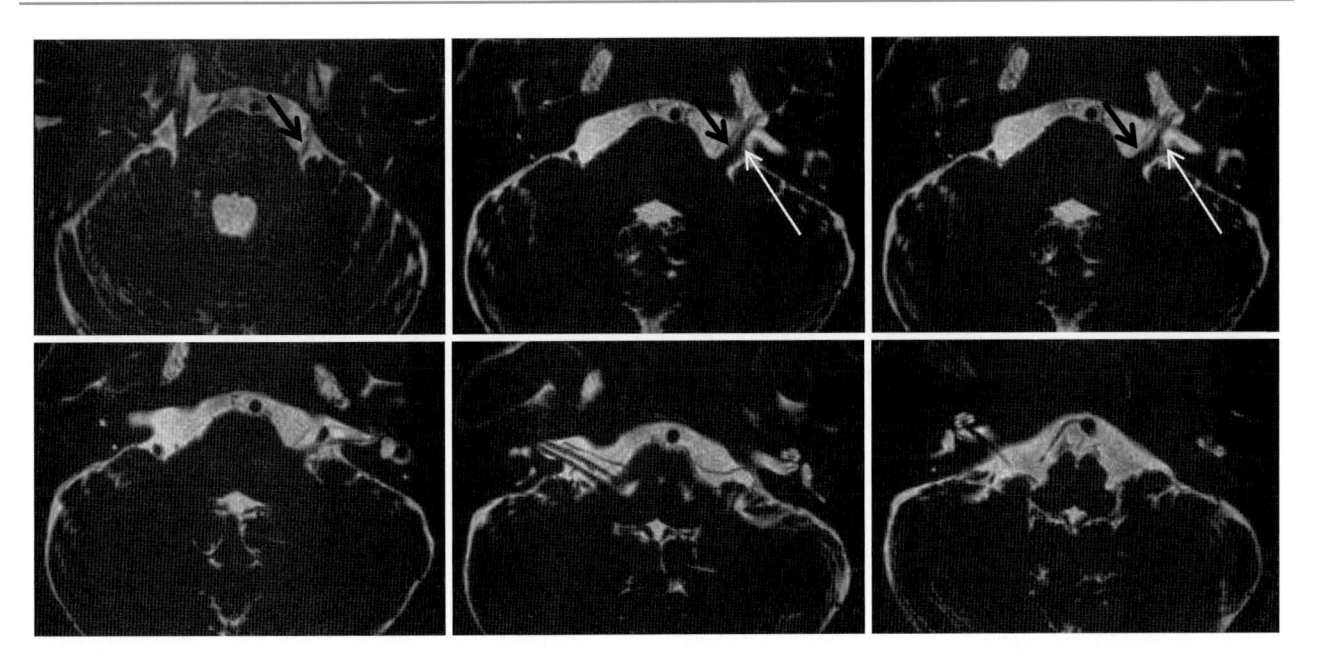

Fig. 59 Axial reconstructions from a 3D CISS MR acquisition in a 28-year-old man with a deaf ear on the left show agenesis of the left cochlear nerve and an abnormal origin of the left facial nerve (*white arrows*) emerging from the lateral pons together with the trigeminal nerve (*black arrows*). The cisternal V is displaced laterally and the IAC is much smaller compared to the normal contralateral side. Diagnosis: Cochlear nerve agenesis and joint origin of the trigeminal and facial nerves emerging from the same trunk at the lateral midpons. (*Courtesy of Prof. B. de Foer*)

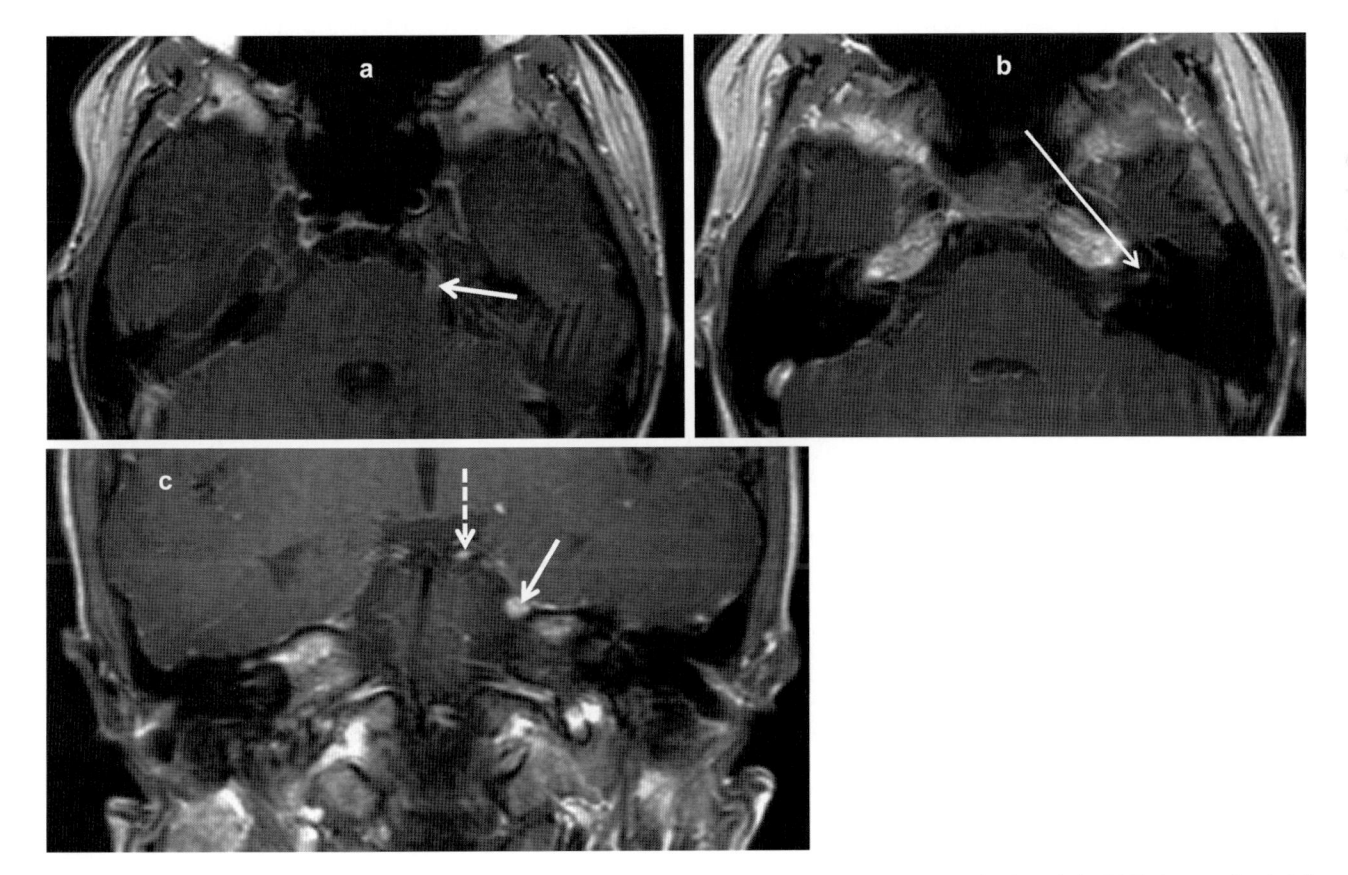

Fig. 60 Post gadolinium axial (**a** and **b**) and coronal (**c**) T1 W MR images in a 11-year-old girl presenting with facial nerve palsy on the left show abnormal enhancement along the cisternal course of the oculomotor nerve (*dashed arrow* in **c**), trigeminal nerve (*short white arrows* in **a** and **c**) and at the fundus of the IAC close to the facial nerve meatus (*long white arrow* in **b**) on the left side. Diagnosis: Lyme's disease (*Courtesy of Prof. M. Lemmerling*)

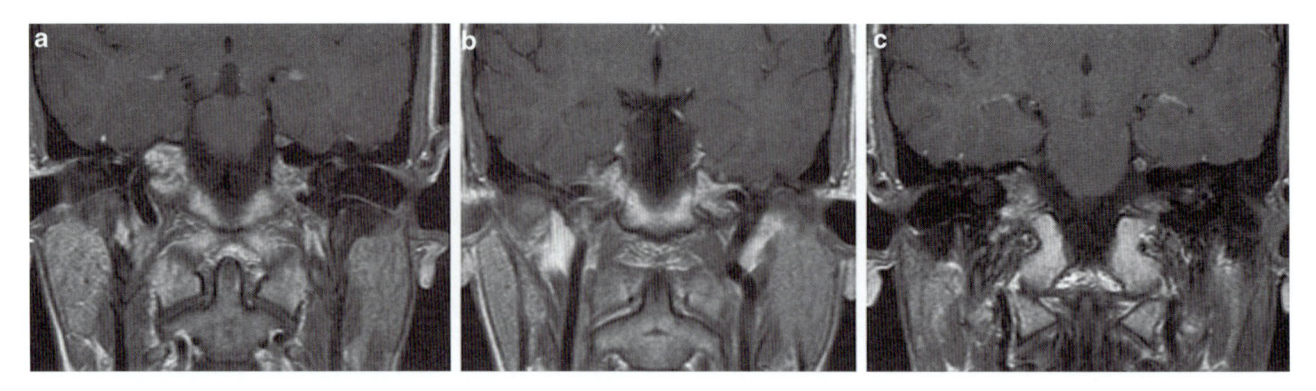

Fig. 61 Post-gadolinium coronal T1 W images (**a**, **b,** and **c**), show abnormal enhancement along in a 6 year old girl presenting with FNP. Prior history of a tick bite was elicited and serology was positive for Borrelia burgdorferi. Diagnosis: Lyme's disease (*Courtesy of Prof. B. de Foer*)

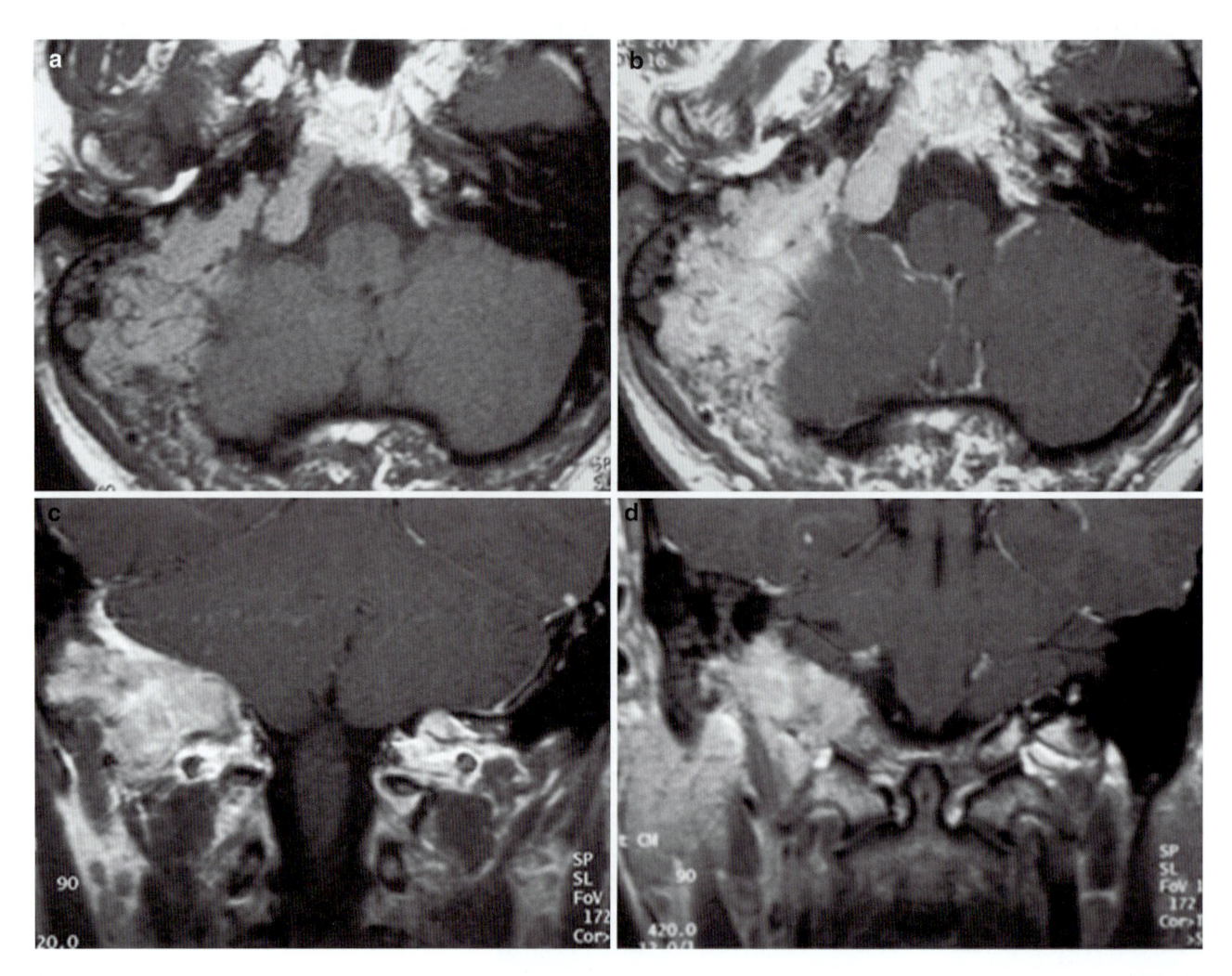

Fig. 62 Axial pre (**a**) and axial (**b**) and coronal (**c** and **d**) post-gadolinium T1 W images show a large lobulated mass replacing the mastoid bone and basi-occiput on the right with intermediate signal intensity on T1 W and showing vivid enhancement after gadolinium. The lesion involves the mastoid segment of the facial nerve canal and abuts the stylomastoid foramen. Diagnosis: Malignant teratoma in a child

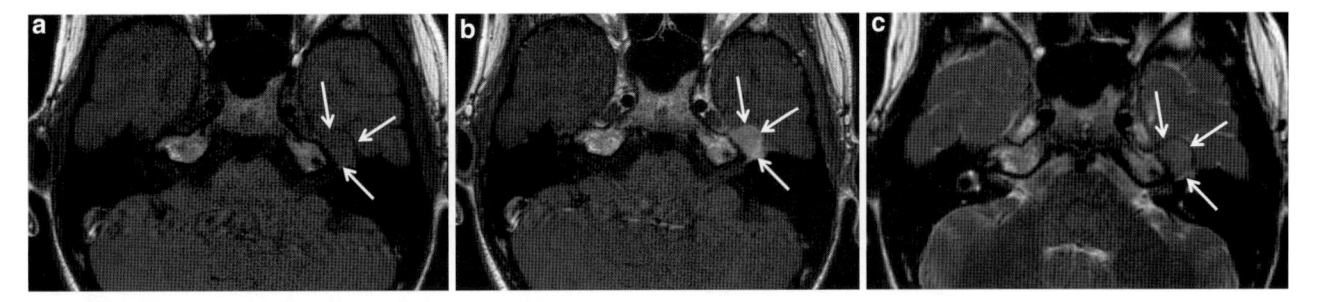

Fig. 63 Axial pre (**a**) and post-gadolinium (**b**) T1 W images and axial T2 W images through the temporal bone in a 11-year-old girl with left facial nerve palsy lasting for several months, show a well-defined lesion involvig the distal labyrinthine segment of the facial nerve and geniculate ganglion fossa (*white arrows*). The lesion is hypointense on T1 W, intermediate in signal intensity on T2 W and shows moderate homogeneous enhancement. A presumed diagnosis of facial nerve schwannoma was made at this point. A follow up CT scan performed 4 months later due to worsening symptoms including pain, show extensive bone destruction with a permeative pattern involving the anterior petrous bone and petrous apex. Note the destruction of the tegmen with tumor growth into the MEC (**d** and **e**) axial and (**f** and **g**) coronal reconstructions. There is also involvement of the labyrinthine and tympanic segments of the facial nerve over the cochlear promontory. The lesion is also shown to grow superiorly into the middle cranial fossa. At this point a follow up MR was obtained showing a striking increase in the size of the tumor mass (*white arrows*). Axial T1W (**h**), coronal T2W (**i**) and post gadolinium axial (**j**) and coronal (**k**) T1W images. Surgical excision disclosed Ewing's sarcoma on pathology and the patient was started on chemotherapy. (*Courtesy of Prof. B. de Foer*)

Fig. 63 continued

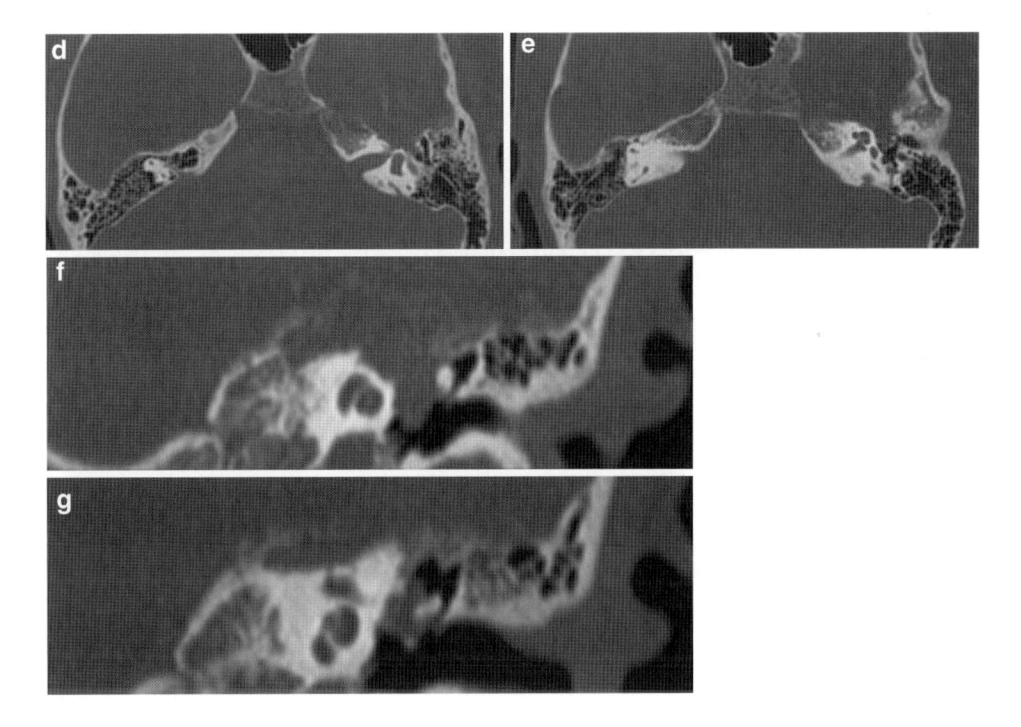

Many causes of congenital deafness course with abnormalities of the facial nerve and therefore one should always evaluate the entire course of the facial nerve in these patients particularly when a surgical intervention is being considered. Atresia of the EAC is associated with anterior displacement of the mastoid segment of the facial nerve which can be damaged when drilling the mastoid (Gassner et al. 2004) (Fig. 56). Mondini malformations, incomplete partition and agenesis/hypoplasia of the cochlear nerve are commonly associated with an abnormal course of the facial nerve (Figs. 58 and 59) (Curtin et al. 1982).

In children, other than neonates, the most common cause of FNP is infection with viral infection and Lyme's disease leading the list of pathogens involved (Pavlou et al. 2011; Burgio et al. 2000). In the USA, Lyme's disease (Figs. 60 and 61) has been reported as responsible for 50 % of all FNP in children (Siwula and Mathieu 2002). Common viral etiologies include herpetic gengivo-stomatitis, herpes

Fig. 63 continued

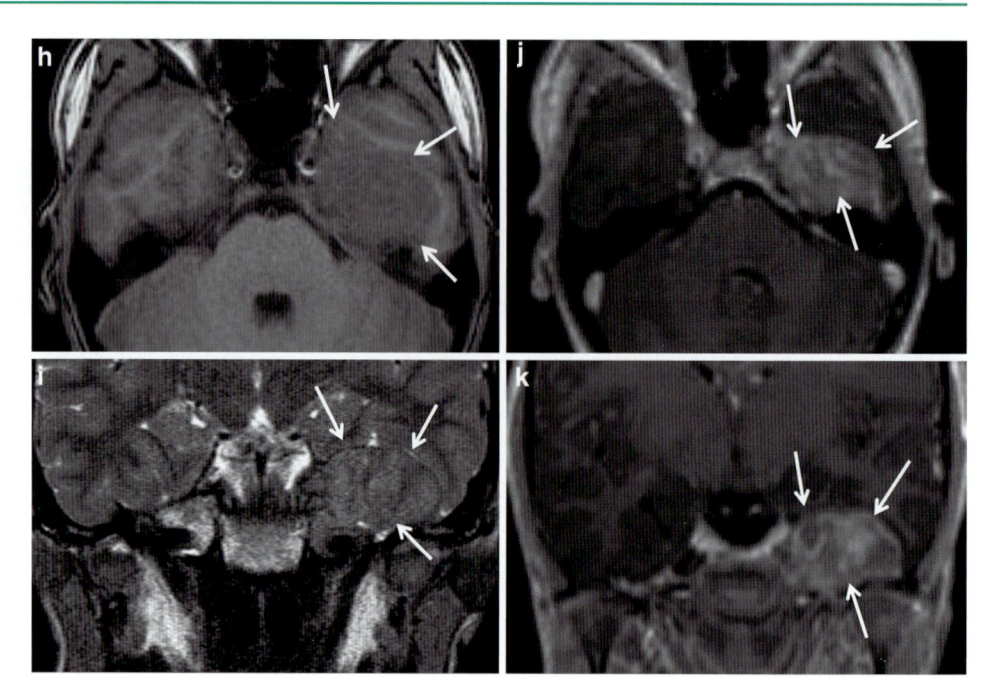

zoster, varicella zoster, mumps, rubeolla, cossackievirus and HIV. FNP may also be secondary to acute or chronic otitis media or meningitis, such as in adult patients.

FNP secondary to neoplasm is rare (Figs. 62 and 63). When present, one should suspect Langerhans cell histiocytosis, hematologic malignancies, rhabdomyosarcoma and metastatic neuroblastoma (Pavlou et al. 2011; Shargorodsky et al. 2010). Facial nerve palsy in histiocytosis may be secondary to involvement of the temporal bone by histiocytic masses or from leptomeningeal coating of the cisternal segment of the facial nerve.

Other rare causes in children include Guillain-Barré syndrome, sarcoidosis and Melkersson-Rosenthal syndrome (Ferriby et al. 1998). The latter is a rare neuromucocutaneous disease coursing with recurrent facial nerve palsy, facial edema, and a fissured tongue, often presenting during childhood or adolescence. A genetic predisposition has been reported as well as an association with Chron's disease and sarcoidosis (Ferriby et al. 1998).

7 Bilateral Facial Nerve Paralysis

Bilateral facial nerve palsy or facial diplegia is rare and is often an ominous sign ((Kim et al. 2008). It is a typical feature of Mobius syndrome and may also be seen is certain acute polyneuropathies such as Guillain-Barré and Miller Fisher syndromes and infections such as in Lyme's disease and several viral neuronitis (Coddington et al. 2010; Atsumi et al. 2004; Yardimci et al. 2009; Balatsouras et al. 2007). Nuclear lesions affecting the pontine tegmentum can also course with facial diplegia such as brainstem encephalitis, pontine neoplasms and post-traumatic tegmental pontine hemmorrhages. Diffuse basilar meningitis, of infectious or noninfectious etiology, may involve the cisternal segment of both facial nerves and lead to bilateral palsy. These comprise tuberculous and cryptococal meningitis, sarcoidosis, histiocytosis, and leptomeningeal carcinomatosis including involvement by hematologic malignancies (Ferrari et al. 2004; Mohebbi et al. 2011; Ozaki et al. 2011). Facial diplegia has also been reported in diabetes, systemic lupus, Kawasaki disease, and bulbospinal neuronopathy (Lim et al. 2009; Price and Fife 2002; Fogarty et al. 2006). Although the most common cause of FNP, Bell's palsy is rarely bilateral.

References

Borges A (2005) Trigeminal neuralgia and facial nerve paralysis. Eur Radiol 15(3):511–533
Benecke JE Jr (2002) Facial paralysis. Otolaryngol Clin North Am 35(2):357–365
Rainsbury JW, Aldren CP (2007) Facial nerve palsy. Clin Otolaryngol 32(1):38–40 discussion 41
Roob G, Fazekas F, Hartung HP (1999) Peripheral facial palsy: etiology, diagnosis and treatment. Eur Neurol 41(1):3–9
Syed I, Bhutta M (2008) Facial nerve palsy: assessment and management. Br J Hosp Med (Lond) 69(3):M34–M37
Borges A, Casselman J (2007a) Imaging the cranial nerves: Part I: methodology, infectious and inflammatory, traumatic and congenital lesions. Eur Radiol 17(8):2112–2125
Phillips CD, Bubash LA (2002) The facial nerve: anatomy and common pathology. Semin Ultrasound CT MR 23(3):202–217
Raghavan P, Mukherjee S, Phillips CD (2009) Imaging of the facial nerve. Neuroimaging Clin N Am 19(3):407–425
Finsterer J (2008) Management of peripheral facial nerve palsy. Eur Arch Otorhinolaryngol 265(7):743–752

Jager L, Reiser M (2001) CT and MR imaging of the normal and pathologic conditions of the facial nerve. Eur J Radiol 40(2):133–146

Veillon F et al (2010) Imaging of the facial nerve. Eur J Radiol 74(2):341–348

Sittel C, Stennert E (2001) Prognostic value of electromyography in acute peripheral facial nerve palsy. Otol Neurotol 22(1):100–104

Valls-Sole J (2007) Electrodiagnostic studies of the facial nerve in peripheral facial palsy and hemifacial spasm. Muscle Nerve 36(1):14–20

Yeong SS, Tassone P (2011) Acute unilateral facial nerve palsy. Aust Fam Physician 40(5):296–298

Veillon F et al (2008) Pathology of the facial nerve. Neuroimaging Clin N Am 18(2):309–320 x

Peitersen E (2002) Bell's palsy: the spontaneous course of 2,500 peripheral facial nerve palsies of different etiologies. Acta Otolaryngol Suppl 549:4–30

Al-Noury K, Lotfy A (2011) Normal and pathological findings for the facial nerve on magnetic resonance imaging. Clin Radiol 66(8):701–707

Linder TE, Abdelkafy W, Cavero-Vanek S (2010) The management of peripheral facial nerve palsy: "paresis" versus "paralysis" and sources of ambiguity in study designs. Otol Neurotol 31(2):319–327

Lorch M, Teach SJ (2010) Facial nerve palsy: etiology and approach to diagnosis and treatment. Pediatr Emerg Care 26(10):763–769 quiz 770-3

Kumar A, Mafee MF, Mason T (2000) Value of imaging in disorders of the facial nerve. Top Magn Reson Imaging 11(1):38–51

Kinoshita T et al (2001) Facial nerve palsy: evaluation by contrast-enhanced MR imaging. Clin Radiol 56(11):926–932

Iwai H et al (2000) Consecutive imaging of the facial nerve using high-resolution magnetic resonance imaging. Acta Otolaryngol Suppl 542:39–43

Burmeister HP et al (2010) CT and MR imaging of the facial nerve. HNO 58(5):433–442

Ishibashi M et al (2010) The ability to identify the intraparotid facial nerve for locating parotid gland lesions in comparison to other indirect landmark methods: evaluation by 3.0 T MR imaging with surface coils. Neuroradiology 52(11):1037–1045

Qin Y et al (2011) 3D double-echo steady-state with water excitation MR imaging of the intraparotid facial nerve at 1.5T: a pilot study. AJNR Am J Neuroradiol 32(7):1167–1172

Shelton C (2000) Preoperative identification of the facial nerve achieved using fast spin-echo MR imaging: can it help the surgeon? AJNR Am J Neuroradiol 21(5):805

Tada Y et al (2000) Identification of the intraparotid facial nerve on magnetic resonance imaging. Acta Otolaryngol Suppl 542:49–53

Burmeister HP et al (2009) Improvement of visualization of the intermediofacial nerve in the temporal bone using 3T magnetic resonance imaging: part 1: the facial nerve. J Comput Assist Tomogr 33(5):782–788

Lim HK et al (2012) MR diagnosis of facial neuritis: diagnostic performance of contrast-enhanced 3D-FLAIR technique compared with contrast-enhanced 3D-T1-fast-field echo with fat suppression. AJNR Am J Neuroradiol 33(4):779–783

Gerganov VM et al (2011) Diffusion tensor imaging-based fiber tracking for prediction of the position of the facial nerve in relation to large vestibular schwannomas. J Neurosurg 115(6):1087–1093

Roundy N, Delashaw JB, Cetas JS (2012) Preoperative identification of the facial nerve in patients with large cerebellopontine angle tumors using high-density diffusion tensor imaging. J Neurosurg 116(4):697–702

Borges A (2010) Imaging cranial nerves and the brachial plexus. Eur J Radiol 74(2):287

Borges A, Casselman J (2007b) Imaging the cranial nerves: part II: primary and secondary neoplastic conditions and neurovascular conflicts. Eur Radiol 17(9):2332–2344

Sherman SC, Thompson TM (2005) Pontine hemorrhage presenting as an isolated facial nerve palsy. Ann Emerg Med 46(1):64–66

Agarwal R et al (2011) Pontine stroke presenting as isolated facial nerve palsy mimicking Bell's palsy: a case report. J Med Case Rep 5:287

Novy J et al (2008) Isolated nuclear facial palsy, a rare variant of pure motor lacunar stroke. Clin Neurol Neurosurg 110(4):420–421

Roh JK, Kim BK, Chung JM (1999) Combined peripheral facial and abducens nerve palsy caused by caudal tegmental pontine infarction. Eur Neurol 41(2):99–102

Thomke F et al (2002) Seventh nerve palsies may be the only clinical sign of small pontine infarctions in diabetic and hypertensive patients. J Neurol 249(11):1556–1562

Arnaout OM et al (2009) Posterior fossa arteriovenous malformations. Neurosurg Focus 26(5):E12

Mathai K (2009) The enigma of traumatic, behaviourally benign brainstem bleeds: case report. IJNT 6(2):141–144

Parizel PM et al (2002) Brainstem hemorrhage in descending transtentorial herniation (Duret hemorrhage). Intensive Care Med 28(1):85–88

Oppenheim C et al (2000) False-negative diffusion-weighted MR findings in acute ischemic stroke. AJNR Am J Neuroradiol 21(8):1434–1440

Braga BP et al (2006) Cavernous malformations of the brainstem in infants. Report of two cases and review of the literature. J Neurosurg 104(6 Suppl):429–433

Giliberto G et al (2010) Brainstem cavernous malformations: anatomical, clinical, and surgical considerations. Neurosurg Focus 29(3):E9

Duckworth EA (2010) Modern management of brainstem cavernous malformations. Neurol Clin 28(4):887–898

Zausinger S et al (2006) Cavernous malformations of the brainstem: three-dimensional-constructive interference in steady-state magnetic resonance imaging for improvement of surgical approach and clinical results. Neurosurgery 58(2):322–330 discussion 322-30

Critchley EP (2004) Multiple sclerosis initially presenting as facial palsy. Aviat Space Environ Med 75(11):1001–1004

Carter S, Sciarra D, Merritt HH (1950) The course of multiple sclerosis as determined by autopsy proven cases. Res Publ Assoc Res Nerv Ment Dis 28:471–511

Fukazawa T et al (1997) Facial palsy in multiple sclerosis. J Neurol 244(10):631–633

Schnorpfeil F, Braune HJ (1997) Nuclear facial palsy in multiple sclerosis: a case report. Electromyogr Clin Neurophysiol 37(4):207–211

Telischi FF et al (1991) Hemifacial spasm. Occurrence in multiple sclerosis. Arch Otolaryngol Head Neck Surg 117(5):554–556

Haacke EM et al (2009) Characterizing iron deposition in multiple sclerosis lesions using susceptibility weighted imaging. J Magn Reson Imaging 29(3):537–544

Grabner G et al (2011) Analysis of multiple sclerosis lesions using a fusion of 3.0 T FLAIR and 7.0 T SWI phase: FLAIR SWI. J Magn Reson Imaging 33(3):543–549

Davies RS, Burgin M (1996) MRI appearances of *Listeria rhombencephalitis*. Australas Radiol 40(3):354–356

Alper G, Knepper L, Kanal E (1996) MR findings in *listerial rhombencephalitis*. AJNR Am J Neuroradiol 17(3):593–596

Mori M et al (2008) Bickerstaff's brainstem encephalitis after an outbreak of *Campylobacter jejuni* enteritis. J Neuroimmunol 196(1–2):143–146

Nicolao P et al (2011) Bickerstaff's brainstem encephalitis: case report and Tc99 m brain SPECT findings. Neurol Sci 32(6):1153–1156

Chataway SJ, Larner AJ, Kapoor R (2001) Anti-GQ1b antibody status, magnetic resonance imaging, and the nosology of Bickerstaff's brainstem encephalitis. Eur J Neurol 8(4):355–357

Laigle-Donadey F, Doz F, Delattre JY (2008) Brainstem gliomas in children and adults. Curr Opin Oncol 20(6):662–667

Boop FA (2011) Brainstem gliomas. J Neurosurg Pediatr 8(6):537–538 discussion 538

Leach PA et al (2008) Diffuse brainstem gliomas in children: should we or shouldn't we biopsy? Br J Neurosurg 22(5):619–624

Sedrak P et al (2011) Erdheim-Chester disease of the central nervous system: new manifestations of a rare disease. AJNR Am J Neuroradiol 32(11):2126–2131

Chavin JM (2003) Cranial neuralgias and headaches associated with cranial vascular disorders. Otolaryngol Clin North Am 36(6):1079–1093 vi

Chang JW et al (2002) Role of postoperative magnetic resonance imaging after microvascular decompression of the facial nerve for the treatment of hemifacial spasm. Neurosurgery 50(4):720–725 discussion 726

Chung SS et al (2000) Microvascular decompression of the facial nerve for the treatment of hemifacial spasm: preoperative magnetic resonance imaging related to clinical outcomes. Acta Neurochir (Wien) 142(8):901–906 discussion 907

Fukuda H, Ishikawa M, Okumura R (2003) Demonstration of neurovascular compression in trigeminal neuralgia and hemifacial spasm with magnetic resonance imaging: comparison with surgical findings in 60 consecutive cases. Surg Neurol 59(2):93–99 discussion 99-100

Leal PR, Froment JC, Sindou M (2009) Predictive value of MRI for detecting and characterizing vascular compression in cranial nerve hyperactivity syndromes (trigeminal and facial nerves). Neurochirurgie 55(2):174–180

Leal PR, Froment JC, Sindou M (2010) MRI sequences for detection of neurovascular conflicts in patients with trigeminal neuralgia and predictive value for characterization of the conflict (particularly degree of vascular compression). Neurochirurgie 56(1):43–49

Lutz J et al (2011) Trigeminal neuralgia due to neurovascular compression: high-spatial-resolution diffusion-tensor imaging reveals microstructural neural changes. Radiology 258(2):524–530

Leal PR et al (2011) Structural abnormalities of the trigeminal root revealed by diffusion tensor imaging in patients with trigeminal neuralgia caused by neurovascular compression: a prospective, double-blind, controlled study. Pain 152(10):2357–2364

Bonneville F, Savatovsky J, Chiras J (2007) Imaging of cerebellopontine angle lesions: an update. Part 2: intra-axial lesions, skull base lesions that may invade the CPA region, and non-enhancing extra-axial lesions. Eur Radiol 17(11):2908–2920

Ishikura R et al (2010) High Resolution Three-dimensional T(2)*-weighted Imaging at 3T: Findings of Cerebellopontine Angle Schwannomas and Meningiomas. Magn Reson Med Sci 9(4):177–178

Roche PH, Regis J (2005) Cerebellopontine angle meningiomas. J Neurosurg 103(5):935–937 author reply 937-8

Roser F et al (2005) Meningiomas of the cerebellopontine angle with extension into the internal auditory canal. J Neurosurg 102(1):17–23

Iwai Y, Yamanaka K, Nakajima H (2001) Hemifacial spasm due to cerebellopontine angle meningiomas–two case reports. Neurol Med Chir (Tokyo) 41(2):87–89

Nakamura M et al (2005) Facial and cochlear nerve function after surgery of cerebellopontine angle meningiomas. Neurosurgery 57(1):77–90 discussion 77-90

Revuelta-Gutierrez R et al (2009) Cerebellopontine angle epidermoid cysts. Experience of 43 cases with long-term follow-up Cir Cir 77(4):257-65–241-8

Akhavan-Sigari R et al (2007) Epidermoid cysts of the cerebellopontine angle with extension into the middle and anterior cranial fossae: surgical strategy and review of the literature. Acta Neurochir (Wien) 149(4):429–432

Alaani A et al (2005) Cerebellopontine angle arachnoid cysts in adult patients: what is the appropriate management? J Laryngol Otol 119(5):337–341

Nguyen JB et al (2004) Magnetic resonance imaging and proton magnetic resonance spectroscopy of intracranial epidermoid tumors. Crit Rev Comput Tomogr 45(5–6):389–427

Bohne S et al (2010) Bilateral deafness and unilateral facial nerve palsy as presenting features of Wegener's granulomatosis : a case report. HNO 58(5):480–483

Caldas AR et al (2012) Hypertrophic cranial pachymeningitis and skull base osteomyelitis by pseudomonas aeruginosa: case report and review of the literature. J Clin Med Res 4(2):138–144

Yamashita H et al (2012) Hypertrophic pachymeningitis and tracheobronchial stenosis in IgG4-related disease: case presentation and literature review. Intern Med 51(8):935–941

Vale TC et al (2013) Cranial hypertrophic pachymeningitis secondary to neurocysticercosis. Neurol Sci 34(3):401–403

Christakis PG, Machado DG, Fattahi P (2012) Idiopathic hypertrophic pachymeningitis mimicking neurosarcoidosis. Clin Neurol Neurosurg 114(2):176–178

Pai S et al (2007) Idiopathic hypertrophic spinal pachymeningitis: report of two cases with typical MR imaging findings. AJNR Am J Neuroradiol 28(3):590–592

Lee YC et al (2003) Idiopathic hypertrophic cranial pachymeningitis: case report with 7 years of imaging follow-up. AJNR Am J Neuroradiol 24(1):119–123

Friedman DP, Flanders AE (1997) Enhanced MR imaging of hypertrophic pachymeningitis. AJR Am J Roentgenol 169(5):1425–1428

Spiegel DR, Morris K, Rayamajhi U (2012) Neurosarcoidosis and the complexity in its differential diagnoses: a review. Innov Clin Neurosci 9(4):10–16

Nozaki K, Judson MA (2012) Neurosarcoidosis: clinical manifestations, diagnosis and treatment. Presse Med 41(6 Pt 2):e331–e348

Loor RG, van Tongeren J, Derks W (2012) Multiple cranial nerve dysfunction caused by neurosarcoidosis. Am J Otolaryngol 33(4):484–486

De Diego-Sastre JI, Prim-Espada MP, Fernandez-Garcia F (2005) The epidemiology of Bell's palsy. Rev Neurol 41(5):287–290

Yetiser S et al (2003) Magnetic resonance imaging of the intratemporal facial nerve in idiopathic peripheral facial palsy. Clin Imaging 27(2):77–81

Han DG (2010) Pain around the ear in Bell's palsy is referred pain of facial nerve origin: the role of nervi nervorum. Med Hypotheses 74(2):235–236

Kress BP et al (2002) Bell's palsy: what is the prognostic value of measurements of signal intensity increases with contrast enhancement on MRI? Neuroradiology 44(5):428–433

Kress B et al (2004) Bell palsy: quantitative analysis of MR imaging data as a method of predicting outcome. Radiology 230(2):504–509

Mantsopoulos K et al (2011) Predicting the long-term outcome after idiopathic facial nerve paralysis. Otol Neurotol 32(5):848–851

Kuzma BB, Goodman JM (1997) Pitfalls of facial nerve enhancement on MRI. Surg Neurol 48(6):636–637

Burmeister HP et al (2011) Evaluation of the early phase of Bell's palsy using 3 T MRI. Eur Arch Otorhinolaryngol 268(10):1493–1500

Kondo Y et al (2012) The relationship between Bell's palsy and morphometric aspects of the facial nerve. Eur Arch Otorhinolaryngol 269(6):1691–1695. doi: 10.1007/s00405-011-1835-0

Kaylie DM, Wax MK, Weissman JL (2003) Preoperative facial muscle imaging predicts final facial function after facial nerve grafting. AJNR Am J Neuroradiol 24(3):326–330

Song MH et al (2008) Clinical significance of quantitative analysis of facial nerve enhancement on MRI in Bell's palsy. Acta Otolaryngol 128(11):1259–1265

Hato N et al (2003) Efficacy of early treatment of Bell's palsy with oral acyclovir and prednisolone. Otol Neurotol 24(6):948–951

Sullivan FM et al (2007) Early treatment with prednisolone or acyclovir in Bell's palsy. N Engl J Med 357(16):1598–1607

Fishman JM (2011) Corticosteroids effective in idiopathic facial nerve palsy (Bell's palsy) but not necessarily in idiopathic acute vestibular dysfunction (vestibular neuritis). Laryngoscope 121(11):2494–2495

Oczkowski W (2008) Early treatment with prednisolone, but not acyclovir, was effective in Bell's palsy. Evid Based Med 13(2):44

Gilchrist JM (2009) Seventh cranial neuropathy. Semin Neurol 29(1):5–13

Kinishi M et al (2001) Acyclovir improves recovery rate of facial nerve palsy in Ramsay Hunt syndrome. Auris Nasus Larynx 28(3):223–226

Garcia-Monco JC (2002) Lyme's disease: mimicker and enigmatic. Med Clin (Barc) 119(18):693–694

Siwula JM, Mathieu G (2002) Acute onset of facial nerve palsy associated with Lyme disease in a 6 year-old child. Pediatr Dent 24(6):572–574

Lipsker D (2004) European tick-bite disease and Lyme's disease: historical overview and unsolved questions. Ann Dermatol Venereol 131(6–7 Pt 1):533–536

Larrosa F, Aguilar F, Benitez P (1999) Otoneurological manifestations of Lyme's disease. Acta Otorrinolaringol Esp 50(8):644–648

Djukic M et al (2011) The diagnostic spectrum in patients with suspected chronic Lyme neuroborreliosis–the experience from one year of a university hospital's Lyme neuroborreliosis outpatients clinic. Eur J Neurol 18(4):547–555

Makhani N et al (2011) A twist on Lyme: the challenge of diagnosing European Lyme neuroborreliosis. J Clin Microbiol 49(1):455–457

Abul-Kasim K (2010) Neuroborreliosis with enhancement of the third, fifth, sixth, and twelfth cranial nerves. Acta Neurol Belg 110(2):215

Helms D, Roberge RJ, Kovalick M (2003) Otomastoiditis-related facial nerve palsy. J Emerg Med 25(1):45–49

Kristensen RN, Hahn CH (2012) Facial nerve palsy caused by parotid gland abscess. J Laryngol Otol 126(3):322–324

Roberts J et al (2010) Malignant otitis externa (MOE) causing cerebral abscess and facial nerve palsy. J Hosp Med 5(7):E6–E8

Reiter D, Bilaniuk LT, Zimmerman RA (1982) Diagnostic imaging in malignant otitis externa. Otolaryngol Head Neck Surg 90(5):606–609

Szymanski M et al (2012) The use of MRI DWI-imaging in assessment of cholesteatoma recurrences after canal wall up technique. Otolaryngol Pol 66(4 Suppl):45–48

Hoa M et al (2013) Petrous apex cholesterol granuloma: pictorial review of radiological considerations in diagnosis and surgical histopathology. J Laryngol Otol 127(4):339–348

Hoa M, House JW, Linthicum FH Jr (2012) Petrous apex cholesterol granuloma: maintenance of drainage pathway, the histopathology of surgical management and histopathologic evidence for the exposed marrow theory. Otol Neurotol 33(6):1059–1065

Gore MR et al (2011) Cholesterol granuloma of the petrous apex. Otolaryngol Clin North Am 44(5):1043–1058

Hsu KC, Wang AC, Chen SJ (2008) Mastoid bone fracture presenting as unusual delayed onset of facial nerve palsy. Am J Emerg Med 26(3):386 e1–2

Odebode TO, Ologe FE (2006) Facial nerve palsy after head injury: case incidence, causes, clinical profile and outcome. J Trauma 61(2):388–391

Rotondo M et al (2010) Post-traumatic peripheral facial nerve palsy: surgical and neuroradiological consideration in five cases of delayed onset. Acta Neurochir (Wien) 152(10):1705–1709

Pownder S et al (2010) Computed tomography of temporal bone fractures and temporal region anatomy in horses. J Vet Intern Med 24(2):398–406

Barreau X (2011) Imaging features of temporal bone fractures. J Radiol 92(11):958–966

Rinaldo A, Mondin V, Ferlito A (2002) Immediate facial nerve palsy following stapedectomy. ORL J Otorhinolaryngol Relat Spec 64(5):355–357

Safdar A et al (2006) Delayed facial nerve palsy following tympanomastoid surgery: incidence, aetiology and prognosis. J Laryngol Otol 120(9):745–748

Xu HX et al (2011) Delayed facial nerve palsy after endolymphatic sac surgery. Ear Nose Throat J 90(8):E28–E31

Ciorba A et al (2012) Postoperative complications in cochlear implants: a retrospective analysis of 438 consecutive cases. Eur Arch Otorhinolaryngol 269(6):1599–1603

Stoddart RL, Cooper HR (1999) Electrode complications in 100 adults with multichannel cochlear implants. J Laryngol Otol Suppl 24:18–20

Falcioni M et al (2003) Facial nerve tumors. Otol Neurotol 24(6):942–947

Fabiano AJ, Plunkett RJ, Gibbons KJ (2010) Diagnosis of facial nerve schwannoma by magnetic resonance imaging enhancement of the geniculate ganglion. Arch Neurol 67(1):112–113

Shimizu K et al (2005) Intraparotid facial nerve schwannoma: a report of five cases and an analysis of MR imaging results. AJNR Am J Neuroradiol 26(6):1328–1330

Thompson AL et al (2009) Magnetic resonance imaging of facial nerve schwannoma. Laryngoscope 119(12):2428–2436

Benoit MM et al (2010) Facial nerve hemangiomas: vascular tumors or malformations? Otolaryngol Head Neck Surg 142(1):108–114

Gonzalez-Darder JM, Pesudo-Martinez JV (2007) Facial nerve palsy due to cavernous angioma of the petrous bone. Case report. Neurocirugia (Astur) 18(1):44–46

Salib RJ et al (2001) The crucial role of imaging in detection of facial nerve haemangiomas. J Laryngol Otol 115(6):510–513

Jabor MA, Amedee RG, Gianoli GJ (2000) Primary meningioma of the fallopian canal. South Med J 93(7):717–720

Namdar I, Smouha EE, Kane P (1995) Salivary gland choristoma of the middle ear: role of intraoperative facial nerve monitoring. Otolaryngol Head Neck Surg 112(4):616–620

Michalopoulos K, Bajaj Y, Strachan DR (2008) Recurrent facial nerve palsy caused by a facial cyst. Br J Hosp Med (Lond) 69(8):475

Pertzborn SL et al (2003) Epineurial pseudocysts of the intratemporal facial nerve. Otol Neurotol 24(3):490–493

Kunzel J et al (2012) Paraganglioma of the facial nerve, a rare differential diagnosis for facial nerve paralysis: case report and review of the literature. Eur Arch Otorhinolaryngol 269(2):693–698

Wippold FJ, Neely JG, Haughey BH (2004) Primary paraganglioma of the facial nerve canal. Otol Neurotol 25(1):79–80

Petrus LV, Lo WM (1996) Primary paraganglioma of the facial nerve canal. AJNR Am J Neuroradiol 17(1):171–174

Noujaim SE et al (2000) Paraganglioma of the temporal bone: role of magnetic resonance imaging versus computed tomography. Top Magn Reson Imaging 11(2):108–122

Van den Berg R, van Gils AP, Wasser MN (1999) Imaging of head and neck paragangliomas with three-dimensional time-of-flight MR angiography. AJR Am J Roentgenol 172(6):1667–1673

Martinez-Miravete P et al (2007) Adenocarcinoma of the endolymphatic sac in von Hippel-Lindau disease. A case report. Radiologia 49(4):287–289

Malhotra S et al (2006) Low-grade adenocarcinoma of endolymphatic sac origin. Am J Otolaryngol 27(5):362–365

Mukherji SK, Castillo M (1996) Adenocarcinoma of the endolymphatic sac: imaging features and preoperative embolization. Neuroradiology 38(2):179–180

Yildiz O et al (2011) Facial nerve palsy: an unusual presenting feature of small cell lung cancer. Case Rep Oncol 4(1):35–38

Kundu S, Eynon-Lewis NJ, Radcliffe GJ (2001) Extensive metastatic renal cell carcinoma presenting as facial nerve palsy. J Laryngol Otol 115(6):488–490

Diamond M et al (2011) Peripheral facial nerve communications and their clinical implications. Clin Anat 24(1):10–18

Jungehuelsing M et al (2000) Limitations of magnetic resonance imaging in the evaluation of perineural tumor spread causing facial nerve paralysis. Arch Otolaryngol Head Neck Surg 126(4):506–510

Quesnel AM, Lindsay RW, Hadlock TA (2010) When the bell tolls on Bell's palsy: finding occult malignancy in acute-onset facial paralysis. Am J Otolaryngol 31(5):339–342

Ginsberg LE (2004) MR imaging of perineural tumor spread. Neuroimaging Clin N Am 14(4):663–677

Ginsberg LE (2002) MR imaging of perineural tumor spread. Magn Reson Imaging Clin N Am 10(3):511–525 vi

Ginsberg LE (1999) Imaging of perineural tumor spread in head and neck cancer. Semin Ultrasound CT MR 20(3):175–186

Ginsberg LE, Eicher SA (2000) Great auricular nerve: anatomy and imaging in a case of perineural tumor spread. AJNR Am J Neuroradiol 21(3):568–571

Ozdogmus O et al (2004) Connections between the facial, vestibular and cochlear nerve bundles within the internal auditory canal. J Anat 205(1):65–75

Jethanamest D, Roehm P (2011) Fibrous dysplasia of the temporal bone with complete canal stenosis and cholesteatoma. Otol Neurotol 32(7):e52–e53

Zaytoun GM, Dagher WI, Rameh CE (2008) Recurrent facial nerve paralysis: an unusual presentation of fibrous dysplasia of the temporal bone. Eur Arch Otorhinolaryngol 265(2):255–259

Shonka DC Jr, Kesser BW (2006) Paget's disease of the temporal bone. Otol Neurotol 27(8):1199–1200

Song JJ et al (2005) Monostotic fibrous dysplasia of temporal bone: report of two cases and review of its characteristics. Acta Otolaryngol 125(10):1126–1129

Noorizan Y et al (2009) Parotid abscess: an unusual cause of facial nerve palsy. Med J Malaysia 64(2):172–173

Pavlou E, Gkampeta A, Arampatzi M (2011) Facial nerve palsy in childhood. Brain Dev 33:644–650. doi:10.1016/j.braindev.2010.11.001

Shargorodsky J, Lin HW, Gopen Q (2010) Facial nerve palsy in the pediatric population. Clin Pediatr (Phila) 49(5):411–417

Toelle SP, Boltshauser E (2001) Long-term outcome in children with congenital unilateral facial nerve palsy. Neuropediatrics 32(3):130–135

Rizk EB et al (2005) Facial nerve palsy with acute otitis media during the first 2 weeks of life. J Child Neurol 20(5):452–454

Burgio DL et al (2000) Magnetic resonance imaging of the facial nerve in children with idiopathic facial paralysis. Otolaryngol Head Neck Surg 122(4):556–559

Al Tawil K et al (2010) Traumatic facial nerve palsy in newborns: is it always iatrogenic? Am J Perinatol 27(9):711–713

Duval M, Daniel SJ (2009) Facial nerve palsy in neonates secondary to forceps use. Arch Otolaryngol Head Neck Surg 135(7):634–636

Berker N, Acaroglu G, Soykan E (2004) Goldenhar's syndrome (oculo-auriculo-vertebral dysplasia) with congenital facial nerve palsy. Yonsei Med J 45(1):157–160

Carvalho GJ et al (1999) Auditory and facial nerve dysfunction in patients with hemifacial microsomia. Arch Otolaryngol Head Neck Surg 125(2):209–212

Ferriby D et al (1998) Magnetic resonance imaging of the facial nerve in a case of Melkerson-Rosenthal syndrome. Rev Neurol (Paris) 154(5):426–428

Rahbar R et al (2001) Craniofacial, temporal bone, and audiologic abnormalities in the spectrum of hemifacial microsomia. Arch Otolaryngol Head Neck Surg 127(3):265–271

Lima LM, Diniz MB, dos Santos-Pinto L (2009) Moebius syndrome: clinical manifestations in a pediatric patient. Pediatr Dent 31(4):289–293

Dubrey SW, Patel MC, Malik O (2009) Moebius-Poland syndrome and drug associations. BMJ Case Rep

Fons-Estupina MC et al (2007) Moebius sequence: clinico-radiological findings. Rev Neurol 44(10):583–588

Hillerer C et al (2007) Neuroradiologic findings in Mobius syndrome. Rofo 179(5):532–534

de Greef JC et al (2010) Clinical features of facioscapulohumeral muscular dystrophy 2. Neurology 75(17):1548–1554

Pratap A et al (2007) Congenital unilateral lower lip palsy and eventration of diaphragm. Singapore Med J 48(8):e209–e211

Kobayashi T (1979) Congenital unilateral lower lip palsy. Acta Otolaryngol 88(3–4):303–309

Kobrynski LJ, Sullivan KE (2007) Velocardiofacial syndrome, DiGeorge syndrome: the chromosome 22q11.2 deletion syndromes. Lancet 370(9596):1443–1452

Cure JK et al (2000) Cranial MR imaging of osteopetrosis. AJNR Am J Neuroradiol 21(6):1110–1115

Abadie V et al (2000) Vestibular anomalies in CHARGE syndrome: investigations on and consequences for postural development. Eur J Pediatr 159(8):569–574

Gassner EM, Mallouhi A, Jaschke WR (2004) Preoperative evaluation of external auditory canal atresia on high-resolution CT. AJR Am J Roentgenol 182(5):1305–1312

Curtin HD, Vignaud J, Bar D (1982) Anomaly of the facial canal in a Mondini malformation with recurrent meningitis. Radiology 144(2):335–341

Kim YH et al (2008) Bilateral simultaneous facial nerve palsy: clinical analysis in seven cases. Otol Neurotol 29(3):397–400

Coddington CT et al (2010) Neurological picture. Bilateral facial nerve palsy associated with Epstein-Barr virus infection. J Neurol Neurosurg Psychiatry 81(10):1155–1156

Atsumi M et al (2004) A variant of Guillain-Barre syndrome with prominent bilateral peripheral facial nerve palsy–facial diplegia and paresthesias. Rinsho Shinkeigaku 44(8):549–552

Yardimci N et al (2009) Bilateral facial nerve enhancement demonstrated by magnetic resonance imaging in Guillain-Barre syndrome. Neurol Sci 30(5):431–433

Balatsouras DG et al (2007) Infectious causes of bilateral facial nerve palsy. J Otolaryngol 36(3):E42–E44

Ferrari J et al (2004) Bilateral facial nerve palsy as first indication of relapsing hairy cell leukemia after 36 years. Neurology 63(2):399–400

Mohebbi A, Jahandideh H, Harandi AA (2011) Rare presentation of rhino-orbital-cerebral zygomycosis: bilateral facial nerve palsy. Case Rep Med 2011:216404

Ozaki K et al (2011) Bilateral facial nerve palsy caused by a metastatic malignant lymphoma. Intern Med 50(19):2247

Lim TC et al (2009) Bilateral facial nerve palsy in Kawasaki disease. Ann Acad Med Singapore 38(8):737–738

Price T, Fife DG (2002) Bilateral simultaneous facial nerve palsy. J Laryngol Otol 116(1):46–48

Fogarty GB, Cassumbhoy R, Ball D (2006) Magnetic resonance imaging changes in synchronous bilateral progressive facial nerve weakness. J Thorac Oncol 1(5):487–488

Imaging of the Jugular Foramen

Hervé Tanghe

Contents

1	**Anatomy**	307
2	**Radiological Examination of the Jugular Foramen**......	309
3	**Overview of the Lesions of the Jugular Foramen**	310
4	**Vascular Lesions**...	311
5	**Common Tumours**	311
5.1	Paraganglioma	313
5.2	Schwannoma..	313
5.3	Meningioma...	314
6	**Other Lesions of the Jugular Foramen**	318
6.1	Traumatic lesions	318
7	**Uncommon Tumours (Primary and Secondary)**	318
7.1	Endolymphatic Sac Tumour	318
7.2	Giant Cell Tumour	320
7.3	Metastasis	320
7.4	Chordoma	320
7.5	Nasopharyngeal Carcinoma	321
7.6	Temporal Bone/Middle Ear Carcinoma	322
8	**Infectious Disease**	322
8.1	Malignant External Otitis (Necrotizing External Otitis) ...	322
9	**Lesions of the Jugular Foramen in Children**	324
9.1	Congenital Lesions...	324
10	**Tumours**	324
10.1	Primary Ewing's Sarcoma/Peripheral Primitive Neuroectodermal Tumour	324
10.2	Fibromatosis	325
10.3	Osteosarcoma...	325
10.4	Histiocytosis	325
10.5	Rhabdomyosarcoma	326
References...		326

Abstract

This chapter discusses the jugular fossa with a description of the anatomy, a discussion of the radiological imaging techniques. The emphasis is on the various tumours that can be encountered. Thereafter less common pathologies are discussed. There is a separate paragraph on lesions of the jugular foramen in children.

1 Anatomy

The jugular foramen is an opening in the skull base, located between the temporal and the occipital bone. Asymmetry between the right and left foramen is the rule. The right foramen is the largest in 68 % of the cases, equal to the left in 12 % and smaller than the left in 20 % (Rhoton 2000). This is explained by the asymmetry in the intracranial venous drainage (Fig. 1).

Several anatomical structures goes through the jugular foramen: the sigmoid sinus, jugular bulb, the inferior petrosal sinus, the meningeal branches of the ascending pharyngeal and the occipital arteries, the glossopharyngeal, vagus and accessory nerves, the tympanic branch of the glossopharyngeal nerve (Jacobson's nerve) and the auricular branch of the vagus nerve (Arnold's nerve) (Fig. 2a) (Rhoton 2000; Sen et al. 2001).

Despite several studies, the exact anatomy of the jugular foramen is uncertain, mostly because of the great variations from person to person (Rubinstein et al. 1995). Hovelaque in 1934 described two compartments: the pars nervosa (anteromedial) and the pars venosa (posterolateral). Rhoton (2000) proposes a division in three parts at the intracranial orifice: a small petrosal compartment anteromedially, containing the inferior petrosal sinus, a large lateral sigmoid part containing the sigmoid sinus and an intrajugular part, containing the cranial nerves IX, X and XI. Within the foramen, there is a bony and fibrous septum between the

H. Tanghe (✉)
Section of Neuroradiology and ENT Radiology,
Department of Radiology, Erasmus Medical Centre,
Erasmus University Rotterdam, 's-Gravendijkwal 230,
3015 CE, Rotterdam, The Netherlands
e-mail: h.l.j.tanghe@erasmusmc.nl

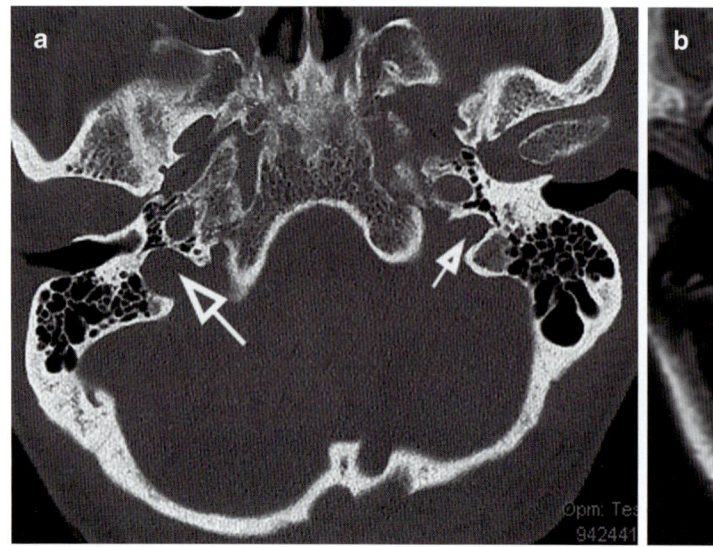

Fig. 1 *Normal asymmetry of the jugular foramen.* **a** CT bone window. The *right* jugular foramen (*large arrow*) is larger than the *left* (*small arrow*, due to the asymmetry of the intracranial venous drainage. **b** MRI 3d GRE T1 W 1 mm without contrast. The left foramen (*large arrow*) is larger than the right foramen (*small arrow*). Notice also the difference in signal intensity of both foramina due to flow-related artefacts

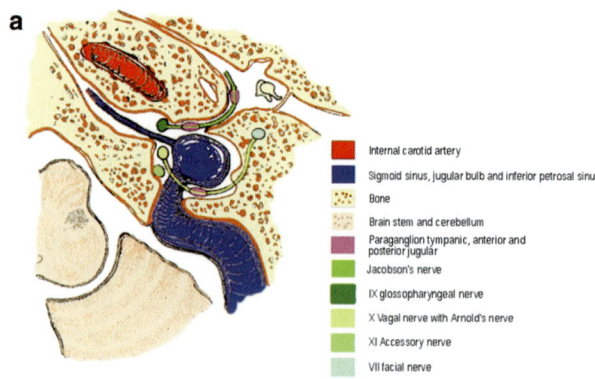

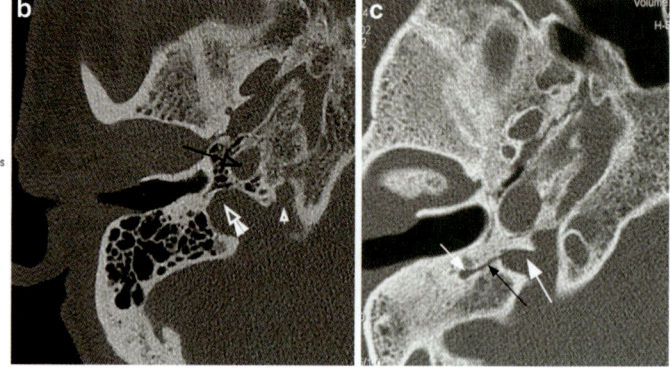

Fig. 2 *Normal anatomy of the jugular foramen.* **a** Scheme; **b** axial CT of the left jugular foramen at the level of the horizontal part of the carotid canal; **c** axial CT at the level of the vertical part of the carotid canal (*black arrow*). The jugular foramen is divided into a medial small pars nervosa (*small with arrow*) and a larger lateral part, the pars vascularis (*large white arrow*), separated by a bony and fibrous septum. In **c** the mastoid canaliculus (*black arrow*), containing the Arnold's nerve, is visible running from the lateral wall of the jugular foramen (*large white arrow*) towards the mastoid segment of the facial canal (*small white arrow*)

sigmoid and petrosal part. It is through this area that the cranial nerves pass (Fig. 2a, b, c).

The nerve of Jacobson is the tympanic branch of the glossopharyngeal nerve, originating at the external orifice of the jugular foramen. It traverses the tympanic canaliculus to enter the tympanic cavity where it gives rise to the tympanic plexus providing the sensory innervation of the middle ear and the parasympathetic innervation via the otic ganglion to the parotid gland (Fig. 2a).

The nerve of Arnold, the auricular cutaneous branch of the vagus nerve, arises at the level of the superior vagal ganglion. This branch goes to the lateral wall of the jugular foramen to enter the mastoid canaliculus (Fig. 2c), and ascends towards the mastoid segment of the facial canal to exit the temporal bone via the tympanomastoid fissure.

The inferior petrosal sinus enters the jugular bulb between the IXth and Xth cranial nerves, as single or multiple venous channels (Sen et al. 2001) (Fig. 3).

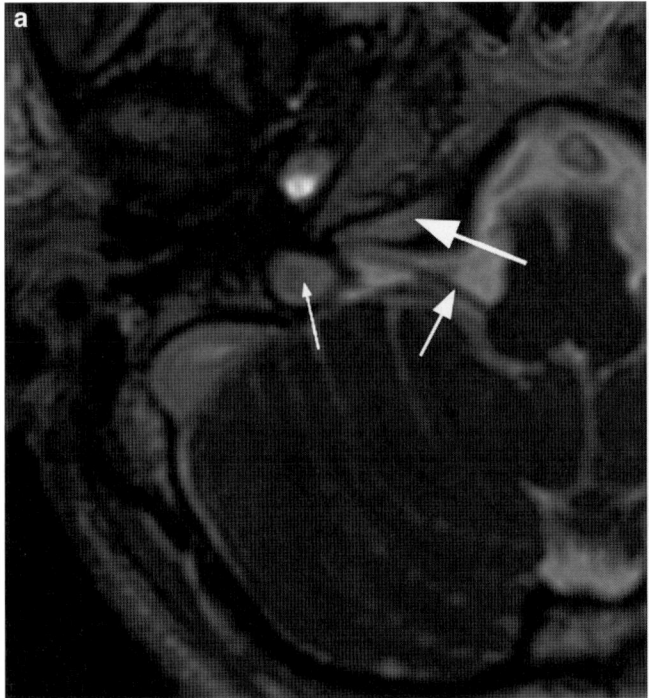

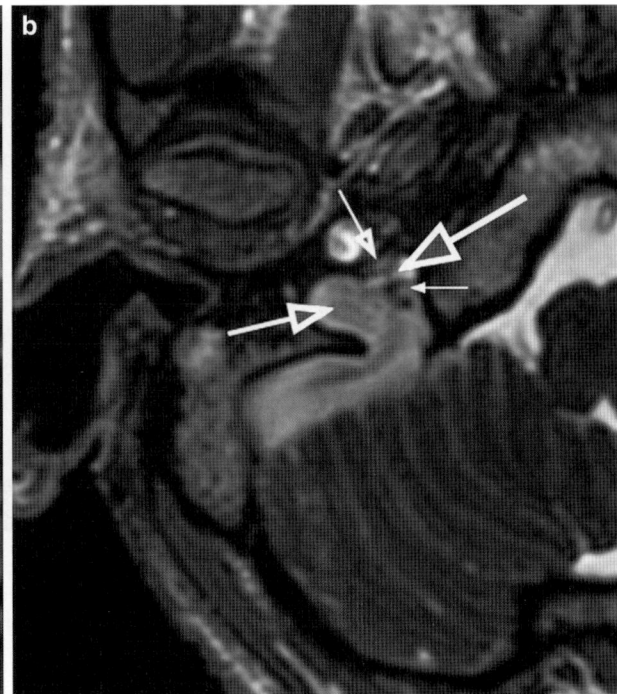

Fig. 3 *The inferior petrosal sinus enters the jugular bulb between the IXth and Xth nerves.* **a** high-level trough inferior petrosal sinus; 3D FIESTA with gadolinium. *Large white arrow* the inferior petrosal sinus. *Small white arrow* the cisternal segment of the IXth nerve, going to the nervosal part of the foramen. *Small white arrow* the jugular bulb in the vascular part of the foramen. **b** entrance of the inferior petrosal sinus in the jugular bulb. 3D FIESTA with gadolinium. The inferior petrosal sinus (*largest white arrow*) enters the jugular bulb (*second largest arrow*) between the IXth (*second smallest arrow*) and Xth nerves (*smallest arrow*)

The cranial nerves remain fasciculated within the foramen, with the vagus nerve containing multiple fascicles and the glossopharyngeal and accessory nerves containing one and two fascicles, respectively (Sen et al. 2001).

2 Radiological Examination of the Jugular Foramen

The evaluation of the jugular foramen and the temporal bone, especially in tumours requires high-quality cross-sectional imaging with both CT and MR to fully answer all the detailed preoperative questions. For the anatomical variants, CT imaging alone is preferable.

The CT examination is best done with a multidetector spiral CT (when available) making ultra thin sections (0.7 mm) in the axial plane with coronal and sagittal reconstructions. When both CT and MR are used, the task of CT is not to explore the soft tissue extension, but to show the bony anatomy, the condition of the bony margins of the foramen and other structures in the neighbourhood, the extend of the bony destruction of the skull base and to detect some lesion characteristic features that are not visible on MR, like the intratumoral calcifications or the hyperostosis of a meningioma.

Modern MR techniques allow the identification of the complex anatomy of the jugular foramen and can demonstrate the cranial nerves IX–XII in the foramen. This can be done by using 3D FIESTA (Fast Imaging Employing Steady-State Acquisition) after gadolinium (General Electric). The enhancement of the jugular vein and associated venous plexus surrounding the cranial nerves provided excellent contrast of the small structures within the jugular foramen on FIESTA images after gadolinium, not obtained on 3D FIESTA without gadolinium (Davagnanam and Chavda 2008; Linn et al. 2009) (Fig. 4). Other useful MR techniques are: contrast-enhanced MR angiography, contrast-enhanced 3D T1W, balanced fast-field echo (b-FFE) (Aydin et al. 2011). The contrast-enhanced 3D T1W sequence is somewhat inferior.

The primary task of MR is to evaluate the soft tissue extension of the disease, to interpret the signal intensity characteristics and to find additional features not visible on CT like the presence of intratumoral vessels in a paraganglioma. Our MR imaging protocol for the jugular foramen (on a GE 1.5 or 3 T) consists of (1) a nonenhanced axial 3D gradient echo T1W sequence with contiguous slice thickness of 1 mm, starting at C2 level until above the internal auditory canal; (2) this sequence is repeated after the administration of gadolinium in the axial plane with coronal reconstructions;

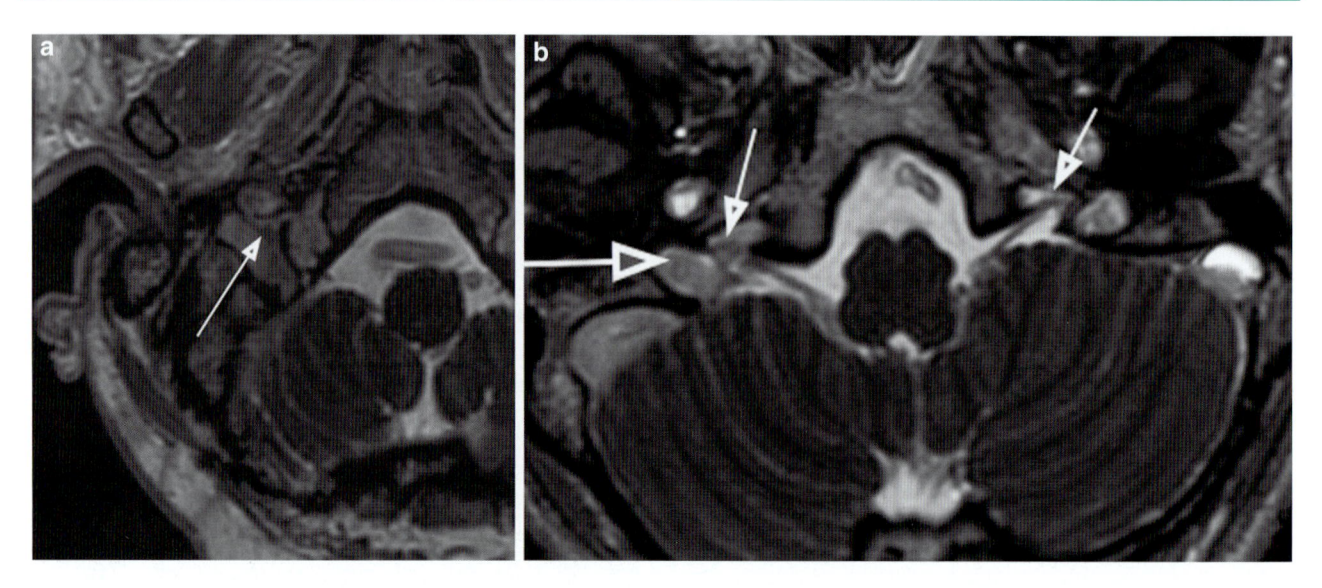

Fig. 4 *The cranial nerves in the jugular foramen.* **a** 3D FIESTA with gadolinium. *Arrow* shows the cranial nerve X in the vascular part of the foramen. **b** 3D FIESTA with gadolinium. *Small arrows* show the cranial nerve IX on the right and left side in pars nervosa of the foramen. *Large arrow* pars vascularis of the foramen

Table 1 "Do not touch lesions/pseudo lesions" of the jugular foramen

1. Normal asymmetrically enlarged jugular foramen on CT
2. Normal asymmetrically enlarged jugular bulb on MRI
3. Flow-related artefacts of the jugular bulb on MRI
4. High jugular bulb on CT or MRI
5. Dehiscent jugular bulb on CT
6. Jugular bulb diverticulum on CT

(3) a 3D FIESTA after gadolinium with slice thickness of 1 mm; (4) a 2D TSE T2 W sequence in the axial plane 3 mm. starting at the level of C2. In addition, an evaluation of the neck can be necessary in case of a paraganglioma, to find multiplicity. MR venography in the coronal plane can be used to study the patency or invasion of the internal jugular vein, and the sigmoid sinus. In the postoperative situation, after an infratemporal approach with filling up the defect with a fat/muscle graft, the use of a fat-saturated contrast-enhanced T1W image is important to detect recurrent paraganglioma. The diagnosis of recurrent paraganglioma in a previous operated patient can be very difficult.

Angiography is seldom needed for diagnostic purposes, but plays a role in the preoperative embolization (see the chapter on the vascular lesions of the temporal bone).

3 Overview of the Lesions of the Jugular Foramen

The jugular foramen is a complex region of the skull base with an extensive differential diagnostic list of possible lesions.

It is important to recognize the "pseudo-lesions" like the normal asymmetry of the foramen, the anatomical vascular variants (see the chapter on vascular temporal bone lesions) and the modality-dependent pitfalls like the flow-related artefacts on MR (Fig. 1b) (Swartz and Loevner 2009) (Table 1).

The true lesions can be divided into primary lesions located in the foramen and secondary extensions to the jugular foramen. (Weber and McKenna 1994; Lowenheim et al. 2006; Vogl and Bisdas 2009; Kang Ong and Fook-Hin Chong 2009). The possibilities are different for adults (Table 2), compared to children (Table 3).

A practical starting point for the differential diagnosis is to look at the dimension and the bony margin of the jugular foramen on CT. There are four possibilities: (1) the jugular foramen is normal; (2) the foramen is enlarged with an intact cortical outline; (3) the foramen is enlarged with an erosion, destruction of its cortical outlines; (4) the foramen has a normal size but its bony margins are destroyed. In the first category, one must think on pseudo lesions like flow-related artefacts on MR, on a dural A-V fistula and on a thrombosis of the jugular bulb or sigmoid sinus. The possibilities in the second category are: normal asymmetry, schwannoma, meningioma, dural A-V fistula, cholesteatoma. The differential diagnostic list in the third category consists of: paraganglioma, metastasis, Ewing sarcoma, giant cell tumour. The lesions of the fourth category are secondary extensions to the foramen from lesion originating elsewhere like: malignant otitis externa, cholesteatoma, metastasis, chondrosarcoma, chordoma, nasopharyngeal carcinoma, endolymphatic sac tumour (Table 4).

Table 2 True lesions of the jugular foramen in adults

Traumatic	Fracture
	CSF lekkage
	Arterial/venous damage
Infectious	Abscess
	Cholesterol granuloma
	Cholesteatoma
	Malignant otitis externa
Tumoral intrinsic	Paraganglioma
	Schwannoma
	Meningioma
	Peripheral primitive neuroectodermal tumour
	Leptomeningeal metastasis
Tumoral extrinsic	Endolymphatic sac tumour
	Chordoma
	Chondrosarcoma
	Giant cell tumour
	Metastasis: bone metastasis
	Osteosarcoma
	Temporal bone carcinoma
	Nasopharyngeal carcinoma

Table 3 True lesions of the jugular foramen in children

Congenital	Craniosynostosis
	Achondroplasia
	Meningocoele
	Congenital vascular variants
Infectious	Abscess
	Cholesteatoma
Tumour	Meningioma
	Osteosarcoma
	Ewing's sarcoma/Peripheral primitive neuroectodermal tumour
	Rhabdomyosarcoma
Vascular	Thrombosis of the jugular bulb
	Dural A-V fistula

4 Vascular Lesions

These are discussed in the chapter on vascular temporal bone lesions.

5 Common Tumours

5.1 Paraganglioma

Paragangliomas, also called glomus tumours, are neuroendocrine neoplasm's composed largely of paraganglion chief cells (Burger and Scheithauer 2007). These tumours arise from glomus bodies also named paraganglia. A paraganglion possesses unique regulatory function and is part of the extra adrenal neuroendocrine system. Normal paraganglia occur in the head and neck region at several places (Table 5), frequently located near nerves and vessels (Petrus and Lo 1992; Rao et al. 1999; Lowenheim et al. 2006). Within the jugular foramen, the paraganglioma can arise from paraganglia located in the adventitia of the jugular bulb or at Jacobson's nerve (nerve IX) or at Arnold's nerve (nerve X). In the middle ear normal paraganglia are found at the cochlear promontory. Of all paragangliomas, 80 % are either glomus jugulare tumours or carotid body tumours (Lowenheim et al. 2006). Glomus jugular tumours are not encapsulated and tend to infiltrate connective tissue planes (Vogl and Bisdas 2009).

Paragangliomas restricted to the middle ear are called glomus tympanicum tumours. Glomus jugulotympanicum and glomus jugulare tumours involve, respectively, the middle ear plus the jugular foramen or the jugular foramen alone. Endocrinological functional activity is rare in head and neck paragangliomas, 93 % of the functioning tumours are pheochromocytomas (also a tumour of paraganglionic tissue) and only 7 % occurs at other sites (Maffe et al. 2000).

Paragangliomas may be multiple, either synchronously or metachronously in 3 % for sporadic cases to 26 % for the familial cases (Fig. 5). They can occur in association with pheochromocytoma, thyroid carcinoma, Carney triad (gastric leiomyosarcoma, pulmonary chondroma and paraganglioma) and other endocrine disorders. Familial paragangliomas have a prevalence of 7–9 %, with 90 % of the cases arising from the carotid body (Rao et al. 1999).

The symptoms depend on the primary site of origin and the extension of the tumour and include: a vascular tympanic membrane, conductive hearing loss, pulsatile tinnitus, bruit, vertigo, sensorineural hearing loss, cranial nerve deficit.

Paragangliomas are benign, but local invasive and very vascular tumours. From its origin in the middle ear, the glomus tympanicum first invades the bone between the hypotympanum and the jugular foramen. With further growth they are indistinguishable from a glomus jugulare, hence the term glomus jugulotympanicum. The differentiation between a simple glomus tympanicum and a glomus jugulotympanicum is an important radiological task, because there is a big difference in the operative approach, with the latter requiring extensive skull base surgery. From the jugular foramen the tumour can extend laterally with destruction of the mastoid segment of the facial canal and invasion of the facial nerve. Anteriorly, the tumour grows into the total middle ear and further along the petrous bone to the foramen lacerum and the cavernous sinus. Inferior spread produces infiltration of the internal jugular vein and further growth in the carotid loge below the skull base. The

Table 4 Differential diagnosis of the jugular foramen lesions, based on the size and the cortical outline of the jugular foramen on CT

A	B	C	D
MR flow-related artefacts	Normal asymmetry	Paraganglioma	Malignant otitis externa
Thrombosis	Schwannoma	Metastasis	Metastasis
Dural A-V fistula	Meningioma	Ewing sarcoma	Chordoma
Leptomeningeal metastasis	Dural A-V fistula	Giant cell tumour	Chondrosarcoma
			Nasopharyngeal carcinoma
			Endolymphatic sac tumour
			Cholesteatoma

A: normal jugular foramen
B: enlarged foramen with an intact cortical outline
C: erosion, destruction of the cortical outline in an enlarged foramen
D: normal sized foramen with bony destruction

Table 5 Locations of the normal paraganglia in the head and neck region. (From Lo et al. 1993; Manski et al. 1997)

Name	Relationship
1. Tympanic	The cochlear promontory in the middle ear
2. Anterior jugular	Jacobson's nerve (IX) in jugular foramen
3. Posterior jugular	Arnold's nerve (X) in jugular foramen
4. Adventitia of the jugular bulb	Jugular bulb in jugular foramen
5. (a) Intravagale (b) Extravagale	Ganglion nodosum of the vagal nerve Along the vagal nerve in the carotid space
6. Facial	Mastoid segment of the facial canal or ganglion geniculi
7. Carotid body	Carotid bifurcation
8. Superior laryngeal	Superior laryngeal nerve
9. Inferior laryngeal	Recurrent laryngeal nerve
10. Orbital	Ganglion ciliare in the orbit
11. Fossa pterygopalatina	Pterygopalatine ganglion
12. Nasopharynx	
13. Buccal mucosa	

Table 6 Classification of glomus temporal tumours (from Fisch and Mattox 1988)

Type	Description
A	Glomus tympanicum confined to the tympanic cavity of the middle ear
B	Glomus tympanicum extending into the the mastoid bone but leaving the cortical outline of the jugular foramen intact
C	Glomus jugulare. The letter C describes the variable extension into the infralabyrinthine portion of the temporal bone and along the carotid canal
C1	Minimal erosion of the vertical segment of the carotid canal
C2	Extensive erosion of the vertical segment of the carotid canal
C3	The erosion extends into the horizontal segment of the carotid canal
C4	The tumours reaches the foramen lacerum and may extend into the cavernous sinus
D	Glomus jugulare with intracranial extension
De1 to De3	Extradural extension, depending on the size
Di1 to Di3	Additional intradural extension, depending on the size. Di3 means inoperable intracranial extension

intracranial extension is first situated extra-axial in the cerebellopontine angle and in advanced cases not only extra-axial, but also intra-axial in the cerebellum. Glomus vagale tumours, arising from the ganglion nodosum or extravagal, may secondary extend into the jugular foramen.

The neuroradiological evaluation requires both CT and MRI (Table 7). Thin section CT in the axial and coronal plane with bone window gives information about the surrounding bony structures, such as the enlargement and erosion of the jugular foramen, the infiltration of the petrous bone, the carotid canal, the facial canal, the hypoglossal canal and the inner ear structures. It also helps in the differential diagnosis with lesions that do not erode the bone like schwannoma, meningioma (Fig. 6). MR shows the soft tissue extension of the tumour in the ear and below the skull base and intracranially (Fig. 7). MR is equally important in the differential diagnosis by showing the characteristic intratumoral vessels (signal void) and the frequent presence of subacute intratumoral haemorrhage with a high signal in the T1W and T2W image. The combination of both features gives a salt and pepper appearance in the T1W images without contrast. This feature is limited to the larger paragangliomas (>1 cm) and is not pathognomonic, as it is also seen in other hypervascular lesions like metastasis. Use of contrast is necessary to find the smaller tumours like the glomus tympanicum and for the demonstration of the soft tissue extent in the larger tumours. All paragangliomas have a strong enhancement. MR venography provides

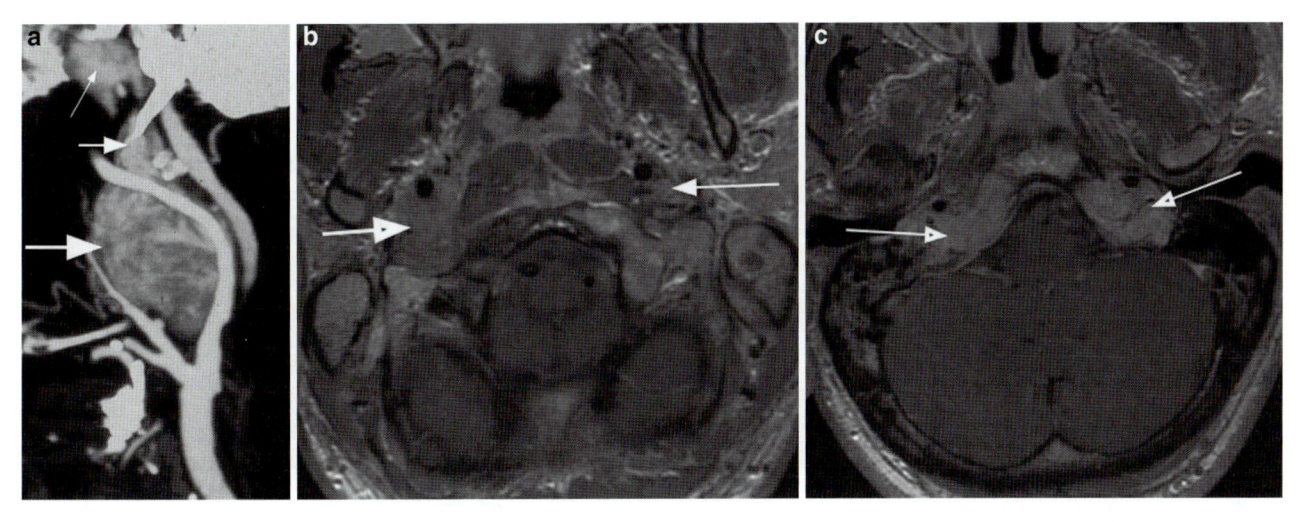

Fig. 5 *Multiple paragangliomas.* **a** CT-angiography, sagittal MIP reconstruction of axial contrast-enhanced thin sections from a multislice spiral CT examination. A large carotid paraganglioma (*large arrow*) is situated at the bifurcation of the common carotid artery, displacing the internal carotid artery backwards and the external carotid artery anteriorly. In the higher cervical region, a small vagal paraganglioma (*midsize arrow*) is typically situated behind the internal carotid artery, witch is displaced anteriorly. At the skull base, a jugular paraganglioma (*small arrow*) is visible with its extension in the carotid loge below the skull base. **b** and **c** MRI axial T1W after gadolinium shows bilateral vagal and jugulotympanical paraganglioma

Table 7 Radiological hallmarks of paraganglioma

Modality	Hallmark	Remark
CT	Enlargement of the foramen	Not in type A & C
	Destruction of cortical outline of the foramen	Contrary to schwannoma
	Isodense without contrast	
	No hyperostosis	Contrary to meningioma
	No intratumoral calcification	Contrary to meningioma
MRI	Intratumoral vessels	Contrary to schwannoma
	No vascular pedicle	Contrary to paraganglioma
	Jugular bulb compression, no invasion	Contrary to paraganglioma, meningioma
CT and MRI	Necrotic parts possible parts	Contrary to meningioma
	Strong enhancement	
	Fixed extension pattern	

information about the jugular vein occlusion and collateral venous drainage. Two hallmarks of this tumour are the bony erosion and the rich vascularisation (Fig. 6). The latter poses special problems of blood loss during operation. Preoperative embolisation is needed in the larger tumours (see the chapter on the vascular lesion of the temporal bone).

In the previous century, Fisch introduced a classification of glomus temporale tumours useful in the planning of the preoperative embolisation and for the selection of the surgical approach (Table 6) (Fisch and Mattox 1988). This classification is based on the location of the tumour in the middle ear or in the jugular foramen, on the relationship between the tumour and the carotid canal and on the possible presence of intracranial extension (Fig. 8).

5.2 Schwannoma

Schwannoma can anatomopathologically be classified as (1) conventional schwannoma; (2) cellular schwannoma; (3) melanotic schwannoma; (4) malignant peripheral nerve sheath tumour (MPNST) and (5) neurofibroma (Burger and Scheithauer 2007).

The conventional schwannoma is a benign tumour, composed entirely of well-differentiated schwann cells. The cellular schwannoma is a benign well-differentiated schwannoma of high cellularity composed largely of Antoni A tissue and devoid of Verocay bodies. The melanotic schwannoma is an often circumscribed nerve sheath tumour composed of melanin-producing schwann cells. The MPNST is a malignant neoplasm arising from or differentiating towards cells intrinsic to peripheral nerves. Specifically, excluded are tumours of epineurial soft tissue and endothelial tumours from the peripheral nerve vasculature. The neurofibroma is a well-differentiated nerve sheath tumour composed predominantly of schwann cells and to a lesser extent fibroblasts and perineural cells (Burger and Scheithauer 2007). Neurofibroma of cranial nerve is extremely rare. Schwannomas (conventional and cellular) are the second most common extra-axial intracranial tumours, preceded only by meningiomas. They constitute 5–10 % of

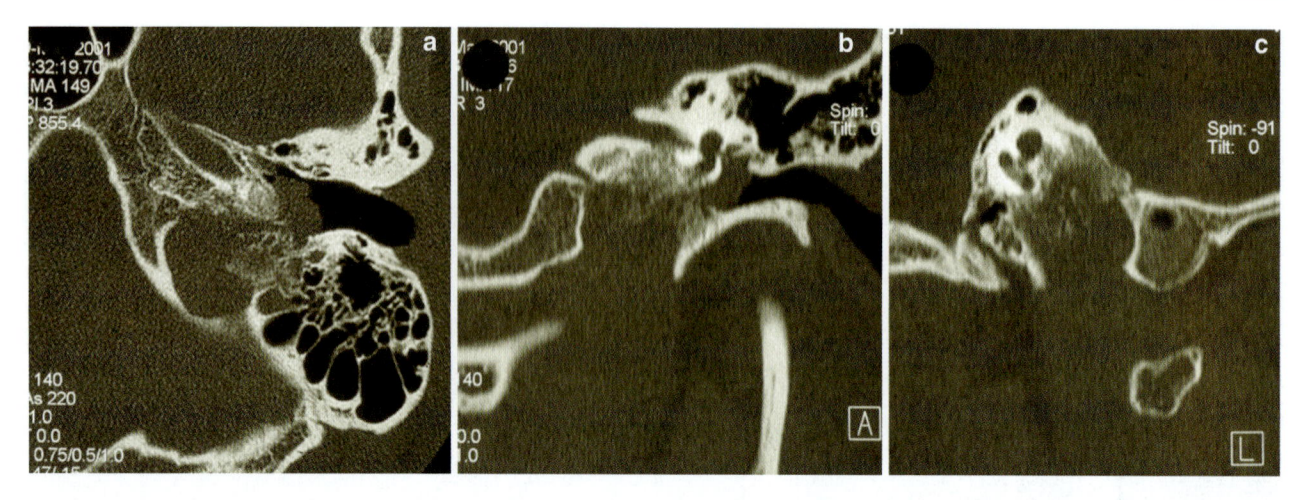

Fig. 6 *Jugulotympanic paraganglioma type C3.* **a** 0.7 mm axial section from a multislice spiral CT examination; **b** coronal reconstruction; **c** sagittal reconstruction, all figures in bone window. The jugular foramen is enlarged. Erosion of the anterior, lateral and superior walls of the foramen with extension of the bony erosion into the medial pars petrosum along the horizontal part of the carotid canal (classification C3). The soft tissue mass invades the bony septum between the jugular foramen and the hypotympanum and extends in the middle ear just to the tympanic membrane. Superiorly, the tumour extends in the bone towards the internal auditory canal and the basal turn of the cochlea. The mastoid segment of the facial canal remains intact

all intracranial neoplasm's. The peak incidence is between the third and sixth decade. Degenerative changes are frequent. Tumour-related cysts can occur in the centre or at the periphery of the tumour. Like their intraspinal counterparts, the intracranial schwannomas show a predilection for the sensory nerves, and most often involve the vestibular division of the eighth nerve. The fifth cranial nerve is the second most common site of origin.

Schwannomas of the cranial nerves three, four and six are rare. Jugular foramen schwannoma may arise from the glossopharyngeal, vagus or accessory nerve or the cervical sympathetic chain within the jugular foramen, although the exact origin of tumour remains undetermined in many cases. The most common nerve of origin was the vagus nerve, followed by the glossopharyngeal nerve. The reason for the predilection of the jugular foramen schwannoma for the glossopharyngeal and vagus nerves may be associated with the presence of their ganglions within the jugular foramen. The presenting symptoms may be similar to those of a vestibular schwannoma, due to the growth in the posterior fossa (Manzzoni et al. 1997) Unilateral hearing loss is the most common presenting symptom in the series of Eldevik et al. 2000. Signs of injury of the vagal or accessory nerve are frequently absent (Eldevik et al. 2000). Samii et al. in 1995 categorised JF neural sheath tumours into four groups: type A, tumours primarily in the cerebellopontine angle with minimal enlargement of the JF; type B, tumours primarily in the JF with intracranial extension; type C, extracranial tumors with extension into the JF (and with clinical signs of XII nerve involvement) and type D, dumbbell-shaped tumours with both intra- and extracranial components. In type A and C, the jugular foramen is not always enlarged (Table 8). Schwannoma is the most common lesion that produces a smooth enlargement of the jugular foramen with sharp contours and often a sclerotic rim, well visible on CT scan with bone window (Fig. 7a). On CT without contrast, the tumour is isodense and sometimes hypodense. On MR, the signal intensity in the T1W image is low and on the T2W image high. The solid part of the tumour enhances strong and usually homogeneous. Intratumoral cysts and necrosis are common and favour the diagnosis of schwannoma against meningioma. Intratumoral calcifications are absent. Bony erosions and intratumoral vessels, like seen in paraganglioma, are absent. Frequently, the tumour has a dumbbell-shaped form with one part in the jugular foramen and the other part in the carotid loge or in the cerebellopontine angle (Fig. 7b, c) (Takahashi et al. 1997; Vogl and Bisdas 2009). Other distinguishing features are the absence of a vascular pedicle (contrary to meningioma) and jugular bulb compression (contrary to invasion with meningioma and paraganglioma) (Vogl and Bisdas 2009). When the tumour has a large intracranial part, confusion with a vestibular schwannoma is possible, especially because the latter can extend into the jugular foramen. But in a vestibular schwannoma, the internal auditory canal is enlarged and in a jugular foramen schwannoma it is normal (Eldevik et al. 2000; Weber and McKenna 1994) (Table 9).

5.3 Meningioma

Meningiomas of the jugular foramen arise from arachnoid villi associated with the jugular bulb or that follow the

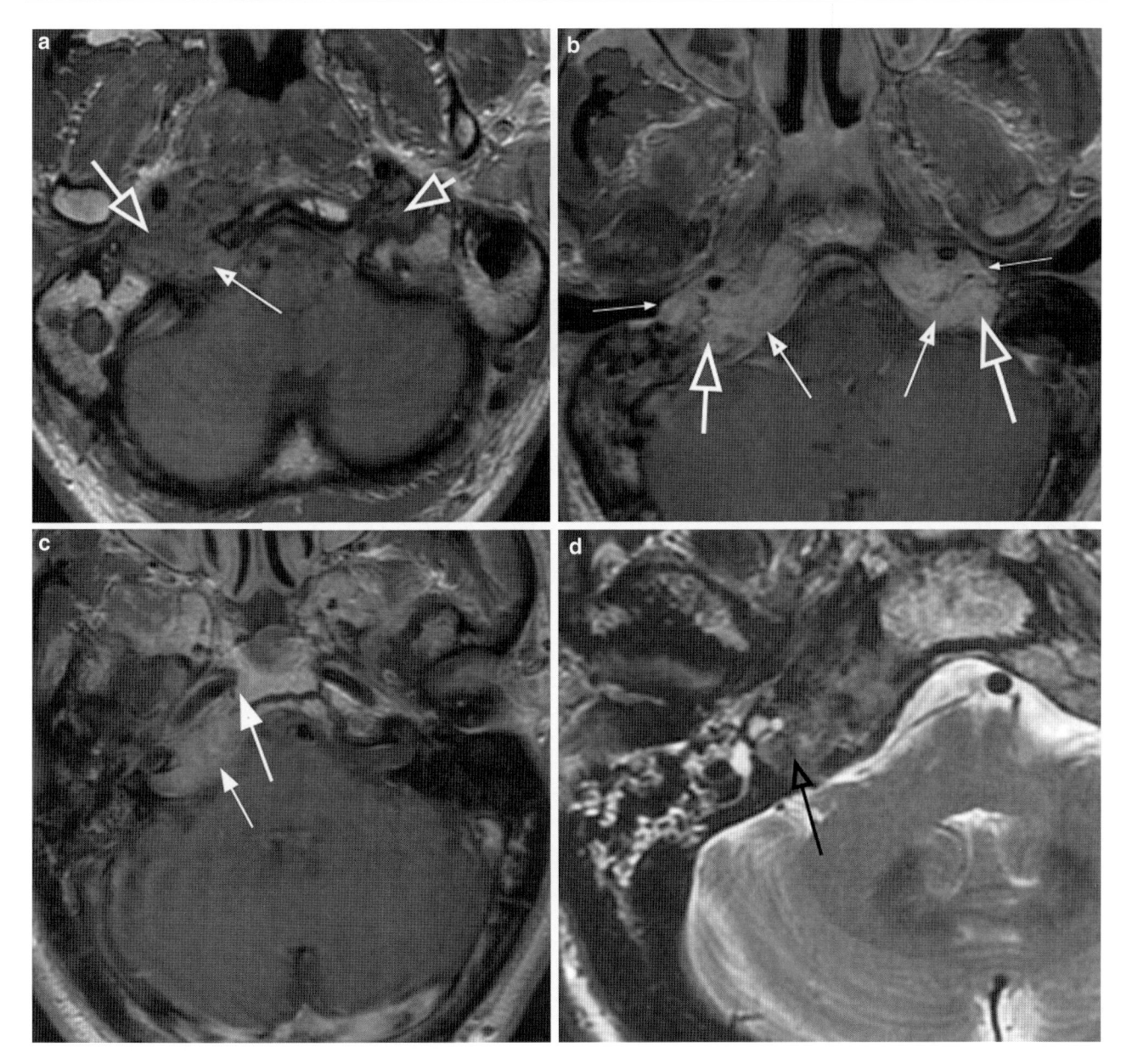

Fig. 7 *Large bilateral jugulotympanic paraganglioma*. Male 31year. Bilateral glomus caroticum (not shown), right glomus vagale (not shown) and bilateral glomus jugulotympanicum: right side classification: type C4De, left side classification: type C3De. **a** 2 mm axial 3D FT gradient echo T1W image without contrast; **b–c** axial T1W after Gd; **d**: axial 3 mm TSE T2W. The location of the tumour on the right side is: jugular foramen (*largest arrow*), medial of the horizontal canal of the carotid artery to the foramen lacerum (*second largest arrow*), intracranial extra-axial (*second smallest arrow*) the middle ear (*smallest arrow*) and the internal auditory canal. The location on the left is different in the relationship to the carotid canal, not reaching the foramen lacerum, in the absence of a location in the internal auditory canal and in the upper border of the extension. MR better shows the soft tissue extension. The intratumoral vessels (puntiforme zone's of signal void) and the salt and pepper appearance are clearly visible. **a** and **d** show the intratumoral vessels

cranial nerves IX–XI into the jugular foramen. Besides this primary meningioma of the jugular foramen, meningiomas may arise within the temporal bone and extend to the jugular foramen. Also, the more common meningioma of the facies posterior of the pars petrosum (cerebellopontine angle meningioma) can grow into the jugular foramen (Russel and Rubinstein 1989).

On CT, a meningioma gives, like a schwannoma, a smooth enlargement of the jugular foramen with an intact cortical outline (Fig. 10a). But cases of primary jugular foramen meningioma can give a diffuse skull base infiltration medial into the jugular tubercle and hypoglossal canal, lateral into the hypotympanum and inferior into the carotid space. The skull base infiltration has a "permeative-sclerotic

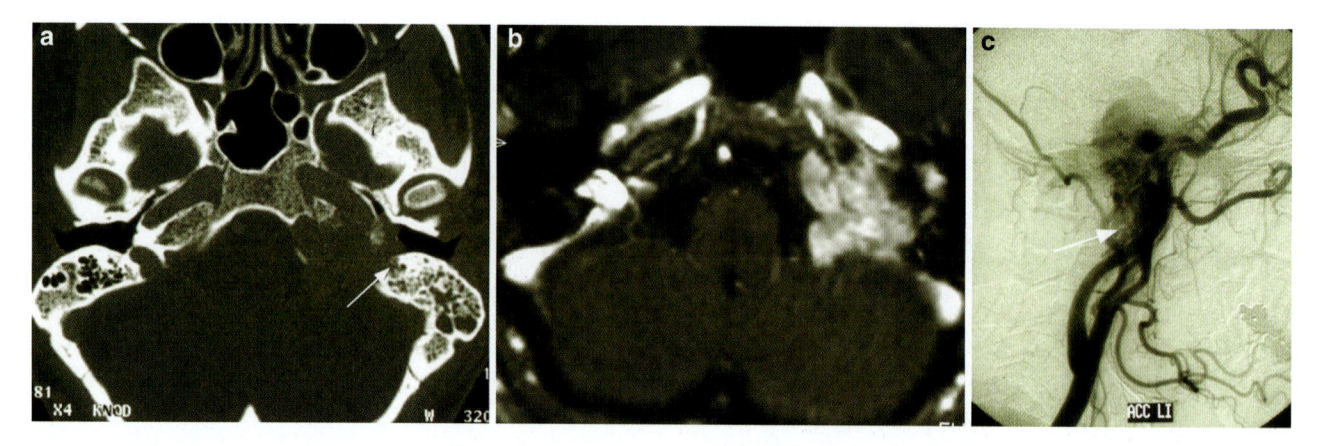

Fig. 8 *Jugulotympanic paraganglioma type C3De.* **a** 1 mm axial CT bone window; **b** 2 mm axial 3D FT gradient echo T1W image after contrast; **c** angiography of the left common carotid artery. The two hallmarks of a paraganglioma of the jugular foramen are the bony erosion (**a**) and the rich vascularisation (**c**). The tumours erodes the medial wall of the mastoid segment of the facial canal (*small arrow*). The intracranial extension remains extra-axial (**b**). The lesion extends below the skull base in the carotid loge until the C2 level (**c**) (*large arrow*)

Table 8 Classification of jugular foramen schwannoma (Samii et al. 1995)

Type A	Tumour primarily in the cerebellopontine angle with minimal location in the jugular foramen, but originating from a lower cranial nerve
Type B	Tumours primarily in the jugular foramen with intracranial extension
Type C	Extracranial tumours of the carotid loge, with intracranial extension
Type D	Dumbbell-shaped tumours with both intra- and extracranial extension

Table 9 Radiological hallmarks of schwannoma

Modality	Hallmark	Remark
CT	Smooth enlargement of the foramen	Not always in type A & C
	Intact cortical outline of the foramen	Contrary to paraganglioma
	Isodense or hypodense without contrast	
	No hyperostosis	Contrary to meningioma
	No intratumoral calcification	Contrary to meningioma, paraganglioma
MRI	No intratumoral vessels	Contrary to paraganglioma
	No vascular pedicle	Contrary to meningioma, paraganglioma
	Jugular bulb compression, no invasion	Contrary to paraganglioma, meningioma
CT and MRI	Frequent solid and cystic parts	Contrary to meningioma
	Location: Dumbbell in foramen and predominantly intracranial	
	Extension pattern	Not the fixed pattern of paraganglioma

appearance on CT and the margins of the jugular foramen become irregular". The medial extension differentiates the meningioma from paraganglioma (MacDonald et al. 2004; Vogl and Bisdas 2009). The presence of a broad dural attachment ("dural tail") is the most important differentiating imaging finding encountered in meningiomas. Nevertheless, in other cases a jugular foramen meningioma may arise from the arachnoid within the lower cranial nerve sheaths and not present a dural tail (Lowenheim et al. 2006). The tumour is isodense or hyperdense in the native CT without contrast. It is the most common tumour in this location that can have intratumoral calcifications (Fig. 10a), and practically the only one with bony sclerosis or hyperostosis. When this signs are absent the differential diagnosis with a paraganglioma can be difficult. On MR, the signal intensity is low in the T1W image and variable in the T2W image. After the administration of gadolinium the enhancement is strong and homogeneous (Fig. 10b, c). Frequently, there is an enhancement of the adjacent dura with gadolinium. This dural tail sign, although not pathognomonic, is very suggestive for meningioma, but it is among other lesions also described in schwannoma (Bourekas et al. 1995). Further features in the differential diagnosis with a paraganglioma are: a meningioma rarely has intratumoral vessels or the same angiographic appearance as a paraganglioma, the local extension pattern is different. Meningiomas do not have cystic components like a schwannoma (Table 10).

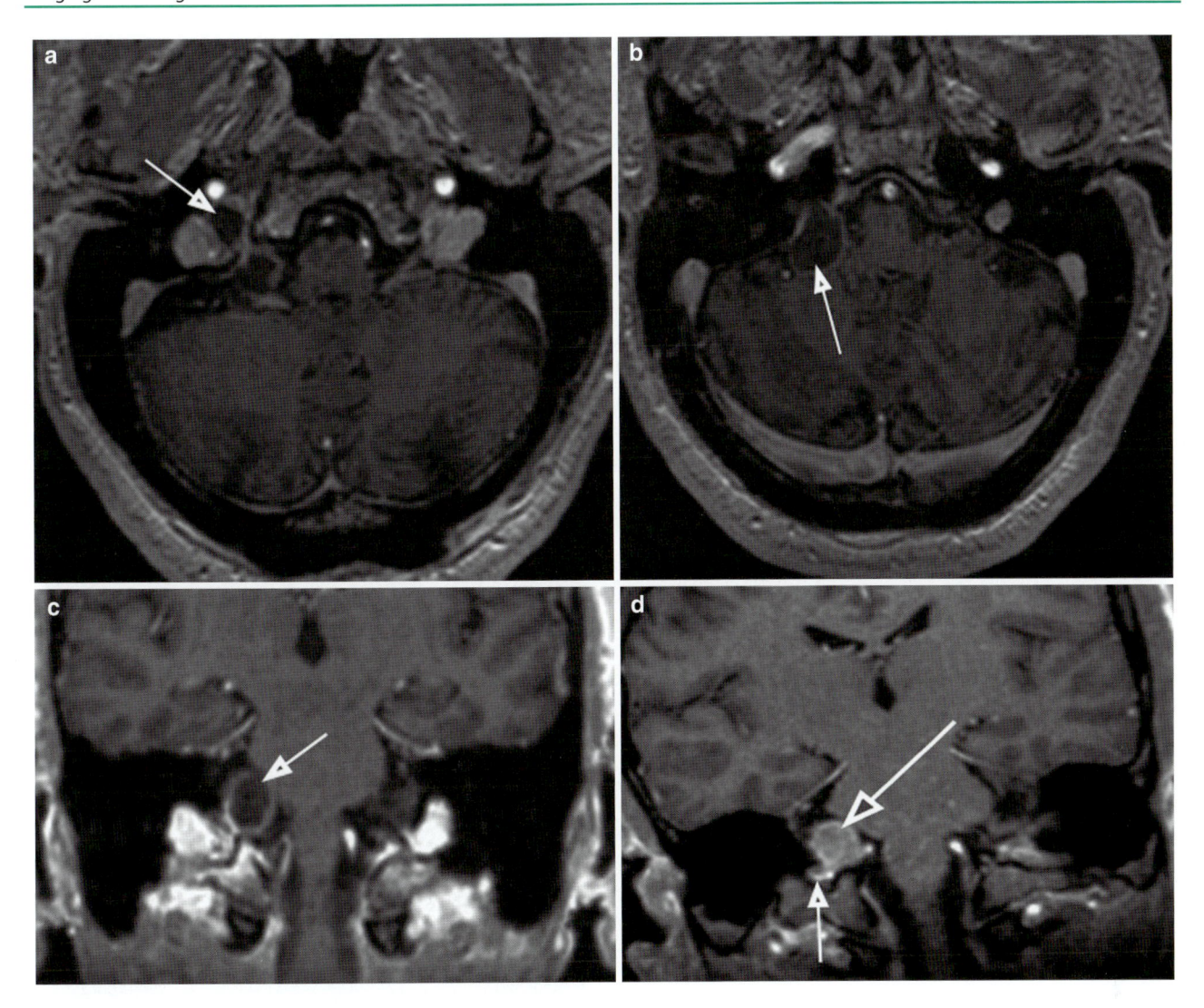

Fig. 9 *Schwannoma of the lower cranial nerves.* **a** axial MRI 3D GRE T1W 2 mm with contrast: smooth enlargement of pars nervosa with cystic tumour in this part (*arrow*). **b** axial MRI 3D GRE T1W with contrast and coronal MRI reconstruction: larger cystic part in the cerebellopontine angle (*arrow*) **c** coronal 3D GRE T1W image after contrast. In **d**, different patient shows a small tumour component in pars nervosa with in enlarged with intact cortical outline. The component in the cerebellopontine angle is larger and completely solid, without a cystic part

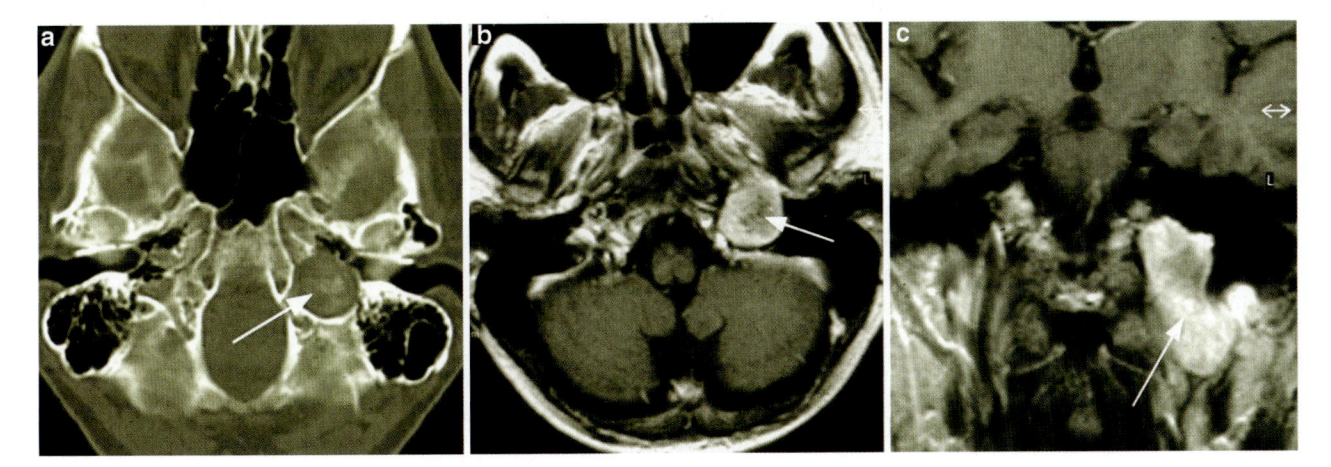

Fig. 10 *Meningioma.* **a** axial CT bone window; **b** and **c** 3 mm axial and coronal SE T1W image after contrast. Smooth enlargement of the jugular foramen with intact bony margins. The intratumoral calcifications (**a** *arrow*) give an important clue to the diagnosis. The tumour extends below the skull base in the carotid loge (**c** *arrow*). The non-enhancing part in **b** and **c** corresponds to the calcifications (*arrow*)

Table 10 Radiological hallmarks of meningioma

Modality	Hallmark	Remark
CT	Secondary meningioma: Smooth enlargement of the foramen with intact cortical outline	
	Primary meningioma: Possible permeative-sclerotic invasion of the walls of the foramen	Contrary to paraganglioma
	Isodense or hyperdense without contrast	
	Hyperostosis possible	Contrary to schwannoma
	Intratumoral calcification possible	Contrary to schwannoma, paraganglioma
MRI	No intratumoral vessels	Contrary to paraganglioma
	Vascular pedicle possible	Contrary to schwannoma, paraganglioma
	Jugular bulb invasion	Contrary to schwannoma
	Dural tail sign	
CT and MRI	No cystic parts	Contrary to schwannoma
	Location: primary in foramen or extension to the foramen from infratentorial	
	Medial extension pattern	Not the fixed pattern of paraganglioma

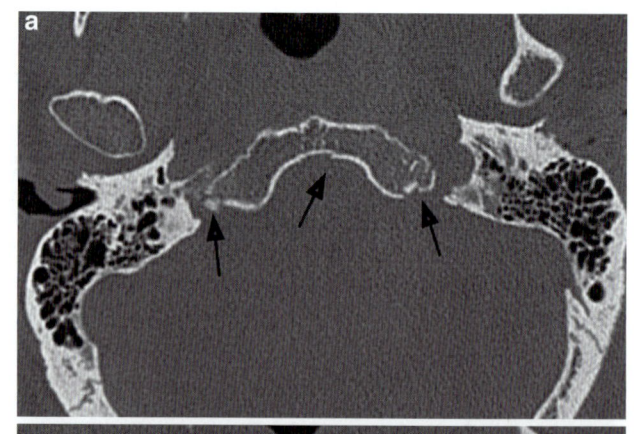

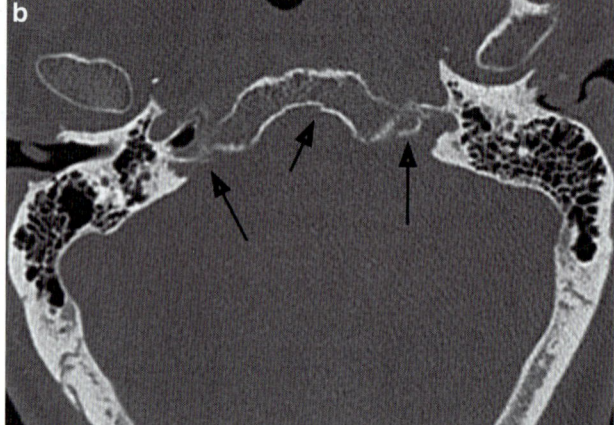

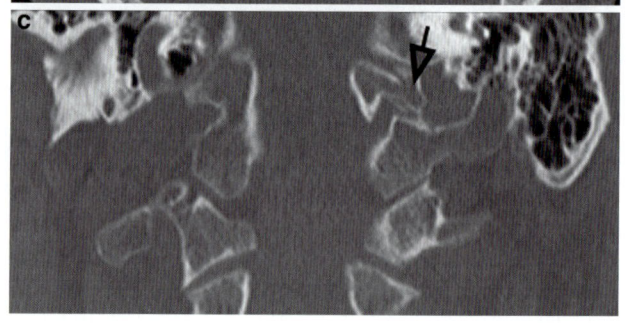

Fig. 11 *Traumatic lesion of the jugular foramen*: fracture CT axial bone window. **a–c** fracture of right and left jugular foramen and the clivus. (Among many other cranio-cerebral lesion, not shown)

6   Other Lesions of the Jugular Foramen

6.1   Traumatic lesions

Traumatic lesion of the jugular foramen occurs in the setting of serious cranio-cerebral trauma with associated skull base fracture or by penetrating trauma (Sacks 1993). Possible traumatic lesions of the jugular foramen are: (1) fracture (Fig. 11), (2) CSF lekkage, (3) Arterial or venous damage.

In the presence of a skull base fracture, with or without a dural tear and cerebrospinal fluid (CSF) leakage, bone-windowed, high-resolution CT with multiplanar reconstructions is the imaging of choice. A suspected dural tear is best evaluated with thin section CT. Contrast administration is not necessary because the fracture indicates where the CSF leak is, unless there is extensive damage or if the precise site of the fracture is in question. In these cases, intrathecal contrast medium may be useful (Vogl and Bisdas 2009).

7   Uncommon Tumours (Primary and Secondary)

7.1   Endolymphatic Sac Tumour

In the late years of the previous century, the endolymphatic sac tumour (ELST) has been recognized as a separate entity. The ELST is an adenomatous neoplasm of the papillary pattern originating from the endolymphatic sac's epithelium. Other possible adenomatous tumours of the temporal bone are metastases, direct extensions from extratemporal lesions and the primary middle ear adenomatous tumours of

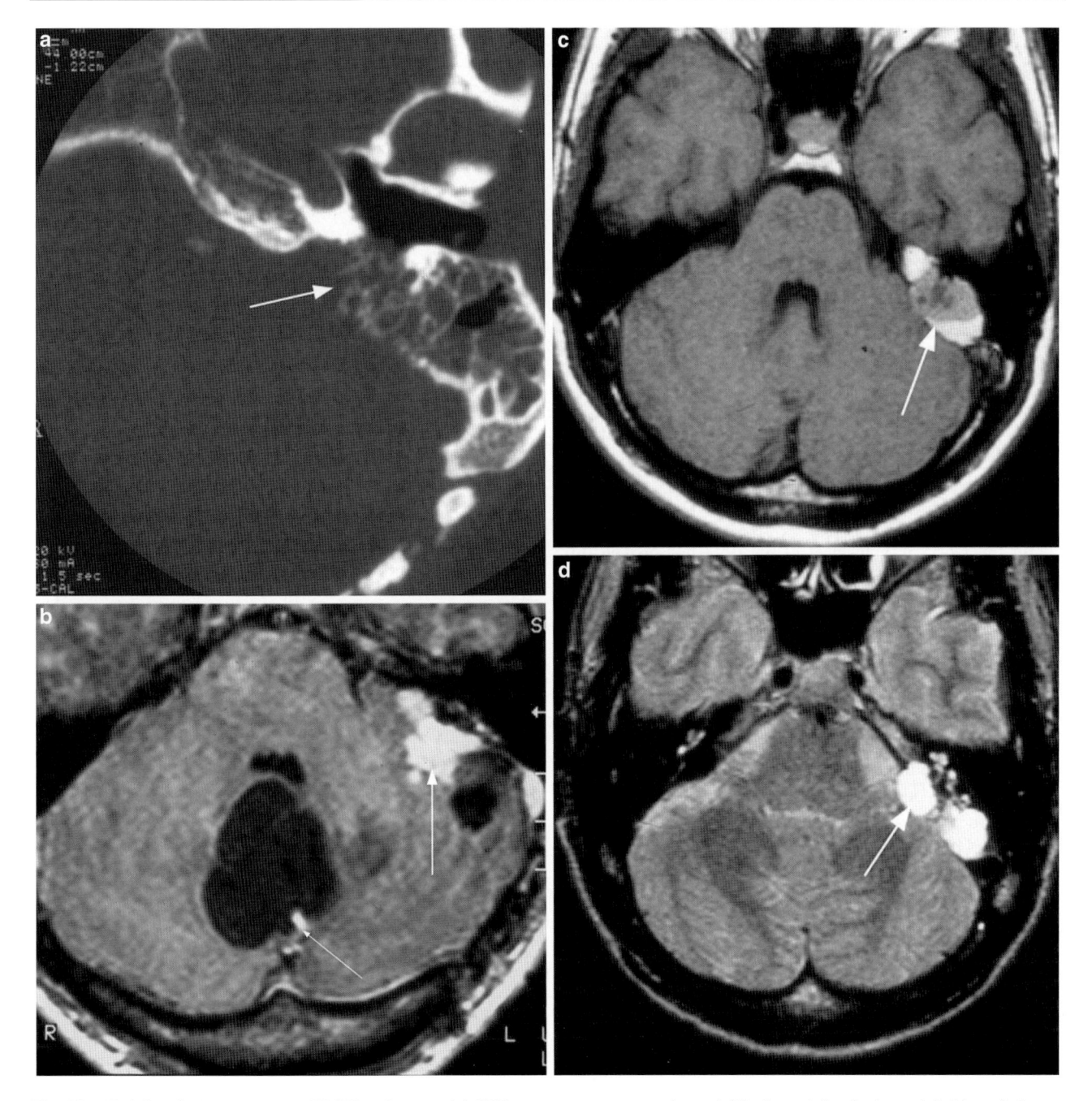

Fig. 12 *Endolymphatic sac tumour (ELST).* **a** 1 mm axial CT bone window and **b** 3 mm axial SE T1 W image after contrast in a patient with Von Hippel-Lindau disease. **c** 3 mm axial non-enhanced SE T1W image and **d** 3 mm axial SE T2W image in a different patient. The CT in **a** in a patient with Von Hippel-Lindau disease shows bony erosions of the jugular foramen and extension along the facies posterior of the pars petrosum (*arrow*). The bony defect in the occipital bone is from a previous operation. The MR in **b** shows the enhancing of the ELST (*large arrow*) and an haemangioblastoma with a large cystic part and a small mural nodule (*small arrow*). The signal intensity of the lesion in the MR of **c** and **d** in a different patient corresponds to blood products with a fluid level in **c** (*arrow*)

the mixed histological pattern (Batsakis and El-Naggar 1993). The endolymphatic sac is the terminal saccular enlargement of the endolymphatic duct and lies between the inner and outer layers of the dura and the facies posterior of the pars petrosum. The ELST is centred between the sigmoid sinus and the internal auditory canal (IAC) around the vestibular aqueduct at the facies posterior. There is frequent involvement of the IAC, the jugular foramen and the posterior fossa. When it extends into the middle ear, it is a rare cause of a vascular mass (Batsakis and El-Naggar 1993). Several isolated reports have suggested a possible association of ELST with the von Hippel-Lindau disease, and

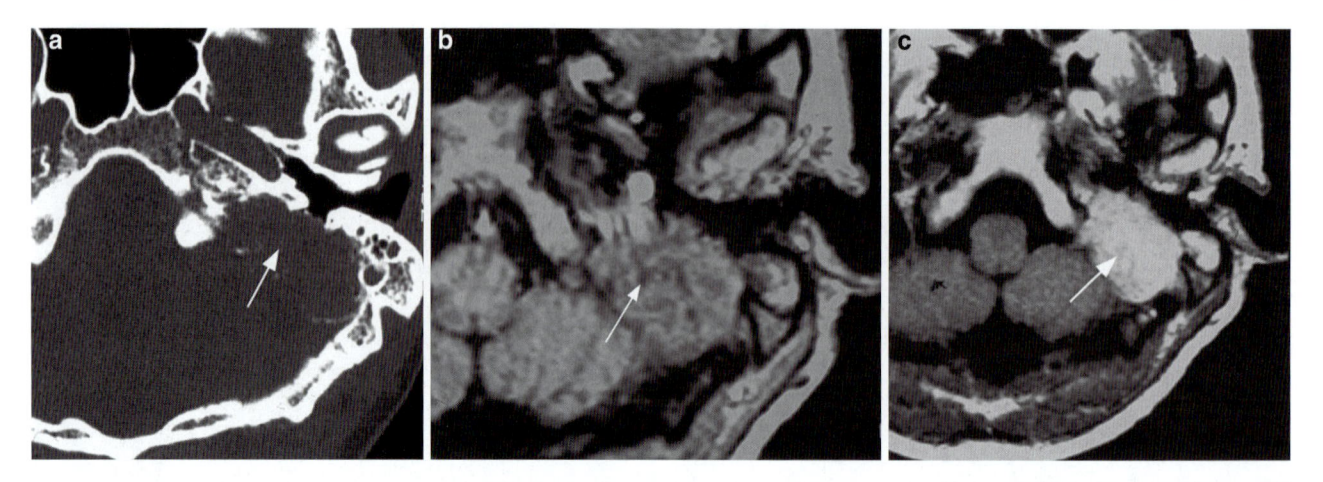

Fig. 13 *Giant cell tumour.* **a** 1 mm axial CT bone window, **b** and **c** 2 mm axial 3D FT gradient echo T1W image without and with contrast. The CT and MR examination shows a destructive lesion in the jugular foramen and pars petrosum (*large arrow* in **a**, **b**), with some intratumoral zones of signal void not due to calcifications (*arrow* in **b**). The tumour was avascular on angiography (not shown). Strong enhancement after contrast (*arrow* in **c**)

finally the work of Manski et al. in 1997 has proven this association (Fig. 9a, b). The prevalence of ELST in the von Hippel-Lindau disease is 6 %, much higher than in the general population (Manski et al. 1997). The ELST is a slow-growing, locally aggressive, hypervascular tumour that do not metastasise. The hallmark of the tumour on CT is bony destruction (Fig. 12a). The lytic bony margins have a geographic or mixed geographic-moth-eaten pattern. Within the lesion there are hyperdense areas, corresponding to intratumoral bone with bone trabeculae, as found on histological sections. On MR, the ELST is a "blood product containing" tumour. In the T1W and T2W images the signal intensity (SI) is heterogeneous, with hyperintens areas corresponding to blood-filled cysts, proteinaceous cysts and subacute haemorrhage. In between are smaller foci of marked hypointensity, representing the tumour bone matrix and/or hemosiderin (Fig. 12c, d). After administration of gadolinium, the enhancement is strong (Fig. 12b). Angiography shows a hypervascular mass, that mimics a paraganglioma (Lo et al. 1993). Although both ELST and paraganglioma cause irregular bone destruction, may involve the jugular foramen and are hypervascular, the differential diagnosis is easy when looking at the primary location of the tumour: ELST is located retrolabyrinthine at the facies posterior, and the glomus tumour primary infralabyrinthine. The typical flow voids on MR of the larger glomus tumours are not seen in the smaller ones and also not in the ELST. The haemangioma, an other tumour with prominent intratumoral bone spiculae in this region has a different location at the IAC, the suprageniculate region or the mastoid genu of the facial canal.

7.2 Giant Cell Tumour

This tumour occurs rarely in the jugular foramen. The radiological features on CT and MR can be indistinguishable from those of a paraganglioma. On angiography, this tumour can be as vascular as a paraganglioma (Rosenbloom et al. 1999), although our own case was avascular (Fig. 13).

7.3 Metastasis

In an early stage, metastases may be indistinguishable from paraganglioma, but they are more aggressive and destructive, evolve faster and the extension pattern is different. The history is usually key to the diagnosis. A metastasis can be lytic, sclerotic or mixed. Figure 14a–d shows a rare case of a primary malignant brain tumour, glioblastoma multiforme with bone metastasis to the jugular foramen and the skull base. Apart from bone metasis to the jugular foramen also leptomeningeal metastasis of the cranial nerves within the foramen can occur (Fig. 14e).

7.4 Chordoma

Chordoma arises from notochord that forms the embryonal axial skeleton. Remnants of the primitive notochord can occur at any position along the neuraxis, but mostly in the sacrococcygeal region and in the spheno-occipital area. In principle, the chordoma of the skull base is a midline tumours arising from the clivus but they can extend to the

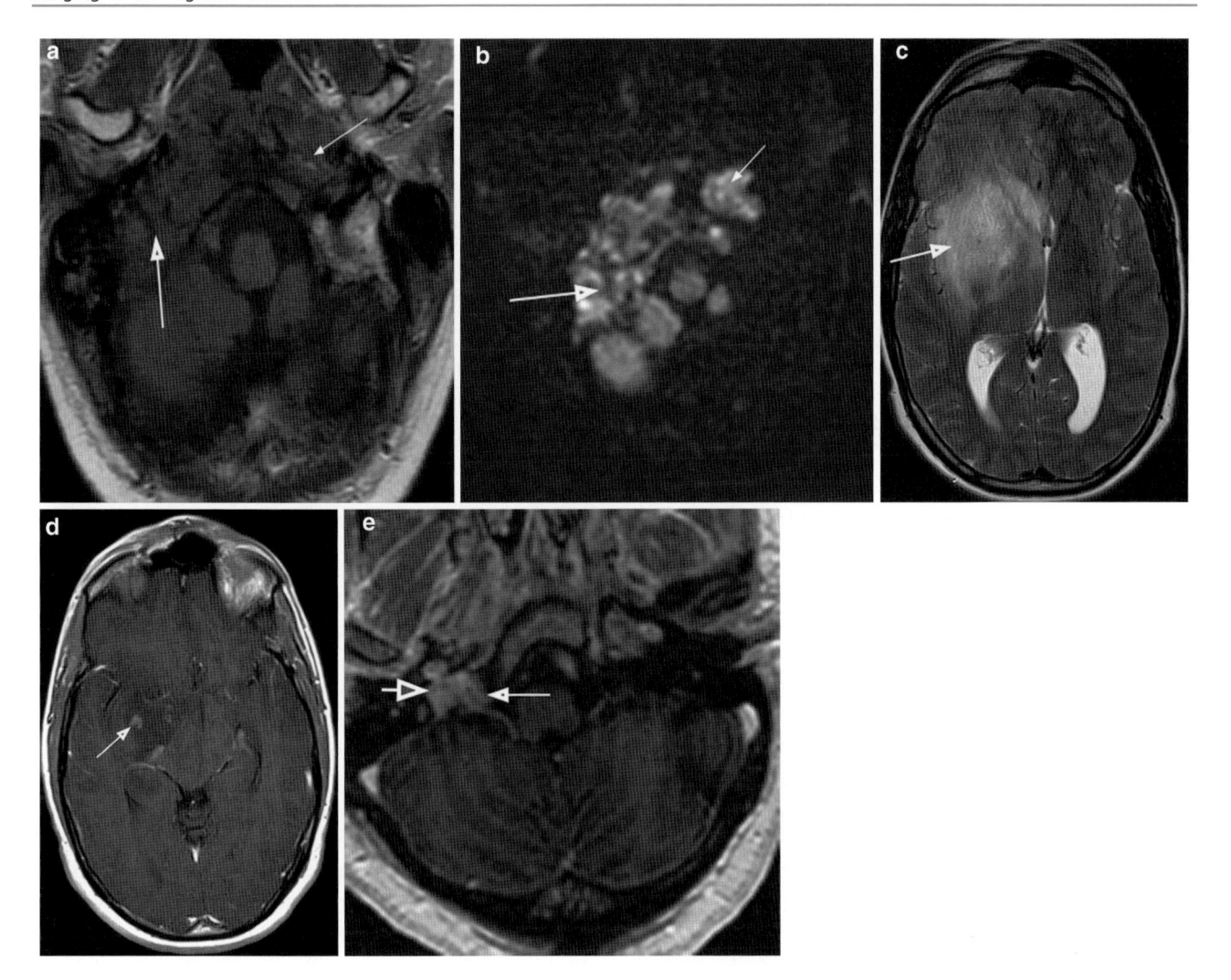

Fig. 14 *Metastasis and leptomeningeal metastasis (two different patients)* **a–d** Man, 38 year, primary malignant brain tumour: glioblastoma multiforme. Rare occurrence of bone metastasis and lymphogenetic metastasis due to a primary brain tumour. **a** axial MRI 3D GRE 2 mm without contrast and **b** axial DWI shows an osteolytic lesion of the right jugular foramen, pars petrosum, clivus, retropharyngeal region, prevertebral muscles (*large arrow*) and extension to the left (*small arrow*). There is a diffusion restriction of the lesion. The primary brain tumour, a glioblastoma multiforme can be seen in **c** axial TSE T2W 5 mm and **d** axial TSE T1W after gadolinium 5 mm (*arrow*) shows an intra-axial mass with pathologic enhancement. **e** Woman, 64 year, mamma carcinoma. Axial 3D GRE T1W after gadolinium, 1 mm thickness. Thickening and abnormal enhancement of the right IXth nerve in the pars nervosa of the jugular foramen as a manifestation of leptomeningeal metastasis (*small arrow*), also present on the facial nerve, not shown. The jugular foramen is not enlarged and not eroded and the pars vascularis is normal (*large arrow*)

jugular foramen. The phenomenon of lateral occurrence of chordomas is embryologically possible, because forking at the rostral end of the embryonic notochord can leave behind some notocordal remnants in these areas. Chordomas arising around the jugular foramen and extending into the carotid space are theoretically possible but extremely rare (Dwivedi et al. 2011). On CT, the tumour shows a lytic bone destruction without sclerosis. Bony sequestra within the tumour mass occur. On MR, the lesion has frequently a heterogeneous signal intensity, because of old intratumoral haemorrhage, high protein mucinous collections and bony sequestra. The enhancement after contrast is moderate to marked (Dwivedi et al. 2011) (Fig. 15).

7.5 Nasopharyngeal Carcinoma

Nasopharyngeal cancer accounts for only a small percentage of all head and neck malignancies. About 85 % are carcinoma, while 10 % are lymphoma. The carcinoma can

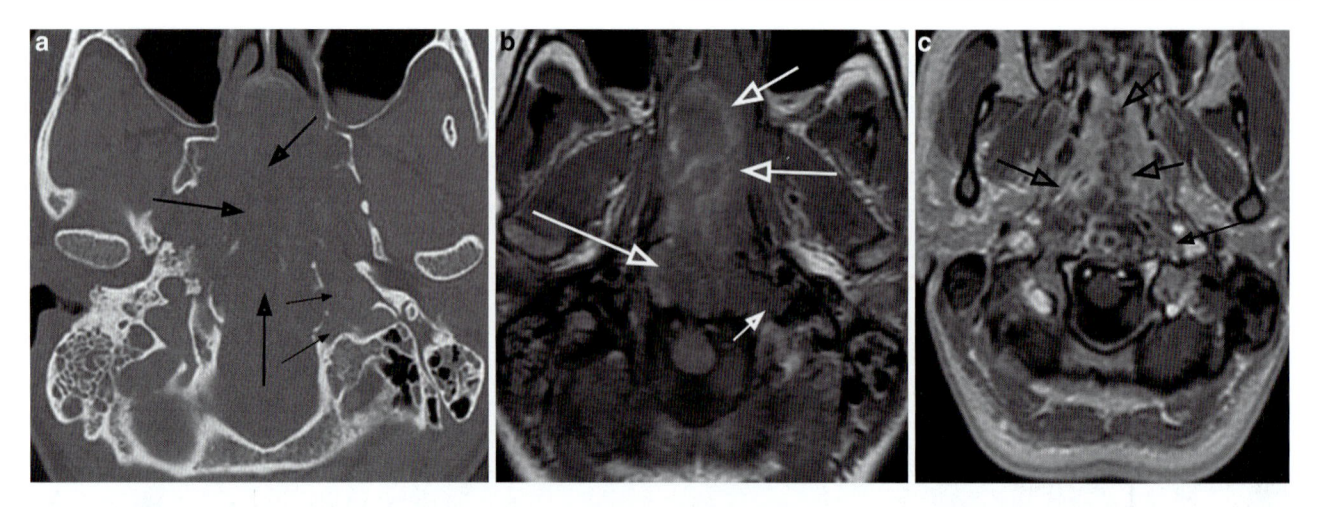

Fig. 15 *Midline chordoma with lateral extension to the left jugular foramen.* **a** axial CT bone window; **b** MRI 3D GRE T1W 1.6 mm without contrast; **c** MRI 3D GRE T1W 1.6 mm with contrast. Extensive bone destruction of the midline skull base with large soft tissue mass (*large arrow*). The left jugular foramen is involved (*small arrow*)

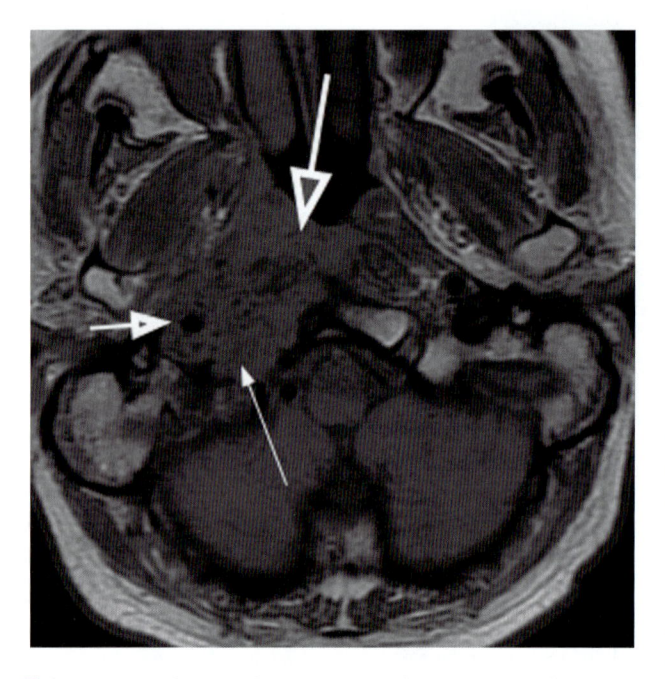

Fig. 16 *Nasopharyngeal carcinoma with extension to the jugular foramen.* Axial TSE T1W without contrast 3 mm. Nasopharyngeal carcinoma with extension to the retropharyngeal space, prevertebral muscles, the clivus (*large arrow*), the pars petrosum, the carotid canal (*middle sized arrow*) and the jugular foramen (*small arrow*)

invade local bony structures like the central skull base, clivus, pars petrosum and the jugular foramen (Mancuso 2011) (Fig. 16).

7.6 Temporal Bone/Middle Ear Carcinoma

Malignant tumours arising from the middle ear are rare. Possible tumour types are: squamous cell carcinoma and benign and malignant salivary gland tumours. These tend to arise from the middle two-thirds of the Eustachian tube and the middle ear. Middle ear carcinoma can be seen in patients with long-standing middle ear inflammation. These lesions are usually extensive at the first time of presentation with growth to the carotid canal, jugular foramen, inner ear, along the facial nerve and intracranially to the dura, venous sinuses, leptomeninges and brain parenchyma. CT shows massive bony destruction in and around temporal bone and possible also the jugular foramen. MRI is needed to demonstrate the soft tissue extension outside the temporal bone. The MRI characteristics are compatible with a soft tissue mass without extensive vascularisation. The extension pattern differs from paraganglioma. For the diagnosis the history of long-standing middle ear disease, combined with the imaging documentation of extensive bony destruction of the surrounding structures is important (Verbist et al. 2011).

8 Infectious Disease

8.1 Malignant External Otitis (Necrotizing External Otitis)

Malignant external otitis (necrotizing external otitis) is a potentially life-threatening infection of the external auditory canal and skull base. The infection occurs mostly in elderly diabetic or immunocompromised patients. The infection begins as a typical external otitis (Fig. 17a) and extends from the external auditory canal inferiorly via the fissures of Santorini to involve the soft tissues around the stylomastoid foramen, causing a facial nerve palsy. With further extension the mastoid, middle ear, the parotis and other soft tissues of the neck becomes involved and with posteromedial extension also the jugular foramen. A diffuse skull base

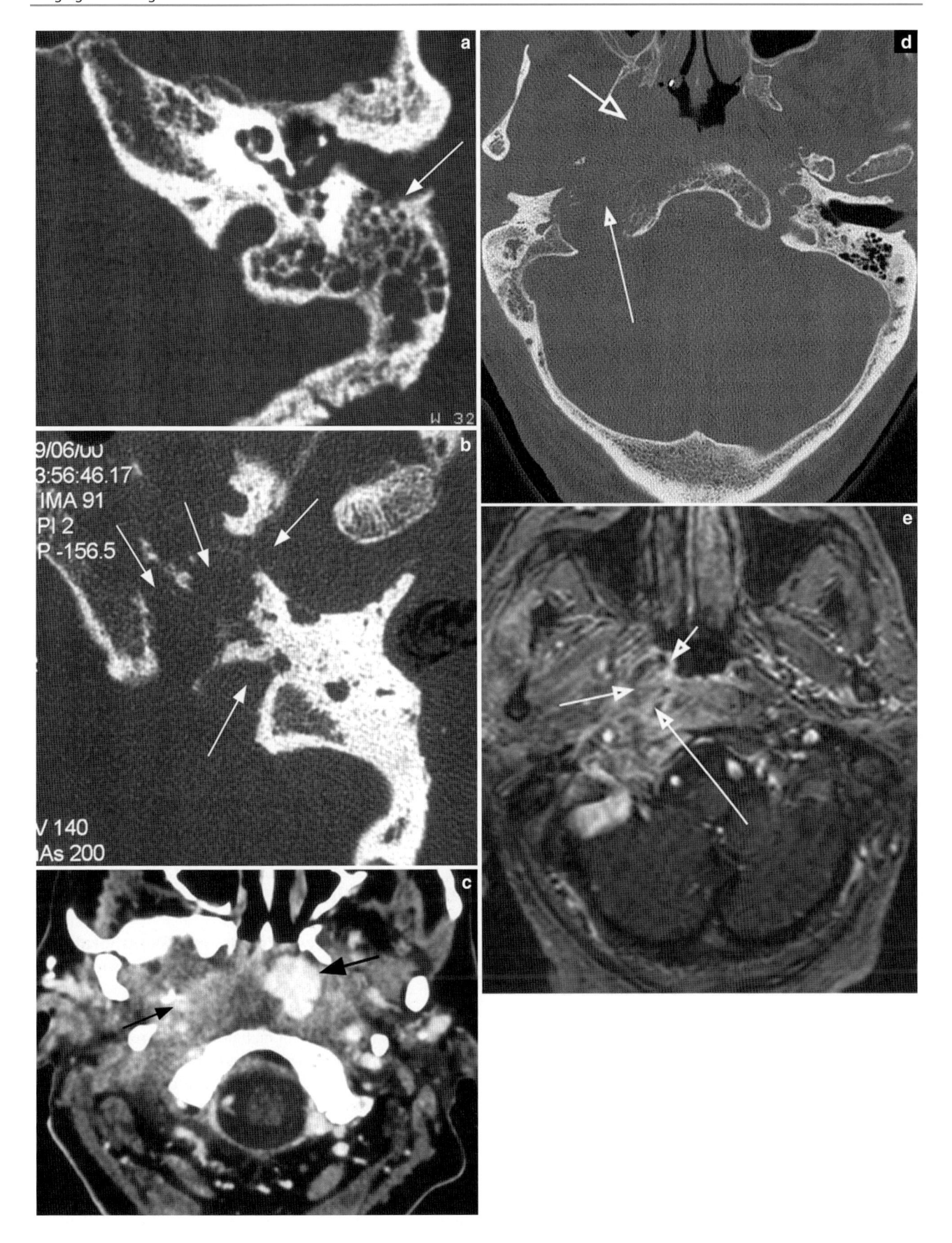

Imaging of the Jugular Foramen   323

◀ **Fig. 17** *Malignant external otitis.* **a** 1 mm axial CT bone window in a patient with an early stadium of the disease. There is a soft tissue mass in the external and middle ear with minimal erosion of the posterior wall of the external auditory canal (*arrow*). No further extension into the skull base and the jugular foramen is intact. **b** and **c** 1 mm axial CT bone window and 2 mm axial CT after contrast in a different patient shows extensive disease with erosion, destruction of large parts of the temporal bone and skull base, including the jugular foramen (*arrows*). The soft tissue extension below the skull base is bilateral with invasion of both carotid loges and bilateral bacterial arteritis. On the right, this leads to a stenosis of the internal carotid artery (*small arrow*) and on the left to a rupture of the artery with a large pseudo aneurysm (*large arrow*). The patient died from a bleeding. **d** and **e** different patient: Axial CT bone window and axial MRI T1W after gadolinium. Extensive bone destruction, osteomyelitis of the skull base, including the temporal bone, clivus and the jugular foramen. Soft tissue extension to prevertebral, retropharyngeal, nasopharyngeal mucosal spaces (*arrows*)

osteomyelitis finally results (Fig. 17b–e). *Pseudomonas aeruginosa* is the most common pathogen. Infections caused by aspergillus are less frequent and typically begins in the middle ear or mastoid.

CT and MRI are used for the initial inventarisation of the extend of the disease. CT shows the bony erosions and the soft tissue extension, but for the latter is MRI better. Neither modalities are suited for the follow up of the osteomyelitis. Nuclear medicine techniques are a better choice for the treatment follow up (Slattery and Brackmann 1996).

9 Lesions of the Jugular Foramen in Children

9.1 Congenital Lesions

9.1.1 Craniosynostosis

Craniosynostosis is defined as a premature closure of 1 or more cranial sutures. There are two types: (1) syndromic, which is associated with other congenital abnormalities as seen in patients with Apert, Crouzon and Pfeiffer syndromes; and (2) nonsyndromic, which is an isolated spontaneous closure of 1 or more cranial sutures. It is a relatively rare congenital defect that occurs in about 1 in 2,500 births. A serious potential complication of craniosynostosis is intracranial hypertension. Booth et al. (2011) found a reduction of 23 % in size of the diameter of the right jugular foramen (not the left) in children with craniosynostosis as the possible cause. Jugular venous outflow obstruction has a major role in the pathogenesis of raised ICP in children with craniosynostosis. The jugular bulb develops after birth and in early infancy, alternative emissary veins have a more important functional role than after establishment of a more adult pattern of jugular venous drainage (Rich et al. 2003). CT is used to document the jugular foramen narrowing (Fig. 18).

9.1.2 Achondroplasia

Achondroplasia is the most common form of dwarfism. It is a congenital disorder of the endochondral ossification and as such it is associated with a variable severe skull base deformity. Achondroplasia follows an autosomal dominant inheritance pattern, although 80 % of cases arise as a result of spontaneous mutations in the fibroblast growth factor receptor 3. Because of the defective endochondral bone formation at the skull base and the craniocervical junction, infants with achondroplasia may have among other deformities a to small foramen magnum, and a stenotic jugular foramen. These combination is considered as the cause of hydrocephalus in children with achondroplasia because of obstruction of the CSF outflow (foramen magnum stenosis) combined with elevated venous sinus pressures (jugular foramen stenosis) (Moritani et al. 2006; Hervey-Jumper et al. 2011).

9.1.3 Meningocoele

A jugular foramen meningocoele occur especially in patients with neurofibromatosis type I. On CT, the jugular foramen is enlarged with a smooth expansion and intact cortical outline. On MRI, the jugular foramen is filled with a cerebrospinal fluid signal intensity, communicating with the cerebellomedullary cistern. The underlying cause is the dural ectasia or dysplastic weakening of the bone, known to occur in neurofibromatosis type I (Siddiqui et al. 2008).

9.1.4 Congenital vascular variants

These are discussed in the chapter on vascular temporal bone lesions.

10 Tumours

10.1 Primary Ewing's Sarcoma/Peripheral Primitive Neuroectodermal Tumour

Ewing's sarcoma (ES)/peripheral primitive neuroectodermal tumour (pPNET) is a malignant small, round, blue cell tumour within the Ewing's sarcoma family of tumours originating from the neural crest. The chromosomal translocations t, q and immunoreactivity for CD99 encoded by the MIC2 gene are reliable diagnostic markers of this neoplasm. These tumours usually occur in the long bones or soft tissues of children and young adults. Approximately 1 % of ES/pPNET tumours arise in the cranium. The skull base region is a far less commonly affected site. ES/pPNET

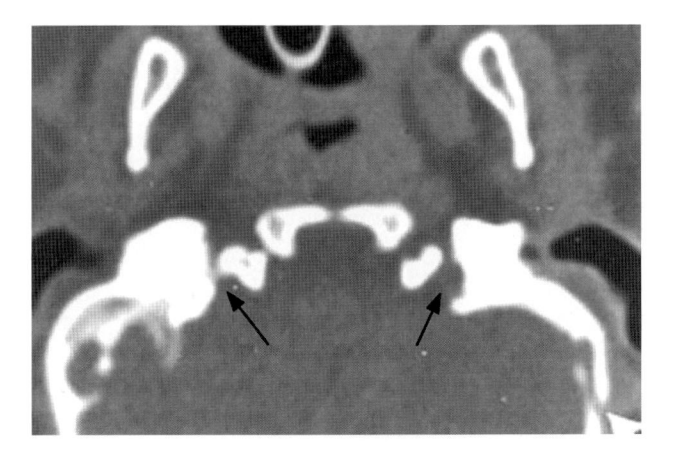

Fig. 18 *Craniosynostosis with bilateral narrowing of the jugular foramen.* Axial CT in a child. Bilateral narrowing of the jugular foramen (*arrows*)

occurs mostly in the second decade of life. On CT with bone window, the jugular foramen is enlarged without bony destruction and without calcifications. On MRI the lesion is on isointense in T1W sequence, moderately hyperintens on T2W sequence. The enhancement after gadolinium is heterogeneously. The differential diagnosis with schwannoma and meningioma can be difficult, but these two lesions occur in another age group (Kobayashi et al. 2008).

10.2 Fibromatosis

Fibromatosis is defined as an infiltrating or aggressive fibroblastic proliferation lacking histologic features of either an inflammatory process or a neoplasm. It is a benign tumor with locally invasive characteristics. It infiltrates surrounding tissues and tends to recur after surgical resection. This behaviour has lead to difficulty in classifying the lesion with synonyms of desmoid tumor, aggressive fibromatosis and inflammatory pseudotumor all used to refer to the same lesion. Perez-Cruet et al. (1998) describe 78 patients with aggressive fibromatosis of the head and neck over a 12-year period and of these, five patients had cranial base involvement. All five were children ranging from 1 to 16 years old. Localisation in the jugular foramen is rare. The neuroradiological characteristics are non-specific.

On CT, the jugular foramen is enlarged with intact cortical outline. The mass can extend below the skull base into the carotid loge. After contrast, there is a ringlioke enhancement with a hypodense centre. On MRI, the signal intensity is hyperintens on T2W sequence and the enhancement is heterogeneous (Madnani et al. 2006).

10.3 Osteosarcoma

Osteosarcoma is the most common primary bone malignancy. It is characterised by osteoid or immature bone production by malignant spindle cells. Osteosarcoma primarily affects the long bones in children and adolescents and has an incidence of approximately 1:100,000 per year. Mostly, 6–10 % of cases present in the head and neck, usually in the mandible or less frequently, in the maxilla. Location in the jugular foramen is very rare. Complete surgical excision is the mainstay of treatment, of course difficult to impossible in the region of the jugular foramen (Chennupati et al. 2007). On CT the jugular foramen is enlarged, initially with an intact cortical outline, later this can be damaged. The surrounding bone shows permeative-sclerotic changes, comparable to the primary meningioma of the jugular foramen. In our case, there were calcifications within the foramen. On MRI, the signal intensity of parts of the lesion are compatible with heavy calcifications. There are no intratumoral vessels. With specialized MR techniques (like 3D FIESTA after gadolinium), the damage to the cranial nerves in and around the jugular foramen can be examined. The enhancement in the few documented cases is homogeneous (Fig. 19).

10.4 Histiocytosis

Langerhans cell histiocytosis occurs predominantly in children (15–60 % of children with the disease) (Rubinstein et al. 1995). Total 86 % of the patients are under the age of 10 years at onset. Approximately 70–80 % have head and neck involvement and 20–30 % of the children have temporal bone involvement. The pathogenesis is not well established, but it is supposed to be caused by an abnormal immune regulation. The disease is not considered as truly neoplastic. This tumour like condition is characterised by a lytic bone destruction, which may be extensive. In the temporal bone the disease primary involves the otic capsule, lateral mastoid or the external auditory canal region. The jugular foramen may be secondarily involved. CT shows a lytic lesion without reactive sclerosis. The soft tissue mass enhances strong and homogeneous (Fig. 19). On MRI, the lesion can have a heterogeneous signal intensity due to the presence of blood degradation products (Bonafé et al. 1994). The radiological differential diagnosis with rhabdomyosarcoma may be difficult, but the occurrence of cranial nerve palsy is less frequent in histiocytosis (Fernandes-Latorre et al. 2000) (Fig. 20).

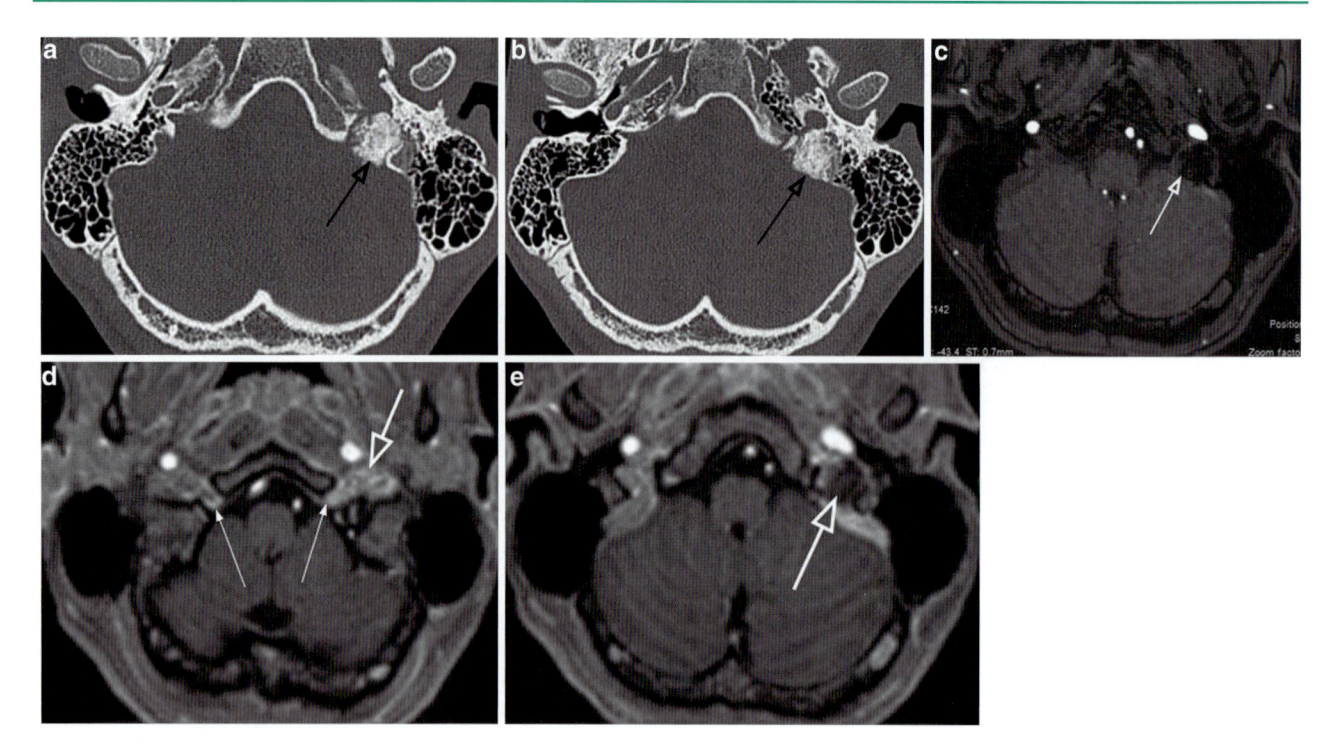

Fig. 19 *Osteosarcoma* Boy 16 year. **a–b** CT bone window. Slight enlargement of the left jugular foramen. Heavely calcification in the foramen with extension to the lateral and posterior wall of the foramen, permeative-sclerotic of character (*arrow*). **c** MRI TOF 3D. Dark signal intensity in the lumen, due to the calcifications (*arrow*). **d–e** MRI 3D GRE T1W after gadolinium Soft tissue enhancement around the calcifications in the foramen (*large arrow*) Occlusion of the jugular bulb. Extension to the canalis hypoglossus and the left nervus hypoglossus cannot identified compared to right side (*small arrows*)

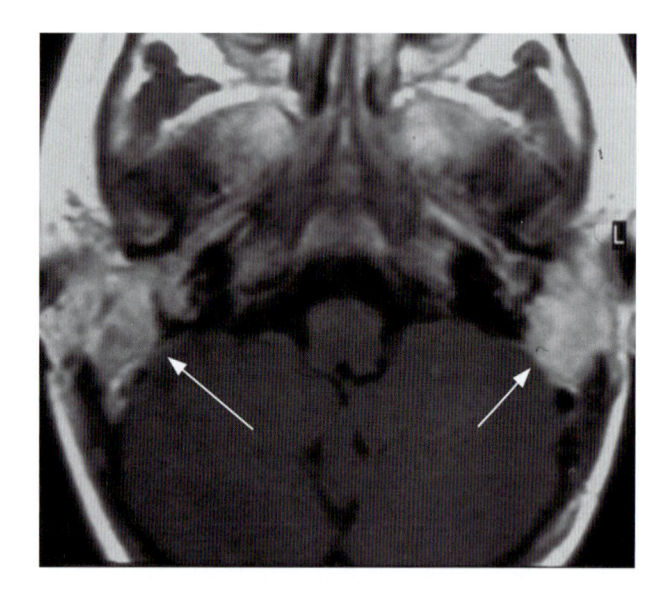

Fig. 20 *Histiocytosis*. MRI 3 mm axial SE T1W image after contrast in a child of 2 year. Bilateral homogeneous enhancing lesion of many parts of the temporal bone, including the jugular foramen (*arrows*)

10.5 Rhabdomyosarcoma

Rhabdomyosarcoma is the most common soft tissue sarcoma in children. About 30–50 % occur in the head and neck region. It is a highly malignant neoplasm thought to arise from primitive mesenchymal cells committed to skeletal muscle differentiation (rhabdomyoblast). Head and neck rhabdomyosarcoma is classified as cranial parameningeal, orbital and non-orbital parameningeal. The temporal bone rhabdomyosarcoma is classified as parameningeal. It can extend to the jugular foramen. CT demonstrates extensive bony destruction. Intratumoral calcifications are rare. The extent of the soft tissue mass is best seen on MRI. The MRI signal characteristics are a non-specific intermediate T1W signal abnormality and hyperintens T2W signal abnormality. The enhancement after gadolinium is intens. The imaging differential diagnosis with Langerhans histiocytosis and other aggressive tumours, like adenocarcinoma and squamous cell carcinoma may be impossible. The age of the patient is an important factor in the differential diagnosis. (McCarvill et al. 2001; Vogl and Bisdas 2009).

References

Aydin H, Altin E, Dilli A, Sipahioglu S, Hekimoglu B (2011) Evaluation of jugular foramen nerves by using b-FFE, T2-weighted DRIVe, T2-weighted FSE and post-contrast T1-weighted MRI sequences. Diagn Intervent Radiol 17:3–9

Batsakis GJ, El-Naggar AK (1993) Papillary neoplasm (Heffner's Tumors) of the endolymphatic sac. Ann Otol Rhinol Laryngol 102:648–651

Bonafé A, Joomye H, Jaeger P, Fraysse B, Manelfe C (1994) Histiocytosis X of the petrous bone in the adult: MRI. Neuroradiology 36:330–334

Booth CD, Figuero RE, Lehn A, Yu JC (2011) Analysis of the jugular foramen in pediatric patients with craniosynostosis. J Craniofac Surg 22:285–288

Bourekas EC, Wildenhain P, Lewin JS, Tarr RW, Dastur KJ, Raji MR, Lanzieri CF (1995) The dural tail sign revisited. AJNR 16:1514–1516

Burger PC, Scheithauer BW (2007) AFIP atlas of tumor pathology series 4: tumors of the central nervous system. ARP, Washington

Chennupati SK, Norris R, Dunham B, Kazahaya K (2007) Osteosarcoma of the skull base: case report and review of the literature. Int J Pediatr Otorhinolaryngol 72:115–119

Davagnanam I, Chavda SV (2008) Identification of the normal jugular foramen and lower cranial nerve anatomy: contrast-enhanced 3D fast imaging steady-state acquisition MR imaging. AJNR 29:574–576

Dwivedi RC, Krishna BK, Mishra A, Youssefi P, Thway K, Sultan Ul Hassan M, Agrawal N, Kazi R (2011) A rare case of jugular foramen chordoma with an unusual extension. Arch Otolaryngol Head Neck Surg 137:513–517

Eldevik OP, Gabrielsen TO, Jacobsen EA (2000) Imaging findings in schwannomas of the jugular foramen. AJNR 21:1139–1144

Fernandez-Latorre F, Menor-SerranoF Alonso-Charterina S, Arenas-Jiminez J (2000) Langerhans' cell histiocytosis of the temporal bone in pediatric patients: imaging and follow-up. AJR 174:217–221

Fisch U, Mattox D (1988) Microsurgery of the skull base. Thieme, New York

Hervey-Jumper S, Garton HJL, Wetjen NM, Maher CO (2011) Neurosurgical management of congenital malformations and inherited disease of the spine. Neuroimaging Clin North Am 21:719–732

Hovelaque A (1934) Osteologie, vol 2. G. Doin, Paris, pp 155–156

Kang Ong C, Fook-Hin Chong V (2009) Imaging of jugular foramen. Neuroimaging Clin North Am 19:469–482

Kobayashi H, Terasaka S, Yamaguchi S, Kubota K, Iwasaki Y (2008) Primary Ewing's sarcoma: peripheral primitive neuroectodermal tumour of the jugular foramen. Acta Neurochir 150:817–821

Linn J, Peters F, Morriggl B, Naidich TP, Bruckmann H, Yuosry I (2009) The jugular foramen: Imaging Strategy and Detailed Anatomy at 3T. AJNR 30:34–41

Lo WWM, Applegate LJ, Carberry JN, Solti-Bohman LG, House JW, Brackmann DE, Waluch V, Li JC (1993) Endolymphatic sac tumors: radiologic appearance. Radiology 189:199–204

Lowenheim H, Koerbel A, Ebner FH, Kumagami H, Ernemann U, Tatagiba M (2006) Differentiating imaging findings in primary and secondary tumors of the jugular foramen. Neurosurg Rev 29:1–11

Madnani DD, Mysiorek D, Wassreman PG, Zahtz G, Mittler M (2006) Jugular foramen fibromatosis in a 3-month-old male. Int J Pediatric Othorhinolaryngol 70:2119–2123

Maffe MF, Raofi B, Kumar A, Muscato C (2000) Glomus faciale, glomus jugulare, glomus tympanicum, glomus vagale, carotid body tumors and simulating lesions. Radiol Clin North Am 38:1059–1076

Manski TJ, Hefner DK, Glenn GM, Patronas NJ, Pikus AT, Katz D, Lebovics R, Sledjeski K, Choyke PL, Zbar B, Linehan M, Oldfield EH (1997) Endolymphatic sac tumors: a source of morbid hearing loss in von Hippel-Lindau Disease. JAMA 277:1461–1466

Manzzoni A, Sanna M, Saleh E, Achilli V (1997) Lower cranial nerve schwannoma involving the jugular foramen. Ann Otol Rhinol Laryngol 106:370–379

MacDonald AJ, Salzman KL, Harnsberger HR, Gilbert E, Shelton C (2004) Primary jugular foramen meningioma: Imaging appearance and differentiating features. AJR 182:373–377

Mancuso AA, Mendenhall WM (2011) Nasopharynx: Malignant tumors. Head and Neck Radiology. Wolters Kluwer/Lippincott Williams Wilkins, Philadelphia

McCarvill MB, Spunt SL, Pappo AS (2001) Pictorial essay Rhabdomyosarcoma in pediatric patient: the good, the bad and the unusual. AJR 176:1563–1569

Moritani T, Aihari T, Oguma E, Makiyami Y, Nishimoto H, Smoker WR, Sato Y (2006) Magnetic resonance venography of achondroplasia: correlation of venous narrowing at the jugular foramen with hydrocephalus. Clin Imaging 3:195–200

Perez-Cruet MJ, Burke JM, Weber R, DeMonte F (1998) Aggressive fibromatosis involving the cranial base in children. Neurosurgery 43:1096–1102

Petrus LV, Lo WMM (1996) Primary paraganglioma of the facial nerve canal. AJNR 17:171–174

Rao AB, Koeller KK, Adair CF (1999) Paragangliomas of the head and the neck: radiologic-pathologic correlation. Radiographics 19:1605–1632

Rich PM, Cox TC, Hayward RD (2003) The jugular foramen in complex and syndromic craniosynostosis and its relationship to raised intracranial pressure. AJNR 24:45–51

Rhoton AL (2000) Jugular foramen. Neurosurgery 47:S276–S285

Rosenbloom JS, Storper IS, Aviv JE, Hacein-Bey L, Bruce JN (1999) Giant cell tumors of the jugular foramen. Am J Otolaryngol 20:176–179

Rubinstein D, Burton BS, Walker AL (1995) The anatomy of the inferior petrosal sinus, glossopharyngeal nerve, vagus nerve, and accessory nerve in the jugular foramen. AJNR 16:185–194

Russel DS, Rubinstein LJ (1989) Pathology of tumours of the nervous system 5th edn. Edward Arnold, London

Sacks AD (1993) Penetrating trauma of the jugular foramen. Ann Otol Rhinol Laryngol 102:485

Samii M, Babu RP, Tatgiba M, Sepehrnia A (1995) Surgical treatment of jugular foramen schwannoma. J Neurosurg 82:924–932

Sen C, Hague K, Kacchara R, Jenkins A, Das S, Catalano P (2001) Jugular foramen: microscopic anatomic features and implications for neural preservation with reference to glomus tumours involving the temporal bone. Neurosurgery 48:838–848

Siddiqui A, Connor S, Gleeson M (2008) Jugular foramen meningocoele in a patient with neurofibromatosis type 1. J Laryngol Otol 122:213–216

Slattery WH, Brackmann DE (1996) Skull base osteomyelitis, malignant otitis externa. Otolaryngol Clincs North Am 29:795–806

Swartz JD, Loevner LA (2009) Imaging of the temporal bone (Fourth Edition). Thieme, New York

Takahashi M, Adachi T, Sako K (1997) Dumbbell-shaped jugular foramen schwannoma. Eur Arch Otorhinolaryngol 254:474–477

Verbist BM, Mancuso AA, Mendenhall WM, Antonelli PJ (2011) Malignant tumors of the external and middle ear and mastoid. Head and Neck Radiology. Wolters Kluwer/Lippincott Williams Wilkins, Philadelphia

Vogl TJ, Bisdas S (2009) Differential diagnosis of jugular foramen lesions. Skull Base 19:3–16

Weber AL, McKenna MJ (1994) Radiologic evaluation of the jugular foramen; anatomy, vascular variants, anomalies and tumors. Neuroimag Clin N Am 4:579–598

Vascular Temporal Bone Lesions

Hervé Tanghe

Contents

1 Definition and Classification of Pulsatile Tinnitus 329
2 Imaging Strategy in PT 330
3 Vascular Anatomical Variants 330
3.1 Arterial Variants 332
3.2 Venous Variants 333
4 Acquired Vascular Lesions 335
5 Vascular Tumors 335
6 Vascular Malformations 337
6.1 Vertebral Arteriovenous Fistula 339
References 340

Abstract

This chapter discusses the possible causes of pulsatile tinnitus (PT). First the possible causes are classified into groups. The imaging strategy is explained, with the otoscopcally findings as starting point. Thereafter, only the vascular etiologies are highlighted in detail. Attention is also given to the neurointerventional treatment of some of these diseases.

1 Definition and Classification of Pulsatile Tinnitus

Tinnitus is a "sound in one ear or both ears, such as buzzing, ringing or whistling, occurring without an external stimulus" (American Heritage Dictionary 2000). Tinnitus can be classified as pulsatile (coinciding with the heartbeat) or continuous, and subjective (perceived only by the patient) or objective (perceptible to another person). Pulsatile tinnitus is less common than continuous tinnitus.

Pulsatile tinnitus (PT) can be caused by (1) vascular anatomical variants; (2) vascular tumors; (3) vascular malformations; (4) acquired vascular lesions; (5) vascularized chronic inflammatory tissue of the middle ear; (6) other diseases like otosclerosis, Paget disease, benign intracranial hypertension. Some other causes may be transient, related to drugs, hypertension, anaemia, and pregnancy (Table 1) (Weissman and Hirsch 2000; Madani and Connors 2009; Vattoh et al. 2010).

Vascular anatomical variants frequently are not associated with symptoms.

H. Tanghe (✉)
Department of Radiology,
Section of Neuroradiology & ENT Radiology,
Erasmus Medical Centre, Erasmus University Rotterdam,
's-Gravendijkwal 230, 3015 CE,
Rotterdam, The Netherlands
e-mail: h.l.j.tanghe@erasmusmc.nl

Table 1 Overview of vascular temporal bone lesions

Pseudo lesions
Vascular anatomical variants
Tumors with rich vascularity
Acquired vascular lesions
Vascularized chronic inflammation tissue
Vascular malformations

Table 2 Imaging strategy in pulsatile tinnitus

Otoscopy: intratympanic mass	Small lesion	Only CT
	Vascular variants	Only CT
	Large lesion	CT and MRI
Otoscopy: no intratympanic mass		CTA and CTV

2 Imaging Strategy in PT

The pre-imaging evaluation of a patient consists of a detailed history, looking for hearing loss, vertigo, headaches, and a medical examination including a neuro-otologic and audiologic evaluation.

There is a wide variation in the reported incidence of structural abnormalities in patients with PT ranging from 44 to 91 % (Madani and Connors 2009). Diagnostic imaging, even performed optimally, fails to find a reason for PT in many patients (Verbist et al. 2011). If an intratympanic mass is seen at otoscopy, then the imaging analysis can start with a CT, thin sections with bone algorithm in the axial and coronal plane, of the temporal bone and adjacent structures of the skull base. The anatomy of the carotid canal and the jugular foramen is carefully studied. For the anatomical vascular variants and small soft tissue masses, like a small glomus tympanicum no further study is needed. For larger masses, an MRI examination is complementary and the CT study can be done without intravenous contrast. Various imaging strategies have been proposed for the investigation of PT in the otoscopically normal patient. Combined CT angiography (CTA) and CT venography (CTV) with a multidetector CT is a good approach for demonstrating arterial, venous, skull base and middle ear disease. MR and MR angiography cannot be trusted to confidently exclude all causes (Krishnan et al. 2006; Mattox and Hudgins 2008; Narvid et al. 2011; Verbist et al. 2011) (Table 2). Our protocol for the imaging analysis op PT consists of an CTA & CTV. The lower scan border is the level of vertebra cervical 7 and the upper border is the end of the skull. The lower border is chosen to include the carotid bifurcation in the protocol. The upper border is chosen for the detection of a possible high flow intracranial AVM, whereby the venous drainage is causing PT. Postprocessing includes maximum intensity projections in the axial, coronal and sagittal planes. There are also separate multiplanar bony algorithm reconstructions of the right and left temporal bone with thin slices of 0.75 mm in the axial and coronal plane to detect an anatomical vascular variant or another intratemporal cause of the PT. For the detection of a dural arteriovenous fistula (DAVF) you have to look to: asymmetric arterial feeding vessels, "shaggy" appearance of a dural venous sinus, transcalvarial venous channels, asymmetric venous collaterals and abnormal size and number of cortical veins. The presence of asymmetrically visible and enlarged arterial feeders has a high sensitivity and specificity for the diagnosis of a DAVF (Fig. 1). A conventional digital subtraction angiography (DSA) is necessary in cases of a negative CTA, but a strong clinical suspicion and in the presence of vascular malformations to demonstrate the angioarchitecture and in case of endovascular treatment (Narvid et al. 2011).

3 Vascular Anatomical Variants

Vascular anatomical variants of the temporal bone are a frequent cause of PT or a vascular retrotympanic mass that often clinically cannot be differentiated from a paraganglioma. This differentiation is important prior to biopsy or therapy. Often these variants are an incidental asymptomatic finding on a CT done for other reasons (Table 3). The radiological diagnosis is possible with MRI, MR angiography, and with CT. For some variants, like the dehiscent jugular bulb, the bone detail, available with CT is important. On MR spin echo sequences, the signal void of the abnormally located artery or vein may be identical to the signal void of the cortical bone and the air in the ear and the anomaly can be missed. A gradient echo sequence gives a high signal from the vessel with better differentiation from the cortical bone.

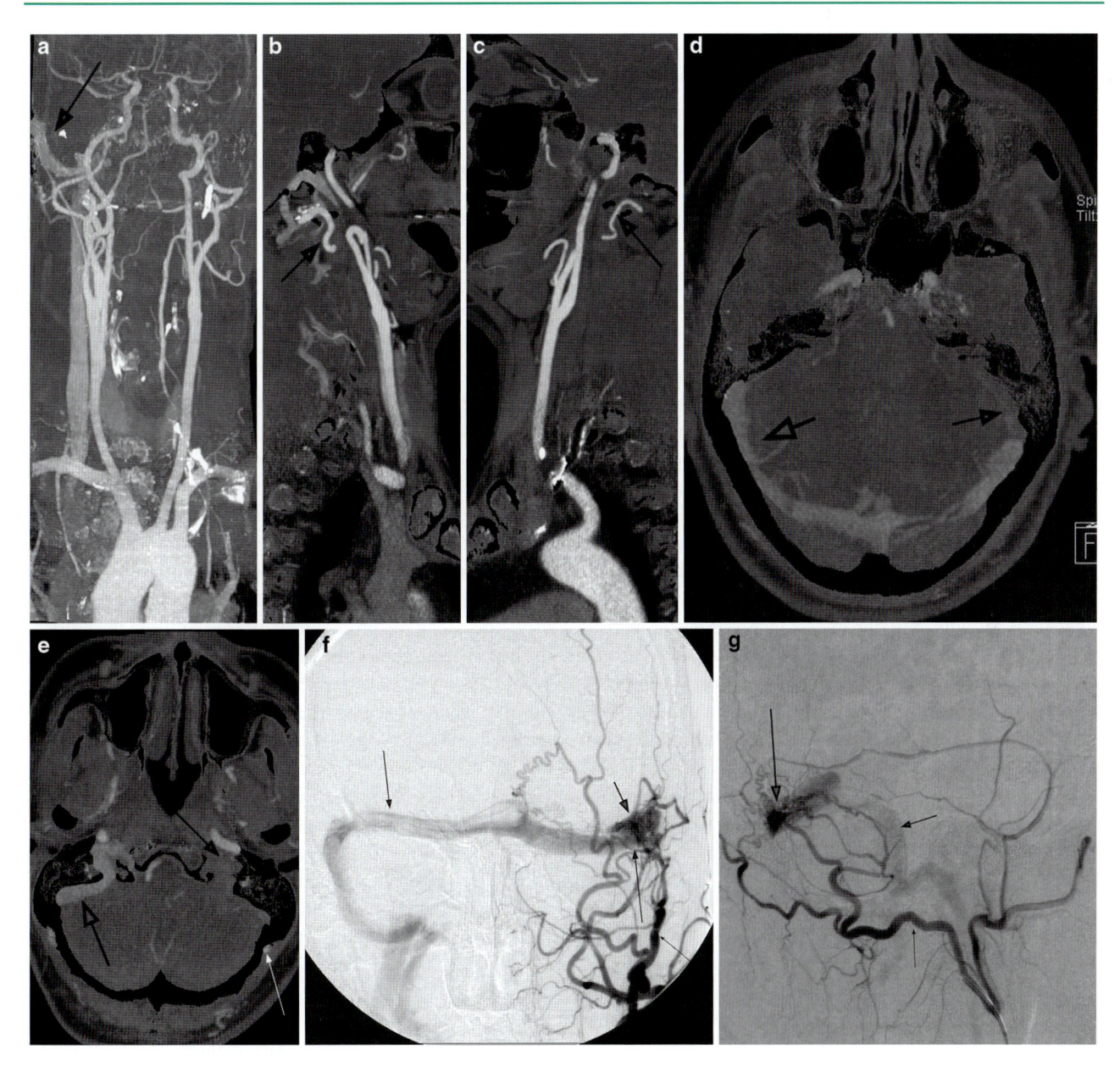

Fig. 1 Use of CTA: dural A-V fistula *left* with contralateral *right* venous drainage. CT Siemens Flash Definition double source/double energy with use of CT-angiography subtraction. **a** CTA- subtraction. Early venous drainage in *right* transverse, sigmoid sinus (*arrow*). **b** *Left* common carotid artery shows hypertrophy of the occipital artery (*arrow*). **c** *Right* common carotid artery with a normal occipital artery (*arrow*). **d–e** Axial reconstruction shows in the arterial phase early venous drainage *left* (*large arrow*), no contrast in *left* sigmoid sinus (*middle-sized arrow*) en hypertrophy of *left* occipital artery (*small arrow*). **f–g** DSA confirms the dural A-V fistula with nidus in the *left* transverse sinus (*large arrow*), the occlusion of the *left* sigmoid sinus (*middle-sized arrow*), the contralateral venous drainage (*middle-sized arrow*) and the feeding vessels, most important the hypertrophied occipital artery (*small arrow*)

Table 3 Vascular anatomical variants

Arterial	Venous
The aberrant ICA	High jugular bulb
Hyostapedial artery variants	Dehiscent jugular bulb
Laterally displaced ICA	Jugular bulb diverticulum
Isolated agenesis of the ICA	
Pharyngo-tympano-stapedial artery	
Splitting of the petrous ICA	

Table 4 CT appearance of the "aberrant ICA"	1	Absence of the vertical part of the carotid canal
	2	Enlarged inferior tympanic canaliculus
	3	The vertical segment of the ICA enters the temporal bone through (2), running more posterior and laterally than normal
	4	Absence of the normal bony posterior margin of the horizontal part of the carotid canal
	5	Soft tissue density in the middle ear at the level of the promontory, joining the horizontal carotid canal through the bony defect mentioned in (4) and simulating a paraganglioma
	6	"Stenosis" at the entry point in the horizontal carotid canal

3.1 Arterial Variants

3.1.1 The Aberrant Internal Carotid Artery

The aberrant internal carotid artery (ICA) also called the aberrant flow of the internal carotid artery in the tympanic cavity (Lasjaunias et al. 2001) enters the skull base through an enlarged inferior tympanic canaliculus with a characteristic narrowing of the vessel. The fundamental cause is a segmental agenesis, absence of the cervical part of the internal carotid artery with the subsequent absence of the vertical part of the bony carotid canal. The ascending pharyngeal artery with its tympanic branch (going through its own enlarged inferior tympanic canaliculus) serves as a collateral pathway to the normal horizontal part of the ICA. At the end of the inferior tympanic canaliculus, the artery enters the middle ear cavity and is located behind the tympanic membrane at the promontorium as a "vascular mass," not covered by bone, before entering the horizontal part of the carotid canal through a bony dehiscence. An aberrant ICA can be associated with a persistent stapedial artery (vide infra; Tanghe 1994; Weisman and Hirsch 2000).

This anomaly can present with objective or subjective pulsatile tinnitus and conductive hearing loss. On otoscopy the ENT surgeon finds a vascular appearing retrotympanic mass that mimics a paraganglioma. A misdiagnosis as a glomus tympanicum must be avoided: the operation can result in a debacle (Tanghe 1994).

The CT features are characteristic (Table 4): (1) absence of a normal-appearing vertical segment of the carotid canal; (2) absence of the bony wall in the posterolateral portion of the horizontal segment of the carotid canal; (3) a round soft tissue mass in the middle ear at the promontorium. Especially in a coronal section this mass can look similar to a glomus tympanicum; (4) on axial CT this mass is in continuity with the horizontal segment of the carotid canal; (5) the aberrant ICA enters the tympanic cavity through an enlarged inferior tympanic canaliculus, located more lateral and posterior compared to a normal vertical ICA segment (Tanghe 1994) (Fig. 2). On conventional MRI, the diagnosis of an aberrant ICA is difficult because of the lack of contrast between the low signal of bone, the signal void of the ICA, and the air in the middle ear and mastoid portion. Flow-sensitive MR images or MR angiography (MRA) allow the diagnosis. Conventional angiography is not necessary for the diagnosis (Weisman and Hirsch 2000).

3.1.2 Partial Persistence of the Stapedial Artery

The so-called "persistent stapedial artery" is in fact a partial persistence of the stapedial artery, different from the full persistent variant which is vary rare (Lasjaunias et al. 2001). The partial persistent variant is an intratympanic origin of the middle meningeal artery. The artery originates from the ICA between the vertical and the horizontal portion of the carotid canal. It enters the middle ear cavity anteroinferiorly, runs along the promontory, passes between the crura of the stapes and enters the tympanic segment of the facial canal causing an enlargement of this canal. At the level of the first genu, it leaves the facial canal through its own foramen and enters the extradural space of the middle cranial fossa, becoming the middle meningeal artery (MMA) (Tanghe 1994). It can be associated with an aberrant ICA (Fig. 3) and with an aneurysmal enlarged ICA (Fig. 4).

This vascular variant is most often an incidental finding at operation or on a CT examination (easily overlooked) and rarely symptomatic with pulsatile tinnitus.

A persistent stapedial artery cannot be diagnosed with MR or even MRA. The CT features are pathognomonic (Tanghe 1994) (Table 5): (1) absence of the foramen spinosum, because there is no MMA to go through; (2) erosion of the promontory; (3) widening of the proximal tympanic segment of the facial canal to accommodate for the artery; and (4) absence of the MMA from the internal maxillary artery on angiography.

3.1.3 Splitting of the Petrous ICA

In this case, two channels carry the flow into the petrous portion. Both channels belong to the ascending pharyngeal artery of the ICA system and the internal carotid artery can still be considered segmentally agenetic (Lasjaunias et al. 2001) (Fig. 5).

3.1.4 The Intrameatal Vascular Loop

The presence of an intrameatal vascular loop of the anterior inferior cerebellar artery (AICA) in the internal auditory canal is a frequent finding on MRI or in cadaver sections (Fig. 6). Some authors consider this as a possible cause of

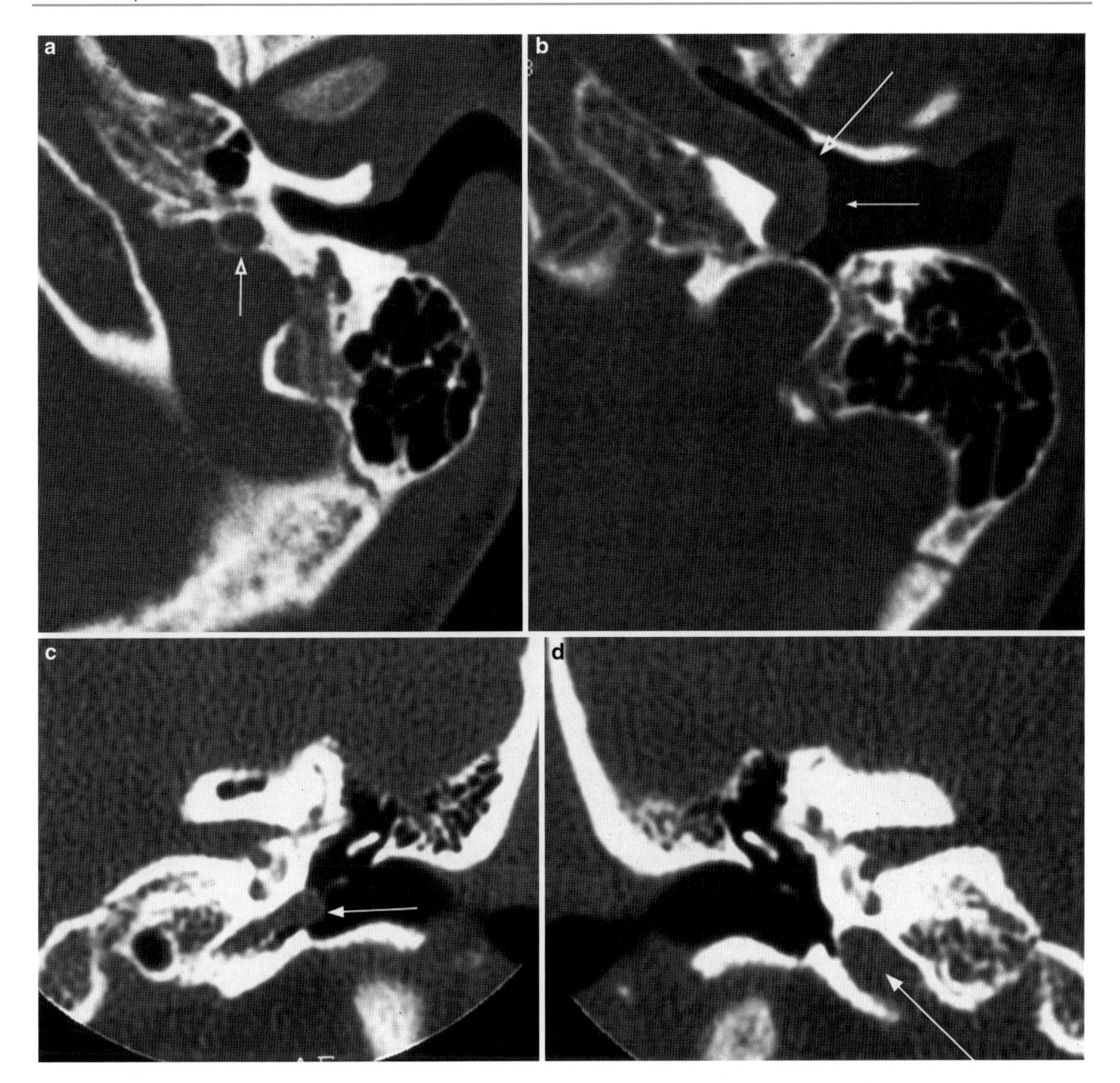

Fig. 2 **Aberrant internal carotid artery. a** Axial CT at the level of the enlarged inferior tympanic canaliculus. This canal is located more lateral and is smaller than the normal vertical part of the carotid canal (*arrow*). **b** Axial CT at the level of the horizontal part of the carotid canal. Part of the lateral bony wall is absent (*large arrow*) and the carotid artery comes close to the tympanic membrane (*small arrow*). **c** Coronal CT at the level of the genu in a different patient. The carotid artery reaches the tympanic membrane (*arrow*). The inferior tympanic canaliculus is smaller than the normal vertical part of the carotid canal at the opposite site in **d** (*arrow*)

PT and advocate a major surgical treatment (De Ridder et al. 2005). However, this intravascular loop is encountered in 40 % of the people. There are many persons with deep vascular loops into the internal auditory canal that do not suffer from pulsatile tinnitus. Conversely, not all patients with pulsatile tinnitus have loops into the IAC. More research and understanding of the underlying mechanisms of pulsatile tinnitus is needed before proposing a craniotomy as a treatment for this symptom.

3.2 Venous Variants

3.2.1 The High or High Riding Jugular Bulb

The jugular bulb is considered high when it extends above the level of the floor of the internal auditory canal. On a T1 W MR sequence after gadolinium this variant can simulate an enhancing tumor in the medial temporal bone. But the bony margins of the jugular foramen are intact and well corticated. In case of doubt a CT with bone algorithm can

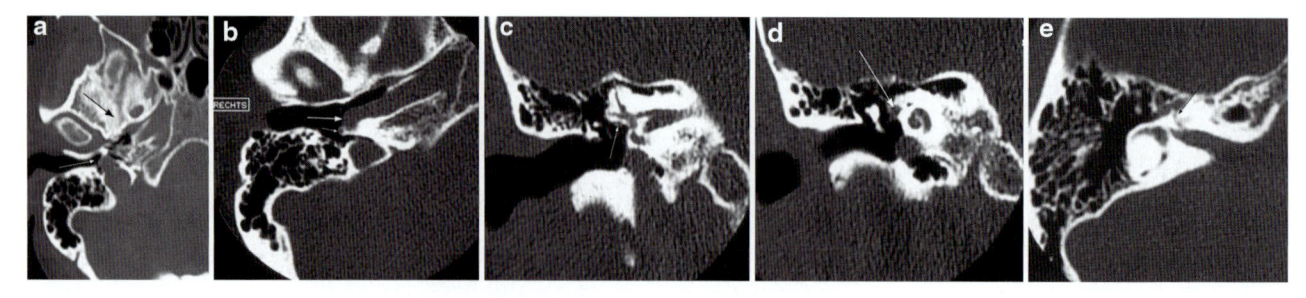

Fig. 3 Persistent stapedial artery, associated with an aberrant internal carotid artery. **a** Axial CT. The foramen spinosum is absent (*large arrow*), compared with the normal left side. The carotid artery is in contact with the tympanic membrane through a bony defect at the end of inferior tympanic canaliculus (*small arrow*). There is no bony margin between the inferior tympanic canaliculus and the jugular foramen. **b** Axial CT. The carotid artery lies in the middle ear with a large bony defect in the horizontal part of the carotid canal (*large arrow*). Notice the origin of the persistent stapedial artery (*small arrow*). **c** Coronal CT at the level of the oval window; **d, e** coronal and axial CT at the level of the proximal tympanic segment of the facial canal. The facial canal at the level of the oval window is still normal in size (*small arrow*), but it is enlarged at his proximal tympanic segment, to accommodate for the persistent stapedial artery (*large arrow*). The labyrinthine segment of the facial canal is normal (*small arrow* in **e**)

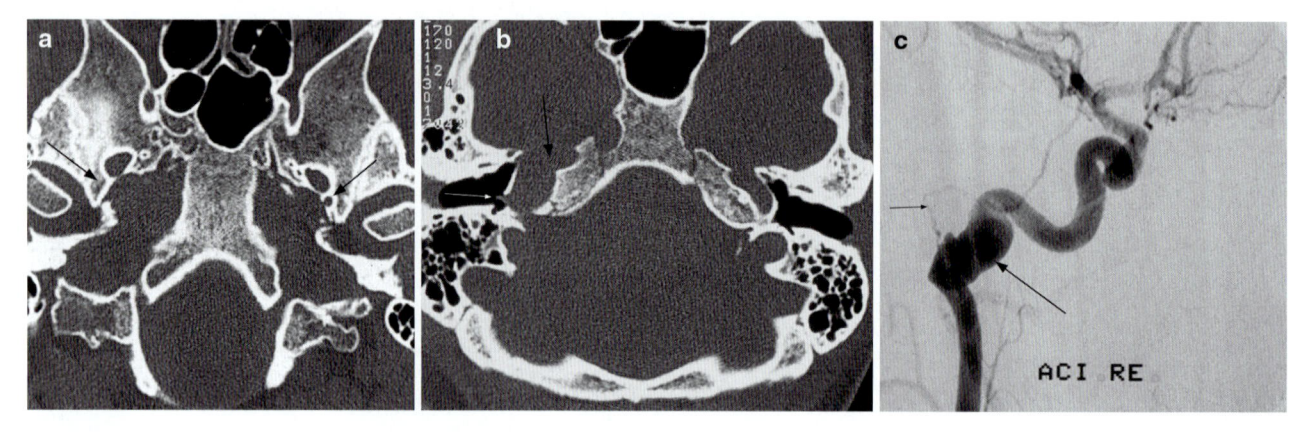

Fig. 4 Persistent stapedial artery, associated with aneurysmal enlargement of the carotid artery. **a** Axial CT of the skull base. The foramen spinosum is absent on the right side (*arrow*) and normal on the *left side* (*arrow*). **b** Axial CT at the level of the horizontal part of the carotid canal. The canal is enlarged (*large arrow*). Also notice the origin of the persistent stapedial artery (*small arrow*). **c** The angiogram in the same patient shows the fusiform aneurysmal enlargement of the carotid artery (*large arrow*) and the persistent stapedial artery (*small arrow*)

Table 5 CT appearance of the partial persistent stapedial artery

1	Absence of the foramen spinosum
2	Erosion of the promontory
3	Widening of the proximal tympanic segment of the facial canal

be done (Tanghe 1994; Weissmann and Hirsch 2000; Vattoh et al. 2010).

3.2.2 The Dehiscent Jugular Bulb

A dehiscent jugular bulb lacks a complete cortical covering and lies in part in the hypotympanum of the middle ear. It usually presents as a vascular retrotympanic mass behind the posteroinferior quadrant of the tympanic membrane (Tanghe 1994; Weissmann and Hirsch 2000; Vattoh et al. 2010).

On MR the diagnosis is difficult because MR cannot demonstrate the presence or absence of the cortical covering of the jugular foramen. The dehiscence can be inferred from a more lateral position of the bulb on coronal images and by the presence of a lateral lobulation.

On CT the dehiscent jugular bulb is visible as a mass low in the medial part of the middle ear. This mass is in continuity with the jugular bulb in the foramen trough a bony defect (Fig. 7).

3.2.3 The Jugular Bulb Diverticulum

A jugular diverticulum is a protrusion of the jugular bulb superior and medial to the jugular foramen which extends above the inferior border of the round window. It does not extend into the middle ear, but can be associated with PT, because of turbulence of the venous flow. The tympanic

Fig. 5 Splitting of the internal carotid artery. Angiogram. The carotid artery is split into two parts (*arrow*) from its origin at the carotid bifurcation, until the horizontal part of the carotid canal

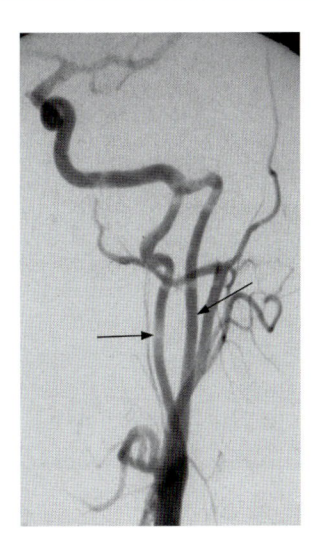

membrane is normal and the anomaly cannot be seen at otoscopy (Weissmann and Hirsch 2000; Madani and Connor 2009; Vattoth et al. 2010) (Fig. 8).

4 Acquired Vascular Lesions

Numerous acquired vascular lesions can cause PT. A detailed description is beyond the scope of this chapter (Lo and Solti-Bohman 1996; Weissmann and Hirsch 2000; Sismanis and Girevendoulis 2008; Madani and Connor 2009) (Table 7).

Aneurysm of the petrous portion of the carotid artery can cause PT but is rare. Intracranial aneurysms are far more frequent (Table 6).

Atherosclerotic stenotic disease at the carotid bifurcation in the neck may produce turbulence of flow but gives only occasionally PT. Despite its high prevalence as a cause of asymptomatic carotid bruit, atherosclerosis is not a common cause of symptomatic pulsatile tinnitus (Sandok et al. 1982).

Fibromuscular dysplasia of the internal carotid artery most frequently gives intracranial ischemia, but PT is the second most frequent manifestation (Sismanis et al. 1994).

Other acquired vascular lesions that can give tinnitus are: spontaneous dissection of the internal carotid artery, idiopathic intracranial hypertension, a vascular compression of the eight nerve in the cerebellopontine angle.

5 Vascular Tumors

Paraganglioma is the most common tumor causing PT or a vascular tympanic membrane (Lasjaunias et al. 2001). Other less common vascular tumors are: meningioma, haemangioma of the facial nerve, endolymphatic sac tumor (see the chapter on imaging of the jugular foramen),

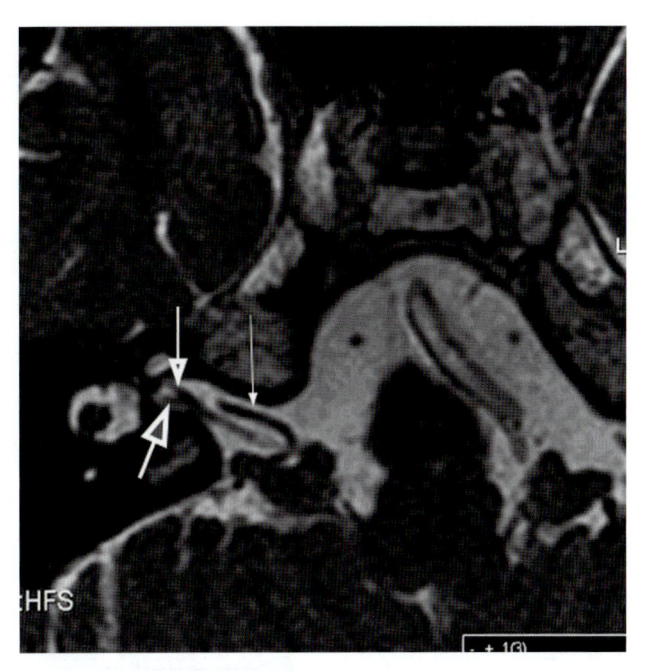

Fig. 6 Intrameatal vascular loop MRI 3D FIESTA. The presence of an intrameatal vascular loop of the anterior inferior cerebellar artery (AICA) (*small arrow*) in the internal auditory canal is a frequent finding on MRI or in cadaver sections. *Middle-sized arrow* cochlear nerve, *large arrow* inferior vestibular nerve

cavernous haemangioma of the middle ear and vascular metastasis like Grawitz tumor (Madani and Connor 2009) (Table 7). A meningioma located in the temporal bone can clinically mimic a paraganglioma. When it protrudes in the middle ear, the ENT surgeon sees on otoscopy a vascular retrotympanic mass, indistinguishable from a paraganglioma. Meningioma is characterized by the presence of sclerotic changes on CT and the absence of flow voids on MR, in contrast to a glomus tumor (Vattoth et al. 2010). Meningioma and metastasis can be as vascular as paraganglioma. For a detailed discussion of the noninvasive imaging features of these tumors, see the chapter on the imaging of the jugular foramen.

An angiography is rarely needed for diagnostic purposes and is usually done to perform a preoperative embolization in cases where an operation is chosen as the treatment.

Paragangliomas have a characteristic angiographic appearance with enlarged feeding arteries, an early and intense tumor blush and early draining veins (Fig. 9a). The intratumoral arterioles in the periphery of the tumor are smaller than those in the centre. There are multiple intratumoral direct communications between arterioles and venules with arterio-venous shunting. Large paragangliomas (type C2 or more, according to the classification of U. Fisch) (Fisch and Mattox 1988) have a lot of feeding vessels and large intratumoral A-V shunts, making them almost impossible to resect without a pre-operative embolization (Connors and Wojak 1999) (Fig. 9b and c).

Fig. 7 Dehiscent jugular bulb.
a Axial CT. The jugular bulb protrudes in the middle ear through a bony defect in the jugular foramen (*arrow*). **b** Axial CT in a different patient: a woman of 19 yr with disease of Crouzon. Same abnormality (*arrow*)

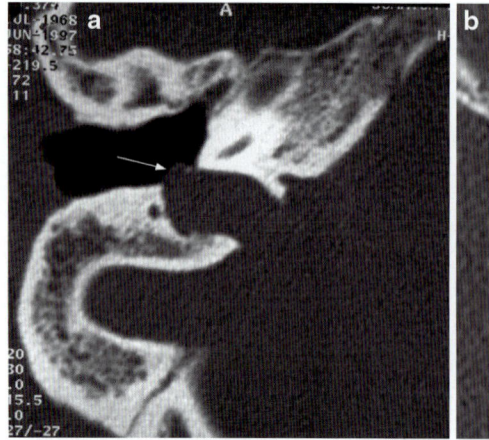

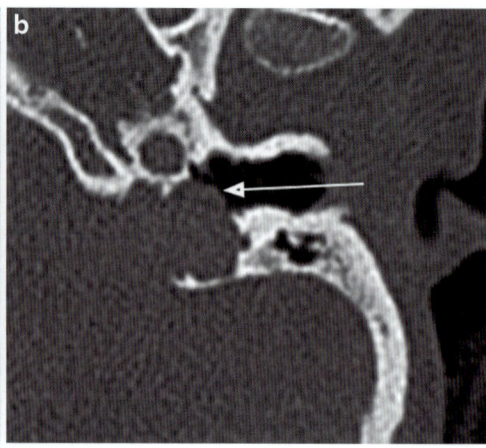

Fig. 8 Jugular bulb diverticulum. Coronal CT. There is a protrusion of the jugular bulb superior and medial to the jugular foramen. Such a protrusion is called a diverticulum (*arrow*). It does not extend into the *middle* ear

Table 6 Acquired vascular lesions

Petrous carotid aneurysm
Atherosclerotic carotid artery disease
Fibromuscular dysplasia
Spontaneous carotid dissection
Thrombosis of dural sinus with intracranial hypertension

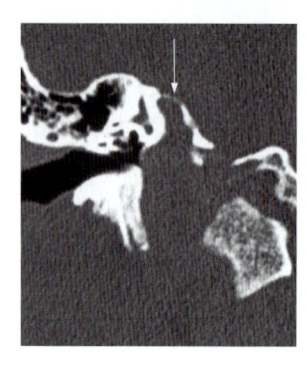

Table 7 Tumors of the temporal bone that may present with pulsatile tinnitus or a vascular retrotympanic mass

Paraganglioma
Haemangioma
Meningioma
Endolymphatic sac tumor
Vascular metastasis

In 75–85 % of the cases the angioarchitecture of a paraganglioma is multicompartmental (Table 8).

The pre-embolization angiographic protocol consists of a study of the ICA, the vertebral, internal maxillary, occipital and ascending pharyngeal artery. It is further important to look at the relationship of the tumor to the internal jugular vein, the inferior petrosal sinus and the other dural sinus. Especially the detection of extraluminal compression or intraluminal tumor extension is important for the surgeon. This information can be obtained from the venous phase of the vertebral and carotid angiography and from the CT and MRI.

The embolization is carried out with a microcatheter with superselective catheterisation of the different feeding vessels. As embolisation material can be used particles polyvinyl alcohol (PVA), with a size of 150–250 μ or Onyx. In case of a good intratumoral catheter position smaller particles, less than 90 μ, can be used to reach the centre of the tumor trough the small-sized peripheral intratumoral arterioles. To prevent complications, the dangerous anastomoses among the vertebral, internal carotid and external carotid arteries must be known (Moret et al. 1982; Connors and Wojak 1999; Lasjaunias et al. 2001) (Fig. 10). Furthermore, it is important to remember that several cranial nerves receive their blood supply by the vessels we intend to embolize: the IX, X, XI and XII cranial nerve by the ascending pharyngeal artery, the facial nerve by the middle meningeal and accessory meningeal artery, the III, IV, V, VI cranial nerve by the accessory meningeal artery. Use of too small particles or of glue in conjunction with an improper catheter position can result in definitive cranial nerve palsy.

Until early in this millennium microsurgical resection, endovascular embolization, conventional radiation therapy, or any combination of these, were the only treatment modalities for glomus jugulare tumors. However, with the establishment of effectiveness of stereotactic radiotherapy

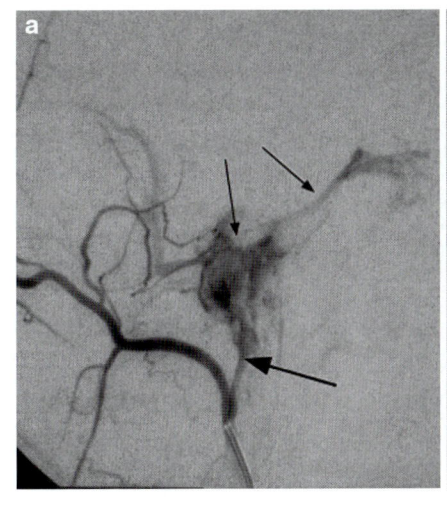

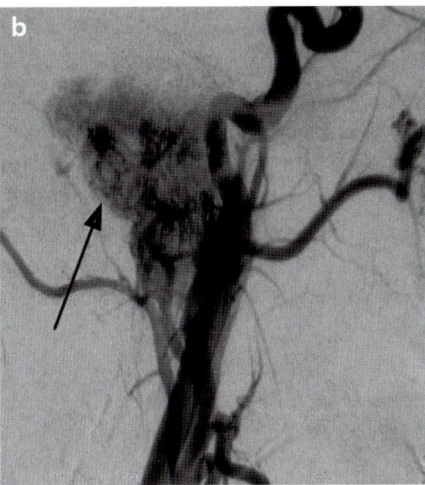

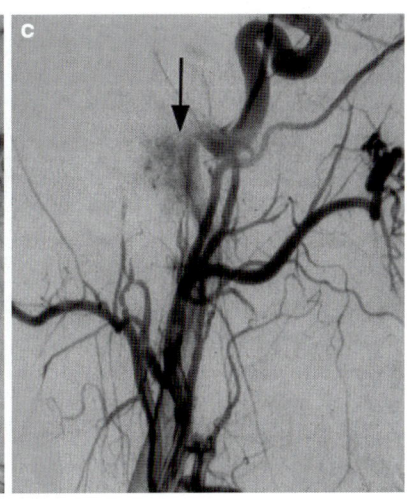

Fig. 9 **Glomus jugulotympanicum. a** Occipital artery. The posterior part of the tumor is fed by the stylomastoid artery (*large arrow*). The angiographic appearance is characteristic, with an enlarged feeding artery, an early and intense tumor blush and early draining veins (*small arrow*). **b, c** Angiogram of the common carotid artery before and after embolization. The tumor is very vascular with an intens tumor blush (*arrow* in **b**). The small tumor blush *left*, after embolization, comes from feeding from the internal carotid artery via the caroticotympanic ramus (*arrow* in **c**). This vessel usually cannot be catheterized selectively

Table 8 Angioarchitecture of paraganglioma: compartment and feeding vessels (Krishnan et al. 2006). For each compartment the feeding vessels are arranged starting from the principal vessel to additional feeding vessels with increasing volume of that tumor compartment

Compartment	Feeding vessels
Infero-medial	Inferior tympanic branch (ascending pharyngeal artery)
	Neuromeningeal trunk (ascending pharyngeal artery)
	Lateral clival branch of the ICA
	Meningeal branches of the vertebral artery
Postero-lateral	Stylomastoid artery (occipital artery or posterior auricular artery)
	Meningeal branches of the occipital artery
	Meningeal branches of the vertebral artery
Anterior	Anterior tympanic artery (internal maxillary artery)
	Caroticotympanic artery (ICA)
	Cavernous branches of the ICA
Superior	Middle meningeal artery
	Accessory meningeal artery

(SRT) in the treatment of cerebral arteriovenous malformations and in other highly vascular brain tumors, the vascular character of paragangliomas made them appropriate targets for SRT. Compared with conventional radiotherapy, SRT has fewer complications, and shorter course of treatment and hospital stay (Genc et al. 2010; Ivan et al. 2011). Other authors demonstrated that gross total resection of large paraganglioma (type C and D) is possible with low mortality and may be curative (Makiese et al. 2012).

6 Vascular Malformations

Vascular malformations may cause PT, usually objective and sometimes subjective. Often the patient has in addition an audible bruit or a pulsatile thrill. When these signs are present, the angiography can be the initial imaging study. It is important to know that not only intracranial or skull base vascular malformations, but also cervical vascular lesions like vertebral arteriovenous fistula can cause PT. Every high

Fig. 10 Dangerous anastomosis. a Selective injection of the inferior tympanic artery with the microcatheter, shows the tumor blush in the *middle* ear. There is also a visualisation of the vertebral artery (*large arrow*) at the C2–3 level via the dens arcade (*small arrow*). **b** After closure of the dens arcade with a microcoil (*arrow*), the feeding artery can safely be embolized

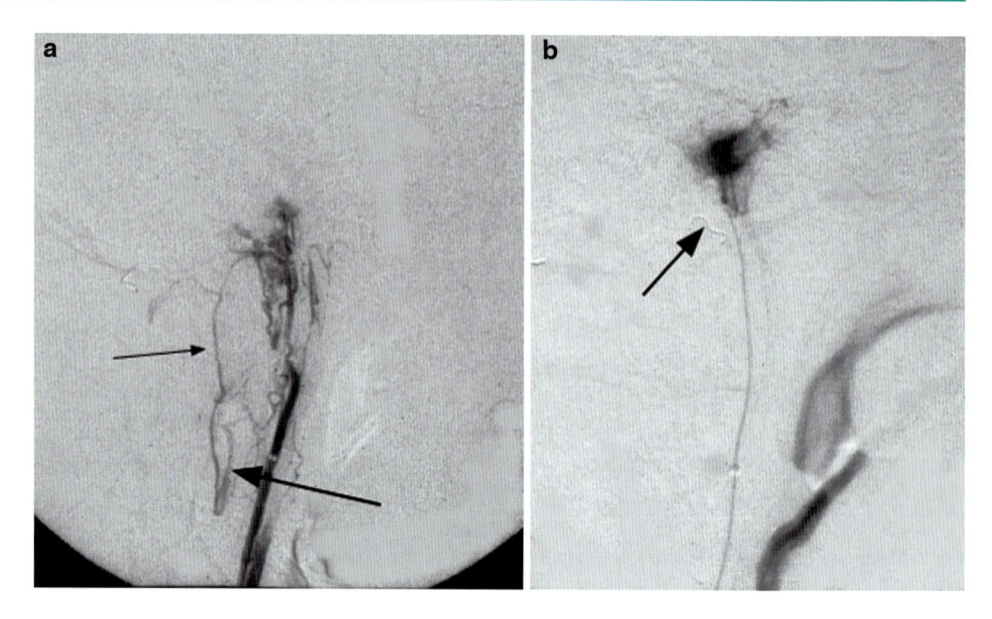

Table 9 Vascular malformations that can cause pulsatile tinnitus

Dural arteriovenous fistula
Carotid-cavernous fistula: direct or dural
Vertebral arteriovenous fistula
External carotid fistula
Brain AVM

Table 10 Classification of dural arteriovenous fistula (DAVF) according to the type of venous drainage (Cognard et al. 1995)

Type I	Antegrade into the venous sinus
Type IIa	Into the venous sinus with reflux in the sinus or retrograde into the sinus
Type IIb	Antegrade into the venous sinus with cortical venous drainage
Type IIa + b	Retrograde into the venous sinus with cortical venous drainage
Type III	Direct cortical venous drainage
Type IV	Type III with venous ectasia
Type V	Spinal perimedullary venous drainage

flow vascular lesion of which the venous drainage comes through or near the jugular bulb can cause PT (Table 9). Therefore, the angiographic protocol should not only include the internal and the external carotid artery but also the vertebral artery. In some cases, the vascular lesion can be located contralateral to the side of the PT. For example, a left-sided dural carotid-cavernous fistula can drain through the right cavernous sinus into the right inferior petrosal sinus to the jugular bulb. Both cavernous sinus plexuses exist anteriorly and posteriorly (Lasjaunias et al. 2001).

Dural arteriovenous fistula's (DAVF) are the most common cause of objective PT in the patient with a normal otoscopic examination (Weissman and Hirsch 2000). DAVF are abnormal shunts located in the dura. They can occur at any site in the dura, but most frequently they are located near a venous sinus. They are classified according to their location, or to the type of venous drainage. The criterion standard to diagnose and classify cranial DAVFs is DSA. This is an invasive, relatively expensive, and time-consuming procedure. A noninvasive alternative is CTA although it may not

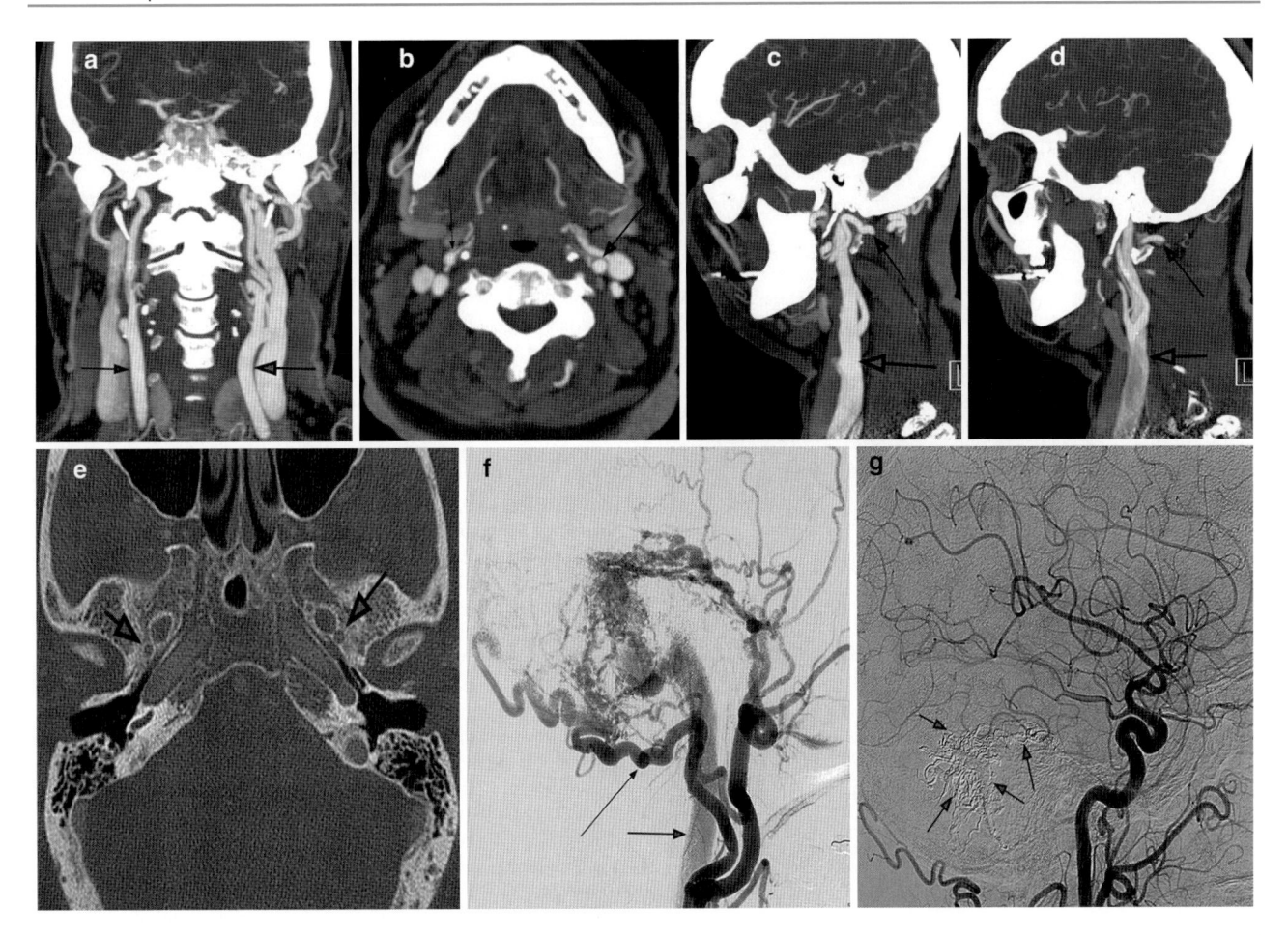

Fig. 11 Dural arteriovenous fistula of the transverse sinus type I. a–d CT-angiography, e–f DSA with embolisation with Onix. **a** The *left* common carotid artery (*large arrow*) is larger than the *right* (*small arrow*). **b** The *left* external carotid artery (*large arrow*) is larger than the *right* (*small arrow*). **c** *Left* sagittal view. The *left* occipital artery is hypertrophied (*small arrow*), and also the *left* jugular vein (*large arrow*). **d** *Right* sagittal view. Normal *right* occipital artery (*small arrow*) and jugular vein (*large arrow*). **e** Because of the hypertrophy of the feeding *left* meningeal artery, the *left* foramen spinosum is enlarged compared to the *right* (*arrow*). **f** DSA before embolization: feeding occipital artery (among others) (*small arrow*). Draining transverse sinus (*large arrow*). **g** DSA after embolization. The radio-opaque Onix. is visible (*arrow*). The fistula is closed

rule out a small slow-flow DAVF (Willems et al. 2011). The classification is important for determining the natural history, the prognosis and the indication for treatment (Cognard et al. 1995; Ghandhi et al. 2012) (Table 10). Type I lesions have a benign natural history and these lesions are only treated when the pulsatile tinnitus cannot be tolerated by the patient. Type IIa lesions are less benign with intracranial hypertension occurring in 20 % of the cases. In type IIb the risk for an intracranial bleeding is 10 %, in type III the risk is 40 % and in type IV 65 %. Patients with a DAVF type V developed progressive myelopathy in 50 % of the cases. Figure 11 gives an example of the possibilities of CT-A in the diagnosis of DAVF, with a lot of abnormalities you can find in the CT-A.

The treatment of choice is endovascular, via the arterial or via the venous route. It is beyond the scope of this chapter to go further in detail into the endovascular treatment. Surgery is an option in case of failure of the endovascular treatment. When the nidus of the DAVF is small, than stereotactic radiosurgery is an option.

6.1 Vertebral Arteriovenous Fistula

Vertebral arteriovenous fistula (VAF) are less common lesions. The most frequent cause is trauma, but they may also occur spontaneously, sometimes associated with fibromuscular dysplasia and neurofibromatosis type I. The clinical manifestations can vary: spinal cord or vertebrobasilar ischemia, spinal cord compression, nerve root compression, and pulsatile tinnitus. A bruit is present in nearly 100 % of the cases. The treatment of choice is endovascular (Lasjaunias et al. 2001) (Fig. 12).

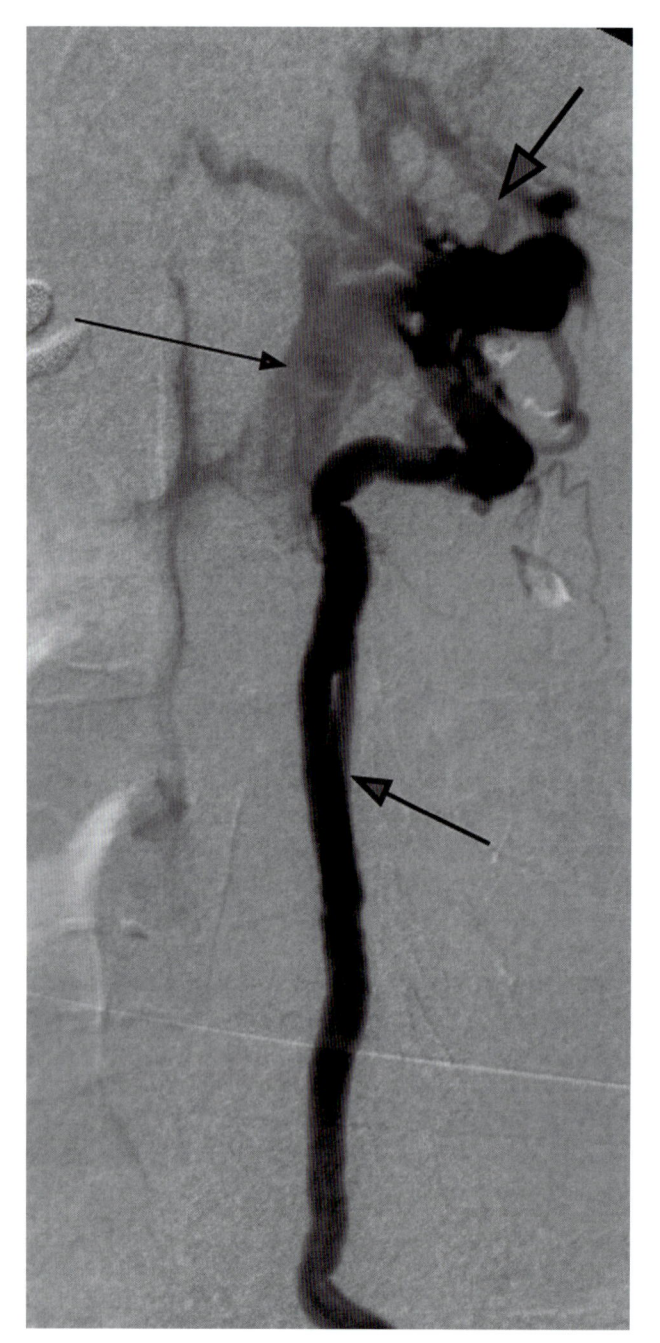

Fig. 12 Vertebro-jugular fistula. Patient with PT caused by a lesion just below the skull base. DSA *left* vertebral artery frontal view. High flow vertebra-jugular fistula. Hypertrophied feeding vertebral artery (*middle-sized arrow*). The fistel place is high cervical, just beneath the jugular foramen (*large arrow*). Early filling of draining veins, also epidural veins (*small arrow*)

References

American Heritage Dictionaries (2000) The American heritage dictionary of the english language, 4th edn. American Heritage Dictionaries, Boston

Cognard C, Gobin YP, Pierot L, Bailly AL, Houdart E, Casasco A, Chiras J, Merland JJ (1995) Cerebral dural arteriovenous fistulas: clinical and angiographic correlation with a revised classification of venous drainage. Radiology 194:671–680

Connors JJ III, Wojak JC (1999) Paragangliomas. In: Connors JJ III, Wojak JC (eds) Interventional Neuroradiology. Strategies and Practical Techniques, Saunders, Philadelphia

De Ridder M, De Ridder L, Nowé V, Thierens H, Van de Heyning P, Moller A (2005) Pulsatile tinnitus and the intrameatal vascular loop: why do we not hear our carotids? Neurosurgery 57:1213–1217

Fisch U, Mattox D (1988) Microsurgery of the skull base. Thieme, New York

Genc A, Bicer A, Abacioglu U, Peker S, Pamir M, Kilic T (2010) Gamma knife radiosurgery for the treatment of glomus jugulare tumors. J Neurooncol 97:101–108

Ghandi D, Chen J, Pearl M, Huang J, Gemmete JJ, Kathuria S (2012) Intracranial dural arteriovenous fistula: classification, imaging findings and treatment. Am J Neuroradiol 33:1007–1013

Ivan ME, Sughrue ME, Clark AJ, Kane AJ, Aranda D, Barani IJ, Parsa AT (2011) A meta-analysis of tumor control rates and treatment-related morbidity for patients with glomus jugulare tumors. J Neurosurg 114:1299–1305

Krishnan A, Mattox DE, Fountain AJ, Hudgins PA (2006) CT arteriography and Venography in pulsatile tinnitus: preliminary results. Am J Neuroradiol 27:1635–1638

Lasjaunias P, Berenstein A, Ter Brugge KG (2001) Surgical neuro-angiography, vol 1, 2nd edn. Springer, Berlin

Lo WWM, Solti-Bohman LG (1996) Vascular tinnitus. In: Som PM, Curtin HD (eds) Head and Neck Imaging, 3rd edn. Mosby—Year Book Inc, St. Louis

Madani G, Connor SEJ (2009) Imaging in pulsatile tinnitus. Clin Radiol 64:319–328

Makiese O, Chibbaro S, Marsella M, Tran Ba Huy P, George B (2012) Jugular foramen paraganglioma: management, outcome and avoidance of complications in a series of 75 cases. Neurosurg Rev 35:185–194

Mattox DE, Hudgins P (2008) Algorithm for evaluation of pulsatile tinnitus. Acta Oto-Laryngolocica 128:427–431

Moret J, Delvert JC, Bretonneau CH, Lasjaunias P, de Bicetre CH (1982) Vascularization of the ear: normal-variations-glomus tumors. J Neuroradiol 3:209–260

Narvid J, Do HM, Blevins NH, Fischbein (2011) CT angiography as a screening tool for dural arteriovenous fistula in patients with pulsatile tinnitus: feasibility and test characteristics. Am J Neuroradiol 32:446–453

Sandok BA, Whisnant JP, Furlan AJ (1982) Carotid artery bruits: prevalence survey and differential diagnosis. Mayo Clin Proc 57:227–230

Sismanis A, Girevendoulis A (2008) Pulsatile tinnitus associated with internal carotid artery morphologic abnormalities. Otol Neurotol 29:1032–1036

Sismanis A, Stamm MA, Sobel M (1994) Objective tinnitus in patients with atherosclerotic carotid artery disease. Am J Otol 15:404–407

Tanghe H (1994) Congenital malformations and anatomic variations of the ear. Rivista di Neuroradiologica 7:417–422

Vattoth S, Shah R, Curé JK (2010) A compartment-based approach for the imaging evaluation of pulsatile tinnitus. Am J Neuroradiol 31:211–218

Verbist BM, Mancuso AA, Antonelli PJ (2011) Pulse synchronous (pulsatile) tinnitus. In: Macuso AA, Hanafee WN, Verbist BM, Hermans R (eds) Head and neck radiology. Wolters Kluwer, Philadelphia

Weissman JL, Hirsch BE (2000) Imaging of tinnitus: a review. Radiology 216:342–349

Willems PWA, Brouwer PA, Barfett JJ, terBrugge KG, Krings T (2011) Detection and classification of cranial dural arteriovenous fistulas using 4D-CT angiography: initial experience. Am J Neuroradiol 32:49–53

Post-operative Temporal Bone Imaging

Luc van den Hauwe, Christoph Kenis, Bert De Foer, and Jan Walther Casselman

Contents

1 Introduction 343
2 **Surgery in Chronic Middle Ear Disease** 344
2.1 Mastoidectomy 345
2.2 Tympanoplasty: Ossicular Reconstruction 347
2.3 Failure/Recurrence 348
3 **Stapes Surgery in Otosclerosis Patients** 354
4 **Vestibular Schwannoma Surgery** 356
4.1 Conservative Management 357
4.2 Radiosurgery 357
4.3 Surgery 357
4.4 Complications: Recurrences 360
5 **Conclusion** 362
References 362

L. van den Hauwe (✉)
Department of Radiology, AZ Klina, Augustijnslei 100, 2930 Brasschaat, Belgium
e-mail: lucvdhauwe@mac.com

L. van den Hauwe
Department of Radiology, Antwerp University Hospital, Wilrijkstraat 10, 2650 Edegem, Belgium

C. Kenis · J. W. Casselman
Department of Radiology, AZ Sint Jan Hospital, Ruddershove 10, 8000 Brugge, Belgium

B. De Foer · J. W. Casselman
Department of Radiology, GZA Sint Augustinus Hospital, Oosterveldlaan 24, 2610 Wilrijk, Belgium

J. W. Casselman
University of Ghent, Gent, Belgium

Abstract

Three categories of patients are referred for follow-up imaging after temporal bone surgery. The first group consists of patients with (complicated) chronic middle ear disease, including cholesteatoma. For this group, the imaging algorithm has changed enormously for the last 10 years. Multidetector computed tomography (MDCT) and more recently cone beam CT (CBCT) are ideally suited to demonstrate the bony details after mastoidectomy and to assess the integrity of the ossicular chain reconstruction when prosthetic failure is suspected. To evaluate the middle ear and/or mastoid cavity for the presence of residual cholesteatoma, MR imaging (MRI) has become the first choice diagnostic modality. Non-EPI diffusion-weighted imaging (DWI) has proven to be the most sensitive and specific technique and has higher diagnostic performance than delayed contrast-enhanced MR-imaging. After stapes surgery in patients with otosclerosis, imaging studies are rarely required. When prosthetic failure is suspected, MDCT and CBCT can be performed. In patients with postoperative vertigo and sensorineural hearing loss (SNHL), MR imaging may be needed to look for labyrinthine abnormalities (hemorrhage, infection, …) if CT is not contributive. In the follow-up of patients with vestibular schwannoma, MR imaging is the modality of choice, whether a conservative ('wait and scan') management, radiosurgery or surgey has been chosen.

1 Introduction

Post-operative changes can be very subtle, especially after ossicular chain reconstruction, or very complex as in middle ear and mastoid surgery for chronic middle ear disease, including cholesteatoma. Therefore, comprehensive information regarding the surgical procedure(s) performed and the motivation for the examination should be addressed to the radiologist. Also, clinical information and the results of paraclinical testing (audiometry, auditory brainstem responses (ABR), …) can be helpful to analyse the post-operative changes in these patients. Preferably, previous pre- and/or post-operative examinations—sometimes realised in other institutions—should be available for comparison.

It is obvious that plain radiography and polytomography have become obsolete in the evaluation of patients with conductive (CHL) or sensorineural hearing loss (SNHL), tinnitus and vertigo.

For many years Computed Tomography (CT) has been the imaging modality of choice in the evaluation of the post-operative middle ear because of its widespread availability and its ability to depict discrete bony abnormalities, and to assess the re-aeration of the middle ear cleft. Helical CT (Hermans et al. 1995) and especially multidetector CT (MDCT) have been a breakthrough (Williams et al. 2000). Improved spatial resolution in the z-axis and scan speed result in fast, high-quality CT examinations. Sagittal and coronal reformatted images as well as three-dimensional renderings of the MDCT data can be realised almost routinely. Endoluminal views of the tympanic cavity can be obtained and virtual endoscopy can be performed to exclude ossicular chain disruption (Klingebiel et al. 2001). To confirm the correct position of the electrode array after cochlear implantation, however, plain radiography and especially digital radiography are used routinely. Cone beam CT (CBCT) plays due to its low dose and high resolution an increasing role in the pre-operative evaluation of the temporal bone and post middle ear surgery and cochlear implantation (CI) patients (Ruivo et al. 2009).

Magnetic resonance (MR) imaging is still the imaging modality of choice in patients with vestibulocochlear schwannoma (VS), not only in the diagnostic work-up of patients with SNHL, but also in the follow-up and after surgery. In patients with chronic middle ear disease and cholesteatoma, MR imaging has now an important role to play since the introduction of non-EPI diffusion-weighted imaging (DWI) sequences whether or not supplemented with delayed post-gadolinium T1-weighted imaging (De Foer et al. 2010). The capability of non-EPI DWI to demonstrate residual cholesteatoma with high sensitivity, specificity, positive predictive and negative predictive values allows us to use this technique as a screening tool (De Foer et al. 2008, 2010; Rajan et al. 2010; Jindal et al. 2011; Dremmen et al. 2012; Corrales and Blevins 2013).

Most middle ear prostheses are not a contraindication for MR imaging at 1.5T (Shellock and Schatz 1991). Results of published 1.5T field studies should not be used directly for safety recommendations in a 3T MR unit. Heat, voltage induction and vibration during exposure to the magnetic resonance fields should be considered as additional possible safety issues. Preference should be given to platinum and titanium implants in manufacturing processes and surgical selection (Fritsch and Gutt 2005). Prostheses made from titanium are safe, neither deflecting nor heating during magnetic resonance examinations conducted at 3T (Martin et al. 2005).

The presence of a functioning cochlear implant (CI) has been considered as an absolute contraindication to MR examination for many years and most radiologists remain reluctant when patients with CI are referred for MR imaging. It has been demonstrated, however, that most of the electromagnetic interferences between the CI and the MR system remain within acceptable limits. But, MR imaging should be performed only if there is a strong medical indication and after assessment of the relative risks involved (Teissl et al. 1998). Demagnetisation of the CI magnet is high on 3T, which necessitates operative removal of the CI magnet before the MR examination and post-examination replacement. Therefore, it is best to work with 1.5T when examining the CI patient. A strongly administered compression bandage over the CI components is needed to avoid damage to the overlying soft-tissues.

2 Surgery in Chronic Middle Ear Disease

Chronic otitis media (COM) indicates irreversible middle ear pathology. Manifestations of COM include middle ear effusion—also known as secretory otitis media (SOM)—tympanic membrane retractions, acquired cholesteatoma, granulation tissue, cholesterol granuloma, ossicular erosion and ossicular fixation due to tympanosclerosis (Swartz and Harnsberger 1998). Often, the mastoid is poorly pneumatised. Eustachian tube dysfunction with subsequent decreased intratympanic pressure is one of the causes responsible for COM. Tympanostomy tubes or transtympanic ventilating tubes can be placed to normalise intratympanic pressure and they are used in patients with recurrent acute otitis media and long-standing SOM. They are available in various types of plastics or stainless steel. Most of these tympanostomy tubes have a diabolo shape and their CT appearance is mostly characteristic (Swartz et al. 1983) (Fig. 1).

The primary goal of the surgical treatment of chronic otitis media with cholesteatoma is the complete eradication of the disease (no residual disease), whereas secondary goals are the prevention of recurrent disease, the improvement of the hygienic status of the ear and the preservation or improvement of hearing (Shelton and Sheehy 1990).

Residual and recurrent cholesteatoma should not be confused. The latter is developing from recurring retraction pockets or defects in the tympanic membrane reconstruction, takes usually more time to develop and are larger at detection (Sheehy et al. 1977). Residual cholesteatoma refers to the presence of small cholesteatoma pearls that are

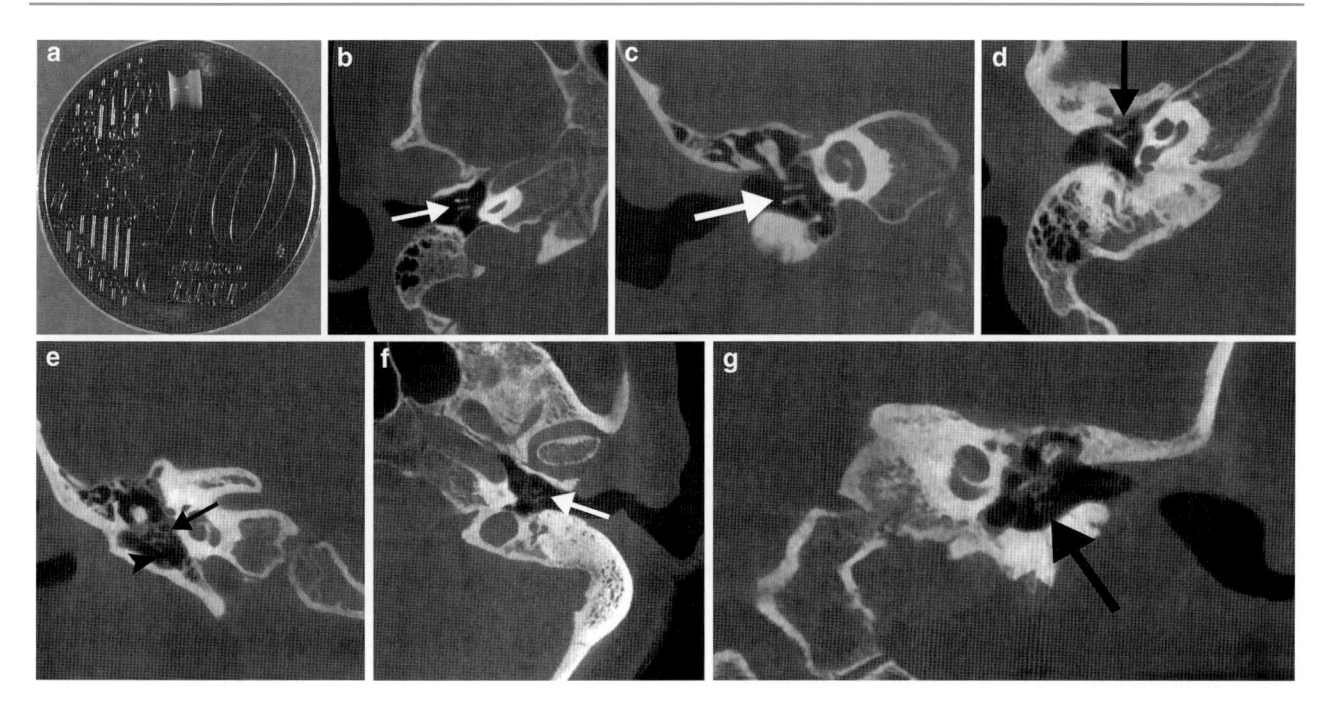

Fig. 1 Tympanostomy tubes. **a** Relationship of a plastic grommet to a 10 cent euro coin. **b** Axial CBCT image and **c** coronal reformatted image of the right ear shows a normally positioned grommet (*arrow*) centered on the anteroinferior part of the pars tensa. **d** Axial and coronal **e** CBCT image of the right ear demonstrates an anteromedially displaced grommet (*arrow*). Note the myringotomy site (*arrowhead* in **e**). **f** Axial and coronal **g** CBCT image of the left ear shows a laterally displaced grommet (*arrow*) lying against the tympanic membrane

accidentally left behind at first-stage surgery. They can be found anywhere in the middle ear and/or resection cavity and are usual very small at detection during second-look surgery. In 90 % of cases, the location of the residual however is found to be that of the primary cholesteatoma. This suggests that the residual cholesteatoma is induced by insufficient local resection of the epidermal matrix. Especially residual cholesteatoma in the anterior attic is a problem in canal-wall-up (CWU) mastoidectomy. While recurrences can be diagnosed otoscopically, residual disease cannot be detected by a simple clinical examination (Venail et al. 2008) and only surgical revision can determine the diagnosis; this is the rationale behind the second-look operation (Gaillardin et al. 2012). The challenge for radiologists is to offer an imaging technique that is able to depict residual and recurrent cholesteatoma with high sensitivity and specificity, to avoid unnecessary surgery (De Foer et al. 2008, 2010).

2.1 Mastoidectomy

CT findings in the different surgical procedures performed in chronic middle ear disease including cholesteatoma have been well illustrated by Mukherji et al.; diagrams of the procedures are shown below, courtesy of the author (Mukherji et al. 1994). Surgical procedures for cholesteatoma can be broadly classified as closed cavity or canal-wall-up (CWU) mastoidectomy/tympanoplasty or open cavity or canal-wall-down (CWD) mastoidectomy depending on whether the posterior wall of the external auditory canal (EAC) is preserved. The choice of technique is usually determined by the extent of the disease and the experience and personal preferences of the surgeon (Majithia et al. 2012; Ayache et al. 2012). Defining the true extent of cholesteatoma and staging disease using non-EPI DWI can help the surgeon with his choice of surgery and surgical approach (Majithia et al. 2012). Both types of procedure have their advantages and disadvantages (Khemani et al. 2011). When possible, CWU is the procedure of choice for the treatment of cholesteatoma for most otologic surgeons (Brackmann 1993). CWU techniques preserve the anatomy of the posterior canal wall, eliminating the need for periodic bowl cleaning and avoiding the risk of recurrent bowl infections. The mastoid air cells including Koerner's septum are removed. In this manner, communication of the surgically created cavity (mastoid bowl) with the antrum and epitympanum is established (Fig. 2). A major disadvantage of CWU procedures is less wide surgical exposure with a subsequent higher rate of residual (35 %) and recurrent (18 %) cholesteatomas (Stasolla et al. 2004). In children, these percentages may be even higher as a more aggressive behaviour of cholesteatomas is observed. Another disadvantage of CWU mastoidectomy is the limited possibility of clinical and otoscopical evaluation. This is why some institutions promote a more rigorous follow-up and a rapid second-look surgery (Plouin-Gaudon et al. 2010a). In case of

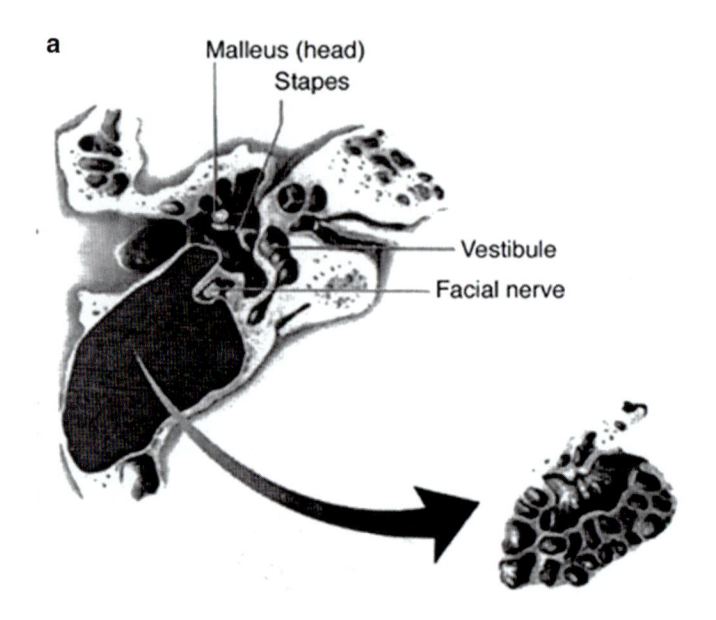

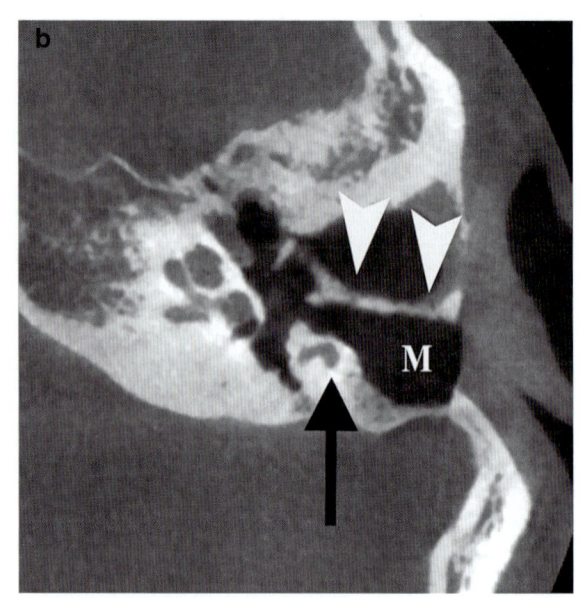

Fig. 2 Canal-wall-up (CWU) mastoidectomy. **a** Diagram shows removal of the mastoid air cells with preservation of the posterior wall of the right external auditory canal (EAC). (From Mukherji et al. 1994. With permission). **b** Axial CBCT image demonstrating CWU mastoidectomy defect (*M*) in the left ear. The posterior wall of the EAC is preserved (*arrowheads*). Note the position of the mastoid segment of the facial nerve canal (*arrow*)

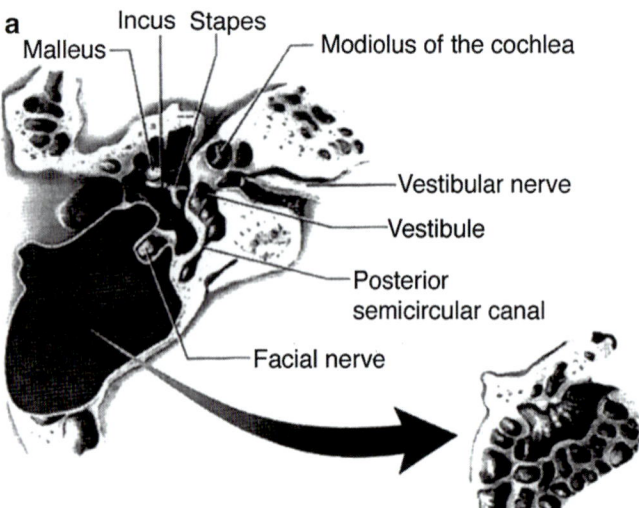

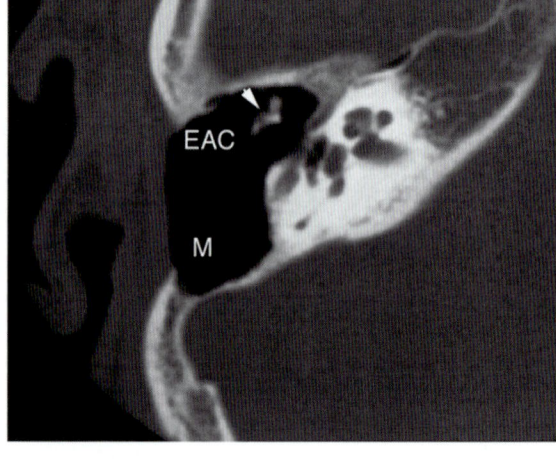

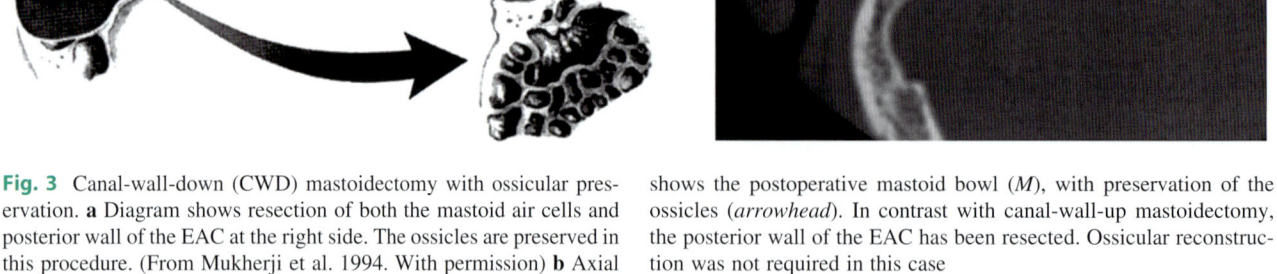

Fig. 3 Canal-wall-down (CWD) mastoidectomy with ossicular preservation. **a** Diagram shows resection of both the mastoid air cells and posterior wall of the EAC at the right side. The ossicles are preserved in this procedure. (From Mukherji et al. 1994. With permission) **b** Axial multidetector CT (MDCT) image at the level of the mesotympanum shows the postoperative mastoid bowl (*M*), with preservation of the ossicles (*arrowhead*). In contrast with canal-wall-up mastoidectomy, the posterior wall of the EAC has been resected. Ossicular reconstruction was not required in this case

CWD mastoidectomy, the posterosuperior wall of the EAC is removed, allowing communication between the mastoid cavity and the EAC. Further access to the middle ear cavity is created, depending on the extent of disease encountered. If disease is limited to the epitympanum, only the scutum needs to be resected and the ossicular chain can be preserved (Fig. 3). When the ossicular chain is involved in the disease process, a radical mastoidectomy is performed. The tympanic membrane is detached from its annulus and the mastoid segment of the facial nerve canal is skeletonised allowing wide access to the middle ear cavity (Fig. 4). However, the stapes superstructure is left in place whenever possible. Complete posterior canal wall removal provides exposure of the entire attic and middle ear, helping to ensure complete disease eradication. This approach can reduce the residual and recurrence rate to as low as 2 %. The CWD procedure is

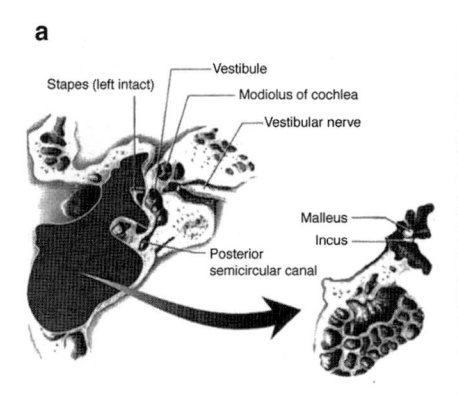

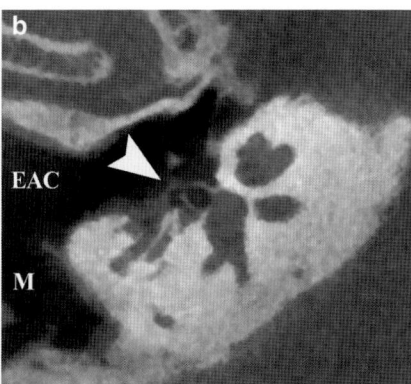

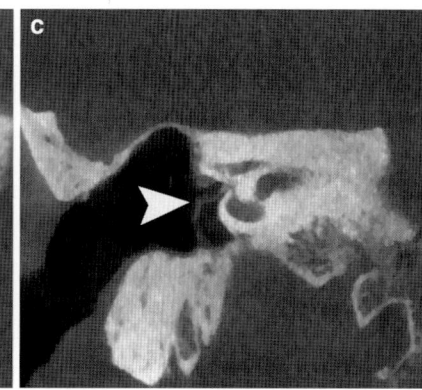

Fig. 4 Canal-wall-down mastoidectomy with removal of malleus and incus. **a** Diagram shows exenteration of the mastoid air cells, posterior wall of EAC, malleus and incus. The stapes superstructure is preserved. (From Mukherji et al. 1994. With permission). **b** Double-oblique reformatted and coronal (**c**) CBCT image of the right ear shows a CWD mastoidectomy defect with communication between the EAC and mastoid (*M*). The tympanic membrane graft (*arrowhead*) is located on the stapes capitulum (type III tympanoplasty)

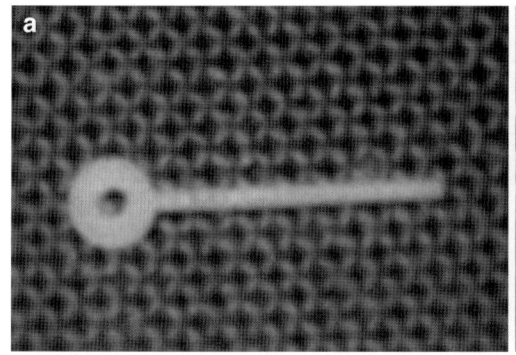

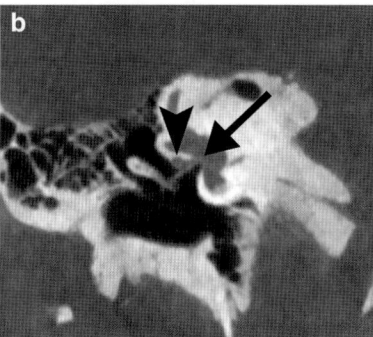

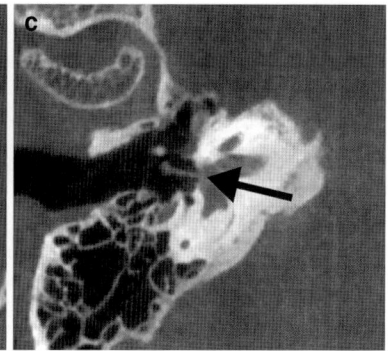

Fig. 5 Stapes prosthesis. **a** Photograph shows a Teflon type polymer stapes prosthesis. **b** Coronal CBCT image of the right ear demonstrates the Teflon prosthesis located underneath the tympanic segment of the facial canal and in contact with it (*arrowhead*) and with its tip on the stapes footplate (*arrow*). This correct position is confirmed on the double-oblique reformatted CBCT image (*arrow*). Not the hook of the prosthesis around the long apophysis of the incus

nowadays preserved for repeatedly recurrent disease with difficult to treat cholesteatoma and for patients with high risk of getting lost in follow-up. A major disadvantage of the CWD technique is the accumulation of debris in the exteriorised mastoid cavity, requiring periodic cleaning and, on occasion, water restrictions to prevent bowel infections. The CWD technique also provides for removal of the nitrogen-absorbing mucosa of the mastoid. After surgery, the new epithelial lining of the mastoid bowl is a stratified keratinizing epithelium. In the CWU procedure, the mastoid retains its native cuboidal nitrogen-absorbing epithelium. Eustachian tube dysfunction could result in reaccumulation of secretory middle ear effusion and retraction of the posterior superior quadrant of the tympanic membrane, causing recurrent cholesteatoma (Gantz et al. 2005). In order to avoid this problem, a bony obliteration technique has been advocated. The advantages of the procedure include providing increased intraoperative exposure (similar to a CWD technique), removal and obliteration of the nitrogen absorbing mastoid epithelium with bone pâté, and reconstruction of the posterior canal wall. The procedure is designed to prevent development of post-operative retraction pockets and recurrences by obliterating the mastoid cavity and isolating the tympanum from the attic and mastoid using bone chips and bone pâté (Mercke 1987). Although primary bony obliteration provides excellent results with low recurrence rates, it also carries with it the risk of obliterating and obscuring residual cholesteatomas. Follow-up by means of imaging using non-EPI DWI MRI is mandatory to prevent late complications after possible obliteration of residual cholesteatomas (De Foer et al. 2007, 2010).

2.2 Tympanoplasty: Ossicular Reconstruction

Tympanoplasty is a technique to reconstruct the conductive hearing system, i.e. the tympanic membrane and/or the ossicles. Five types of tympanoplasty have been defined by

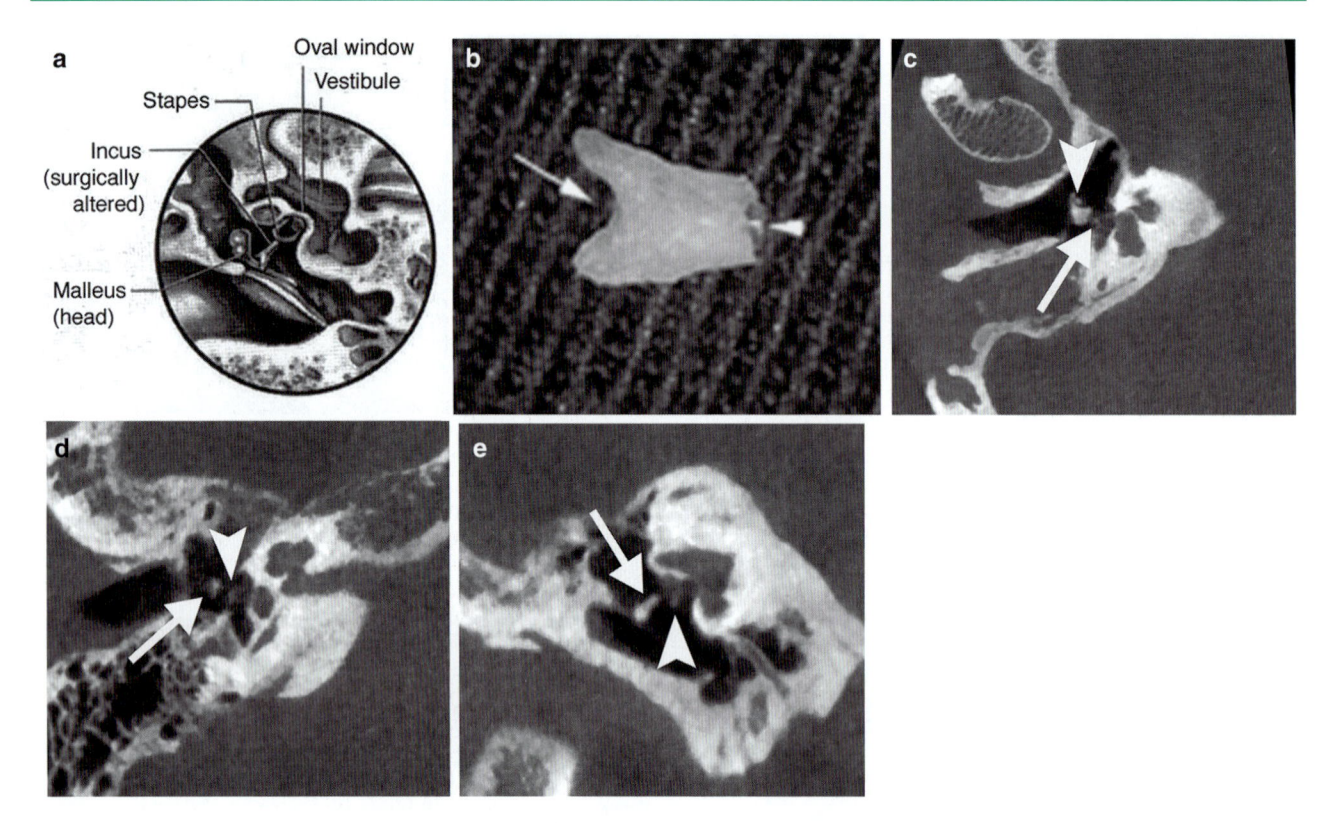

Fig. 6 Incus interposition **a** Diagram shows a surgically altered incus that has been placed between the malleus and stapes in an attempt to maintain ossicular function. (From Mukherji et al. 1994. With permission) **b** Photograph shows an example of a sculptured autologous incus interposition graft. The notch (*arrow*) will fit under the handle of the malleus and the circular groove (*arrowhead*) will be placed on the head of the stapes. Incus interposition homograft. **c** Axial CBCT image of the right ear shows a remodelled incus in contact with the tympanic membrane and malleus manubrium (*arrowhead*) and the stapes capitulum (*arrow*). **d** Double-oblique reformatted and coronal **e** CBCT image of the right ear in another patient show a remodelled incus (*arrow*) dislocated from the stapes capitulum (*arrowhead*), causing the conductive hearing loss

Wullstein (Swartz and Harnsberger 1998). Routine postoperative imaging studies are not required after simple myringoplasty (type I tympanoplasty). However, when imaging is performed within the first weeks after the procedure, a thickening of the tympanic membrane can be noticed, as well as a middle ear effusion. In type II tympanoplasty the malleus is bypassed and the graft connects directly to the body of the incus. In type III tympanoplasty the graft attaches to the capitulum of the stapes, in type IV tympanoplasty to the footplate of the stapes and in type V tympanoplasty the graft attaches to the oval window.

Ossicular reconstructions are commonly performed in patients with extensive cholesteatoma with involvement of the ossicular chain, as well as in patients with tympanosclerosis, otosclerosis or congenital ossicular malformations. Initially, cartilage and temporalis fascia have been used, before the introduction of allografts. Allografts gained wide acceptance, especially in Europe. The main reason for using allografts is their excellent biocompatibility. However, they require time and skill for sculpting and availability may be a problem. Moreover, they may harbour foci of cholesteatoma and a growing risk of transmitting infectious diseases, such as Creutzfeld-Jacob and AIDS, have been mentioned (Stone et al. 2000). For all these reasons, synthetic prostheses have been developed. Prostheses most commonly used for ossicular reconstructions include stapes prostheses for otosclerosis (Fig. 5), incus interposition auto- or homografts (Fig. 6), partial ossicular replacement prostheses (PORP) and total ossicular replacement prostheses (TORP) (Fig. 7).

Otological evaluation of patients who have undergone ossicular reconstruction is often difficult. CT can be helpful in demonstrating prosthetic failure (recurrent cholesteatoma, granulation tissue, adhesions or mechanical problems) that may cause post-operative CHL and identify patients in whom revision surgery must be considered (Stone et al. 2000).

2.3 Failure/Recurrence

2.3.1 Conventional Imaging Techniques

Clinical follow-up in CWD procedures is easy. In CWU, however, clinical and otoscopic diagnosis of residual (and recurrent) disease is unreliable, so second-look procedure is

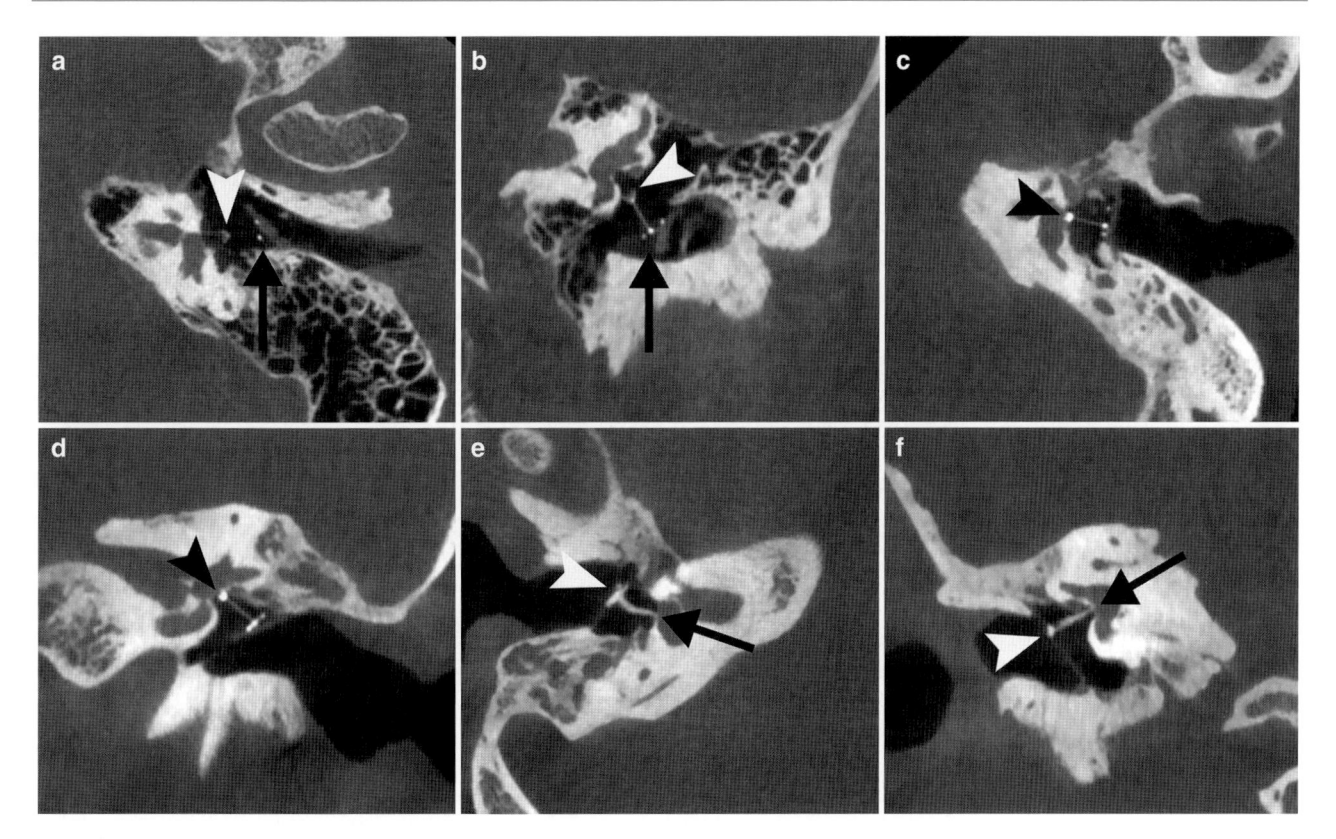

Fig. 7 Partial **a, b** and total **c–f** ossicular prostheses. **a** Para-axial double oblique and para-coronal **b** CBCT reformatted image of the left ear shows a normally positioned partial ossicular prosthesis with base (*arrow*) on a piece of cartilage placed on the tympanic membrane and tip on the stapes capitulum (*arrowhead*). **c** Para-axial double oblique and para-coronal **d** CBCT reformatted image of the left ear shows a total ossicular prosthesis with tip located on the stapes footplate (*arrowhead*). **e** Para-axial double oblique and para-coronal **f** CBCT reformatted image of the right ear shows a total ossicular allograft prosthesis with base on the tympanic membrane and malleus manubrium (*arrowhead*) and tip on the footplate (*arrow*)

considered as an integral part of the CWU procedure by many authors. Imaging has an important role in the management of the post-operative middle ear (Williams and Ayache 2004). To avoid systematic second-look surgery and to better select the true surgical indications after CWU, imaging protocols have been developed with increasing accuracy, safety, and reliability. The primary goal of imaging in the management of postoperative cholesteatoma is to detect any residual or recurrent disease. Whatever imaging technique that is used to do so, if it wants to replace second-look surgery, it should be able to correctly differentiate granulation tissue, fibrosis, inflammatory tissue, fluid, from eventually residual cholesteatoma (Khemani et al. 2011). Until recently, no ideal imaging technique proved to be efficient enough to adequately confirm or eliminate a residual or recurrent cholesteatoma (Plouin-Gouan et al. 2010a).

CT has low sensitivity and low specificity, not allowing to differentiate between the different postoperative tissues such as recurrence, scar tissue or inflammation (Blaney et al. 2000). Therefore, it is now widely accepted that in the follow-up of patients after CWU mastoidectomy or bone obliteration technique (BOT), CT is useful only when it shows complete absence of a soft mass tissue within the post-operative cavity, or the evidence of a cholesteatomatous lesion filling the cavity, i.e. a nodular or lobulated enlarging soft tissue mass associated with osteolytic foci of the bony walls of the tympanomastoid cavity, or with ossicular displacement or destruction (Williams et al. 2003). In the vast majority of cases, however, a partially soft tissue opacification of the middle ear and mastoidectomy cavity is observed, and CT is not able to differentiate cholesteatoma from inflammation, scar tissue, granulation tissue or cholesterol granuloma (Tierney et al. 1999; Blaney et al. 2000) (Fig. 8). Therefore, MRI has become the imaging technique of choice.

Conventional MR imaging in the post-operative evaluation for cholesteatoma consists of T1, T2 and Gd-enhanced T1-weighted images, where cholesteatoma is most often hyperintense on T2-weighted images, hypointense on T1-weighted images and does not enhance on postcontrast images, whereas chronic inflammation will show contrast enhancement. A typical rim enhancement may be seen around the cholesteatoma (Mark and Casselman 2002). It has been proven that also conventional MR imaging is not a valid alternative to second-look surgery in the case of

Fig. 8 Value of CT imaging in the post-operative evaluation of cholesteatoma. **a** Axial CBCT image of the right ear show a status post CWU mastoidectomy and a soft tissue mass in the middle ear with convex borders (*arrow*). There is a medial displacement of the ossicles and subtle erosion of the malleus head (*arrowhead*). These features are highly suspicious of cholesteatoma which is confirmed by the high signal intensity (*arrowhead*) on the non-EPI DWI image **b** and by surgery. **c** Coronal CBCT image of a post-operative left ear with bony obliteration technique (*asterisk*) shows convex borders of a non-specific soft tissue mass (*arrow*) in the middle ear cavity. There is a remodelled incus (*arrowhead*) on the tympanic membrane. **d** The coronal non-EPI MR image shows isointense material consistent with granulation tissue (*arrowhead*). No cholesteatoma can be demonstrated

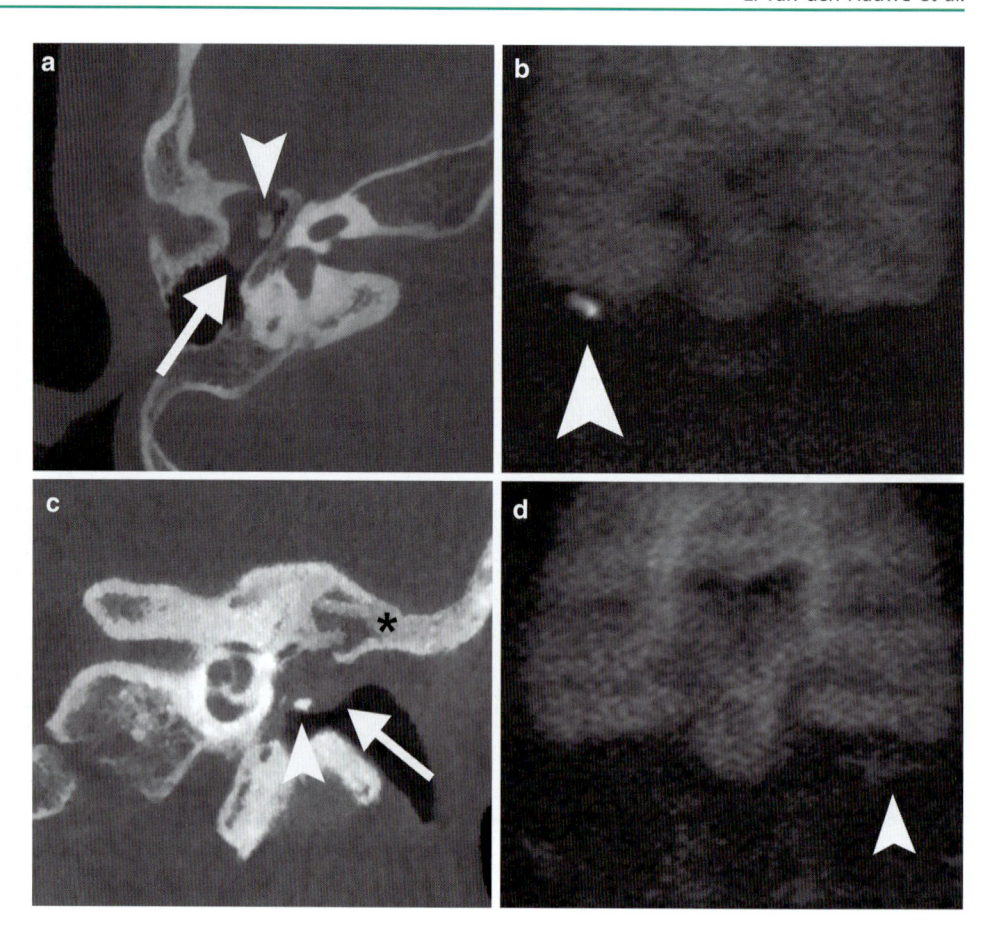

cholesteatoma treated by CWU tympanoplasty (Van den Abeele et al. 1999).

The introduction of new imaging protocols including delayed contrast-enhanced MR imaging and especially the use of non-EPI DWI has totally changed the imaging strategy in the follow-up of patients after CWU mastoidectomy and BOT for cholesteatoma (Figs. 9 and 10) (De Foer et al. 2010).

2.3.2 Delayed Contrast-Enhanced MR Imaging

The initial results of delayed contrast-enhanced MR imaging in the detection of residual cholesteatoma were published in 2003 (Williams et al. 2003) and later confirmed in a larger series of patients by the same group (Ayache et al. 2005). A typical imaging delay after the intravenous injection of gadolinium of some 30–45 minutes is advocated. The protocol is based on the different vascularisation characteristics of cholesteatoma and other post-operative tissues: cholesteatoma is strictly avascular and scar tissue is poorly vascularised (possibly due to microvascular thrombosis). On delayed contrast-enhanced images, enhancement is typical centripetal; it eventually reaches the centre of the scar tissue mass 30–45 min after the contrast medium administration (Williams et al. 2003). With the use of delayed contrast-enhanced MRI residual cholesteatoma as small as 3 mm could be detected. Smaller pearls were probably missed due to signal averaging when a small cholesteatoma pearl is surrounded by granulation tissue (Williams et al. 2003). One could argument that there is probably no important risk to leave such a small residual cholesteatoma pearl for a few months if a close clinical and imaging follow-up is performed. It can be expected that this lesion will be detected on follow-up MRI performed 9–12 months later (Ayache et al. 2005). Although delayed contrast-enhanced MR imaging performs better than HRCT and conventional MR imaging, the sensitivity and specificity are relatively poor (Khemani et al. 2012). Moreover, drawbacks of this technique are poor spatial resolution (when compared to CT), long duration of the imaging protocol and need for intravenous injection of contrast media which make it more expensive and less practical to be used in children (Plouin-Gouan et al. 2010a).

2.3.3 Diffusion-Weighted MR Imaging

At the same time, the potential role of DWI in differentiating cholesteatoma from granulation tissue was suggested in a case report (Maheshwari and Mukherji 2002). The first series reporting on the high signal on DWI in primary

Fig. 9 Post-operative MRI of a patient surgically treated for cholesteatoma. The exclusion cavity was filled up with fat. **a** Axial postcontrast T1-weighted MR image shows a hypointense nodular area (*arrow*) within the surrounding fat tissue which does not show restricted diffusion on the coronal non-EPI DWI image (*arrowhead* in **b**) consistent with granulation tissue. **c** Axial postcontrast T1-weighted MR image in the same patient more caudally demonstrates another nodular area (*arrow*) extending in the external auditory canal which is more hypointense than the area in **a**. **d** Coronal non-EPI DWI MR image confirms a recurrent cholesteatoma (*arrowhead*)

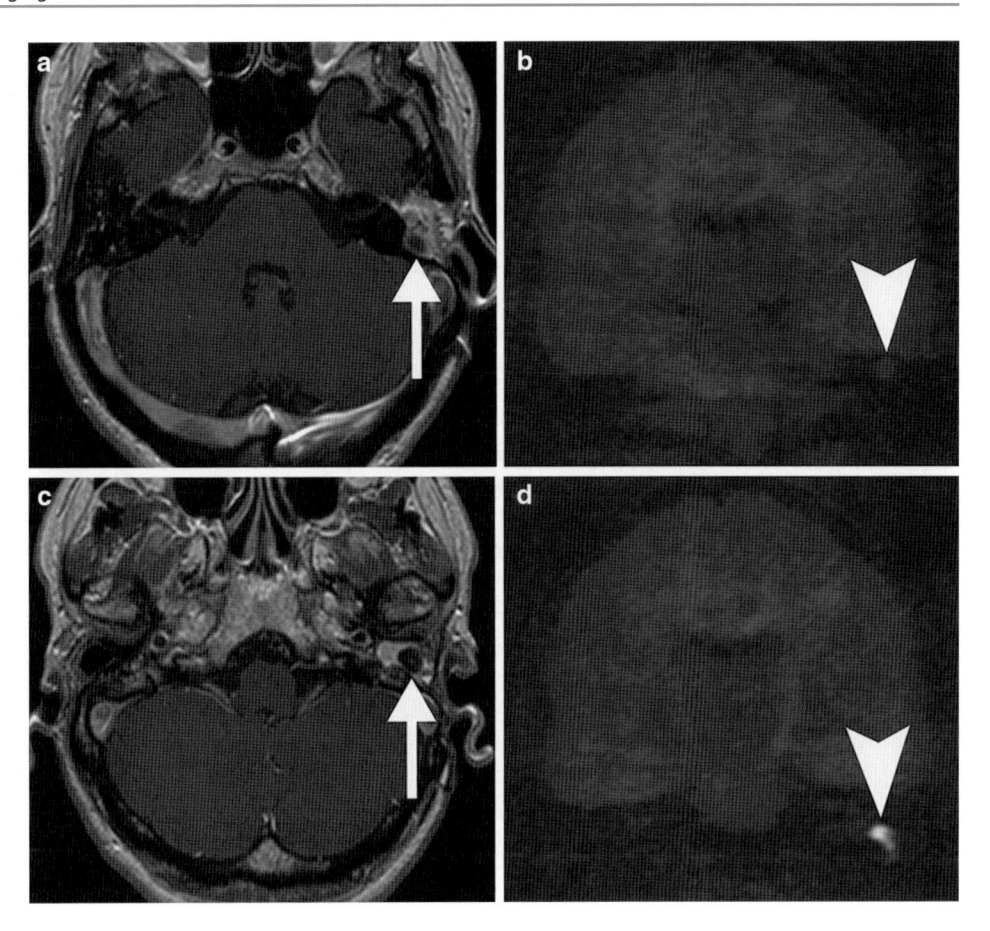

cholesteatomas (Fitzek et al. 2002) and residual or recurrent cholesteatomas (Aikele et al. 2003) followed soon. Cholesteatoma is characterised by a high signal intensity on EPI and non-EPI DWI images with high b-values. The high signal intensity of cholesteatoma on the b-1000 diffusion images allows them to be differentiated from other lesions like fluid, inflammatory tissue, cholesterol granuloma, … which all have a low signal intensity (Figs. 9 and 10). The exact cause of this high signal intensity on DWI is still not completely understood. One explanation could be the decreased mobility of the water molecules in the residual cholesteatoma, so-called diffusion restriction. Another explanation for the increased intensity could be the T2-shine-through effect (Khemani et al. 2012).

Two different diffusion-weighting techniques are in use for detection of post-operative cholesteatoma: traditional spin-echo echo planar (EPI) and non-echo-planar (non-EPI) DWI.

EPI DWI is a very fast pulse sequence that can usually be performed in less than 1-2 minutes. EPI DWI fails to detect small cholesteatomas under 5 mm (Vercruysse et al. 2006). This may be explained by several reasons, among them susceptibility artefacts at the bone–air interface of the tegmen tympani, a low imaging matrix with relatively thick sections. Another limitation of the EPI DWI technique in demonstrating small cholesteatoma pearls are motion artefacts, which are responsible for smearing the hyperintense signal over different voxels (Stasolla et al. 2004). An overall sensitivity and specificity for detecting residual or recurrent cholesteatoma of 13–86 and 73–100 % has been described.

The large variation in sensitivity and specificity may be explained by differences in patient population and patient selection between various studies (i.e. patient selection based on CT findings or not, residual versus recurrent cholesteatoma). Stasolla et al. and Aikele et al. included in their series residual and recurrent cholesteatoma (Aikele et al. 2003; Stasolla et al. 2004), whereas Vercruysse et al. and Venail et al. selected patients with residual cholesteatoma only (Vercruysse et al. 2006; Venail et al. 2008). Incorporating both residual and recurrent cholesteatoma will result in a higher number of cholesteatoma of a larger size which may explain the higher sensitivities in these studies. Including only residual cholesteatoma on the other hand will result in a high number of smaller lesions, typically less than 5 mm, which explains the lower sensitivity in these studies (De Foer et al. 2011). Another explanation for the differences observed between studies could be the delay between MR imaging and surgery (Venail et al. 2008). Nevertheless, EPI DWI had higher specificity when compared to delayed contrast-enhanced MRI, despite its lower specificity (Venail et al. 2008). Several authors advocated

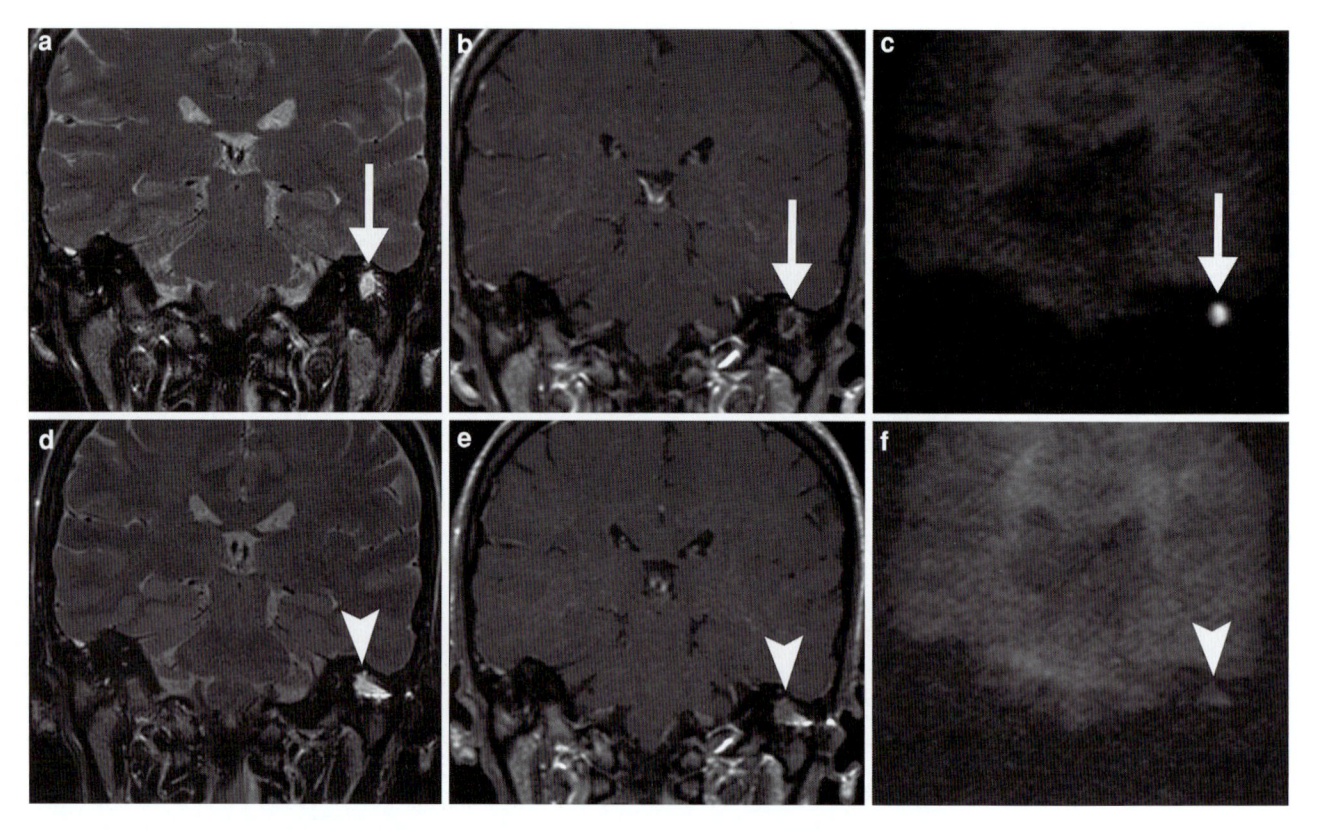

Fig. 10 Pre-operative **a–c** and post-operative **d–f** MRI of a patient with cholesteatoma 1 year after surgery. **a** Coronal T2-weighted MR image shows a homogeneous, sharply delineated mass in the mastoid (*arrow*). **b** On the coronal postcontrast T1-weighted MR image, the lesion has a non-enhancing centre with an enhancing rim (*arrow*) suspicious for cholesteatoma, which is confirmed on the coronal non-EPI DWI MR image (*arrow* in **c**). **d** Post-operative coronal T2-weighted MR image in the same patient again shows a homogeneous, sharply delineated mass in the same region of the previously located cholesteatoma (*arrowhead*). **e** The coronal postcontrast T1-weighted MR image shows that the centre of the lesion is more intense than pre-operatively (*arrowhead*) and does not show a high signal on the coronal non-EPI DWI MR image (*arrowhead* in **f**), which is compatible which protein-rich fluid or granulation tissue

therefore concurrent use of both these techniques for best diagnostic performance (Vercruysse et al. 2006; Venail et al. 2008; Lemmerling et al. 2008).

Technical improvements in sequence design have shifted from using EPI DWI sequences towards the use of non-EPI DWI sequences. Non-EPI techniques are less vulnerable to susceptibility artefacts and have higher spatial resolution due to the use of thinner slices and an increased imaging matrix, yielding sensitivities in the 90–100 % range for lesions as small as 2 mm (De Foer et al. 2008; Pizzini et al. 2010; Más-Estellés et al. 2012). Also, the estimated size correlated well with the operative findings, with all measurements having a discrepancy of no greater than 1 mm (Dheppnorrarat et al. 2009). On a technical note, De Foer et al. were the first to describe the use of a non-EPI single-shot turbo spin-echo (TSE) DWI sequence, i.e. a half-Fourier acquisition single-shot TSE (HASTE, Siemens Medical Systems, Erlangen, Germany) (De Foer et al. 2006). HASTE DWI is now the most reported non-EPI DWI sequence in detecting cholesteatoma (Jindal et al. 2011; Li et al. 2012). HASTE DWI allows the use of thinner sections (down to 2 mm slice thickness), a higher imaging matrix, with a complete lack of susceptibility artefacts (Dheppnorrarat et al. 2009). The non-EPI sequence from Philips is a multishot FSE DWI sequence (Philips Medical Systems, Best, The Netherlands, Dubrulle et al. 2006). PROPELLER DWI (Periodically Rotated Overlapping Parallel Lines with Enhanced Reconstruction) is the multishot non-EPI DWI sequence developed by General Electric (GE Healthcare, Milwaukee, WI, USA). The value of PROPELLER DWI in cholesteatoma was first evaluated on 3T (Lehmann et al. 2009) and more recently on 1.5T (Kasbekar et al. 2010; Más-Estellés et al. 2012). BLADE DWI (Siemens Medical Systems, Erlangen, Germany) is a similar multishot technique, based on a PROPELLER k-space trajectory. Multishot techniques are potentially susceptible to motion artefacts as multiple echoes contribute to a single diffusion measurement. To solve this problem, k-space is acquired through several radially orientated 'propellers' or 'blades'. As the blades overlap at the centre of the k-space, there is relative oversampling resulting in an image with higher signal intensity and with reduced motion artefacts. Relative drawbacks of these techniques is that acquisition time is longer than with HASTE DWI and that the images can only be acquired in the axial plane, potentially resulting in poor visualisation of the tegmen tympani, which can be better evaluated on coronal images (Khemani et al. 2012). BLADE DWI has increased spatial resolution compared with the HASTE DWI technique (Schwartz et al. 2011). Both sequences may be included in post-operative cholesteatoma protocols. Because of its superior signal-to-noise ratio, the HASTE DWI sequence is often preferred since small recurrent cholesteatomas are sometimes more difficult to depict on BLADE DWI and better seen on HASTE DWI (Lane 2012).

HASTE DWI and PROPELLOR DWI have both been shown to have a higher diagnostic performance than delayed contrast-enhanced MR imaging in detecting cholesteatoma prior to second-look surgery (De Foer et al. 2010; Lehmann et al. 2009). Moreover, De Foer et al. compared delayed contrast-enhanced MR imaging with the HASTE DWI—alone and in combination—in the evaluation of cholesteatoma patients. They concluded that the HASTE DWI sequence can be used as a stand-alone screening sequence in cholesteatoma patients and that gadolinium administration is no longer required (De Foer et al. 2010). Similar findings have been reported by other groups (Dheppnorrarat et al. 2009; Huins et al. 2010; Pluoin-Gouan et al. 2010a; Rajan et al. 2010) and the routine use of non-EPI DWI for cholesteatoma screening is fast becoming a widely accepted practice within the radiological community. Many institutions have changed their imaging protocols, where delayed gadolinium-enhanced T1-weighted sequences are no longer used and axial and coronal T2-weighted sequences are added for orientation purposes. Plouin-Gouan et al. investigated the use of fusion of the DWI and HRCT images for more precise localisation of cholesteatomas (Pluoin-Gouan et al. 2010b). These new imaging protocols result in a substantial shortening of imaging time, cost saving for the healthcare system and a higher patient throughput for MR imaging (De Foer et al. 2010). As scanning time is very short (within 2 minutes), sedation or general anesthesia is usually not required in children (Rajan et al. 2010). Many institutions therefore now use non-EPI DWI for screening after CWU surgery and limit second-look surgery to patients with positive DWI (Khemani et al. 2012). Since cholesteatoma pearls less than 3 mm may be missed, further follow-up by MR imaging should be performed annually for 5 years (Geoffray et al. 2012). In our institutions, MRI follow-up is provided after 1, 3 and 5 years.

In a recently published meta-analysis of 342 patients, Li et al. concluded that non-EPI DWI may help to stratify patients into groups of who would benefit from early second-look surgery and who could be closely observed (Li et al. 2012). The overall pooled sensitivity was 94 % and specificity was 94 %. A total of 30 false negatives and 8 false positives were described. The majority of false negative results were due to cholesteatoma pearls measuring less than 3 mm in size, thus exceeding the lower limit of reliability of current imaging technology. Apart from cholesteatoma size, false-negative cases were also attributed to auto-evacuating retraction pockets (aka mural cholesteatomas) and image degradation from motion artefacts. In these cases of empty cholesteatoma pockets—either by auto-evacuation or by suction cleaning—no typical solid 'onionlike mass' filled with keratin debris was present at the moment of revision surgery. Instead, these lesions had the appearance of a deep retraction pocket, with a macroscopically epithelial lining but lacking the presence of firm keratin. Since DWI detects the keratin content of a cholesteatoma, it is unlikely to detect these recurrent retraction pockets without keratin or residual matrix (Dheppnorrarat et al. 2009; Rajan et al. 2010; De Foer et al. 2011; Jeunen et al. 2008). Another false-negative case was a DWI hypointense lesion, hypointense in T2 and hyperintense in T1 without postcontrast enhancing that was interpreted as a subacute or recurrent bleeding in the tissue (Profant et al. 2012).

False positive findings with hyperintensities not corresponding to a cholesteatoma have been described in various situations: after recent surgery (residual haemorrhage), in ears containing silastic sheets and prosthesis (Venail et al. 2008; Geoffray et al. 2012), bone powder (Dubrulle et al. 2006) or a fat plug (Dremmen et al. 2012), scar tissue (Venail et al. 2008; Jeunen et al. 2008), cerumen in the EAC (Kasbekar et al. 2010), cholesterol granuloma (Kösling and Bootz 2001), middle ear or mastoid abscesses (Dremmen et al. 2012; Profant et al. 2012), endocrine adenoma (Barath et al. 2011) and artefacts due to metallic dental braces (Pluoin-Gouan et al. 2010a; Más-Estellés et al. 2012). When non-EPI DWI sequences are not available, susceptibility artefacts on EPI DWI may be a cause for false positive findings (Cimsit et al. 2010).

Clinical and otoscopic findings as well as details from the surgical intervention may help to avoid these pitfalls. In most cases, conventional MRI-sequences (T1, T2, Gd-T1) will be able to differentiate fat plugs and cholesterol granuloma from cholesteatoma (Dremmen et al. 2012). When in doubt, ADC values can be measured; ADC values are usually much higher in cholesterol granuloma than in cholesteatomas. Also, to discriminate abscesses from cholesteatomas, ADC measurements may be helpful; lesions containing pus show very low ADC values ($<0.5 \times 10^{-3}$ mm^2/s). These values have been reported to be higher in cholesteatomas and intermediate when cholesteatoma and infection coexist (Thiriat et al. 2009; Lingam et al. 2013). When DWI suggests recurrence, some institutions add delayed contrast-enhanced imaging to confirm the recurrence and only these children undergo surgery (Geoffray et al. 2012).

Although MR imaging at 3T is becoming more common and available, data on the value and/or benefits of 3T over 1.5T in imaging the petrous bone are scarce and mostly related to imaging of diseases involving the inner ear, such as Menière's disease (Naganawa and Nakashima 2009). Theoretical advantages of 3T over 1.5T are increased signal-to-noise ratio, faster imaging which is less sensitive to patient motion (e.g. in children), and increased spatial and contrast resolution. Disadvantages are increase in RF deposition (SAR) and increased susceptibility artefacts (Schmitz et al. 2005). To the best of our knowledge only two papers have been published using 3T in the evaluation of middle ear cholesteatoma. Similar results comparing EPI DWI and non-EPI PROPELLER DWI on 3T were observed (Lehmann et al. 2009). The resolution power of HASTE on 3T was 2 mm (Pizzini et al. 2010), which is the same as on 1.5T.

3 Stapes Surgery in Otosclerosis Patients

Many diseases and dysplasias can affect the osseous components of the temporal bone. Some diseases such as otosclerosis are limited to the temporal bone and do not occur elsewhere in the body (Hasso et al. 1996). The term 'otosclerosis' was introduced by Adam Politzer, who described the histopathological findings in 1894 (Declau et al. 2001). Otosclerosis occurs in two phases: an early, active phase, during which bone resorption occurs (otospongiotic stage) and a later, inactive phase (sclerotic stage). Diagnosis of otosclerosis is based on clinical findings, audiometric testing and family history, but medical imaging is often demanded to confirm the diagnosis (Nowé et al. 2004). The typical clinical features of otosclerosis are gradually increasing hearing loss (HL), most frequently occurring between the third and fifth decades. Although usually both ears are affected, often there is an asymmetry in HL with one ear showing a greater conductive impairment. Tinnitus is a common symptom and it may become louder as the HL progresses. The origin of the tinnitus is not clear but it may be the result of cochlear degeneration or an abnormal degree of vascularity within the labyrinthine capsule. Vertigo is rare and is probably the effect of toxic enzymes on the vestibular labyrinth (de Bruijn 2000). In otosclerosis, three major patterns of involvement are discerned: fenestral, retrofenestral and mixed. First, a purely fenestral type, which involves the oval window, most commonly the anterior aspect in the approximate location of the embryologic fissula ante fenestram. The second type is a retrofenestral (cochlear) form, primarily involving the cochlea, with SNHL as a result. Both types of otosclerosis may coexist in one patient, resulting in mixed hearing loss (d'Archambeau et al. 1990).

Although stapes surgery is considered nowadays the treatment of choice, hearing aids or BAHA may be a good alternative in those cases, where surgery is not desirable or possible (Raut et al. 2002). The administration of sodium fluoride, to stabilise cochlear deterioration remains a matter of controversy, partly due to the unknown toxic effect of long-term medication (de Bruijn 2000).

Currently, stapes surgery consists of the traditional stapedectomy—introduced by Shea in 1958—in which the footplate is totally or near-totally removed, and stapedotomy in which a small fenestra is made through the central portion of the footplate. Small fenestra stapedotomy, first popularised by Marquet et al. is the operation of choice since this technique has less early complications, including vertigo and reparative granuloma formation (Marquet et al. 1972).

A wide variety of different stapes prostheses is available. They differ in size, shape and weight. Materials most often used for prostheses are a Teflon type polymer, stainless steel, titanium and platinum. Teflon is still the most favoured piston in the UK, although combinations with platinum and stainless steel are increasingly being used in some centres (Raut et al. 2002). The main differences in the design of stapes prostheses are at the point of connection with the incus. The attachment to the incus consists of either a loop that surrounds the incus or a cup into which the lenticular process fits.

In the majority of cases (more than 90 %), post-operative results are good and no further imaging studies are required. However, unsuccessful outcomes (persistent or recurrent CHL, vertigo and fluctuating SNHL) may be observed. Follow-up CT examination is performed in these patients to demonstrate abnormalities that may require re-intervention. Abnormal findings on CT to identify are incorrect stapes prosthesis position, inflammatory changes, perilymphatic fistula (PLF) and regrowth of otosclerosis (Williams et al. 2000) (Figs. 11, 12, 13 and 14).

According to Causse et al., three categories of complications after otosclerosis surgery can be discerned: intra-operative complications, immediately post-operative and delayed post-operative complications (Causse et al. 1983). Vertigo immediately after the surgical procedure can be explained by the sudden drop in intralabyrinthine pressure while opening the oval window, especially in cases of pre-existing hydrops. Other causes of vertigo include intra-operative contamination of the labyrinth with blood and compression of the saccule when the shaft of the prosthesis enters the vestibule (Fig. 11). Prosthesis displacement is the most common cause of CHL recurrence or persistence after surgery (Fig. 12).

CT visualisation of the prosthesis depends on its material (Chakeres and Mattox 1985). Thin metallic or teflon prostheses, may be more difficult to identify (Kösling and Bootz

Fig. 11 Double-oblique reformatted **a** and coronal **b** CBCT image demonstrates a piston prosthesis protruding into the vestibule in a patient without hearing benefit after stapedotomy

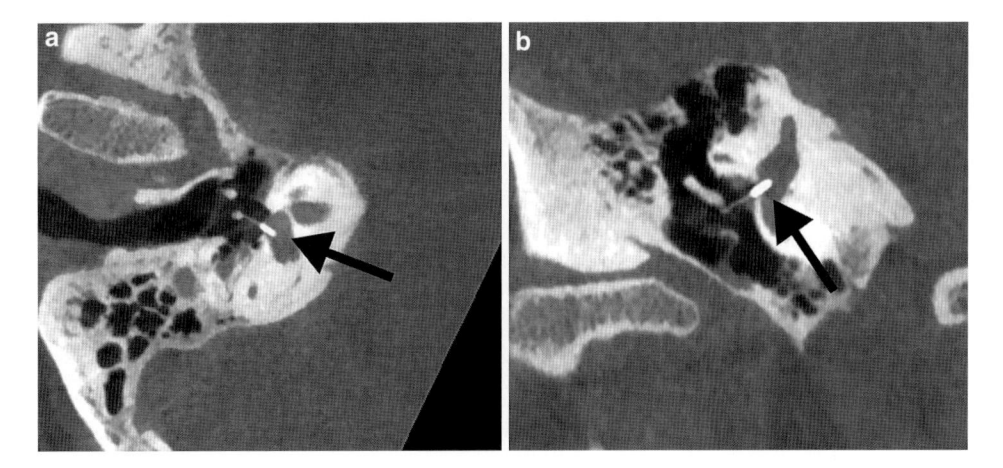

Fig. 12 Dislocated stapes prosthesis. Axial **a** and coronal **b** CBCT image showing a dislocated Teflon stapes prosthesis lying against the posterolateral wall of the tympanic cavity (*arrowhead*)

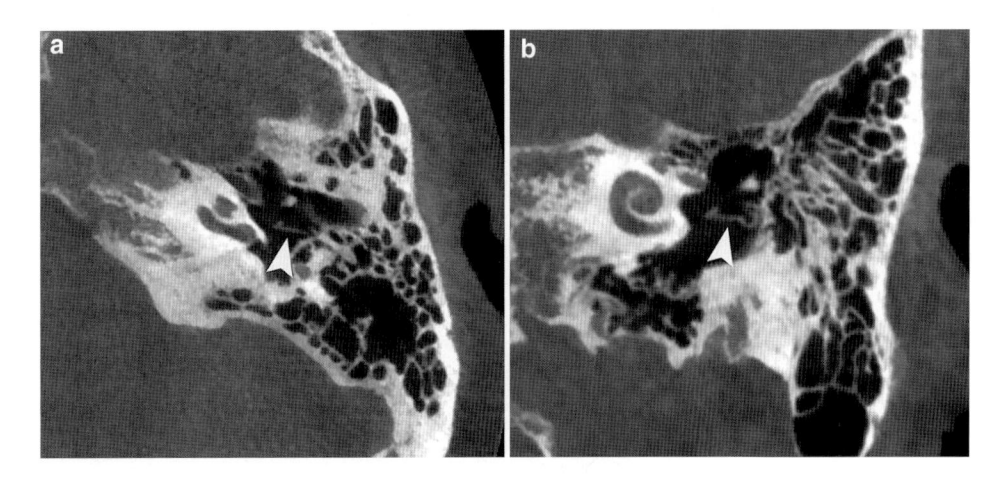

2001). Prosthetic position in the middle ear can be determined with HRCT, especially when helical or even better MDCT is used (Rangheard et al. 2001). Conventional CT is limited by the obliquity of the prosthesis relative to the conventional scan planes. Helical CT yields high-resolution reformatting in oblique planes along the main axis of the prosthesis, allowing a more accurate depiction of the prosthesis status. Multiplanar reconstructions provided by helical CT acquisition greatly improve imaging accuracy by showing the full length of the prosthesis on single axial or coronal reformatted images. Nevertheless, the resolution of reformatted images remains insufficient to determine the type of surgical procedure that has been performed (Williams et al. 2000). The dislocation of the prosthesis of the stapes footplate may be limited to an inframillimetric gap between the footplate plane and the tip of the prosthesis. In such cases, the medial end of the prosthesis may appear to be in the correct position on conventional CT, but oblique multiplanar reconstructions accurately show the abnormal location of the prosthesis (Fig. 13). Cone-beam CT (CBCT) volumetric scanning allows a thinner slice thickness of 0.15 mm compared to a multi-detector scanner (MDCT) slice thickness of 0.5–0.625 mm, at a reduced dose exposure. CBCT is routinely used for dental applications, and it now has become available for scanning temporal bones (Peltonen et al. 2007; Miracle and Mukherji 2009; Penninger et al. 2011). Other advantages of CBCT are less metal artefacts when imaging prostheses and better image quality in other planes due to isotropic voxel. Especially, double-oblique reformats are of value when evaluating the stapes and prostheses.

Fixation of the prosthesis can be caused by post-operative fibrous adhesions. CT scan shows a soft tissue mass around the prosthesis or the ossicles and may cover the oval window. PLF is a more serious complication that counts for 10 % of all stapedectomy failures. Fluctuations of hearing and vertigo are the most common clinical symptoms associated with PLF. Tiny air bubbles at the end of the stapes prosthesis detected with CT are indicative of a pneumolabyrinth, which is the most important indirect sign of PLF. However, a pneumolabyrinth cannot be expected in all patients with PLF (Kösling et al. 1995). CT may also identify small fluid collections immediately outside the oval window and abnormal fluid collections in the middle ear and the mastoid cells in these patients (Pickuth et al. 2000). Proliferation of the otosclerotic focus may cause the impairment of a prosthesis.

Fig. 13 Malpositioned tip of a stapes prosthesis. Double-oblique reformatted **a** and coronal **b** CBCT image shows that the tip of the stainless steel prosthesis is not touching the stapes footplate (*arrow*). This patient only had limited conductive hearing loss, suggesting that some fibrous connection between the prosthesis tip and footplate is present

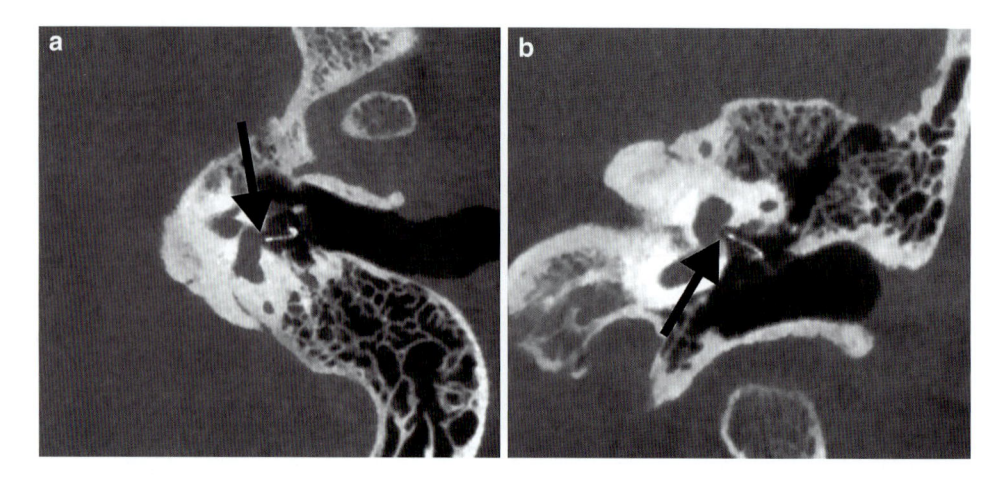

Fig. 14 Otospongiotic proliferation on the stapes prosthesis. Double-oblique reformatted **a** and coronal **b** CBCT image showing an obliteration of the oval window niche by otospongiotic proliferation (*arrow*), lifting up the Teflon prosthesis

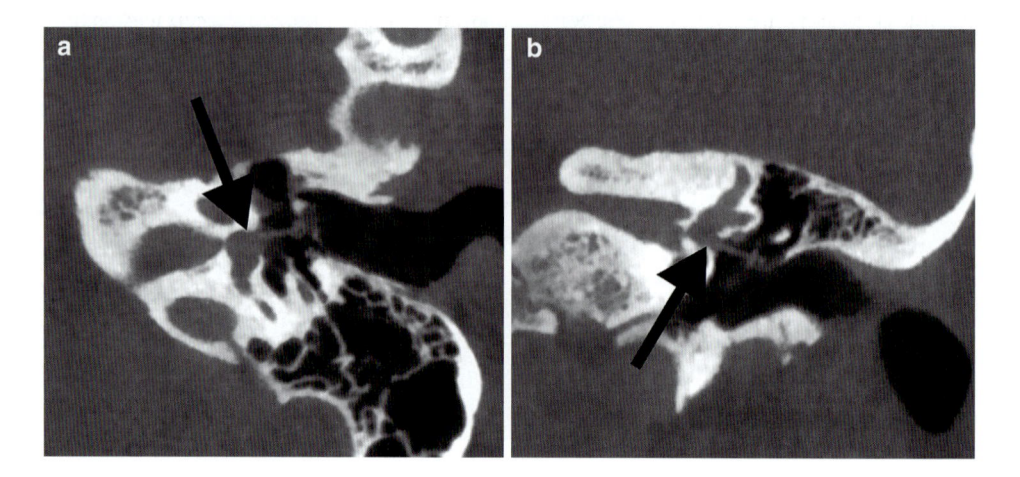

A slightly hyperdense calcified space-occupying mass in the oval window niche, surrounding the medial end of the prosthesis may be observed in these patients (Fig. 14).

Acute labyrinthitis and secondary endolymphatic hydrops are two other causes of vertigo after stapes surgery. These conditions have no pathognomonic CT manifestations (Pickuth et al. 2000). Therefore, if CT is not contributive to the origin of SNHL and vertigo, MR imaging may be helpful to demonstrate reparative intravestibular granuloma, intralabyrinthine haemorrhage and labyrinthitis. High signal intensity of the labyrinth on T1- and T2-weighted is indicative for post-operative haemorrhage. A combination of low signal intensity on T2-weighted images and strong enhancement after injection of gadolinium is noticed in patients with fibrous obliteration of the labyrinth as in reparative granuloma and suppurative labyrinthitis. (Rangheard et al. 2001). Labyrinthine—and especially cochlear—enhancement may also be a possible sign of PLF (Mark and Fitzgerald 1993).

The attachment of the prosthesis to the long process of the incus plays an important role concerning the gain in hearing and the development of late complications such as incus erosion and necrosis (Kwok et al. 2002).

Decreased thickness in the long process of the incus as seen on coronal CT scans may indicate incus necrosis. This is a late complication of stapes surgery and generally occurs after 3 or more years (Kösling and Bootz 2001).

4 Vestibular Schwannoma Surgery

Vestibulocochlear schwannoma (VS)—frequently also referred to as acoustic schwannoma—is a benign tumour of the vestibulocochlear nerve (N. VIII).

They constitute approximately 7–8 % of all primary intracranial neoplasms and approximately 90 % of the cerebellopontine angle (CPA) tumours. Symptoms of VS are variable and are related to the site of origin—internal auditory canal (IAC) versus CPA—and on the size of the tumour. Symptoms related to VS include SNHL, tinnitus, vestibular dysfunction and other symptoms that are related to compression of the cranial nerves in the CPA cistern, or brainstem. MR imaging replaced CT for the detection of VS in the early 1990s, when the use of gadolinium made MR the most sensitive method to demonstrate these lesions (Mulkens et al. 1993). Careful analysis of the high-resolution T2-weighted images (CISS, GRASS, DRIVE, …) may allow in some cases to determine from which branch of the vestibulocochlear nerve the tumour is arising (Sartoretti-Schefer et al. 2000) and virtual endoscopy may demonstrate the anatomical relationships of the tumour with the facial nerve (Nowé et al. 2004).

Once the diagnosis of VS is made on MR, different treatment options are available. Surgery, radiation therapy or a conservative approach can be chosen, depending on patients' health and age, hearing status, facial nerve function and others. Also, MR imaging features may influence the decision of the surgeon. Therefore, size, location and growth of the tumour, extension of VS into the fundus, signal intensity of the cerebrospinal fluid (CSF) in the IAC distal to the tumour, and intralabyrinthine signal intensity on T2-weighted images should be evaluated carefully (Casselman 2001).

4.1 Conservative Management

Several publications have shown that VS are slowly growing tumours with an annual growth rate of 1–2 mm/year (Charabi et al. 1998). Therefore, some authors consider conservative management—'wait and scan'—a reasonable option for selected patients instead of radiation or surgery, especially in elderly (Hoistad et al. 2001) (Fig. 15). However, an increased number of newly diagnosed small tumours has been observed (Charabi et al. 1998). Besides an increased awareness of otolaryngologists and earlier screening with ABR, this is above all due to the more widespread use of MR imaging. These patients with small VS have a significant better change of hearing preservation after surgery (Irving et al. 1995). It has been published that adopting the wait-and-scan policy, these tumours will grow and candidates for hearing preservation surgery will lose their eligibility (Charabi et al. 1998). On the other hand, many VSs followed with periodic MR imaging studies do not grow (Fucci et al. 1999). Therefore, close follow-up in these patients is mandatory and if tumour growth is observed on repetitive MR studies, patients should be operated on (Van de Heyning 2002) (Fig. 16). Evaluation of tumour volume on serial MR examinations can be done with 1-mm-thick contrast-enhanced T1-weighted gradient echo images (MPRAGE, FSPGR, 3D TFE, …). Surface measurements in square millimetres, performed on all images on which the VS can be seen, will eventually allow calculation of the tumour volume (Casselman 2001) (Figs. 15, 16).

4.2 Radiosurgery

Gamma knife therapy has been considered as a safe and effective management for VSs, especially in preventing facial function and hearing. It can be applied as primary treatment in selected patients (e.g. patients in poor clinical condition with a growing VS), but is also an option as additional treatment for regrowing residual VS (Bertalanffy et al. 2001). The purpose of irradiation in patients with VS is to provide maximal local tumour control while minimizing complications such as cranial nerve injuries. Excellent local control can be obtained when treatment is administered in moderate doses and reduction in the tumour dose may increase the hearing preservation rate in the future (Bush et al. 2002). The possible induction of secondary neoplasia in the treatment field and the possibility of malignant transformation of benign neoplasia, even after 30–40 years should not be minimalised (Malis 2000).

Regular follow-up MR examinations are to be performed, most oftenly at 6-month intervals. The tumour volume, as evaluated on serial MR studies, should preferably decrease or at least remain stable. However, a transient volume increase has been reported and should not be confounded with tumour growth and treatment failure (Prasad et al. 2000). Tumour volume reduction after radiotherapy can have a delay of 24 months.

Another feature that has to be evaluated on serial MR examinations is tumour enhancement. A central loss of contrast enhancement is frequently observed within 6–12 months after radiosurgery; probably it represents central radiation necrosis. (Prasad et al. 2000). A significantly higher incidence of central non-enhancement has been observed in tumours that exhibited an early increase in size (Prasad et al. 2000). The true significance of these changes still needs to be established, since, interestingly enough, facial and vestibulocochlear nerve deficiency occur after this same time interval.

4.3 Surgery

Familiarity with the anatomic alterations of each surgical procedure makes it easier to the radiologist to interpret the post-operative findings. Most common approaches in VS surgery include a translabyrinthine (TL) approach, a retrosigmoid (RS) suboccipital craniotomy and middle fossa temporal (MFT) craniotomy. There is a great deal of controversy about the ideal approach for the removal of VS

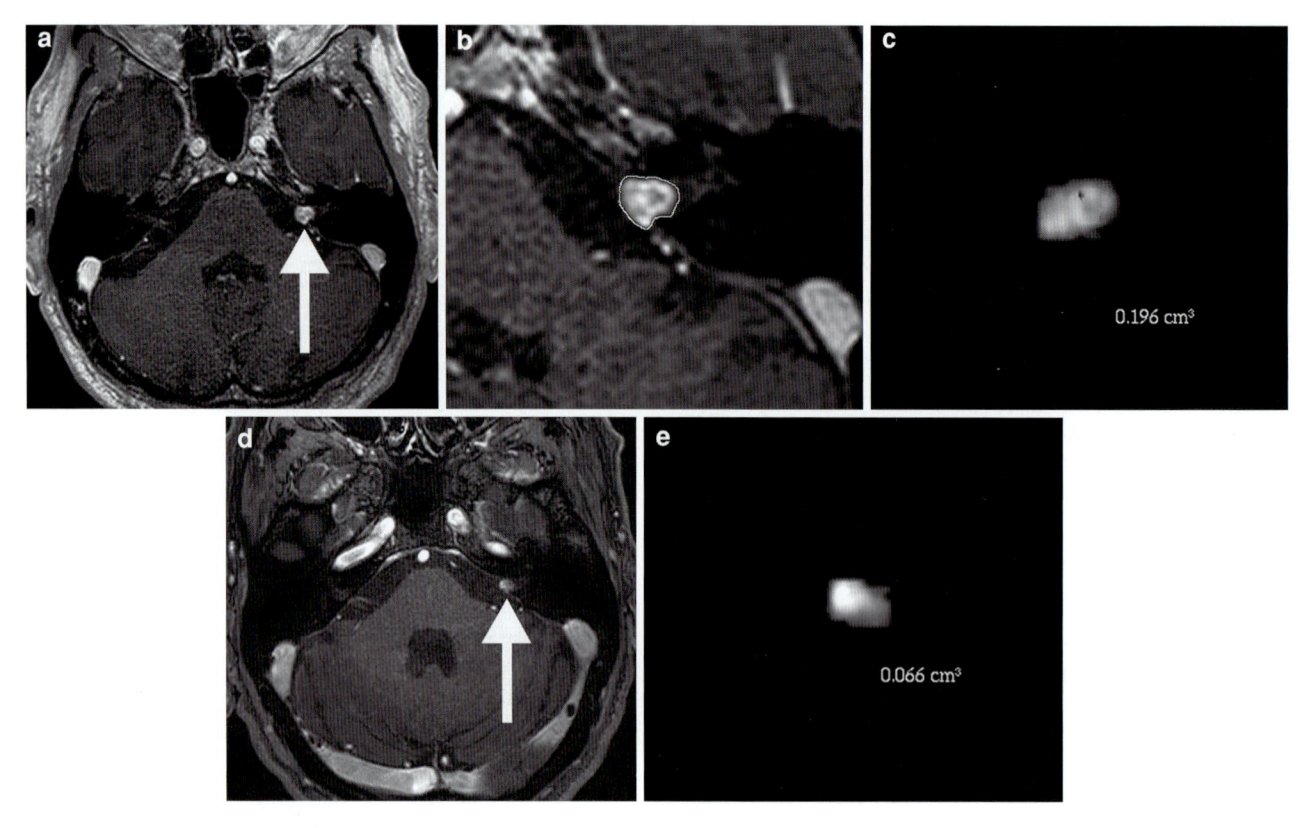

Fig. 15 'Wait and scan' conservative management of a 61-year-old male patient with a vestibular schwannoma (VS). **a** Axial postcontrast T1-weighted MR image demonstrates a small vestibular schwannoma (*arrow*) at the left porus of the internal auditory canal. **b** Volumetric analysis requires delineation of the tumour on all images. **c** Volumetric calculation of the tumour volume was 0.196 cm^3. **d** Axial postcontrast T1-weighted MR image in the same patient after 9 years of follow-up reveals a tumour volume reduction (*arrow*). **e** This was confirmed on the volumetric analysis. Interval follow-up in this patient was yearly the first 5 years, then once two-yearly and finally once after 3 years. The tumour volume loss was only visible on the last 3 scans. Less than 1 % of VS show a spontaneous loss of volume

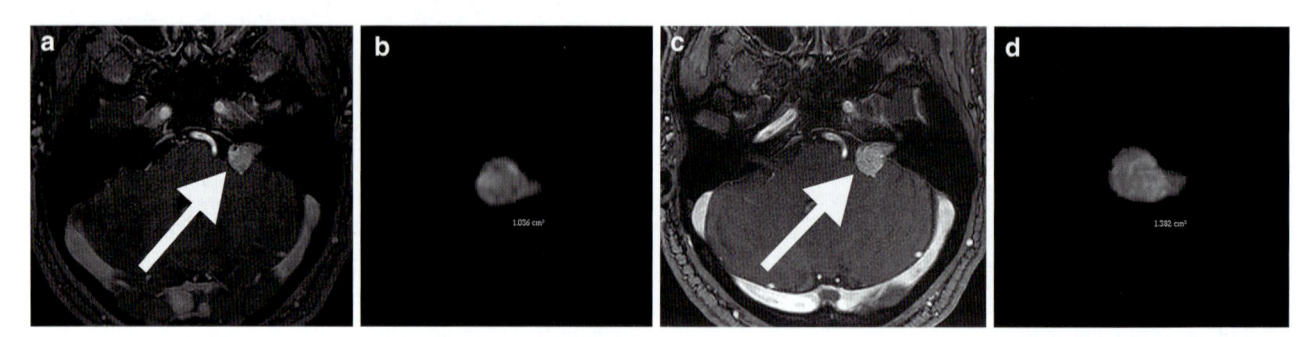

Fig. 16 'Wait and scan' conservative management of 61-year-old male patient with a vestibular schwannoma. **a** Axial postcontrast T1-weighted MR image shows a large vestibular schwannoma in the left IAC and CPA (arrow). **b** Volumetric calculation measured a tumour volume of 1.036 cm^3. **c** Axial postcontrast T1-weighted MR image after 6 months of follow-up period demonstrated increased tumour volume noticed at the level of the middle cerebellar peduncle (*arrow*). **d** This volume increase was confirmed on the volumetric calculation (Volume = 1.382 cm^3) and the patient subsequently underwent surgery

(Haberkamp et al. 1998). In addition to personal favours and experience of the surgeon, factors determining the surgical approach include patients' health and age, size of tumour, hearing status, and location of tumour in the IAC and the CPA. Careful reporting of the MR examination by the radiologist may help the surgeon in this perspective. If fluid is still present between the VS and the fundus of the IAC, an RS suboccipital or MFT approach can be used. If no fluid is left, a TL approach is preferred, leaving however the patient deaf (Somers et al. 2001). Another important sign is the signal intensity on T2-weighted images of the CSF between the VS and the fundus, and the signal intensity of the intralabyrinthine fluid (Casselman 2001). Hearing preservation is achieved four times more often when normal

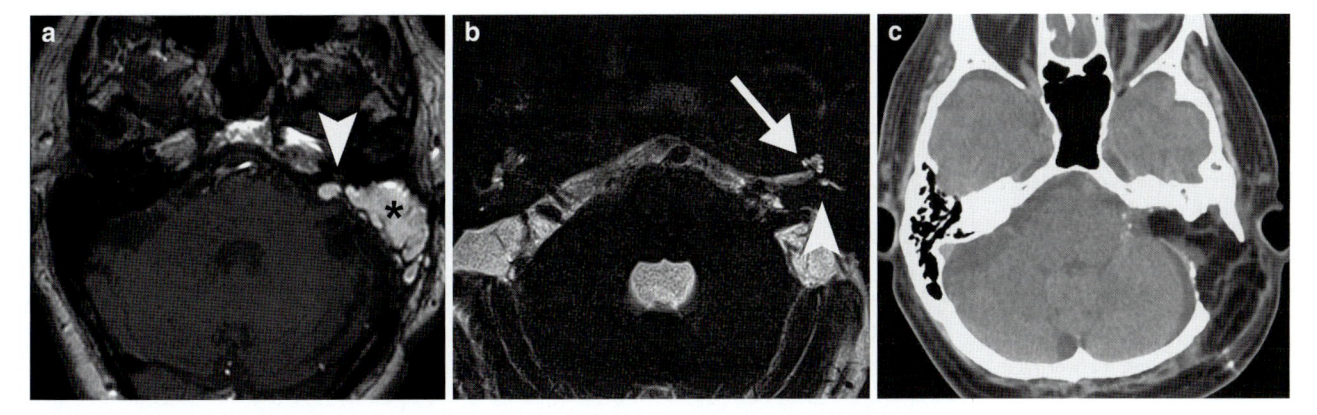

Fig. 17 Post-operative findings after translabyrinthine schwannoma resection. **a** Axial unenhanced T1-weighted MR image shows homogeneous hyperintense material (*asterisk*) in the left petrous bone, compatible with a fat plug. Note the slightly intense signal in the residual cochlea (*arrowhead*) **b** Axial 3D TSE T2-weighted MR image demonstrate shows the loss of the high signal intensity of the fluid in the vestibule (*arrowhead*) following the translabyrinthine resection. The cochlea was not destroyed (*arrow*) which is not always the case with this surgical procedure. **c** Axial CT image confirms the fat density of the abdominal fat-plug (*asterisk*) used to fill up the surgical defect

signal intensity of these fluids is found than when the signal intensity of the fluid is decreased (Somers et al. 2001). It should however be noted that this signal changes on T2-weighted images can best be appreciated with the 3DFT-CISS sequence (Siemens Medical Systems, Erlangen, Germany) and to a lesser extent on 3D-TSE (Siemens Medical Systems, Erlangen, Germany) and DRIVE (Philips Medical Systems, Best, The Netherlands) sequences. When in doubt, MIP reconstructions can aid in the evaluation.

4.3.1 Translabyrinthine Approach

The TL approach, the most direct route to the CPA, allows wide opening of the IAC for complete gross tumour removal and early identification of the facial nerve at the lateral limit of the IAC, with little or no cerebellar retraction (Brackmann 1992). Indications for TL resection are lesions of the IAC and CPA which are not amenable to hearing preservation, or intracanalicular tumours without serviceable hearing. A TL approach to the IAC is a transtemporal labyrinthectomy; it provides complete exposure of the IAC including the fundus, which facilitates tumour removal but destroys any residual hearing (McElveen et al. 1993). The mastoidectomy cavity and the translabyrinthine craniotomy can be secured with fat to prevent cerebrospinal fluid leaks. Also, the eustachian tube and aditus ad antrum can be packed with temporalis muscle, oxidised regenerated cellulose (Surgicel) or both. On high-resolution T2-weighted images, the high signal from the normal fluid-filled membraneous labyrinth may be (partially) absent. A large area of high signal on T1-weighted images from the fat, filling the mastoidectomy, may be the clue to the radiologist to determine which procedure has been performed (Fig. 17). In this case, a T1-weighted image with fat saturation is mandatory.

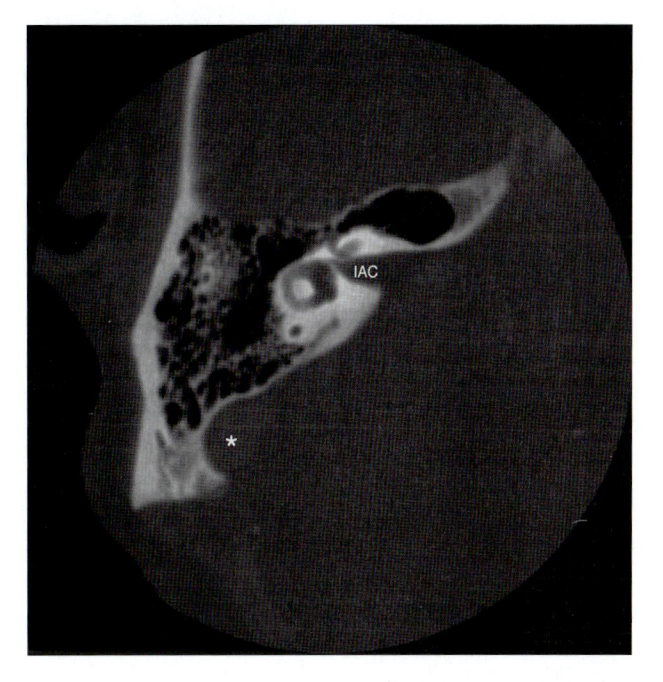

Fig. 18 Retrosigmoid approach for VS in a 59-year-old man. Axial CT scan at the level of the internal auditory canal (IAC) shows a retrosigmoid (* indicates sigmoid sinus) suboccipital craniotomy

4.3.2 Retrosigmoid Suboccipital Craniotomy

The RS approach of the IAC is a frequently used technique to remove VS when hearing-preservation is the issue. A suboccipital craniotomy is performed just behind the sigmoid sinus (Fig. 18). The cerebellum is gently pushed away to reach the pontocerebellar cistern. To reach the most lateral portion of the tumour, the posterior wall of the IAC is progressively drilled away (Van de Heyning 2002). It has been described in the literature that this technique is

Fig. 19 Post-operative follow-up after a retrosigmoid schwannoma resection. **a** Pre-operative axial postcontrast T1-weighted MR image of a vestibular schwannoma (*arrow*) centred on the porus of the left IAC. **b** Post-operative axial postcontrast T1-weighted MR image 6 months after surgery shows a nodular enhancing lesion (*arrow*) in the left IAC, suspicious of residual tumour. **c** Axial postcontrast T1-weighted MR image made 6 months later than **b** shows a volume decrease of the lesion and a less nodular appearance (*arrow*). **d** Axial postcontrast T1-weighted MR image made 6 months later than **c** demonstrates a further decrease in volume of the lesion (*arrow*) excluding tumour recurrence

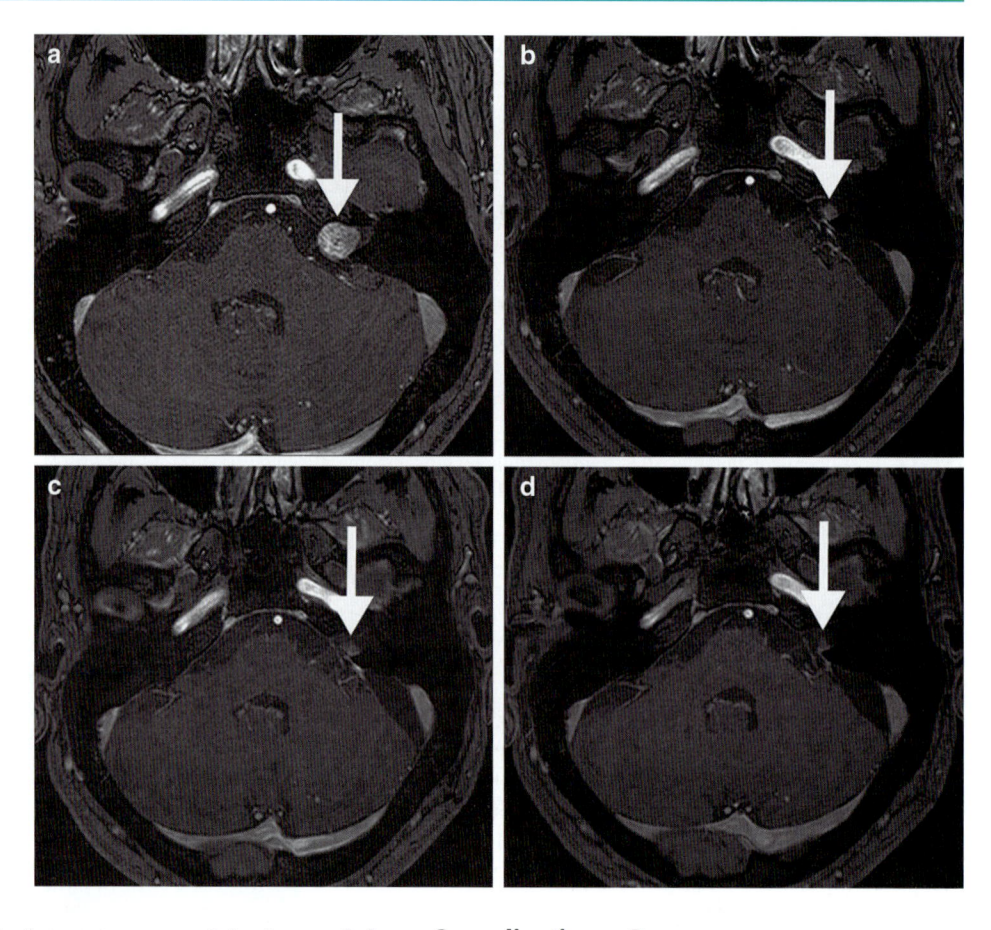

hampered by the fact that final tumour removal is done without direct visualisation of the fundus, with potential for tumour recurrence; and that therefore, close follow-up is mandatory when nodular or masslike enhancement is noticed on post-operative MR studies in these patients (Haberkamp et al. 1998) (Fig. 19). Once again, it should be noticed that post-operative results depend for a great part on the experience of the surgeon.

4.3.3 Middle Fossa Temporal Craniotomy

Deep extension of the tumour into the IAC can make hearing preservation difficult when a retrosigmoid craniotomy is used. Therefore an MFT approach has been advocated (Selesnick et al. 2001). Also in patients with small tumours and normal or nearly normal hearing, this approach can be considered. Almost complete exposure of the IAC including the fundus can be obtained performing a craniotomy at the level of the temporal squamosa. The operative defect that is created is closed with fascia, muscle or both. A scar in the subcutaneous fat above the EAC is noticed on MR. Intense linear enhancement along the roof of the IAC indicates the use of a fascia graft to close the bony defect. Although the exposure of the fundus of the IAC is likely greater through the middle fossa approach, this factor may potentially lead to recurrences, particularly when the tumour arises from the inferior vestibular nerve (Haberkamp et al. 1998).

4.4 Complications: Recurrences

4.4.1 Complications

Reported complications of VS surgery in the literature include facial nerve paresis, CSF leak, meningitis that may be associated with a CSF leak (Fig. 20), injury to the anterior inferior cerebellar artery (AICA), posterior fossa haemorrhage and haematoma at the CPA which may cause hydrocephalus due to fourth ventricle compression. Uncommon complications include late cerebellar abscess, supratentorial subcortical white matter haemorrhages and incomplete tumour removal if the tumour is densely adherent to the AICA or to the brainstem (Wiet et al. 1992). In our institutions, immediate post-operative CT to rule out haemorrhage is not performed routinely anymore (Fig. 21) (Horowitz et al. 1996).

4.4.2 Recurrences

Tumour recurrences large enough to re-operate are rare, since regrowth after removal is rare and residual tumour tends to grow slowly (Lye et al. 1992). Tumour growth after surgery is presumed to represent residual rather than recurrent tumour, since microscopic foci of tumour may be left inadvertent or deliberately to preserve facial nerve function or hearing (Cass et al. 1991).

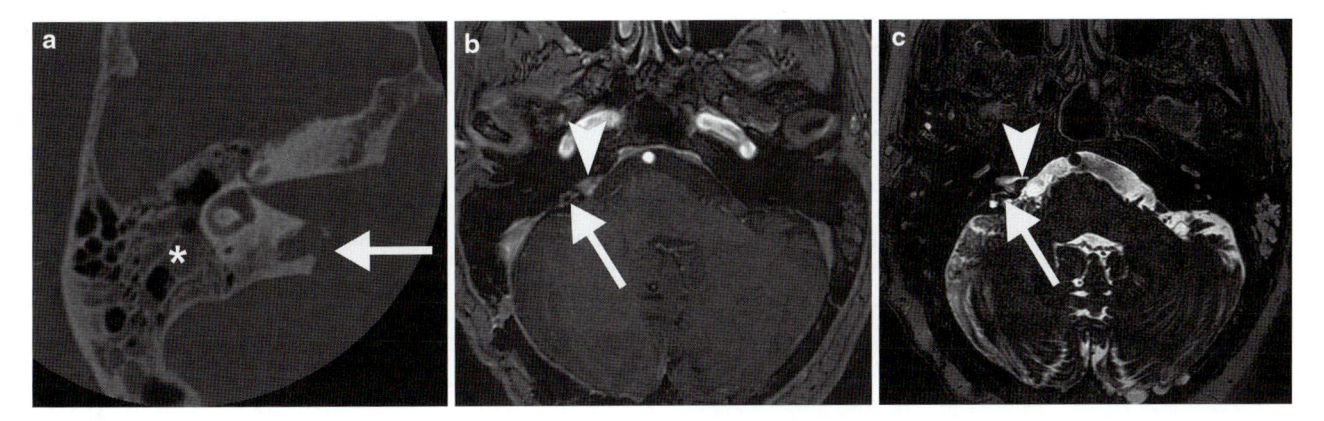

Fig. 20 Post-operative cerebrospinal fluid (CSF) leakage following retrosigmoid vestibular schwannoma surgery. **a** Post-operative axial CT image of the right ear in a patient with post-operative CSF rhinorrhea shows a defect in the medial petrous bone wall behind the IAC (*arrow*) and non-specific opacification of the mastoid cells (*asterisk*). **b** Axial postcontrast T1-weighted MR image and **c** axial DRIVE T2-weighted MR image after revision surgery shows a fat plug in the petrous bone defect (*arrow*) and post-operative fibrous tissue at the porus of the IAC (*arrowhead*)

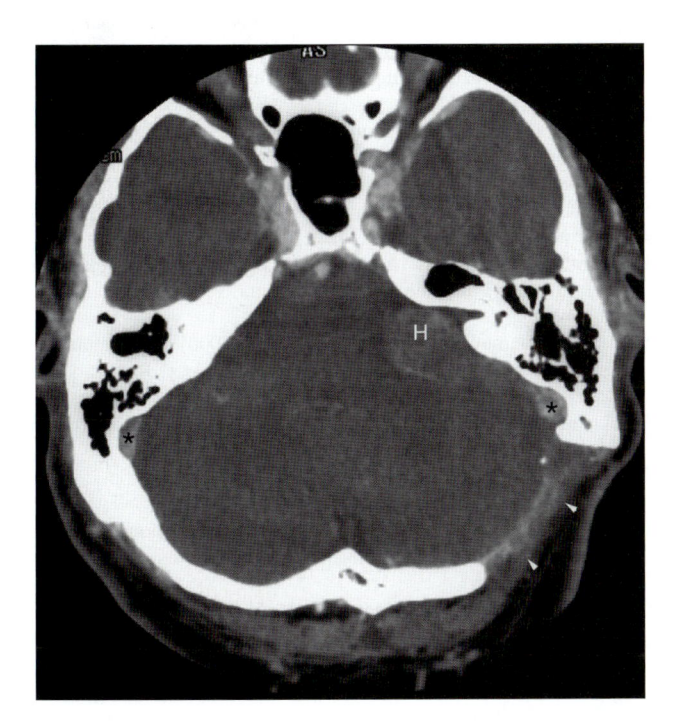

Fig. 21 Routine immediate post-operative CT within 24 h following resection of a VS to rule out complications. A retrosigmoid approach (*arrowheads*) (* indicates sigmoid sinus) has been chosen to gain access to the left cerebellopontine angle cistern. A haematoma (H) can be observed. There is no significant mass effect on the brainstem

Intracranial enhancement after various neurosurgical procedures has been described in up to 100 % of post-operative patients (Millen and Daniels 1994). It may be the result of disruption of the blood–brain barrier (blood–nerve barrier), chemical meningitis from subarachnoid haemorrhage, development of granulation tissue, and inflammation around resorbable surgical materials (e.g. absorbable gelatin powder and sponge etc.). Cass et al. admitted that it is difficult to distinguish postoperative changes from residual tumour (Cass et al. 1991). Weissman et al. described four different patterns of enhancement in the IAC after VS surgery: thin and thick linear enhancement, nodular enhancement and masslike enhancement (Weissman et al. 1997). Thin and thick linear enhancement in the IAC is probably normal after surgery (Fig. 22). However, it may be difficult to differentiate thick linear enhancement from nodular enhancement; thickened leptomeninges may retract over time creating a nodular appearance that could mimic recurrent tumour. Masslike enhancement is difficult to interpret; therefore nodular and masslike enhancement require close follow-up to monitor growth of residual tumour. Especially nodular enhancement in the fundus on postoperative studies after RS craniotomy merits our special attention (Fig. 19).

Also, the membranous labyrinth may show postsurgical alterations. High signal on T1-weighted images from the labyrinth, most frequently observed in the cochlea, is frequently encountered and may reflect blood metabolites (e.g. extracellular methemoglobin) (Weissman et al. 1997).

Hearing preservation surgery is often not possible, and the surgeon cannot always rely on subjective accounts of hearing loss or changes in the audiogram to monitor growth of potential residual tumour. Therefore, MR imaging is indispensable in the post-operative management of VS patients. There are currently no uniform guidelines concerning the timing of post-operative MR studies. Weissman et al. developed a post-operative imaging algorithm. Within 6 months after surgery—but no sooner than 1 month—a first MR examination that may serve as a baseline study is performed. If the baseline study shows only linear enhancement, MR examination is repeated after 1 year and subsequently after 3 years when no intervening changes appear. Nodular or masslike enhancement on the baseline

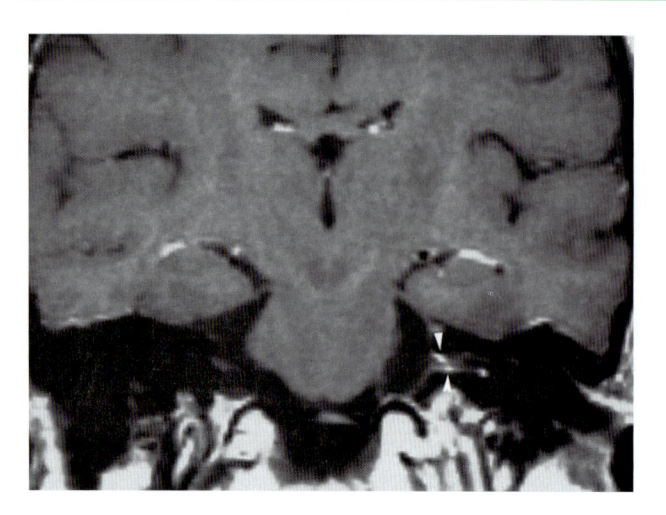

Fig. 22 Linear enhancement in the IAC following VS resection. Coronal postcontrast T1-weighted MR image 6 months after surgery shows thin linear enhancement along the walls of the IAC (*arrowheads*). No residual tumour can be observed

study warrants closer follow-up at intervals of 6 months. If the enhancement regresses, the interval may be increased to 1 year (Weissman et al. 1997).

5 Conclusion

When otoscopic examination and audiological findings fail to demonstrate the reason why surgery has been unsuccessful, patients are often sent to the radiologist for imaging of the temporal bone. Motivation for the examination, comprehensive information regarding the surgical procedure, previous examinations for comparison are indispensable to allow correct analysis of the imaging findings.

Helical CT or MDCT and recently especially CBCT is the imaging modality of choice in the evaluation of patients who had middle ear surgery for COM and otosclerosis. Cholesteatoma is a benign disease and small residual pearls are unlikely to cause any significant problems, especially in the absence of clinical symptoms. In case of a doubtful MRI scan, a repeat MR examination 6–12 months later could be advised and if there was a tiny residual cholesteatoma pearl (2–3 mm), it would have enlarged by now. This pragmatic approach may enable the ENT surgeon to better select patients for second-look procedures and thus avoid some unnecessary routine second-look operations. Financial costs associated with repeat MR imaging far outweigh the risks and inconveniences of a routine second-look surgery (Jindal et al. 2010). CBCT is nowadays preserved for preoperative assessment of ossicular damage and is used for a surgical roadmap.

Also, rare complications after stapes surgery may require further MR imaging, when CT is not contributive.

MR imaging is the imaging modality of choice in the follow-up and after surgery in patients with VS.

Acknowledgements The author wishes to acknowledge his colleagues P.M. Parizel, MD, PhD, J.W. Van Goethem, MD, PhD and O. d'Archambeau, MD, Department of Radiology, Universitair Ziekenhuis Antwerpen—University of Antwerp for their kind readiness to share their imaging files. Thanks also to all colleagues of the Department of ENT Surgery (Chairman: P.H. Van de Heyning, MD, PhD), Universitair Ziekenhuis Antwerpen—University of Antwerp for their clinical input.

References

Aikele P, Kittner T, Offergeld C et al (2003) Diffusion-weighted MR imaging of cholesteatoma in pediatric and adult patients who have undergone middle ear surgery. AJR 181:261–265

Ayache D, Williams MT, Lejeune D et al (2005) Usefulness of delayed postcontrast magnetic resonance imaging in the detection of residual cholesteatoma after canal wall-up tympanoplasty. Laryngoscope 115:607–610

Ayache D, Darrouzet V, Dubrulle F et al (2012) Imaging of non-operated cholesteatoma: clinical practice guidelines. Eur Ann Otorhinolaryngol Head Neck Dis 129:148–152

Barath K, Huber AM, Stämpfli P et al (2011) Neuroradiology of cholesteatomas. AJNR 32:221–229

Bertalanffy A, Dietrich W, Aichholzer M et al (2001) Gamma knife radiosurgery of acoustic neurinomas. Acta Neurochir (Wien) 143:689–695

Blaney SP, Tierney P, Oyarazabal M et al (2000) CT scanning in "second look" combined approach tympanoplasty. Rev Laryngol Otol Rhinol 121:79–81

Brackmann DE (1992) Middle fossa approach for acoustic tumor removal. Clin Neurosurg 38:603

Brackmann DE (1993) Tympanoplasty with mastoidectomy: canal wall up procedures. Am J Otol 14(4):380–382

Bush DA, McAllister CJ, Loredo LN et al (2002) Fractionated proton beam radiotherapy for acoustic neuroma. Neurosurgery 50:270–273

Cass SP, Kartush JM, Wilner HI et al (1991) Comparison of computerized tomography and magnetic resonance imaging for the postoperative assessment of residual acoustic tumor. Otolaryngol Head Neck Surg 104:182–190

Casselman JW (2001) MRI aids evaluation of temporal bone disease. Diagn Imaging March/April:60–65

Causse JB, Causse JR, Wiet RJ et al (1983) Complications of stapedectomies. Am J Otol 4:275–280

Chakeres DW, Mattox DE (1985) Computed tomographic evaluation of non-metallic middle-ear prostheses. Invest Radiol 20:596–600

Charabi S, Thomsen J, Tos M, Charabi B, Mantoni M, Børgesen SE (1998) Acoustic neuroma/vestibular schwannoma growth: past, present and future. Acta Otolaryngol 118(3):327–332

Corrales CE, Blevins NH (2013) Imaging for evaluation of cholesteatoma: current concepts and future directions. Curr Opin Otolaryngol Head Neck Surg 21:461–467

d'Archambeau O, Parizel PM, Koekelkoren E et al (1990) CT diagnosis and differential diagnosis of otodystrophic lesions of the temporal bone. Eur J Radiol 11:22–30 de Bruijn AJG (2000) Clinical and audiological aspects of stapes surgery in otosclerosis. PhD thesis, Amsterdam University

Declau F, Van Spaendonck M, Timmermans JP et al (2001) Prevalence of otosclerosis in an unselected series of temporal bones. Oto Neurotol 22:596–602

De Foer B, Vercruysse JP, Pilet B et al (2006) Single-shot, turbo spin-echo, diffusion-weighted imaging in the detection of acquired middle ear cholesteatoma. AJNR 27:1480–1482

De Foer B, Vercruysse JP, Bernaerts A, Deckers F, Pouillon M, Somers T, Casselman J, Offeciers E (2008) Detection of postoperative residual cholesteatoma with non-echo-planar diffusion-weighted magnetic resonance imaging. Otol Neurotol 29:513–517

De Foer B, Vercruysse JP, Bernaerts A et al (2010) Middle ear cholesteatoma: non-echo-planar diffusion-weighted MR imaging versus delayed gadolinium-enhanced T1-weighted MR imaging—value in detection. Radiology 255:866–872

De Foer B (2011) The value of magnetic resonance imaging in the preoperative evaluation and the postoperative follow-up of middle ear cholesteatoma. PhD thesis, Leuven University Press

Dhepnorrarat RC, Wood B, Rajan GP (2009) Postoperative non-echo-planar diffusion-weighted magnetic resonance imaging changes after cholesteatoma surgery: implications for cholesteatoma screening. Otol Neurotol 30:54–58

Dremmen MHG, Hofman PAM, Hof JR et al (2012) The diagnostic accuracy of non-echo-planar diffusion-weighted imaging in the detection of residual and/or recurrent cholesteatoma of the temporal bone. AJNR 33:439–444

Dubrulle F, Souillard R, Chechin D et al (2006) Diffusion-weighted MR imaging sequence in the detection of postoperative recurrent cholesteatoma. Radiology 238:604–610

Fitzek C, Mewes T, Fitzek S et al (2002) Diffusion-weighted MRI of cholesteatomas of the petrous bone. J Magn Reson Imaging 15:636–641

Fucci MJ, Buchman CA, Brackmann DE, Berliner KI (1999) Acoustic tumor growth: implications for treatment choices. Am J Otol 20(4):495–499

Fritsch MH, Gutt JJ (2005) Ferromagnetic movements of middle ear implants and stapes prostheses in a 3-T magnetic resonance field. Otol Neurotol 26:225–230

Gantz BJ, Wilkinson EP, Hansen MR (2005) Canal wall reconstruction tympanomastoidectomy with mastoid obliteration. Laryngoscope 115(10):1734–1740

Gaillardin L, Lescanne E, Morinière S, Cottier J-P, Robier A (2012) Residual cholesteatoma: prevalence and location. Follow-up strategy in adults. Eur Ann Otorhinolaryngol Head Neck Dis 129(3):136–140

Geoffray A, Guesmi M, Nebbia JF, Leloutre B, Bailleux S, Maschi C (2012) MRI for the diagnosis of recurrent middle ear cholesteatoma in children—can we optimize the technique? Preliminary study. Pediatric Radiology

Haberkamp TJ, Meyer GA, Fox M (1998) Surgical exposure of the fundus of the internal auditory canal: anatomic limits of the middle fossa versus the retrosigmoid transcanal approach. Laryngoscope 108(8 Pt 1):1190–1194

Hasso AN, Opp RL, Swartz JD (1996) Otosclerosis and dysplasias of the temporal bone. In: Som PM, Curtin HD (eds) Head and neck imaging, 3rd edn. Mosby-Year Book, St. Louis, pp 1432–1448

Hermans R, Marchal G, Feenstra L et al (1995) Spiral CT of the temporal bone: value of image reconstruction at submillimetric table increments. Neuroradiology 37:150–154

Horowitz SW, Leonetti JP, Azar-Kia B et al (1996) Postoperative radiographic findings following acoustic neuroma removal. Skull Base Surg 6:199–205

Hoistad DL, Melnik G, Mamikoglu B et al (2001) Update on conservative management of acoustic neuroma. Otol Neurotol 22:682–685

Huins CT, Singh A, Lingam RK et al (2010) Detecting cholesteatoma with non-echo planar (HASTE) diffusion-weighted magnetic resonance imaging. Otolaryngol Head Neck Surg 143:141–146

Irving RM, Beynon GJ, Viani L et al (1995) The patient's perspective after vestibular schwannoma removal: quality of life and implications for management. Am J Otol 16:331–337

Jeunen G, Desloovere C, Hermans R, Vandecaveye V (2008) The value of magnetic resonance imaging in the diagnosis of residual or recurrent acquired cholesteatoma after canal wall-up tympanoplasty. Otol Neurotol 29(1):16–18

Jindal M, Doshi J, Srivastav M et al (2010) Diffusion-weighted magnetic resonance imaging in the management of cholesteatoma. Eur Arch Otorhinolaryngol 267:181–185

Jindal M, Riskalla A, Jiang D, Connor S, O'Connor AF (2011) A systematic review of diffusion-weighted magnetic resonance imaging in the assessment of postoperative cholesteatoma. Otol Neurotol 32:1243–1249

Kasbekar AV, Scoffings DJ, Kenway B, Cross J, Donnelly N, Lloyd SWK, et al (2010) Non echo planar, diffusion-weighted magnetic resonance imaging (periodically rotated overlapping parallel lines with enhanced reconstruction sequence) compared with echo planar imaging for the detection of middle-ear cholesteatoma. J Laryngol Otol 125(04):376–380. Available from: http://eutils.ncbi.nlm.nih.gov/entrez/eutils/elink.fcgi?dbfrom=pubmed&id=21110910&retmode=ref&cmd=prlinks

Khemani S, Singh A, Lingam RK et al (2011) Imaging of postoperative middle ear cholesteatoma. Clin Radiol 66:760–767

Khemani S, Lingam RK, Kalan A et al (2012) The value of non-echo planar HASTE diffusion-weighted MR imaging in the detection, localisation and prediction of extent of postoperative cholesteatoma. Clin Otolaryngol 36:306–312

Klingebiel R, Bauknecht HC, Kaschke O et al (2001) Virtual endoscopy of the tympanic cavity based on high-resolution multislice computed tomographic data. Otol Neurotol 22:803–807

Kösling S, Woldag K, Meister EF et al (1995) Value of computed tomography in patients with persistent vertigo after stapes surgery. Invest Radiol 12:712–715

Kösling S, Bootz F (2001) CT and MR imaging after middle ear surgery. Eur J Radiol 40:113–118

Kwok P, Fisch U, Strutz J et al (2002) Stapes surgery: how precisely do different prostheses attach to the long process of the incus with different instruments and surgeons? Otol Neurotol 23:289–295

Lane J (2012) HASTE DWI versus HASTE DWI on 1.5T and 3T systems. Personal communication

Lehmann P, Saliou G, Brochart C, Page C, Deschepper B, Vallée JN, et al (2009) 3T MR imaging of postoperative recurrent middle ear cholesteatomas: value of periodically rotated overlapping parallel lines with enhanced reconstruction diffusion-weighted MR imaging. Am J Neuroradiol 30(2):423–427

Lemmerling MM, De Foer B, Vandevyver V et al (2008) Imaging of the opacified middle ear. Eur J Radiol 66:363–371

Li PMM, Linos E, Gurgel RK et al (2012) Evaluating the utility of non-echo-planar diffusion-weighted imaging in the preoperative evaluation of cholesteatoma: a meta-analysis. Laryngoscope 33(9):1573–1577

Lingam RK, Khatri P, Hughes J, Singh A (2013) Apparent diffusion coefficients for detection of postoperative middle ear cholesteatoma on non-echo-planar diffusion-weighted images. radiology Jun 25. [Epub ahead of print]

Lye RH, Pace-Balzan A, Ramsden RT et al (1992) The fate of tumour rests following removal of acoustic neuromas: an MRI Gd-DTPA study. Br J Neurosurg 6:195–202

Maheshwari S, Mukherji SK (2002) Diffusion-weighted imaging for differentiating recurrent cholesteatoma from granualtion tissue after mastoidectomy: case report. AJNR 23:847–849

Majithia AA, Lingam RKR, Nash RR, Khemani SS, Kalan AA, Singh AA (2012) Staging primary middle ear cholesteatoma with non-echoplanar (half-Fourier-acquisition single-shot turbo-spin-echo) diffusion-weighted magnetic resonance imaging helps plan surgery in 22 patients: our experience. Clin Otolaryngol 37(4):325–330

Malis L (2000) Gamma surgery for vestibular schwannoma. Letter to the editor. J Neurosurg 92:892–894

Mark AS, Fitzgerald DC (1993) Segmental enhancement of the cochlea on contrast-enhanced MR: correlation with the frequency of hearing loss and possible sign of perilymphatic fistula and autoimmune labyrintihtis. AJNR 14:991–996

Mark AS, Casselman JW (2002) Anatomy and disease of the temporal bone. In: Atlas SW (ed) Magnetic resonance imaging of the brain and spine, 3rd edn. Lippincott Williams & Wilkins, Philadelphia, pp 1363–1432

Marquet J, Greten WL, Van Camp KJ (1972) Considerations about the surgical approach in stapedectomy. Acta Otolaryngol 74:406–410

Más-Estellés F, Mateos-Fernández M, Carrascosa-Bisquert B, Facal de Castro F, Puchades-Román I, Morera-Pérez C (2012) Contemporary non-echo-planar diffusion-weighted imaging of middle ear cholesteatomas. Radiographics 32(4):1197–1213

Martin AD, Driscoll CL, Wood CP et al (2005) Safety evaluation of titanium middle ear prostheses at 3.0 tesla. Otolaryngol Head Neck Surg 132:537–542

McElveen JT Jr, Wilkins RH, Molter DW et al (1993) Hearing preservation using the modified translabyrinthine approach. Otolaryngol Head Neck Surg 108:671–679

Mercke U (1987) The cholesteatomatous ear one year after surgery with obliteration technique. Am J Otol 8:534–536

Millen SJ, Daniels DL (1994) The effect of intracranial surgical trauma on gadolinium-enhanced magnetic resonance imaging. Laryngoscope 104:804–813

Miracle AC, Mukherji SK (2009) Conebeam CT of the head and neck, part 2: clinical applications. AJNR Am J Neuroradiol 30:1285–1292

Mukherji SK, Mancuso AM, Kotzur IM et al (1994) CT of the temporal bone: findings after mastoidectomy, ossicular reconstruction, and cochlear implantation. AJR 163:1467–1471

Mulkens TH, Parizel PM, Martin J-J et al (1993) Acoustic schwannoma: MR findings in 84 tumors. AJR 160:395–398

Naganawa S, Nakashima T (2009) Cutting edge of inner ear MRI. Acta Oto-laryngol 129:15–21

Nowé V, Verstreken M, Wuyts FL, Van de Heyning P, De Schepper AM, Parizel PM (2004) Enhancement of the otic capsule in active retrofenestral otosclerosis. Otol Neurotol 25(4):633–634

Peltonen LI, Aarnisalo AA, Kortesniemi MK, Suomalainen A, Jero J, Robinson S (2007) Limited cone-beam computed tomography imaging of the middle ear: a comparison with multislice helical computed tomography. Acta Radiol 48:207–212

Penninger RT, Tavassolie TS, Carey JP (2011) Cone-beam volumetric tomography for applications in the temporal bone. Otol Neurotol 32:453–460

Pickuth D, Brandt S, Berghaus A et al (2000) Vertigo after stapes surgery: the role of high resolution CT. BJR 73:1021–1023

Pizzini FB, Barbieri F, Beltramello A et al (2010) HASTE diffusion-weighted 3-Tesla magnetic resonance imaging in the diagnosis of primary and relapsing cholesteatoma. Otol Neurotol 31:596–602

Plouin-Gaudon I, Bossard D, Fuchsmann C et al (2010a) Diffusion-weighted MR imaging for evaluation of pediatric recurrent cholesteatomas. Int J Pediatr Otorhinolaryngol 74:22–26

Plouin-Gaudon I, Bossard D, Ayari-Khalfallah S et al (2010b) Fusion of MRIs and CT scans for surgical treatment of cholesteatoma of the middle ear in children. Arch Otolaryngol Head Neck Surg 136:878–883

Prasad D, Steiner M, Steiner L (2000) Gamma surgery for vestibular schwannoma. J Neurosurg 92:745–759

Profant M, Sláviková K, Kabátová Z, Slezák P, Waczulíková I (2012) Predictive validity of MRI in detecting and following cholesteatoma. Eur Arch Otorhinolaryngol 269(3):757–765

Rajan GP, Ambett R, Wun L et al (2010) preliminary outcomes of cholesteatoma screening in children using non-echo-planar diffusion-weighted magnetic resonance imaging. Int J Pediatr Otorhinolaryngol 74:297–301

Rangheard AS, Marsot-Dupuch K, Mark AS et al (2001) Postoperative complications in otospongiosis: usefulness of MR imaging. AJNR 22:1171–1178

Raut VV, Toner JG, Kerr AG et al (2002) Management of otosclerosis in the UK. Clin Otolaryngol 27:113–119

Ruivo J, Mermuys K, Bacher K, Kuhweide R, Offeciers E, Casselman JW (2009) Cone beam computed tomography, a low-dose imaging technique in the postoperative assessment of cochlear implantation. Otol Neurotol 30:299–303

Sartoretti-Schefer S, Kollias S, Valavanis A (2000) Spatial relationship between vestibular schwannoma and facial nerve on three-dimensional T2-weighted fast spin-echo MR images. AJNR 21:810–816

Selesnick SH, Rebol J, Heier LA et al (2001) Internal auditory canal involvement of acoustic neuromas: surgical correlates to magnetic resonance imaging findings. Otol Neurotol 22:912–916

Shea JJ Jr (1958) Fenestration of the oval window. Ann Otol Rhinol Laryngol 67:932–951

Sheehy JL, Brackmann DE, Graham MD (1977) Cholesteatoma surgery: residual and recurrent disease. A review of 1,024 cases. Ann Otol Rhinol Laryngol 86(4 Pt 1):451–462

Shellock FG, Schatz CJ (1991) Metallic otologic implants: in vitro assessment of of ferromagnetism at 1.5 T. AJNR 12:279–281

Shelton C, Sheehy JL (1990) Tympanoplasty: review of 400 staged cases. Laryngoscope 100(7):679–681

Stasolla A, Magliulo G, Parrotto D et al (2004) Detection of postoperative relapsing/residual cholesteatomas with diffusion-weighted echo-planar magnetic resonance imaging. Otol Neurotol 25:879–884

Somers T, Casselman J, de Ceulaer G, Govaerts P, Offeciers E (2001) Prognostic value of magnetic resonance imaging findings in hearing preservation surgery for vestibular schwannoma. Otol Neurotol 22(1):87–94

Stone JA, Mukherji SK, Jewett BS et al (2000) CT evaluation of prosthetic ossicular reconstruction procedures: what the otologist needs to know. RadioGraphics 20:593–605

Swartz JD, Wolfson RJ, Russell KB et al (1983) High resolution computed tomography of the middle ear and mastoid. Part III: surgically altered anatomy and pathology. Radiology 148:461–464

Swartz JD, Harnsberger HR (1998) The middle ear and mastoid. In: Swartz JD, Harnsberger HR (eds) Imaging of the temporal bone, 3rd edn. Thieme, New York, pp 47–169

Schwartz KM, Lane JI, Bolster BD et al (2011) The utility of diffusion-weighted imaging for cholesteatoma evaluation. AJNR 32:430–436

Teissl C, Kremser C, Hochmair ES et al (1998) Cochlear implants: in vitro investigation of electromagnetic interference at MR imaging—compatibility and safety aspects. Radiology 208: 700–708

Thiriat S, Riehm S, Kremer S, Martin E, Veillon F (2009) Apparent diffusion coefficient values of middle ear cholesteatoma differ from abscess and cholesteatoma admixed infection. Am J Neuroradiol 30(6):1123–1126

Tierney PA, Pracy P, Blaney SP et al (1999) An assessment of the value of the preoperative computed tomography scans prior to otoendoscopic 'second look' in intact canal wall mastoid surgery. Clin Otolaryngol 24:274–276

Van de Heyning PH (2002) Personal communication

Van den Abeele D, Coen E, Parizel PM et al (1999) Can MRI replace a second look operation in cholesteatoma surgery? Acta Otolaryngol 119:555–561

Venail F, Bonafe A, Poirrier V, Mondain M, Uziel A (2008) Comparison of echo-planar diffusion-weighted imaging and delayed postcontrast T1-weighted MR imaging for the detection of residual cholesteatoma. Am J Neuroradiol 29(7):1363–1368

Vercruysse JP, De Foer B, Pouillon M et al (2006) The value of diffusion-weighted MR imaging in the diagnosis of primary acquired and residual cholesteatoma: a surgical verified study of 100 patients. Eur Radiol 16:1461–1467

Vercruysse JP, De Foer B, Somers T, Casselman J, Offeciers E (2010) Long-term follow up after bony mastoid and epitympanic obliteration: radiological findings. J Laryngol Otol 124:37–43

Weissman JL, Hirsch BE, Fukui MB et al (1997) The evolving MR appearance of structures in the internal auditory canal after removal of an acoustic neuroma. AJNR 18:313–323

Wiet RJ, Teixido M, Liang JG (1992) Complications in acoustic neuroma surgery. Otolaryngol Clin North Am 25:389–412

Williams MT, Ayache D, Elmaleh M, Héran F, Elbaz P, Piekarski JD (2000) Helical CT findings in patients who have undergone stapes surgery for otosclerosis. AJR 174:387–392

Williams MT, Ayache D (2004) Imaging of the postoperative middle ear. Eur Radiol 14(3):482–495

Willliams MT, Ayache D, Alberti C et al (2003) Detection of postoperative residual cholesteatoma with delayed contrast-enhanced MR imaging: initial findings. Eur Radiol 13:169–174

MultiPlanar Reformation in CT of the Temporal Bone

John I. Lane

Contents

1 Technical Considerations 368
2 Middle Ear 369
3 Inner Ear 372
4 Conclusion 380
References 380

Abstract

Recent advances in multi-detector ct (mdct) technology allow for the acquisition of volumetric data with isotropic voxel size permitting reconstructions in any plane of section. These post-processing techniques have proven to be of benefit in the evaluation of temporal bone pathology. This chapter demonstrates some of the optimal imaging planes that can be used to display normal anatomy as well as pathology involving the middle and inner ear. Most of the multiplanar reconstructions employed in this chapter are slight modifications of the standard imaging planes utilized in the days of multiplanar tomography (sagittal, coronal, Pöschl, and stenvers planes).

Since the advent of computed tomography (CT), the physical limitations of gantry angle and patient positioning have restricted the plane of section in temporal bone imaging to standard axial and coronal projections. Most anatomic structures of the middle and inner ear are not optimally profiled in these planes. In the days of temporal bone polytomography, complex oblique views such as Pöschl and Stenvers projections were often employed to show certain anatomic structures of the middle and inner ear to better effect. Recent advances in multi-detector CT (MDCT) technology allow for the acquisition of volumetric data with isotropic voxel size permitting reconstructions in any plane of section. These post-processing techniques have proven to be of benefit in the evaluation of both middle and inner ear pathology (Hans et al. 1999; Belden et al. 2003; Henrot et al. 2005; Lane et al. 2006; Ozgen et al. 2008; Bin et al. 2008; Krombach et al. 2006; Naganawa et al. 1995; Lane and Witte 2010). This chapter demonstrates some of the optimal imaging planes that can be used to display normal anatomy as well as pathology involving the middle and inner ear.

In one sense, all two-dimensional images reproduced from volumetric acquisitions are multiplanar reconstructions (MPR). Many radiologists have adopted the convention of

J. I. Lane (✉)
Division of Neuroradiology, Department of Radiology,
Mayo Clinic College of Medicine,
200 First St. SW, Rochester, MN, USA
e-mail: lane.john@mayo.edu

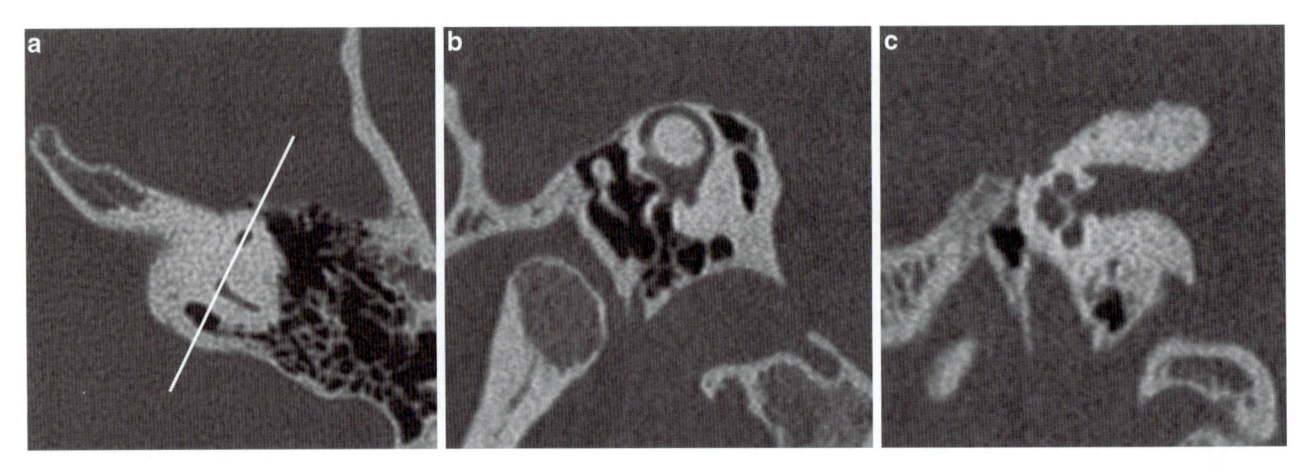

Fig. 1 *Pöschl's Plane*. Single Oblique Reconstruction in the Plane of the Superior Semicircular Canal (SSC) (Short Axis of the Temporal Bone). **a** Axial reference image demonstrating plane of reconstruction (*white line*) intersecting the anterior and posterior limbs of the SSC. **b** Multiplanar reconstruction (MPR) in Pöschl's plane at the level of the SSC. **c** Pöschl MPR through internal auditory canal and cochlea

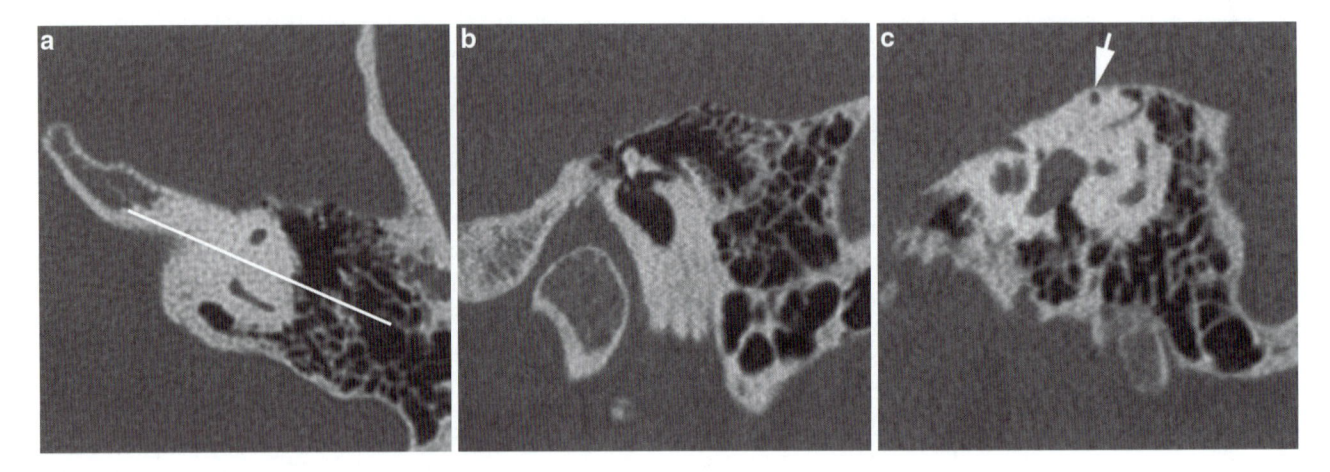

Fig. 2 *Stenvers' Plane*. Single Oblique Reconstruction perpendicular to the Plane of the SSC (Long Axis of the Temporal Bone). **a** Axial reference image demonstrating plane of reconstruction (*white line*) perpendicular to the plane of the SSC. **b** Multiplanar reconstruction in the Stenvers Plane through the middle ear at the level of the incudomalleolar joint. **c** Stenvers MPR through the inner ear at the level of the apex of the SSC (*white arrow*)

displaying axial images reconstructed in the plane of the lateral semicircular canal with the corresponding coronal images reconstructed perpendicular to the lateral canal. Two additional MPR volumes can supplement these standard two-dimensional volumes: one oriented in the plane of the short axis of the temporal bone (Pöschl's Plane) and the second oriented in the plane of the long axis of the temporal bone (Stenvers Plane). Pöschl's plane can be reconstructed by using a single oblique plane parallel to the superior semicircular canal (SSC) (Fig. 1). Stenvers' plane is reconstructed perpendicular to the plane of the SSC (Fig. 2). Both of these supplemental projections were considered as part of the standard examination in the days of temporal bone polytomography (Buckingham and Valvassori 1973; Brunner 1969; Pimontel-Appel and Ettore 1980).

Additional targeted MPRs can be employed to investigate particular anatomic structures in a more detailed manor. Most of the targeted MPRs employed in this chapter are slight modifications of standard imaging planes used in temporal bone polytomography (sagittal, coronal, Pöschl, Stenvers planes). It is often useful to have the capability of performing reconstructions in two independent oblique planes (double oblique reconstruction) in order to optimally profile specific anatomic structures, in particular the auditory ossicles.

1 Technical Considerations

In general, the higher the number of detector rows employed by a particular MDCT scanner, the more isotropic the voxel size and the greater the resolution of the MPRs. All MPR images included in this chapter were reconstructed from volumetric data sets acquired on a 64-slice MDCT yielding a voxel size of 0.4 mm^3. Supplemental short axis

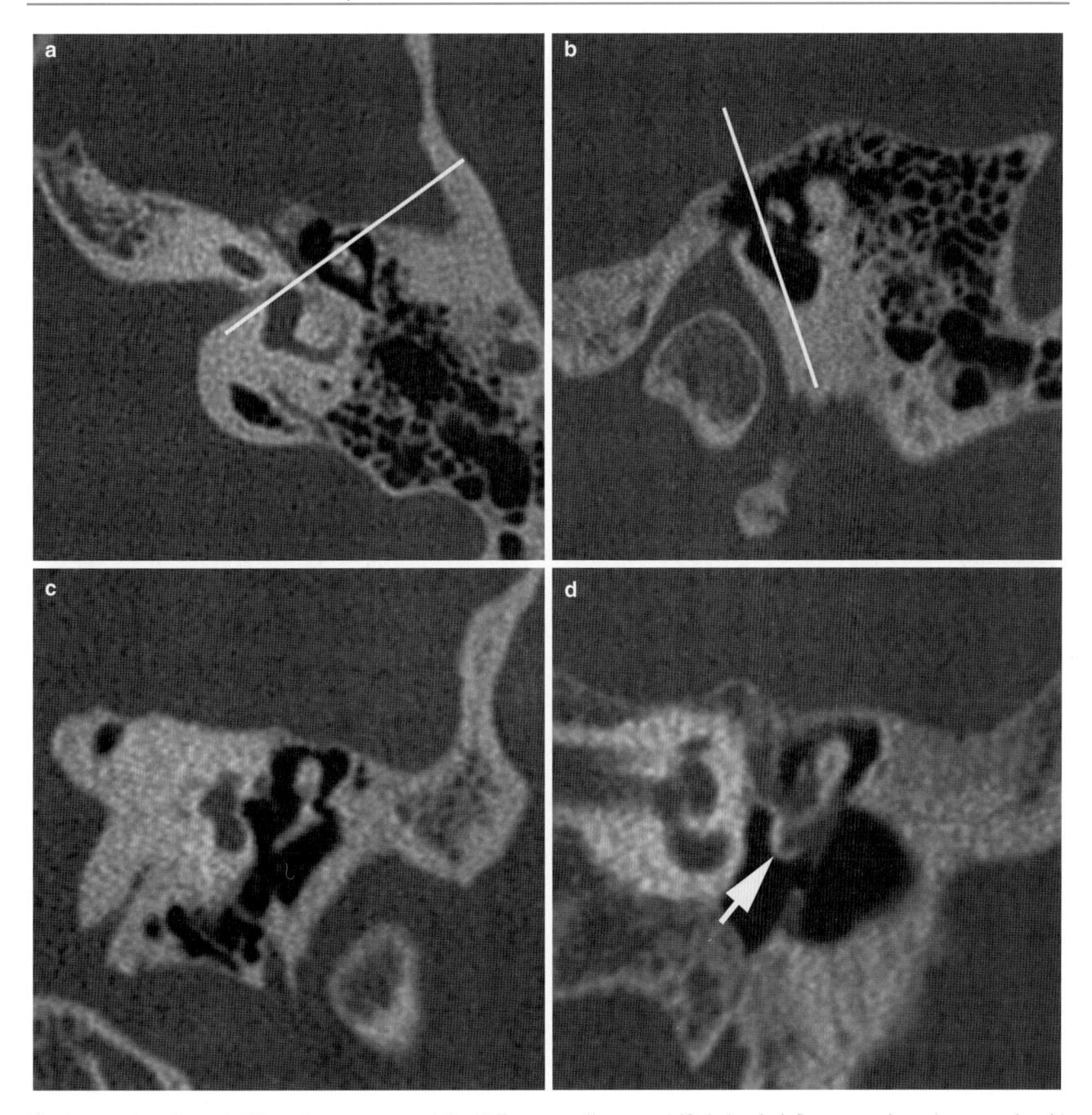

Fig. 3 *Long Axis Coronal Oblique Reconstruction of the Malleus.* **a** Axial and **b** sagittal references images demonstrating multiplanar reconstruction plane required for the coronal long axis view of the malleus. **c** Multiplanar reconstruction (MPR) of the malleus from MDCT data set. **d** MPR demonstrates fixation of the manubrium of malleus to calcified chronic inflammatory tissue (tympanosclerosis) (*arrow*) in this patient with conductive hearing loss. [Reprinted with permission from Springer (Lane & Witte, Temporal Bone: An Imaging Atlas, Springer)]

(Pöschl) and long axis (Stenvers) MPR volumes can be routinely reconstructed at the CT console using the previously mentioned anatomic landmarks at the request of the interpreting radiologist. Any additional targeted MPRs are reconstructed from the volumetric data set at a separate workstation, preferably one that is capable of producing MPRs using at least two independent planes of obliquity.

2 Middle Ear

Long axis MPRs and maximum intensity projections (MIPs) of the ossicles can be useful in assessment of ossicular integrity (Bin et al. 2008). In the clinical setting of conductive hearing loss. Chronic inflammatory disease with or

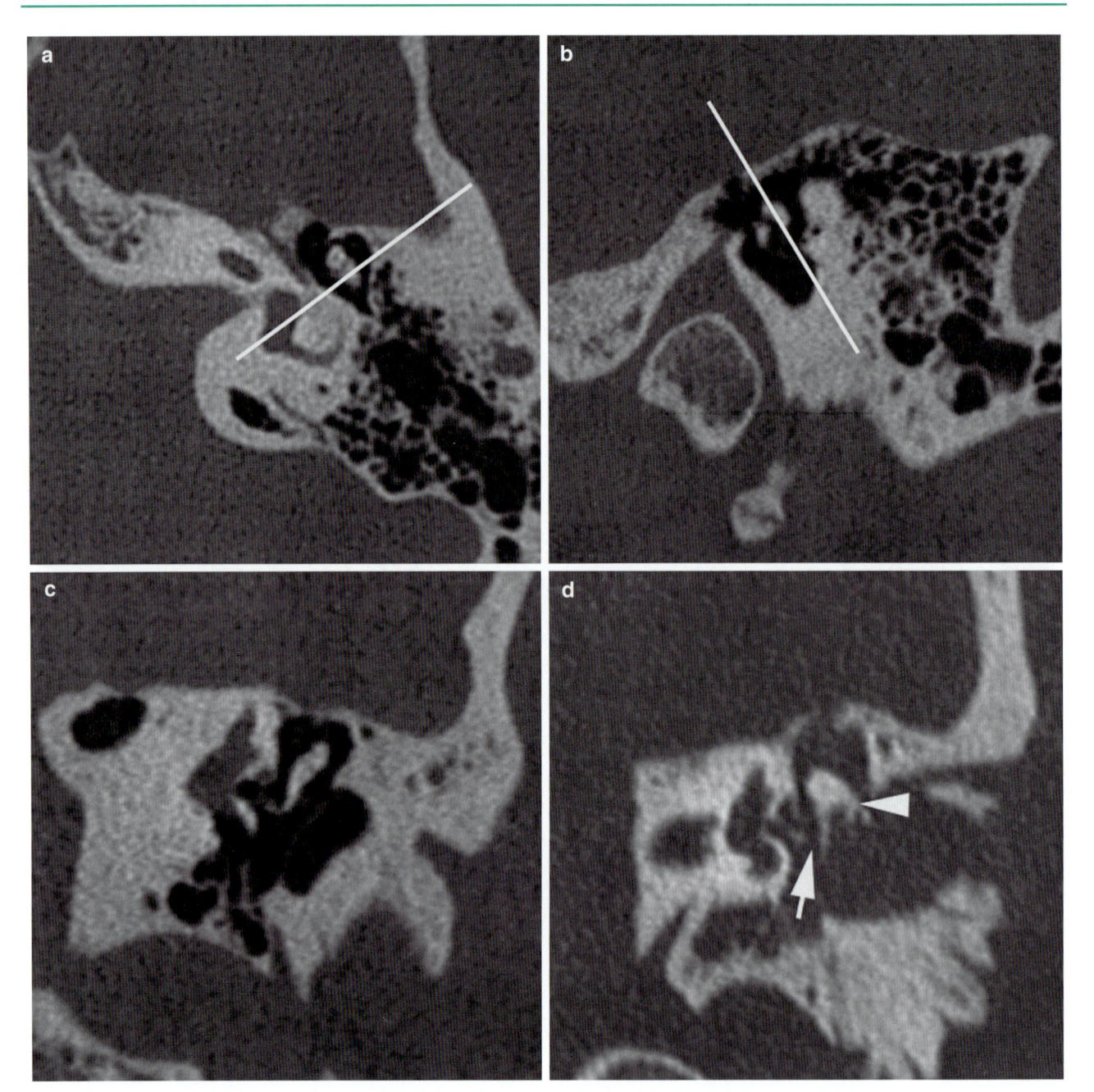

Fig. 4 *Long Axis Coronal Oblique Reconstruction of the Incus.* **a** axial and **b** sagittal references images demonstrating multiplanar reconstruction planes required for the coronal long axis view of the incus. **c** multiplanar reconstruction (MPR) of the incus from MDCT data set. **d** MPR demonstrates incudostapedial disarticulation (*arrow*) with rotational dislocation of the incus. Note short process is rotated laterally from its normal posterior orientation (*arrowhead*) in this patient with acute longitudinal fracture of the left temporal bone. [Reprinted with permission from Springer (Lane & Witte, Temporal Bone: An Imaging Atlas, Springer)]

without cholesteatoma, temporal bone fracture, or congenital anomalies such as aural atresia or microtia can produce various ossicular pathologies to include fixation, erosions, and disarticulations. Since the standard axial and coronal orientations do not display the ossicles to best advantage, the integrity of the ossicular chain can be confirmed with long axis MPRs of each individual ossicle (Figs. 3, 4, 5). Occasionally MPRs in the plane of the short axis of the stapes can be useful, particularly in the setting of stapes footplate fixation secondary to early otospongiotic plaque along the anterior edge of the oval window in the vicinity of the fissula ante fenestram (Fig. 6).

An oblique sagittal MPR can be employed to profile the incudomalleolar joint and at the same time inspect the integrity of the manubrium of the malleus and long process of the incus, recreating the old "Molar Tooth" tomographic

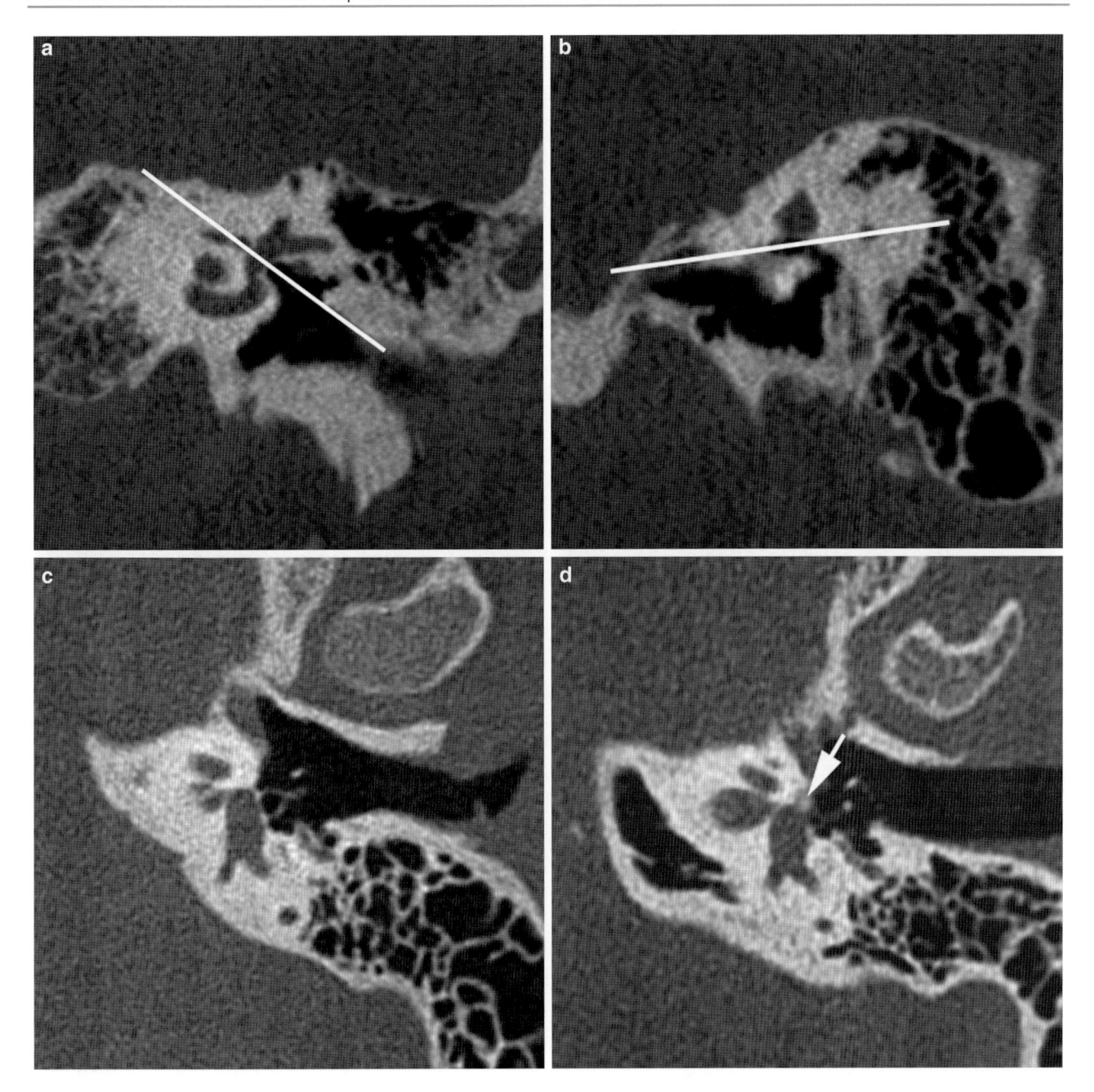

Fig. 5 *Long Axis Axial Oblique Reconstruction of the Stapes.*
a Coronal and **b** sagittal references images demonstrating multiplanar reconstruction plane required for the long axis oblique axial view of the stapes. **c** multiplanar reconstruction (MRP) of the normal stapes. **d** MPR demonstrates fixation of the footplate and anterior crus of the stapes secondary to fenestral otospongiosis. Note stapes seen in long axis with demineralized, otospongiotic bone arising from the region of the fissula ante fenestram and encasing the anterior edge of the footplate and anterior crus (*arrow*). [Reprinted with permission from Springer (Lane & Witte, Temporal Bone: An Imaging Atlas, Springer)]

appearance (Fig. 7). Since the malleus and incus differ slightly in their lateral to medial angulation, a 2–3 mm MIP in the oblique sagittal plane can be quite helpful in producing a more complete assessment of these ossicles (Fig. 7c). This perspective can be useful in confirming any suspicion of malleoincudal luxation seen on axial or coronal images in patients with conductive hearing loss following trauma (Fig. 7e, f). Erosions of the long process of the incus, a relatively common complication of middle ear inflammatory disease, can be nicely demonstrated in this plane with both MPR and MIP images (Fig. 7g, h). Additionally, Pöschl plane reconstructions of the ossicles provide an ideal depiction of both the incudomalleolar and incudostapedial articulations (Fig. 8). Pöschl MPR and MIP images can be useful in confirming incudostapedial disarticulation following trauma or as a result of chronic inflammatory disease (Fig. 8d).

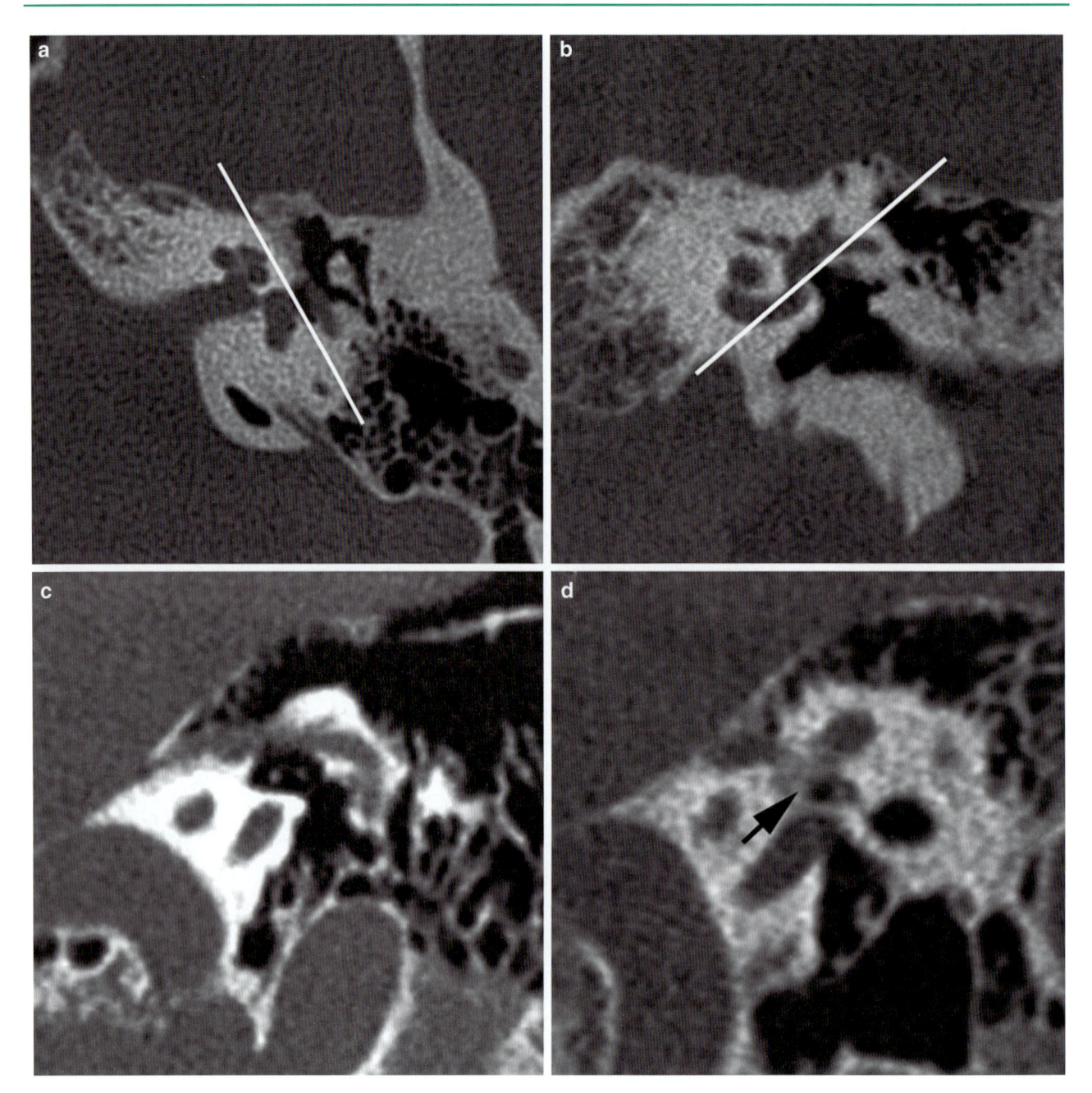

Fig. 6 *Short Axis Sagittal Oblique Reconstruction of the Stapes.* **a** Axial and **b** coronal references images demonstrating multiplanar reconstruction planes required for the short axis oblique sagittal view of the stapes. **c** multiplanar reconstruction (MPR) of the stapes demonstrating anterior and posterior crura in the oval window niche. **d** MPR demonstrates fixation of the footplate and anterior crus of the stapes secondary to fenestral otospongiosis. Note stapes seen in short axis with demineralized, otospongiotic bone arising from the region of the fissula ante fenestram and encasing the anterior crus (*black arrow*). Note that the posterior crus is not involved. [Reprinted with permission from Springer (Lane & Witte, Temporal Bone: An Imaging Atlas, Springer)]

3 Inner Ear

Although inner ear disease is more commonly imaged using MR, MDCT can be useful in the detecting labyrinthine pathology in various clinical settings.

MDCT is useful in demonstrating the dystrophic calcification that accompanies end-stage inner ear inflammation (labyrinthitis ossificans). This information can be critical to the surgical approach used for the insertion of the electrode array. MPRs oriented in the sagittal oblique and axial oblique planes through the cochlea can be helpful in

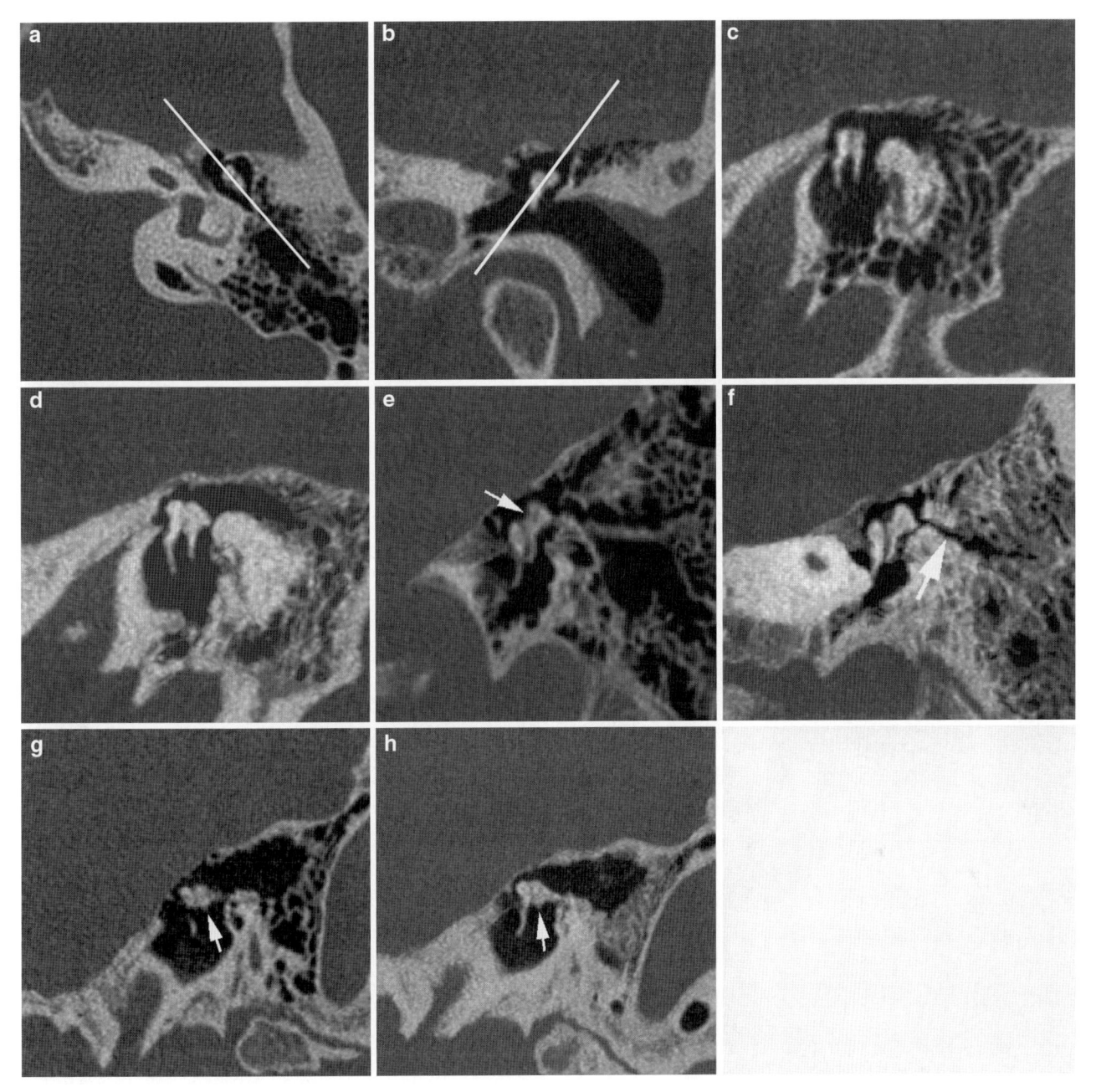

Fig. 7 *Long Axis Sagittal Oblique Reconstruction of the Malleus and Incus (Molar Tooth View).* **a** Axial and **b** coronal references images demonstrating multiplanar reconstruction plane required to view the sagittal long axis of the malleus and incus. **c** multiplanar reconstruction (MPR) of the malleus and incus from multidetector CT data set. Note normal relationship of malleus anterior to incus with mallear head articulating with articular facet of Incus. **d** Maximum intensity projection (MIP) (2 mm slab) of malleus and incus. **e** MPR of disarticulated malleus and incus in patient with conductive hearing loss following remote trauma. Note 'empty' articular facet of the incus (*arrow*) with inferiorly displaced malleus relative to incus. **f** MIP (2 mm slab) of disarticulated malleus and incus. Note ununited fracture plane (*arrow*). **g** MPR demonstrates erosion of the long process of the incus (*arrow*) on MPR and, **h** on MIP (2 mm slab). [Reprinted with permission from Springer (Lane & Witte, Temporal Bone: An Imaging Atlas, Springer)]

localizing the distribution of calcification in relation to the spiral lamina, the incomplete bony partition that separates the anterior scala vestibuli from the posterior scala tympani (Figs. 9, 10). The sagittal oblique MPR is a slight modification of Pöschl plane. Accurate separation of the cochlear scala in the axial plane requires a plane of section perpendicular to the spiral lamina, a requirement not met by routine axial images obtained in the plane of the lateral semicircular canal. Both oblique MPR planes can be useful in determining if the extent of luminal calcification involves

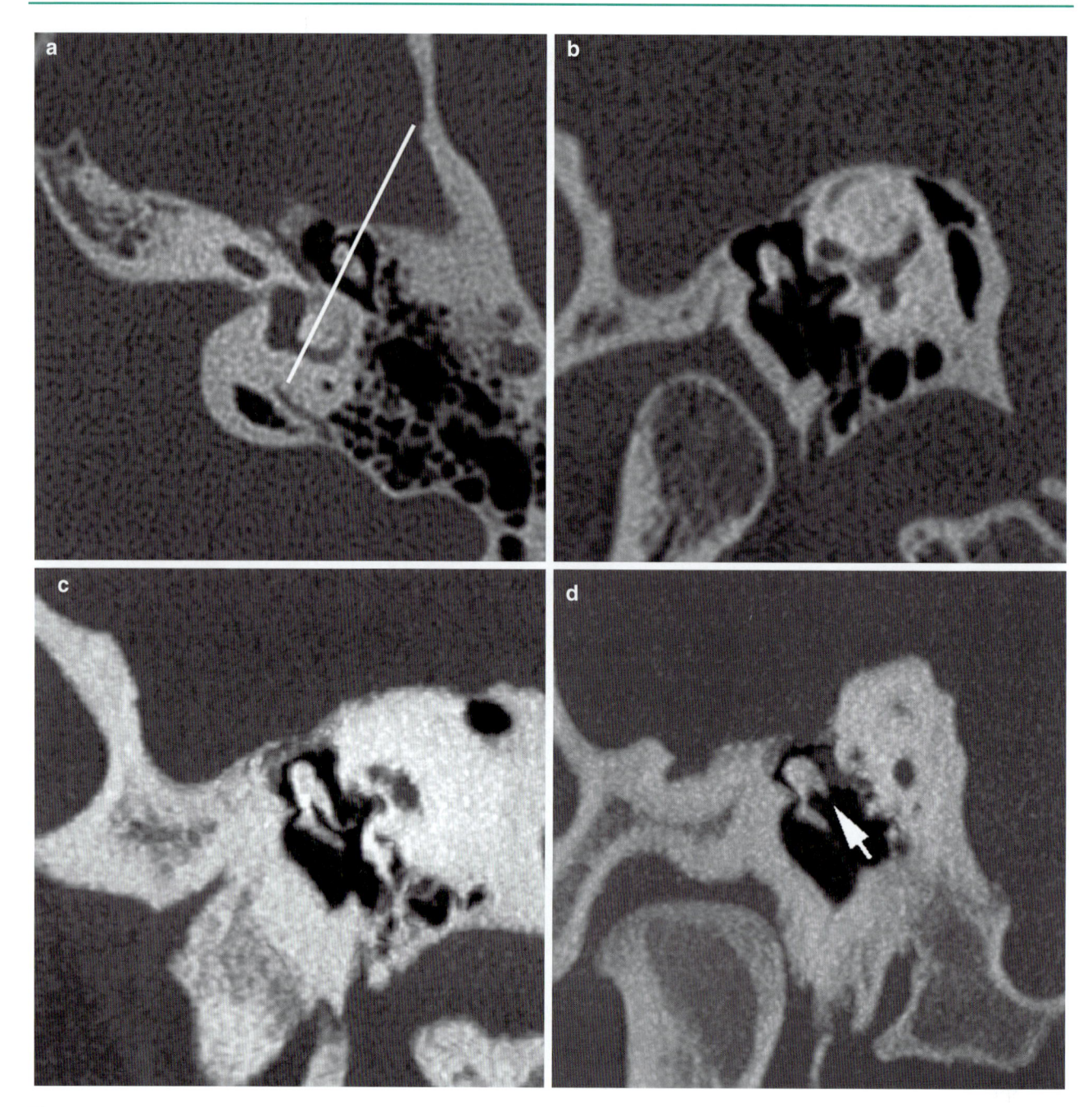

Fig. 8 *Pöschl's plane Reconstruction of the incudomallear and incudostapedial articulations.* **a** Axial reference image demonstrating multiplanar reconstruction in the plane of the short axis of the temporal bone required for this reconstruction. **b** Multiplanar reconstruction (MPR) of the ossicles in Pöschl's plane. **c** Maximum intensity projection (MIP) (2 mm slab) of normal ossicular articulations. **d** MIP (2 mm slab) of eroded long process of the incus (*arrow*) with disarticulation of the incudostapedial joint in a patient with conductive hearing loss. [Reprinted with permission from Springer (Lane & Witte, Temporal Bone: An Imaging Atlas, Springer)]

one or both perilymphatic scala. This information may cause the cochlear implant surgeon to modify placement of the cochlosteomy prior to electrode array insertion in order to target the noncalcified scala (Figs. 9c and 10c).

Bony labyrinthine anomalies associated with congenital deafness or early sensorineural hearing loss can be readily depicted on MDCT. MPRs oriented in the sagittal oblique plane (long axis of the cochlea) can be useful in

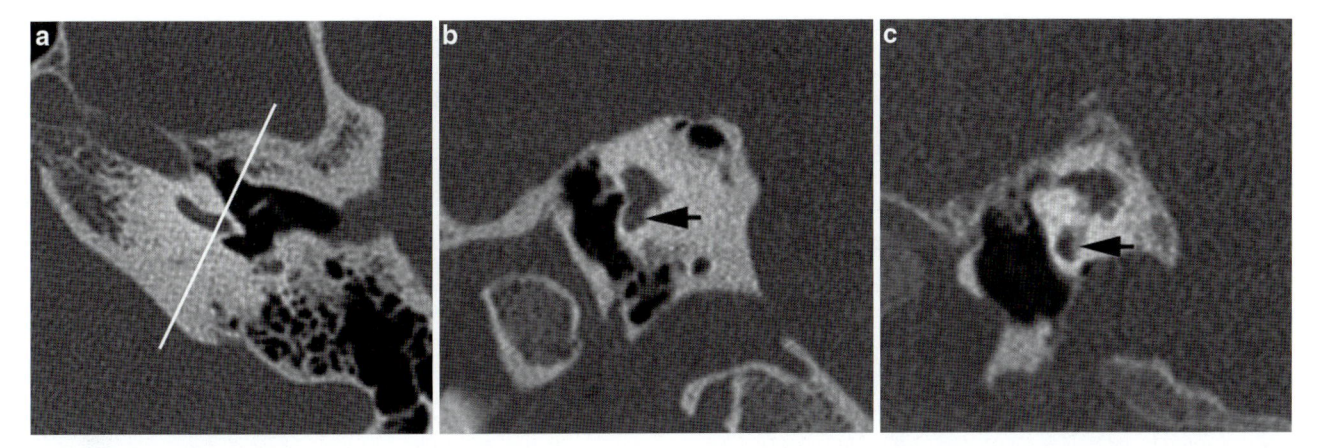

Fig. 9 *Sagittal Oblique Reconstruction of the Basal Turn of the Cochlea.* **a** Axial reference images demonstrating multiplanar reconstruction plane required for the oblique sagittal view trough the basal turn cochlea. Angle of reconstruction is a minor variation of Pöschl's plane. **b** multiplanar reconstruction (MPR) through the basal turn demonstrates patent lumen of the basal turn (*black arrow*). **c** MPR from preoperative MDCT for cochlear implant demonstrates ossification of the scala tympani (*arrow*) within the posterior portion of the basal turn secondary to remote labyrinthitis (labyrinthitis ossificans). Recognition of ossification limited to scala tympani of the basal turn may convince surgeon to modify surgical approach in order to place electrode array more anteriorly into patent scala vestibuli. [Reprinted with permission from Springer (Lane & Witte, Temporal Bone: An Imaging Atlas, Springer)]

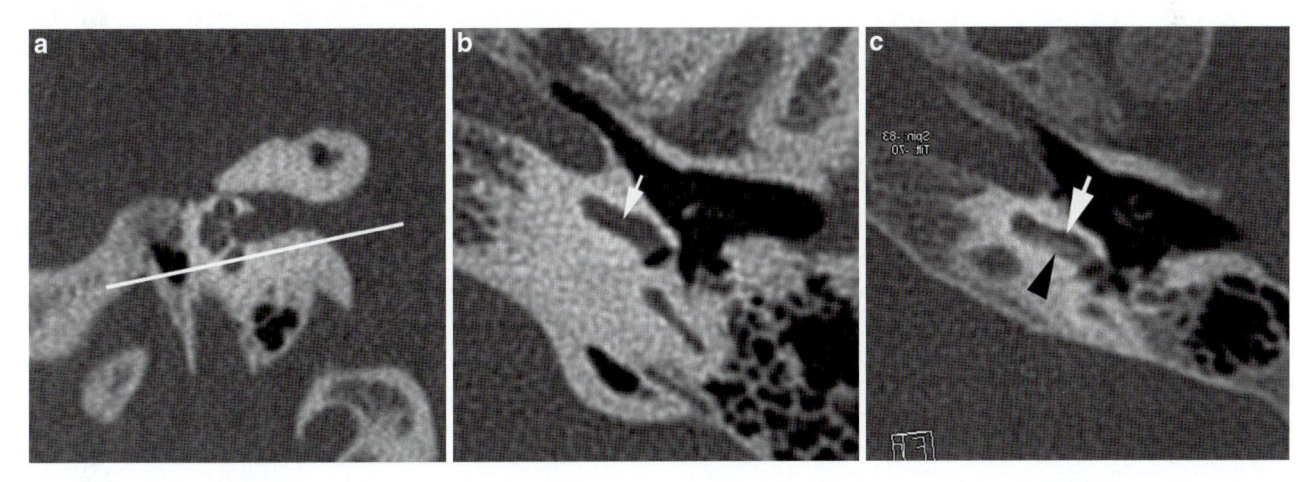

Fig. 10 *Axial Oblique Reconstruction of the Basal Turn of the Cochlea.* **a** Sagittal reference image demonstrating reconstruction plane required for the oblique axial view of the basal turn of the cochlea. **b** Multiplanar reconstruction (MPR) through the basal turn from MDCT data set. Note position of the spiral lamina (*arrow*) partitioning the cochlea into anterior scala vestibuli and posterior scala tympani. **c** MPR from pre-operative MDCT for cochlear implant demonstrates ossification of the scala tympani (*arrow*) within the posterior portion of the basal turn secondary to remote labyrinthitis (labyrinthitis ossificans). Recognition of ossification limited to scala tympani of the basal turn may convince surgeon to modify surgical approach in order to place electrode array more anteriorly into patent scala vestibuli. [Reprinted with permission from Springer (Lane & Witte, Temporal Bone: An Imaging Atlas, Springer)]

demonstrating the integrity of the modiolus (Fig. 11), which is often deficient in the presence of cochlear anomalies (Fig. 11c). MPRs oriented in the coronal oblique plane (short axis of the cochlea) accurately depict the integrity and patency of the cochlear lumen (Fig. 12). MPRs in this plane can be useful in ascertaining the insertion depth of the electrode array and in identifying the electrode closest to the labyrinthine segment of the facial nerve canal in patients with facial nerve stimulation following implant activation (Fig. 12f). In such instances, facial stimulation can be eliminated by selectively turning off the offending electrode or decreasing its current without significant loss of overall implant function (Kelsall et al. 1997).

MPRs in the planes of the semicircular canals can be useful in confirming pathologies suspected on routine axial and coronal images (Figs. 13, 14, 15). Patients with

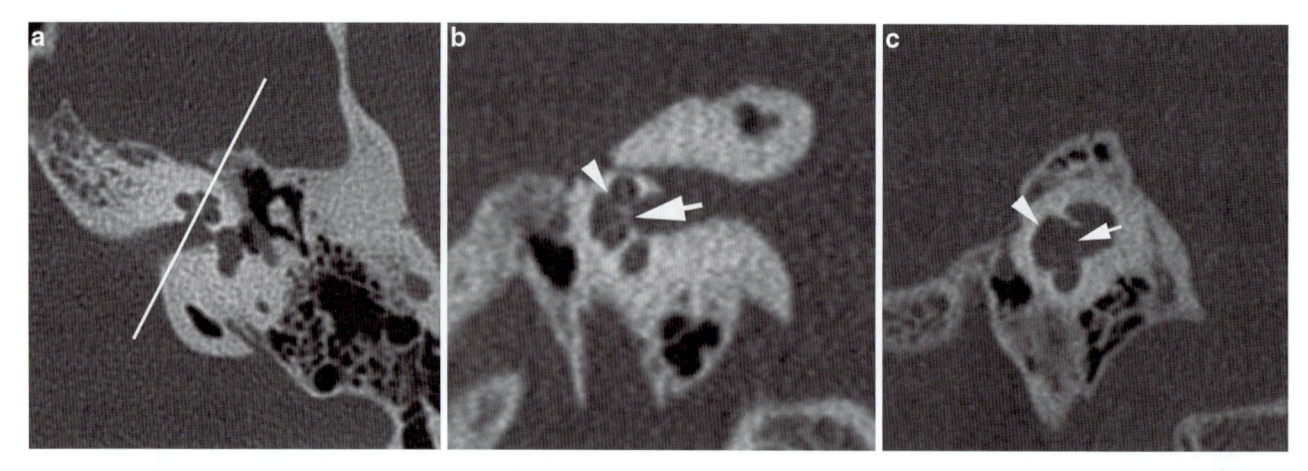

Fig. 11 *Sagittal Oblique Reconstruction of the Modiolus of the Cochlea.* **a** axial reference images demonstrating multiplanar reconstruction plane required for the oblique sagittal view trough the modiolus of the cochlea. Angle of reconstruction is identical to Pöschl's plane. **b** multiplanar reconstruction (MPR) through the modiolus from MDCT data set. Note modiolus (*arrow*) and notched indentation to the superior contour of the cochlea at the site of the interscalar septum, separating basal from middle turns (*arrowhead*). **c** MPR in child with Mondini malformation and profound sensorineural hearing loss demonstrates deficient modiolus (*arrow*). Note partition anomaly of the cochlea evidenced by loss of the normal notched indentation of the superior contour of the cochlea (*arrowhead*). These findings are typical of Mondini malformation. [Reprinted with permission from Springer (Lane & Witte, Temporal Bone: An Imaging Atlas, Springer)]

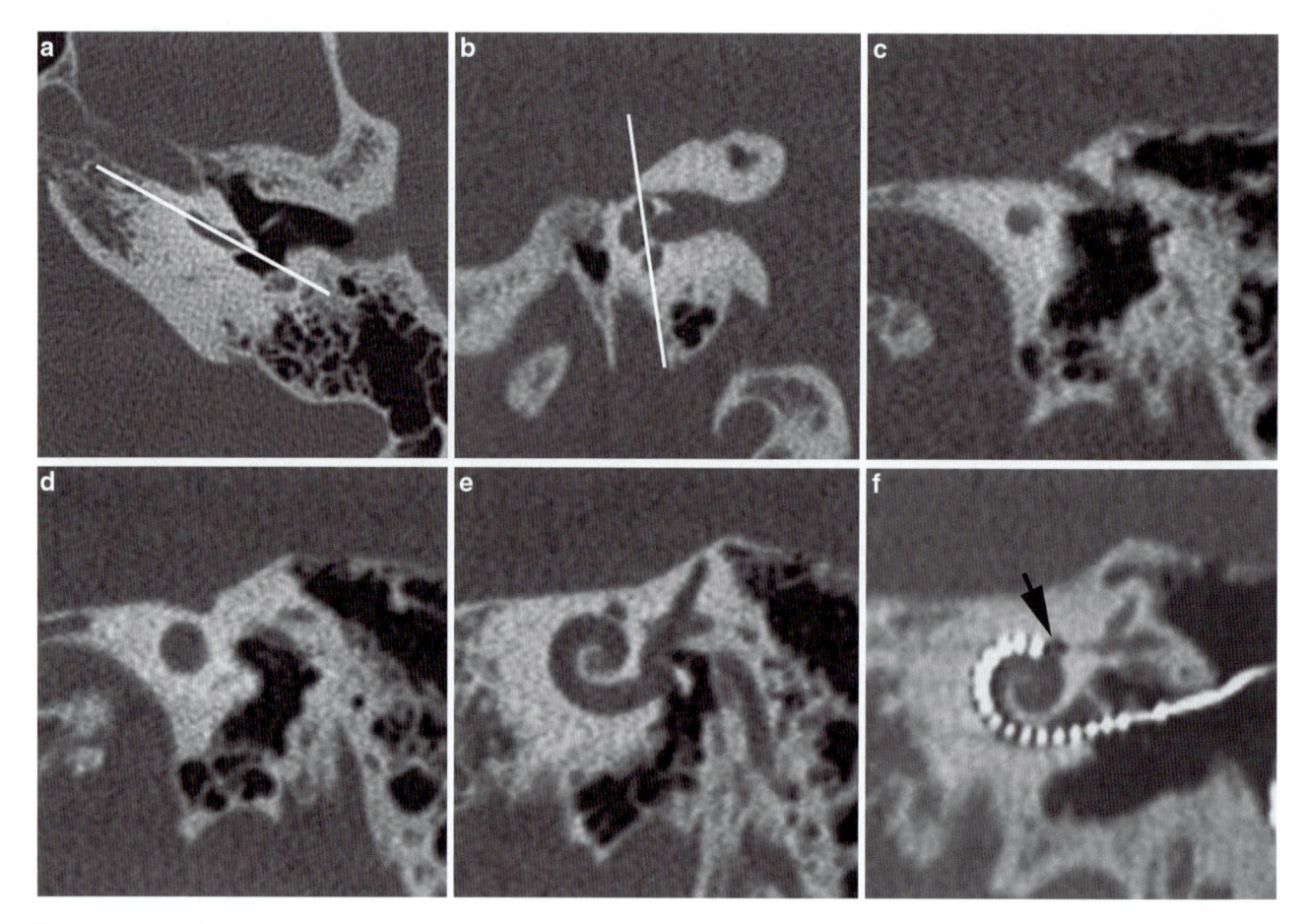

Fig. 12 *Coronal Oblique Reconstruction of the Cochlea.* **a** Axial and **b** Sagittal reference images demonstrating multiplanar reconstruction plane required for the oblique coronal views trough the turns of the cochlea. Angles of reconstruction are slight modifications of Stenvers plane. Multiplanar reconstructions (MPRs) through the cochlea MDCT data set at the level of the apical turn (**c**), middle turn (**d**) and basal turn (**e**). **f** MPR from postoperative MDCT after cochlear implantation. This view of cochlea is ideal for measuring depth of insertion of electrode array in patients with cochlear implant. This patient was experiencing facial stimulation after implant insertion. The distal electrode is noted adjacent to labyrinthine segment of facial nerve (*arrow*). After MDCT demonstrated this relationship, the distal electrode was selectively turned off and symptoms resolved. [Reprinted with permission from Springer (Lane & Witte, Temporal Bone: An Imaging Atlas, Springer)]

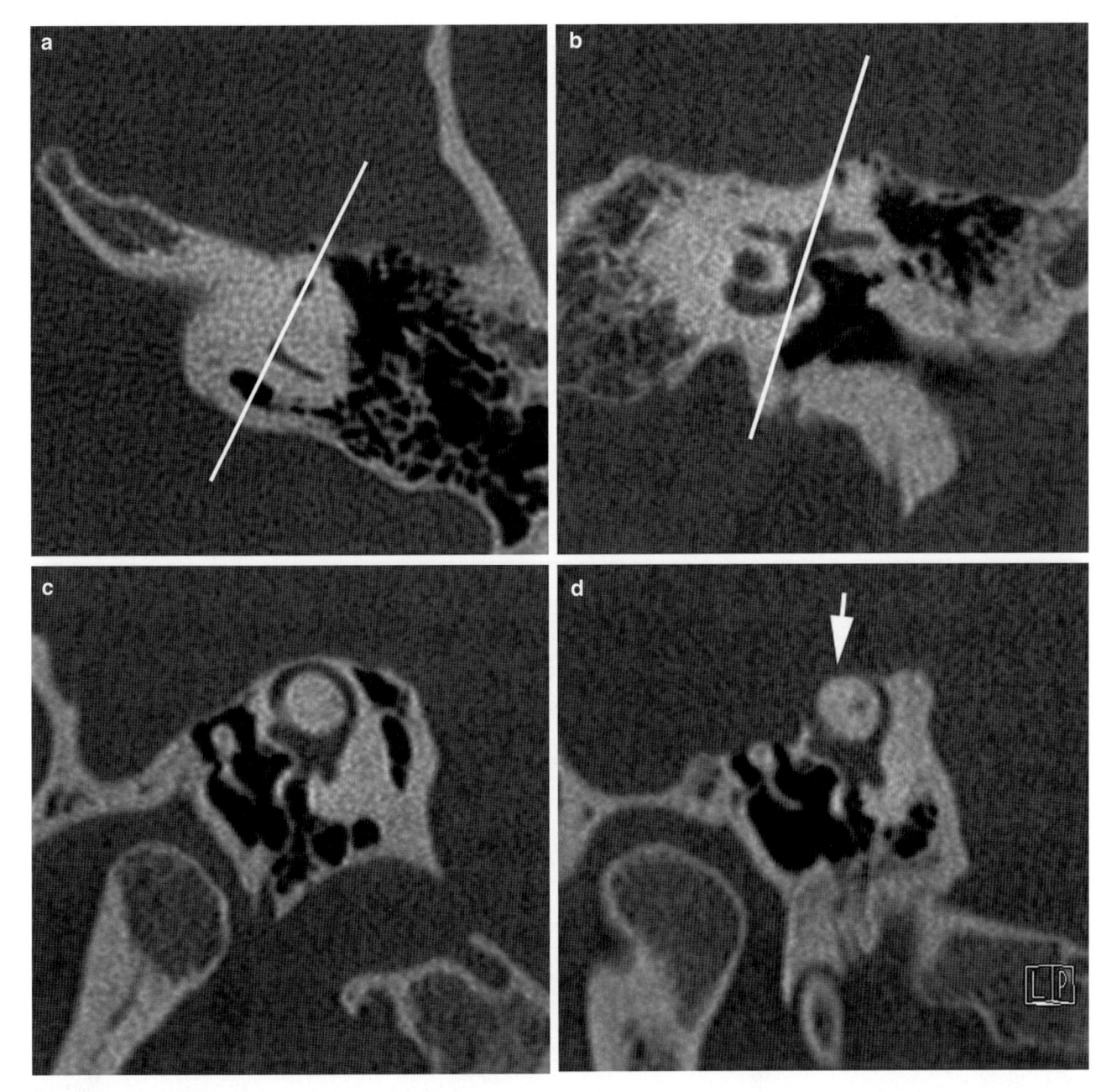

Fig. 13 *Sagittal Oblique Reconstruction of SSC.* **a** Axial and **b** coronal reference images demonstrating multiplanar reconstruction plane required for the oblique sagittal view of the SSC. Plane of reconstruction is identical to Pöschl's plane. **c** Multiplanar reconstruction (MPR) of the SSC from MDCT data set. **d** MPR in patient presenting with vertigo precipitated by loud sounds (Tullio's phenomenon). Note dehiscence of the roof of the canal (*arrow*) allowing the defect to act as a "third window." In these patients, the fluid wave generated at the oval window (*first window*) can decompress at the site of the dehiscence rather than at the round window (*second window*). This abnormal route of fluid wave propagation stimulates the vestibular apparatus resulting in vertigo. [Reprinted with permission from Springer (Lane & Witte, Temporal Bone: An Imaging Atlas, Springer)]

dehiscence of the SSC may present clinically with Tullio's Phenomenon (vertigo precipitated by loud noise) or other types of vestibulopathy (Merchant and Rosowski 2008). These bony defects can be confirmed with MDCT to include MPRs in the plane of the SCC (Fig. 13d). Occasionally, dehiscence of the posterior semicircular canal may present with identical symptomatology (Fig. 14d) (Vanspauwen et al. 2006). Perilymph fistula from lateral semicircular canal

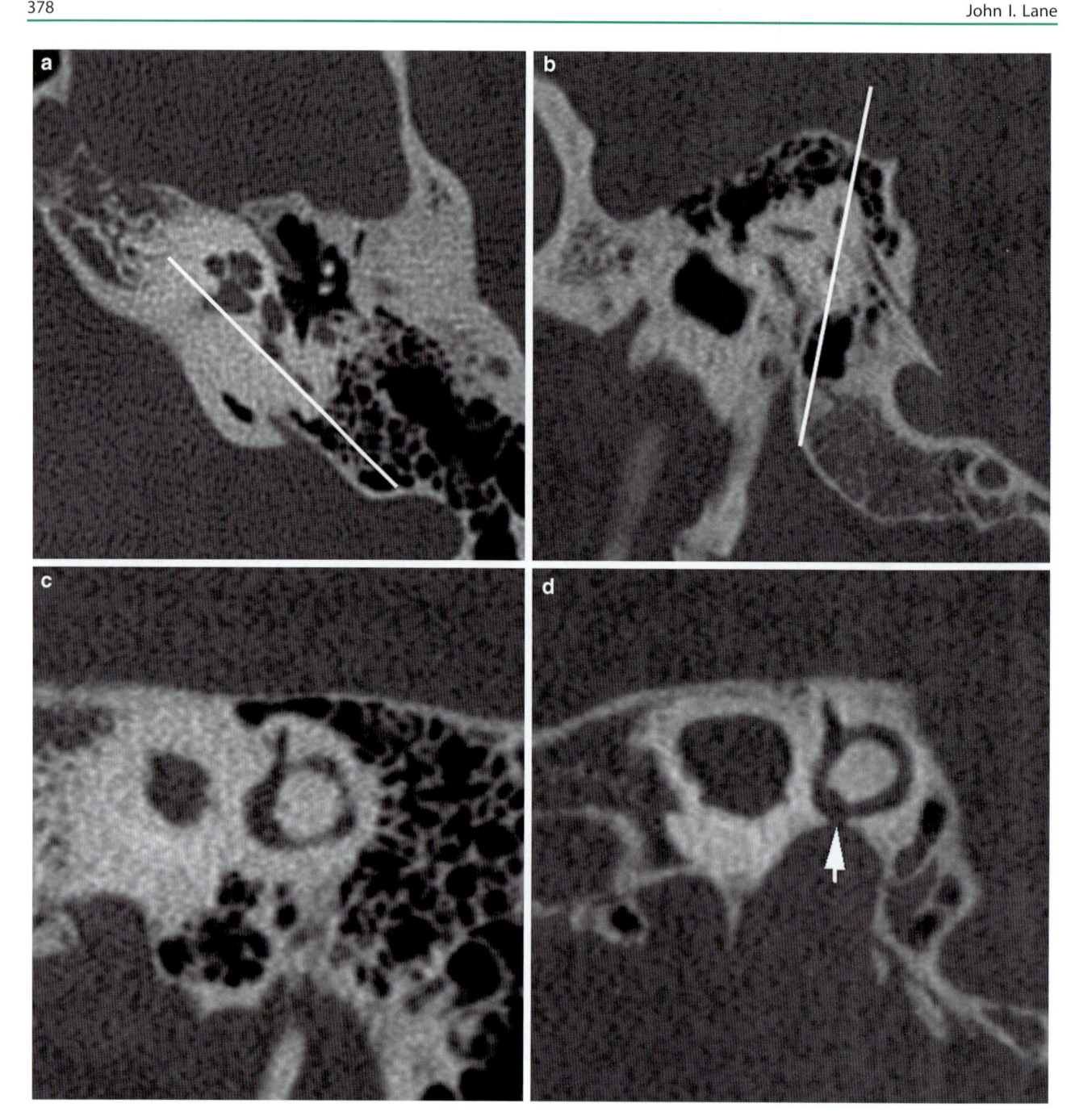

Fig. 14 *Coronal Oblique Reconstruction of Posterior Semicircular Canal.* **a** Axial and **b** oblique sagittal reference images demonstrating multiplanar reconstruction plane required for the oblique coronal view of the posterior semicircular canal. This reconstruction is a slight modification of Stenvers plane. **c** Multiplanar reconstruction (MPR) of the posterior semicircular canal from MDCT data set. **d** MPR in patient presenting with vestibular symptoms. Note focal dehiscence of the bony partition between the inferior wall of the ampulla of the posterior semicircular canal (*arrow*) and adjacent jugular bulb

erosion in the setting of middle ear cholesteatoma can be depicted with MPRs in the plane of the LSC (Fig. 15d). Obviously, these additional MPRs are unnecessary if the routine axial series is prescribed in this plane.

The vestibular aqueduct extends inferiorly from the posterior wall of the vestibule, just anterior and medial to the common crus, to the posterior surface of the petrous portion of the temporal bone, lateral to the porus

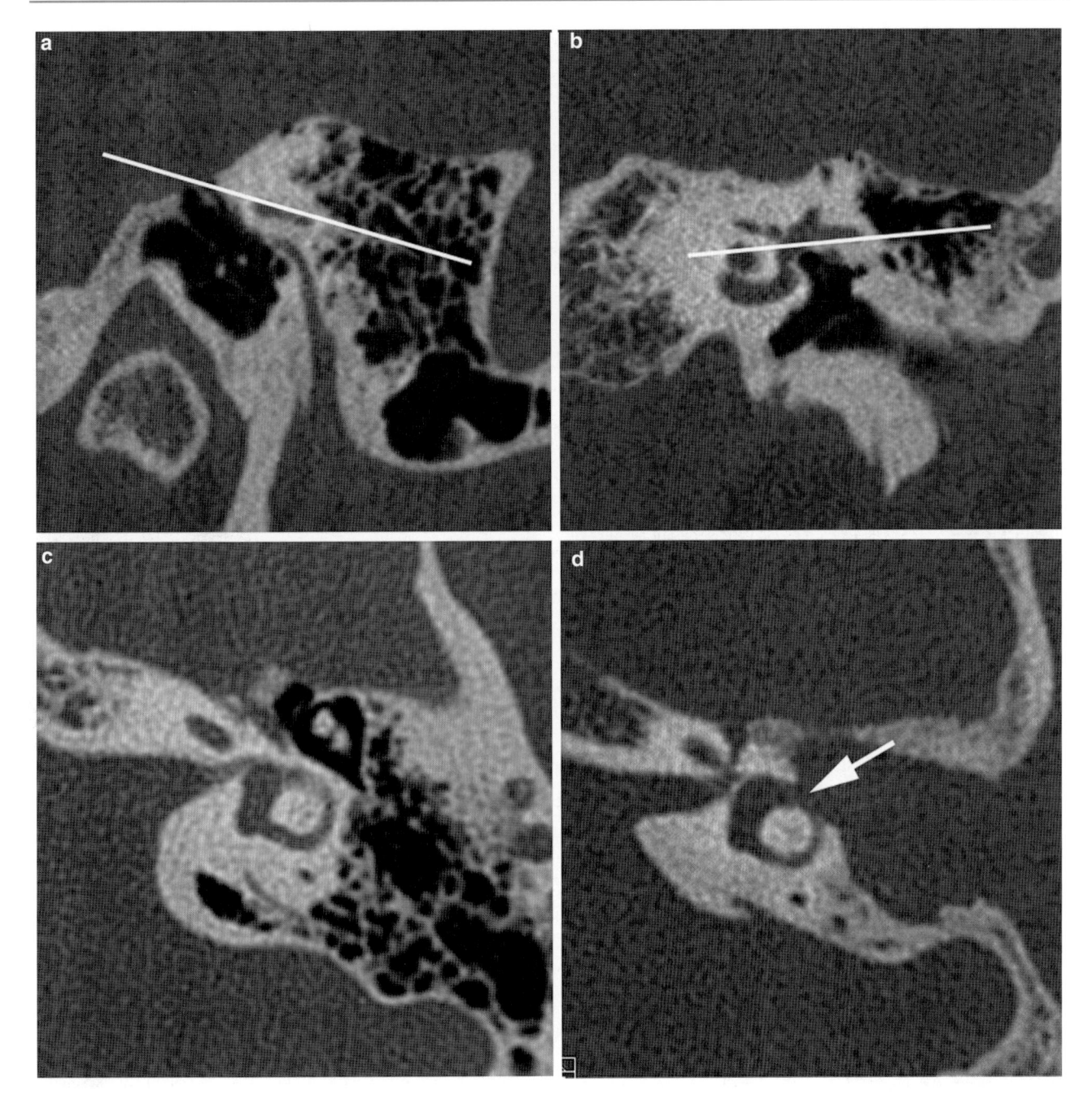

Fig. 15 *Axial Oblique Reconstruction of Lateral Semicircular Canal.* **a** Coronal and **b** sagittal reference images demonstrating multiplanar reconstruction plane required for oblique axial view of the lateral semicircular canal. This reconstruction is obviated if standard axial images are reconstructed in the plane of the lateral canal. **c** Multiplanar reconstruction (MPR) of the lateral semicircular canal from MDCT data set. **d** MPR in patient presenting with positional vertigo related to cholesteatoma with perilymph fistula. Note erosion of the anterior limb of the lateral canal (*arrow*)

acusticus. An MPR oriented in a sagittal oblique plane between the common crus and the aperture of the aqueduct best demonstrates its course and caliber, which in the normal state is no larger than the adjacent semicircular canals measured at its midpoint (Fig. 16) (Mafee et al. 1992). A dilated vestibular aqueduct is the most common anomaly of the inner ear, and most often presents as a progressive sensorineural hearing loss in late first or early second decade (Fig. 16c) (Jackler and De La Cruz 1989).

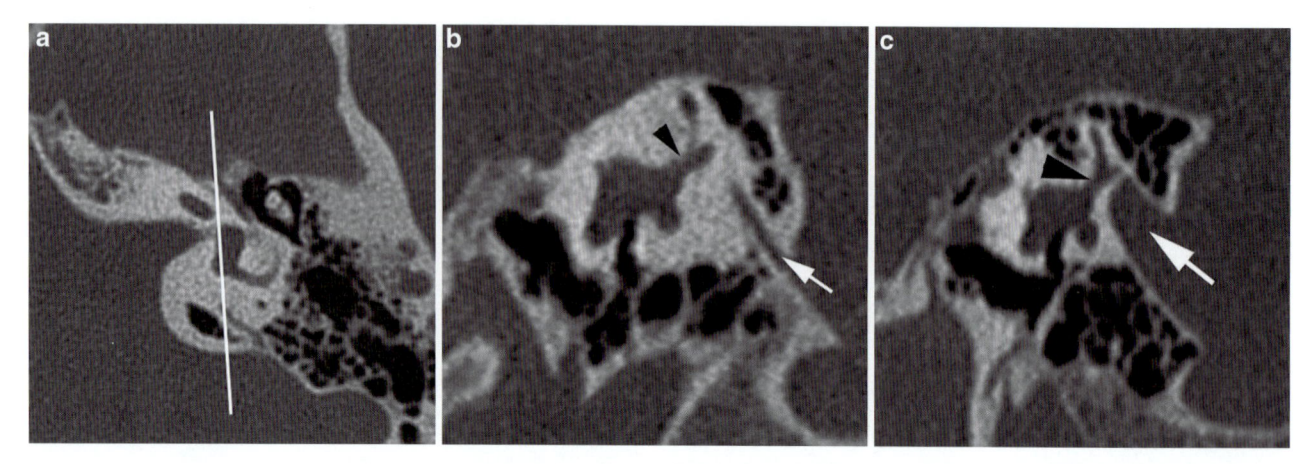

Fig. 16 *Sagittal Oblique Reconstruction of the Vestibular Aqueduct.* **a** Axial reference image demonstrating reconstruction plane required for the oblique sagittal view of vestibular aqueduct. **b** Multiplanar reconstruction (MPR) of the vestibular aqueduct from MDCT data set. Note vestibular aqueduct (*arrow*) transversing anterosuperiorly from the posterior surface of the petrous temporal bone toward the common crus (*arrowhead*). The vestibular aqueduct opens along the medial wall of the vestibule just anterior and inferior to the opening of the common crus. Midportion of the vestibular aqueduct should be no larger in caliber than the adjacent semicircular canals. **c** MPR MDCT demonstrates dilated vestibular aqueduct (*arrow*) in this patient presenting with progressive sensorineural hearing loss. Note relationship to the common crus (*arrowhead*)

4 Conclusion

MDCT of the temporal bone using isotropic volumetric acquisitions permits reconstructions in any plane of section without significant loss of image resolution. This technology allows the radiologist to produce MPRs and MIPs in planes of section that best depict the relevant anatomy and pathology of the middle and inner ear.

References

Belden CJ, Weg N, Minor LB, Zinreich SJ (2003) Ct evaluation of bone dehiscence of the superior semicircular canal as a cause of sound- and/or pressure-induced vertigo [see comment]. Radiology 226(2):337–343

Bin Z, Jingzhen H, Daocai W, Kai L, Cheng L (2008) Traumatic ossicular chain separation: sliding-thin-slab maximum-intensity projections for diagnosis. J Compu Ass Tomogr 32(6):951–954

Brunner S (1969) Tomography in otoradiology. Radiologe 9(2):56–60

Buckingham RA, Valvassori GE (1973) Tomographic anatomy of the temporal bone. Otolaryngol Clin N Am 6(2):337–362

Hans P, Grant AJ, Laitt RD, Ramsden RT, Kassner A, Jackson A (1999) Comparison of three-dimensional visualization techniques for depicting the scala vestibuli and scala tympani of the cochlea by using high-resolution mr imaging. Am J Neuroradiol 20(7):1197–1206

Henrot P, Iochum S, Batch T, Coffinet L, Blum A, Roland J (2005) Current multiplanar imaging of the stapes. Am J Neuroradiol 26(8):2128–2133

Jackler RK, De La Cruz A (1989) The large vestibular aqueduct syndrome. Laryngoscope 99(12):1238–1242; discussion 1242–1233

Kelsall DC, Shallop JK, Brammeier TG, Prenger EC (1997) Facial nerve stimulation after nucleus 22-channel cochlear implantation. Am J Otol 18(3):336–341

Krombach GA, Di Martino E, Martiny S, Prescher A, Haage P, Buecker A, Gunther RW (2006) Dehiscence of the superior and/or posterior semicircular canal: delineation on t2-weighted axial three-dimensional turbo spin-echo images, maximum intensity projections and volume-rendered images. Eur Arch Otorhinolaryngol 263(2):111–117

Lane J, Lindell E, Witte R, DeLone D, Driscoll C (2006) Middle and inner ear: improved depiction with multiplanar reconstruction of volumetric ct data. Radiographics 26(1):115–124

Lane JI, Witte RJ (2010) The temporal bone: an imaging atlas. Springer, Heidelberg

Mafee MF, Charletta D, Kumar A, Belmont H (1992) Large vestibular aqueduct and congenital sensorineural hearing loss. Am J Neuroradiol 13(2):805–819

Merchant SN, Rosowski JJ (2008) Conductive hearing loss caused by third-window lesions of the inner ear. Otol Neurotol 29(3):282–289

Naganawa S, Senda K, Yamakawa K, Fukatsu H, Ishigaki T, Nakashima T, Sugimoto H, Aoki I, Takai H (1995) High resolution mr imaging of the inner ear apparatus using 3d-fast spin echo sequence. Nippon Igaku Hoshasen Gakkai Zasshi—Nippon Acta Radiologica 55(1):81–82

Ozgen B, Cunnane ME, Caruso PA, Curtin HD (2008) Comparison of 45 degrees oblique reformats with axial reformats in ct evaluation of the vestibular aqueduct. Am J Neuroradiol 29(1):30–34

Pimontel-Appel B, Ettore GC (1980) Pöschl positioning and the radiology of meniere's disease. J Belge Radiol 63(2–3):359–367

Vanspauwen R, Salembier L, Van den Hauwe L, Parizel P, Wuyts FL, Van de Heyning PH (2006) Posterior semicircular canal dehiscence: value of vemp and multidetector ct. B-ENT 2(3):141–145

Printing: Ten Brink, Meppel, The Netherlands
Binding: Stürtz, Würzburg, Germany